Kris Nobo

Cellular and Molecular Neuroscience
Charles F. Stevens, editor

Gary Banker and Kimberly Goslin, editors, *Culturing Nerve Cells*, 1991
Gary Banker and Kimberly Goslin, editors, *Culturing Nerve Cells*, second edition, 1998

Culturing Nerve Cells

second edition

edited by Gary Banker and Kimberly Goslin

A Bradford Book
The MIT Press
Cambridge, Massachusetts
London, England

This book was set in Melior and Helvetica on the Monotype "Prism Plus" PostScript Imagesetter by Asco Trade Typesetting Ltd., Hong Kong and was printed and bound in the United States of America.

Library of Congress Cataloging-in-Publication Data

Culturing nerve cells / edited by Gary Banker and Kimberly Goslin. — 2nd ed.
   p. cm.
Includes bibliographical references and index.
ISBN 0-262-02438-1 (alk. paper)
  1. Neurons—Growth—Laboratory manuals. 2. Nerve tissue—Cultures and culture media—Laboratory manuals. I. Banker, Gary.
II. Goslin, Kimberly.
QP363.5.C85 1998
573.8′536—dc21   97-17167
                                                 CIP

Contents

The spectacular advances in biology in the second half of this century have largely resulted from an amazing and rapidly growing array of new experimental methods. Among the most important techniques for many areas of biology, especially for neurobiology, has been the development of methods for growing cells and tissues in culture. Although all culture methods can be difficult and fussy, this is particularly so for neurons and, for this reason, the first edition of this book has played an important role in disseminating culture methods among neurobiologists. Here the neurobiologist who wants to culture neurons and glia can find out what to do and why they are doing it. But like all methods, culture techniques evolve. This second edition provides the latest and best in the how and why of brain cell culturing.

Charles F. Stevens, The Salk Institute

Contributors

Janet Alder

Laboratory of Developmental Neurobiology
Rockefeller University

Hannelore Asmussen

Department of Neuroscience
University of Virginia School of Medicine

Gerard Bain

Department of Anatomy and Neurobiology
Washington University School of Medicine

Gary Banker

Center for Research on Occupational and
Environmental Toxicology
Oregon Health Sciences University

Robert W. Baughman

Division of Fundamental Neurosciences
National Institutes of Health National Institute
of Neurological Disorders and Stroke

Richard P. Bunge

The Miami Project to Cure Paralysis and the
Department of Neurological Surgery
University of Miami School of Medicine

Ann Marie Craig

Department of Cell and Structural Biology
University of Illinois

Matthew E. Cunningham

Department of Pathology
Columbia University College of Physicians and
Surgeons

Dominique Debanne

Brain Research Institute
University of Zurich
Zurich, Switzerland

Stephen E. Farinelli   Department of Pathology
Columbia University College of Physicians and
Surgeons

Michael F. A. Finley   Department of Cell Biology and Physiology
Washington University School of Medicine

Gerald D. Fischbach   Department of Neurobiology
Harvard University School of Medicine

Beat H. Gähwiler   Brain Research Institute
University of Zurich
Zurich, Switzerland

Wei-Qiang Gao   Department of Neuroscience
Genentech, Inc.

Daniel J. Goldberg   Department of Pharmacology
Columbia University College of Physicians and
Surgeons

Kimberly Goslin   Department of Neurology
Oregon Health Sciences University

David I. Gottlieb   Department of Anatomy and Neurobiology
Washington University School of Medicine

Lloyd A. Greene   Department of Pathology
Columbia University College of Physicians and
Surgeons

Mary Beth Hatten   Laboratory of Developmental Neurobiology
Rockefeller University

Dennis Higgins   Department of Pharmacology
State University of New York School of Medicine at
Buffalo

James E. Huettner   Department of Cell Biology and Physiology
Washington University School of Medicine

Kenneth A. Jones   Synaptic Pharmaceutical Corporation

Naomi Kleitman   The Miami Project to Cure Paralysis and the
                          Department of Neurological Surgery
                          University of Miami School of Medicine

Raul Krauss   Department of Neurobiology
                          Harvard University School of Medicine

Ronald M. Lindsay   Regeneron Pharmaceuticals, Inc.

Nagesh K. Mahanthappa   Ontogeny, Inc.

Carol A. Mason   Department of Pathology
                          Columbia University College of Physicians and
                          Surgeons

Margot Mayer-Pröschel   Huntsman Cancer Institute
                          Department of Oncological Sciences
                          University of Utah Health Sciences Center

R. Anne McKinney   Brain Research Institute
                          University of Zurich
                          Zurich, Switzerland

Mary E. Morrison   Department of Pathology
                          Columbia University College of Physicians and
                          Surgeons

Mark Noble   Huntsman Cancer Institute
                          Department of Oncological Sciences
                          University of Utah Health Sciences Center

David S. Park   Department of Pathology
                          Columbia University College of Physicians and
                          Surgeons

Paul H. Patterson   Division of Biology
                          California Institute of Technology

Mu-ming Poo

Department of Biology
University of California at San Diego

Richard T. Robertson

Department of Anatomy and Neurobiology
University of California at Irvine

Samuel Schacher

Center for Neurobiology and Behavior
Columbia University College of Physicians and
Surgeons

Michael M. Segal

Program in Neuroscience
Department of Neurosurgery
Harvard Medical School and Brigham and Women's
Hospital

Carolyn L. Smith

National Institute of Neurological Disorders and
Stroke
National Institutes of Health

Nacira Tabti

Laboratorie de Physiologie
Faculté des Sciences Université Paris XII

Scott M. Thompson

Brain Research Institute
University of Zurich
Zurich, Switzerland

Roseann Ventimiglia

Department of Neuroscience
Pfizer Central Research

Ginger S. Withers

Center for Research on Occupational and
Environmental Toxicology
Oregon Health Sciences University

Patrick M. Wood

The Miami Project to Cure Paralysis and the
Department of Neurological Surgery
University of Miami School of Medicine

Min Yao

Department of Anatomy and Neurobiology
Washington University School of Medicine

I   A User's Guide

1 Getting Started

Gary Banker and Kimberly Goslin

This second edition of *Culturing Nerve Cells*, like the first, is intended for people who want to grow neurons in culture and who want to do it well! In some senses, it is a do-it-yourself manual complete with recipes and protocols. But more than this, it aims to provide an understanding of the principles behind the protocols. Knowing what is done often is less important than knowing why it is done in a particular way and what the alternatives are.

These ideas have led us to develop a book that we believe differs substantially from other volumes on cell culture. One common approach has been to assemble a compendium of methods sections prepared by different experts, one for each cell type you might ever want to culture. The necessarily short chapters of such books rarely provide more information than do the methods sections of individual articles. On the other hand, the books written by a single author are handicapped by the fact that one individual's experience with different cell types and culture conditions is bound to be limited. When it comes to culturing nerve cells, small details can make the difference between success and failure, and first hand knowledge is essential.

Without question, the best way to obtain expertise in such matters is to learn the cultures directly from an expert. As not everybody has this opportunity, we've gathered together a small group of productive and experienced culturists and asked them to write chapters that, in effect, invite you to their labs and provide much of the information that you might obtain from such a visit. All the authors have contributed to the development of unique culture systems that allow them to address the questions of interest to them. In this second edition, we have made a point of selecting new contributors to discuss several of the more commonly used culture systems so as to allow different labs which have also made important contributions—to describe their approaches. Also, we have added chapters on several new systems that we think will be important for addressing important questions in neurobiology. We thank the

authors of both editions for their contributions and for their standards of excellence.

One man, in particular, has defined the discipline of nerve cell culture over the last three decades. That man, Dick Bunge, died last year. His enthusiasm and his generosity helped us to get our start in this field. It is particularly satisfying to be able to include a chapter by Dick and his colleagues in this edition.

We have asked all the contributors to explain to you why they do things as they do—how their experimental goals have shaped their particular cell culture approach and the advantages and disadvantages of the cell culture systems they've developed. They provide detailed protocols explaining how they prepare media and substrates, how they set out cultures, and how they maintain them. We've also asked them to describe their cultures to you in practical terms, from the time the cells are first plated through the various phases of their development. How long should the cells be expected to survive and remain healthy? What do healthy cells actually look like? Finally, they reveal the painful truth that even experts can have problems with their cultures, and they provide information about some of the problems they've experienced and the approaches they use for "trouble shooting."

Nuts and Bolts

In addition to the chapters dealing with the culture of specific types of neurons and glia, introductory chapters offer a brief course on the "nuts and bolts" of culturing neurons. The authors of these chapters discuss the kinds of cultures available and which might be the best for you; the choices you'll have to make, the problems you might face, and the alternatives you might want to consider; what you'll need to do to characterize your cultures so that you can be assured that they're up to snuff. What tissue will you choose, what substrate will you use? What about medium? We've tried to provide a critical discussion of the options available and of the advantages and disadvantages of each. A new chapter on techniques for tranfecting cultured nerve cells is included also.

You can then turn to the individual chapters to see how experienced culturists approach the issues treated in the introduction. You will find detailed methods covering many of the specific procedures used in neuronal culture. In the aggregate, these chapters

represent hundreds of person-years of experience with nerve cell culture and offer a wealth of technical expertise

Getting Started

Though some of you may be coming to this book with experience at culturing nerve cells, others will just be getting started. In the latter case, how should you begin? Before anything else, you need to get healthy cultures growing in your lab. This seems self-evident but the fact is, if you've never seen a healthy pyramidal neuron that has been growing in culture for 24 h, you can't know what to expect. If you've never seen dead and dying neurons (a heart-rending sight), you won't know when your cultures are ailing. Even respected journals, still occasionally publish papers that attempt to draw important conclusions from observations of dying cells. If there is one message that we hope to communicate, it is that you must be willing to evaluate your cultures critically if you hope to perform meaningful experiments. Bad cultures give bad data. The photographs and practical descriptions of cells in this book can serve as standards to help you evaluate your own cultures.

If you plan to grow one of the cell types represented in this book, you will find that the protocols provided here work, they work consistently, and they will work in your lab. If you are inexperienced with neuronal culture, some of these protocols will take practice: They might not work the first time. But we advise you to stick with these protocols until they work consistently (and they will) and only then begin to adapt them for your particular needs.

But this is not an exhaustive treatise. What if you want to culture a cell type that isn't considered at all? Obviously, you'll need to look in the literature to see what success other people have had with the cells of interest. But it's likely that this volume still will be of use to you. The introductory chapters should help you understand the principles of growing nerve cells, the alternative approaches available, and the pluses and minuses of each. The chapters on culturing specific cell types will help as well: Taken together, these chapters describe nearly every common procedure used in culturing nerve cells and include the details that often cannot be gleaned from the methods sections of original articles. Perhaps more important, they provide the rationale underlying the specific approaches that other investigators have taken and may help you with some of the decisions that you must make.

In Defense of Neuronal Cultures

How can information obtained from neurons or glial cells growing under the abnormal conditions of cell culture possibly have relevance for "real" neurons or "real" glia? We've been asked this question more than once, and if you plan to work with neuronal cultures, it's a question you may be asked as well. In some regards, cells in culture *are* abnormal. Neurons are constrained to grow in two dimensions, when they'd certainly prefer to grow in three; they are unable to interact with many of their normal afferents and target cells; and they are forced to exist in a medium and on a substrate alien to them. Similarly, some aspects of glial function undoubtedly depend on the neurons with which they interact, and such interactions are restricted or entirely absent in culture. Nothing of the exquisite architecture of the brain, with its organized layers of cells and fibers, is retained when cells are dissociated and placed in culture. Yet, surprisingly, neurons and glial cells in culture are remarkably similar to neurons and glia in situ. From the properties of the transmitter receptors and ion channels they express, to the organization of their cytoskeletal constituents, to the characteristics of specific synapses and the structure of myelin, nerve cells in culture largely resemble their counterparts in situ. The cell theory lives.

It is equally important to remember that when differentiation in culture is abnormal or incomplete, it is not for metaphysical reasons but more likely because important cell interactions have been disrupted. Thus, even when neurons in culture do not resemble completely their counterparts in situ, cell culture offers an opportunity to dissect out these interactions and to elucidate the mechanisms that underlie them. Use of this approach has made it possible to identify cell interactions whose significance could not have been suspected from in situ studies, to elucidate their mechanisms in culture, and then to show that they are likely to play a similar role in situ. The studies of Patterson and Landis and their colleagues on the change in neurotransmitter phenotype exhibited by sympathetic neurons exemplify the power of this approach (Patterson, 1978; Yamamori et al., 1989; Landis, 1994).

Nevertheless, most culture systems are developed with the goal of obtaining nerve cells in culture that do closely resemble their counterparts in situ. Under these circumstances, it is incumbent to demonstrate that the specific phenomena under study occur appropriately in culture. If this can be shown, it is reasonable to suppose

that the mechanisms that underlie these phenomena in culture are similar to the mechanisms that exist in situ. The success with which cell culture can be used to address scientific problems depends directly on the rigor with which it can be demonstrated that the cell culture model selected accurately mimics the key features of the neurobiological phenomenon under study. All the chapters that follow emphasize the importance of this principle.

2 Types of Nerve Cell Cultures, Their Advantages and Limitations

Gary Banker and Kimberly Goslin

The science of tissue culture, and the application of tissue culture to the problems of neurobiology, began together on the laboratory bench of Ross Granville Harrison (Harrison, 1907, 1910, 1912, 1914). According to Harrison (1914): "Tissues from the chick were incubated at about 39°C. The unusual hot weather which lasted during almost the whole period when the experiments with chick tissues were under way rendered unnecessary any precautions to keep the tissues warm during their preparation and examination." By examining the outgrowth of fibers from fragments of frog and chick neural tube cultured in drops of clotted lymph or plasma, Harrison demonstrated unequivocally that nerve fibers arise as outgrowths from individual nerve cell bodies rather than from the fusion of cells migrating out from the neural tube (figure 2.1). Despite the limited methods then available, some 25 years before the development of the phase-contrast microscope, Harrison also visualized the protoplasmic movement associated with the tips of the elongating fibers, structures whose importance had been inferred by Ramón y Cajal (1890) when he coined the term *growth cone*. Harrison's observations provided the final key evidence for the establishment of the neuron doctrine (Shepherd, 1991) and foreshadowed many issues that continue to preoccupy neurobiologists today.

The demonstration that tissue could survive and grow outside the body created widespread interest, and Harrison's work attracted many followers. Perhaps most prominent among them was the famous surgeon Alexis Carrel, a pioneer in vascular surgery and transplantation, who became a vocal proponent and self-appointed doyen of tissue culture. Harrison and Carrel were a contrast in styles. Carrel's culture of mammalian tissues (Carrel and Burrows, 1910), based on Harrison's methods, was announced with considerable fanfare as a miraculous accomplishment of modern science (box 2.1). For Harrison, the ability to culture tissues outside the body was a natural consequence of the cell theory and, in itself, of

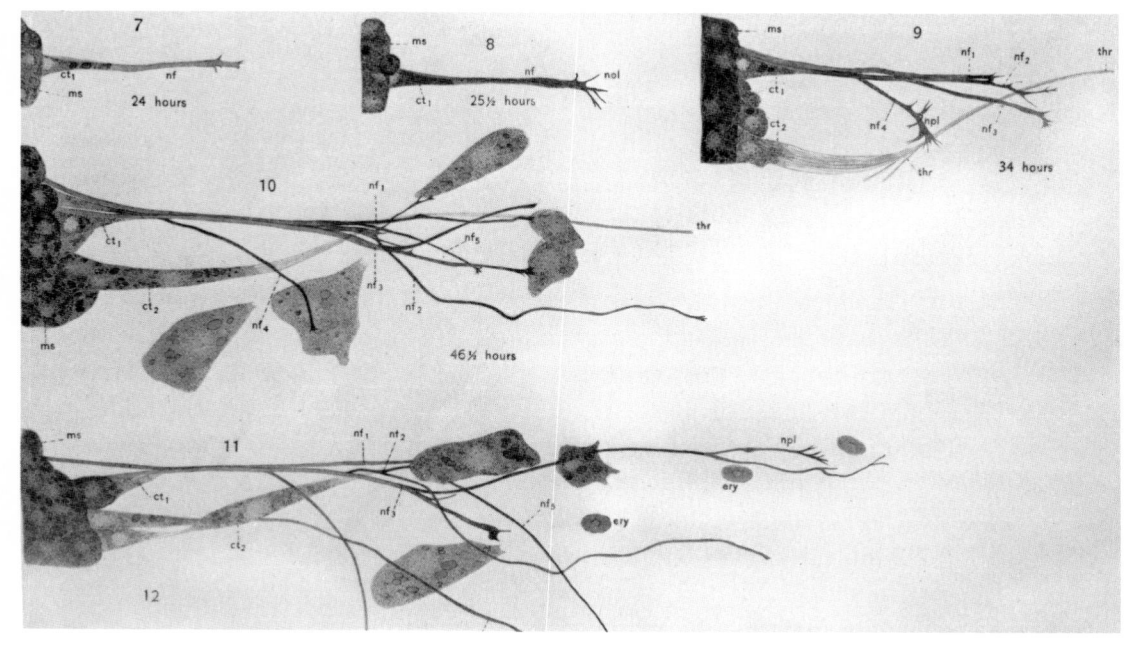

Figure 2.1 Harrison's drawings illustrating nerve fiber outgrowth from an explant of embryonic frog spinal cord cultured in a lymph clot. "The specimen was again examined and found to have undergone remarkable changes. No less than four fibers could then be distinguished diverging from one another in their direction of growth, and each with its characteristic branched end continually undergoing changes in form. Twelve hours later, on the following morning, the change noticed was again very striking . . . Two of the fibers were branched and all had lengthened materially . . . The ends of the fibers continued to show the same activity as before." Ms, main mass of transplanted tissue; nf, nerve fiber; ct, embryonic cell exhibiting independent movement; npl, protoplasmic end of growing nerve; ery, erythrocyte; thr, fibrin threads. (From Harrison, 1910.)

little note; his interest was in using tissue culture to address biological problems. (Which man, do you suppose, has had a lunar crater named in his honor?)

Harrison's observations of neuronal development in culture soon were followed by those of others (for review, see Murray, 1965; Lumsden, 1968). The goal of much of the work in the decades that followed was simply to demonstrate that complex aspects of neuronal maturation, such as synaptogenesis and myelination, could occur in culture (Peterson and Murray, 1955). Other work provided the first, detailed views of the dynamic activities of living nerve cells (Pomerat et al., 1967; see also Nakai, 1956, 1960). It was also during this period that some of the barriers to maintenance of

Box 2.1a   Headline of *New York Times* report of October 20, 1910, describing Carrel and Burrows' article, "Cultivation of adult tissues and organs outside the body," which appeared in the *Journal of the American Medical Association for* October 15, 1910.

BUILD NEW TISSUE OUTSIDE THE BODY

Rockefeller Institute Announces
Success of Experiments Which
May Revolutionize Surgery

MAY BRING A CANCER CURE

Series of Tests Prove That Living
Cells May Be Reproduced and
Multiplied

neurons in long-term culture were overcome. Even so, the techniques for successfully culturing nerve tissue demanded an almost religious dedication, and applying them experimentally was cumbersome. Thus, it is fair to say that tissue culture played a rather small part in the mainstream of neurobiological research during this period.

With the development of two new approaches to nerve cell culture nearly 30 years ago, cell culture began to gain a more prominent and important position in neurobiology. In 1969, two papers described the development of clonal lines of neuroblastoma cells obtained from a neural tumor that had been carried for many years by transplantation from animal to animal (Augusti-Tocco and Sato, 1969; Schubert et al., 1969). When maintained in culture, these cells continued to proliferate but could be induced to stop division and acquire properties characteristic of differentiated neurons (figure 2.2). By comparison with what had gone before, these cell lines offered the possibility of biochemical studies of homogenous populations of neuronal cells uncontaminated by glia. The

Box 2.1b **Excerpt from Harrison's address to the American Association of Anatomists, December 27, 1911, at Princeton, NJ, in opening the symposium on "Tissue Culture" (Harrison, 1912).**

> During the past year we have heard much of the subject of this discussion, and the fact that tissues of the higher animals may be cultivated outside the body has been heralded in the newspapers and magazines as a notable, if not a revolutionary, scientific discovery. When we pause to consider this claim in the light of what has actually been accomplished, we find that there is danger not only of confusing in our minds serveral quite different things, but also that in our enthusiasm for the novelty of the method we may forget the fundamental problems to the solution of which it may be able to contribute—if used critically.
>
> We are taught in every text book of general biology and physiology that the organism is made up of constituent cells, which, while interdependent in the body of the organism, nevertheless have a certain autonomy . . .
>
> While the experiments made with fragments of tissue cultivated *in vitro* show that cells which are entirely isolated or are left together in small aggregates have the faculty of survival in common with whole organs, it is not this, as such, nor is it the fact that we can cultivate animal cells in extraneous media just as we can grow microorganisms, that would entitle the experiments to more than passing interest. Their importance rests, rather, upon the circumstance that they afford a means not only of observing the activities of cells when freed from the entanglements of the organism, but also of studying the conditons which influence these acitivities—activities which constitute morphogenetic as well as maintenance functions of cells and tissues.

following year, two papers described techniques for the culture of dissociated neurons from autonomic and sensory ganglia under conditions that offered unequaled access to individual living nerve cells (Bray, 1970; Yamada et al., 1970). For the first time, it became possible to analyze the elongation of individual neurites and to follow the behavior of their growth cones (figure 2.3). Although both of these developments were foreshadowed by previous findings (e.g., Nakai, 1956, 1960; Goldstein and Pinkel, 1957; Nakai and Kawasaki, 1959) and both were succeeded rapidly by additional work from many other laboratories, they captured the imaginations of neuroscientists and alerted them to new possibilities that nerve cell culture might offer. Since then, technical advances have continued unabated. Many novel methods for deriving clonal cell lines have been developed and, with increasing experience, it has become possible to prepare dissociated cell cultures from virtually every region of the nervous system and from species ranging from slugs to man. Parallel with these advances, tissue culture in general has

become immensely easier. Today it is difficult to imagine what it must have been like to culture cells without such things as laminar flow hoods, sterile filtration, disposable plasticware, and commercially available media. Tissue culture now is an integral part of modern neurobiology. Scanning the contents of current journals brings this point home. Nearly one-third of the papers that currently appear in *Neuron* use nerve cell cultures as an important method.

Primary Cultures Versus Continuous Cell Lines

Most types of tissues, when dissociated into a suspension of single cells and plated into a culture dish, go through a characteristic series of events. First, the cells undergo a period of rapid division, so-called log phase growth. Then, as they approach confluence and form contacts with one another, their rate of division slows and they begin to express a program of differentiation characteristic of their tissue of origin. Muscle cells fuse and acquire cross striations, epithelial cells from the kidney or gut become linked by junctional complexes and transport ions from one surface to another, heart cells begin to beat spontaneously. Glial cells begin to glia.

The situation with neurons is quite different. When cells from the embryonic brain are dissociated and placed into culture, neurons that have completed division in situ will extend processes, form synapses with one another, become electrically active, and so on— just about anything you might want from a neuron. But even if tissue is removed at a time of active neurogenesis, it is rare to observe cells that divide in culture and subsequently acquire a neuronal phenotype. This makes the study of neurons in culture fundamentally different from the study of other cell types. Finally, after many years of active research, exciting advances are being made in understanding the factors that control the proliferation of neuronal progenitors (Gage, Coates, et al., 1995; Vicario-Abejon, Johe, et al., 1995). But it is still likely to be some time before it is routinely possible to grow a flask of neurons from a few precursor cells.

Cultures such as those just described are referred to as *primary cultures*, because they are prepared from cells taken directly from the animal. The cells divide or not, depending on their wont, acquire differentiated characteristics—and ultimately die. For the next experiment, it's back to the animal again to obtain new tissue and to prepare new cultures.

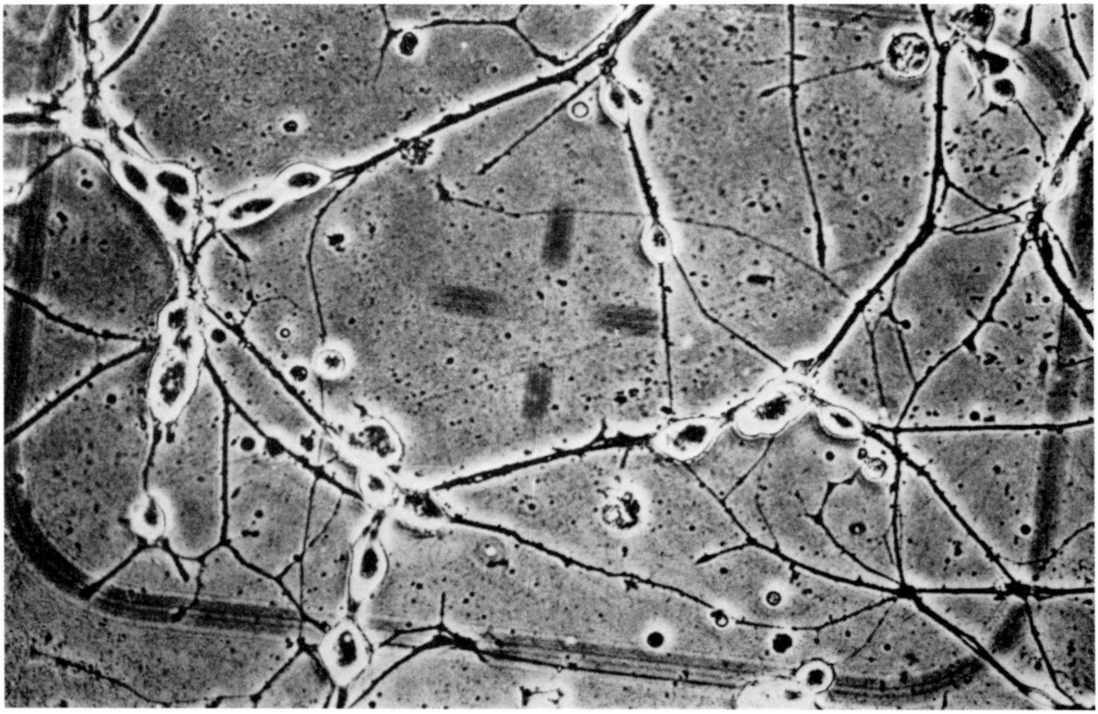

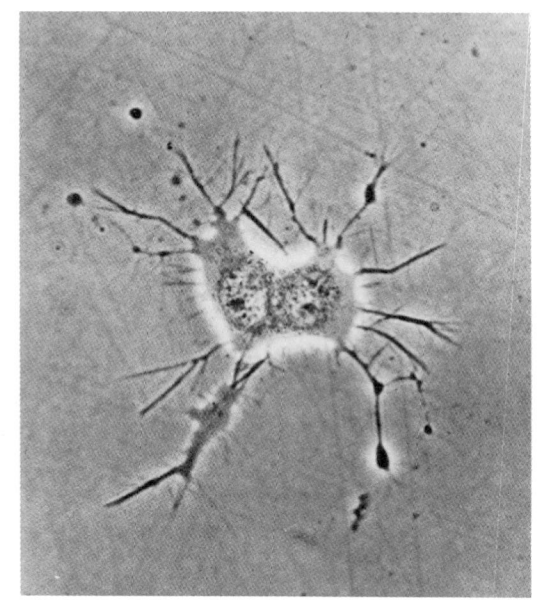

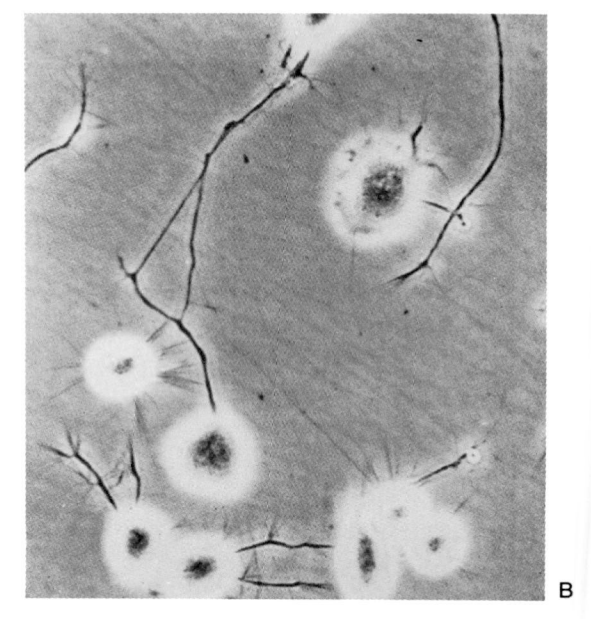

Alternatively, in the case of cells that divide in culture, it is possible to "passage" or "subculture" them by removing them from the substrate, "splitting" them (i.e., diluting them several-fold in media and replating them into new dishes), and allowing them to reenter log-phase growth. However, the properties of the cultured cells often change gradually with passaging, as more rapidly dividing cell populations come to predominate and more "differentiated" cells, which divide more slowly, are lost. Glial cells can be subcultured, at least for a few generations; neurons, of course, cannot.

When cells are subcultured repeatedly, most cease division after a finite number of generations, typically between 20 and 80. The mechanism for this is not understood, but it may be related to the process of senescence that occurs in cells in situ (Orgel, 1973). Cells that can be passaged indefinitely and that express a reasonably stable phenotype are called *established* or *continuous cell lines*. Some cell lines have arisen by spontaneous mutation in normal cells being passaged in culture, but the majority have been obtained by culturing tumor cells. In addition to their infinite life span (their "immortality"), such cell lines frequently share several additional properties that distinguish them from "normal" cells in culture: They divide more rapidly, they lose contact inhibition and, when reintroduced into animals, they form tumors. Cells with these properties sometimes are called *transformed*.

Once a continuous cell line has been established, it is customary to clone the cells to obtain a genetically homogeneous population. Many separate *clonal cell lines*, each exhibiting a different set of properties, can be obtained from a single tumor or tumor cell line. For example, dozens have been derived from the original mouse neuroblastoma tumor C-1300. Over the last two decades, many additional lines of neuroblastoma, glioma, and pheochromocytoma cells have been derived from neural tumors, some from tumors that arose spontaneously, others from tumors induced by mutagenizing agents or x-irradiation. Among the available tumor cell lines are lines that express any of a great variety of neurotransmitters,

Figure 2.2 (*A*) Phase-contrast photomicrograph illustrating neuroblastoma cells derived from the C1300 tumor. (From Augusti-Tocco and Sato, 1969, with permission.) (*B*) Stages in the morphological differentiation of neuroblastoma cells (clone C1), derived from the C1300 tumor line. *B*, left: 5 h; *B*, right: 24 h. (From Schubert et al., 1971, with permission.)

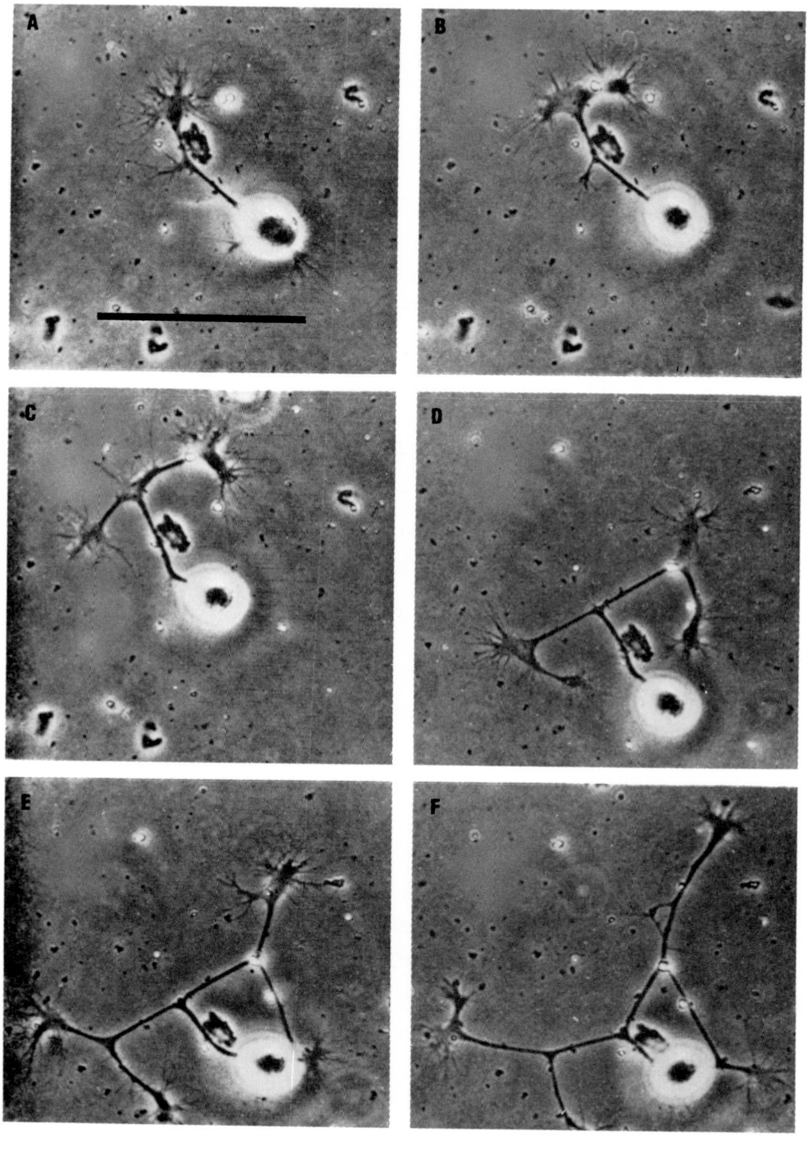

Figure 2.3 Neurite outgrowth from a single dissociated neuron taken from the neonatal rat superior cervical ganglion. The photographs were taken at 30-min intervals. Scale bar: 100 μm. (From Bray [1970], with permission.)

neuropeptides, and receptors (James and Wood, 1992). At the same time, additional approaches have been developed for establishing cell lines from neural tissue (Whittemore and Snyder, 1996).

In principle, cell lines offer many advantages, chief among them their convenience. The cells can be stored indefinitely in liquid nitrogen, grown up whenever needed, and shared with other laboratories throughout the world. When properly handled, the cells will exhibit identical properties time after time, year after year.

Cell lines are such a mainstay of research in other areas of cell biology that someone coming to neurobiology from another discipline must find it peculiar that anyone still works with primary cultures, let alone that these cultures could be the main theme of an entire book. The problem is that the cell lines presently available for neurobiological research do not express some key aspects of neuronal differentiation. Though there are cell lines that express any of a great many of the individual characteristics of differentiated neurons—neurotransmitters, ion channels, receptors, and other neuron-specific proteins—they are not good models for any specific neuronal phenotype. Even PC12 cells, which can come as close as any cell line to mimicking a specific population of differentiated nerve cells, do not develop distinct axons and dendrites or form synapses like the sympathetic neurons they otherwise resemble. The suitability of available cell lines as models for neurons from the central nervous system (CNS) is even more limiting. Presumably this reflects the complexity of the developmental processes that lead to the acquisition of a specific neuronal identity in a tissue with hundreds or thousands of distinguishable neuronal phenotypes.

Primary Cultures

Dissociated-Cell Cultures

The primary cell cultures described in the preceding section usually are termed *dissociated* or *dispersed* cell cultures. These cultures are prepared from suspensions of individual cells obtained by dissociation of neural tissue. When plated onto an appropriate substrate, the neurons begin to extend processes within several hours, ultimately forming a dense network. Under favorable conditions, it is possible to maintain such cultures for months, during

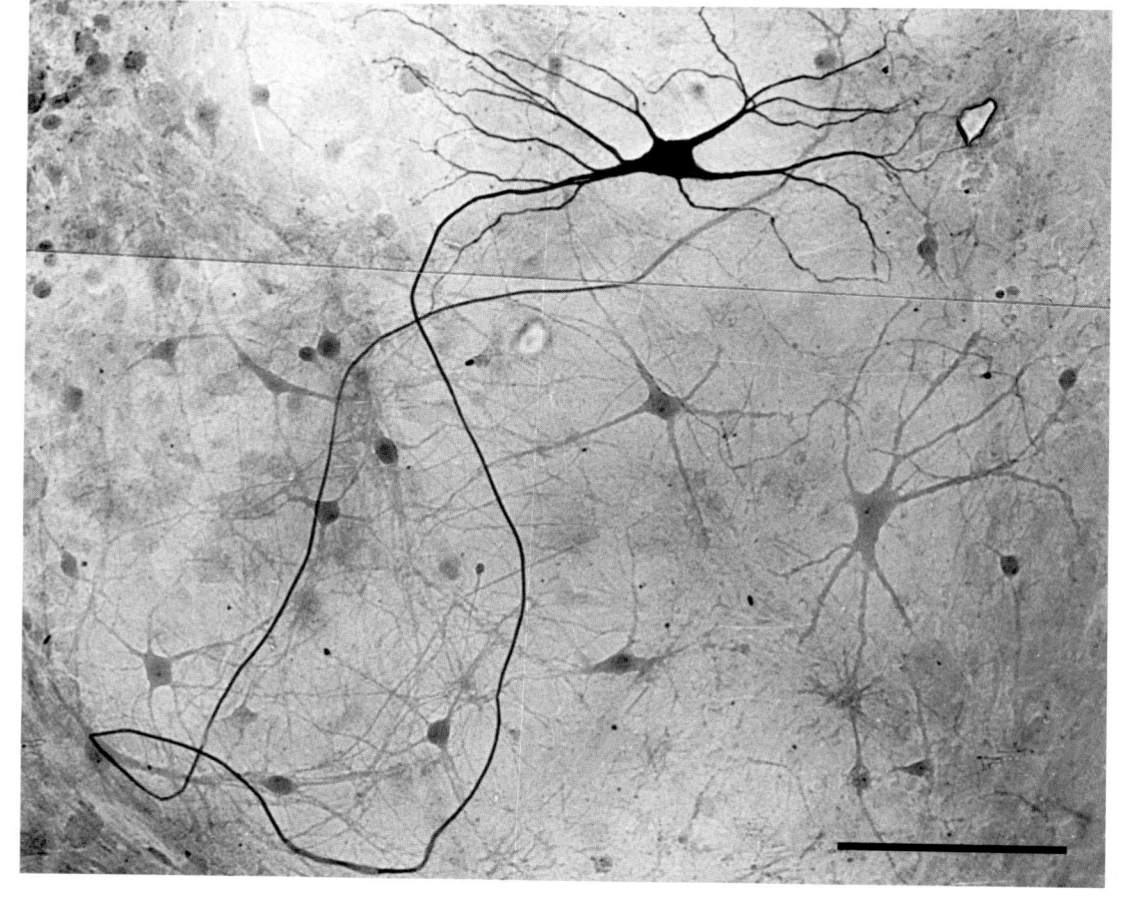

Figure 2.4 Dissociated cell culture from the spinal cord of a fetal mouse (5 weeks in vitro). One cell has been injected with horseradish peroxidase in order to reveal its dendritic arbor and the course of its axon. Scale bar: 200 μm. (From Neale et al. [1978], with permission.)

which time the cells acquire most of the properties of mature neurons (figure 2.4). They develop distinct axons and dendrites, form synapses with one another, and express the receptors and ion channels characteristic of the corresponding cell type in situ. Frequently, considerable spontaneous electrical activity develops, including synaptic potentials that summate to produce action potentials. When cocultured with Schwann cells or oligodendrocytes, axons become myelinated.

Importantly, neurons in dissociated cultures appear to retain their individual identities, presumably because they are postmitotic and committed in their differentiation at the time they are

introduced into culture. Motor neurons express properties reminiscent of motor neurons, Purkinje cells of Purkinje cells, and so on. In a few cases, it has been possible to demonstrate this directly by labeling specific populations of embryonic cells in situ, then examining their properties in culture. For example, embryonic motorneurons have been labeled by injecting retrograde tracers into the muscles they innervate. In culture, the labeled cells develop dendritic arbors and electrical properties that are characteristic of motorneurons (O'Brien and Fischbach, 1986a). They synthesize and release acetylcholine and induce the aggregation of acetylcholine receptors on muscle cells; they express an appropriate population of transmitter receptors on their somata and dendrites; and they receive appropriate synapses from spinal cord interneurons (Role et al., 1985; O'Brien and Fischbach, 1986b,c; Schaffner et al., 1987; Martinou et al., 1989). Similar (although less extensive) experiments have permitted characterization of specific subpopulations of cortical neurons (Huettner and Baughman, 1986; see also chapter 12) and cerebellar neurons (Hockberger et al., 1989; see also chapter 16). In other cases, evidence is less direct. However, in general the morphological and physiological properties of the cell populations present in culture correspond closely to the characteristics of the cell populations present in the tissue of origin (Kriegstein and Dichter, 1983; Banker and Waxman, 1988).

The most obvious advantage of cell culture, and of dissociated cell culture in particular, is that it makes individual living cells accessible. During the first few days in culture, before the neural network becomes too complicated, individual neurons can be visualized in their entirety. This has permitted direct observation of growing axons, their mode of branching (Bray, 1973; Bray and Chapman, 1985; Dotti et al., 1988), and the behavior of their growth cones (figure 2.5; see also chapter 10). In addition, cell culture permits a remarkably precise experimental analysis of these events. Neurites can be cut at defined locations (Shaw and Bray, 1977; Goslin and Banker, 1989), drugs or other agents can be applied to specific sites along growing neurites (Gundersen and Barrett, 1980; Bamburg et al., 1986; Stoop and Poo, 1995; Zheng et al., 1996), and even the tension and adhesive forces generated by single growth cones can be measured (Lamoureux et al., 1989; Zheng et al., 1994). In more mature cultures, dye filling or expression of a reporter gene is necessary to visualize entire cells, because fine ramifications become lost in the neuronal network; only the large branches can

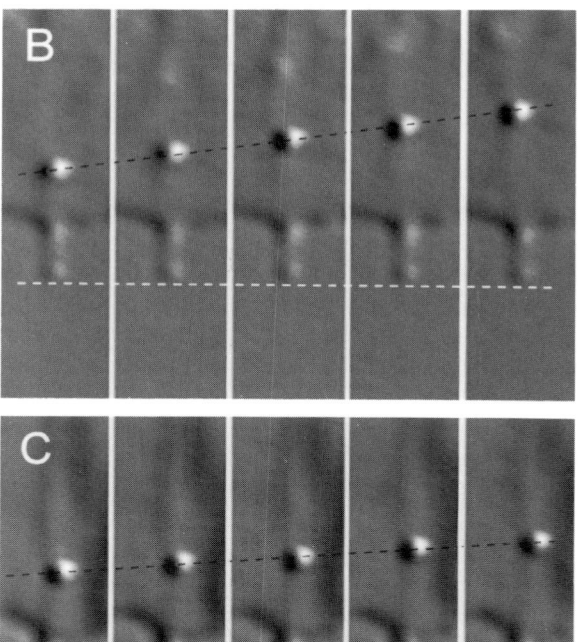

Figure 2.5 Dissociated neurons are a favored preparation for studies of neuronal growth cones. (*A*) The growth cone of a bag cell neuron in a dissociated cell culture from the abdominal ganglion of *Aplysia*. Such preparations allow superb visualization of growth cone dynamics. In this experiment, the movement of beads applied to the growth cone surface was used to measure intracellular actin flow under control conditions (*B*) and in the presence of a drug that inhibits myosin (*C*). Blocking myosin function reduces actin flow and promotes filopodial extension. (From Lin et al., 1996. Copyright 1996 Cell Press.)

be visualized directly by phase contrast or differential interference contrast microscopy. Nevertheless, it is relatively straightforward to map the responsiveness of a cell to a transmitter applied at specific loci along its cell body and dendrites (O'Brien and Fischbach, 1986c), even to determine the classes of receptors associated with individual presynaptic specializations (Bekkers and Stevens, 1989) and to identify individual presynaptic boutons by electron microscopy (Neale et al., 1978).

All in all, primary dissociated neuronal cultures are particularly amenable to study using morphological and physiological techniques, which can be applied on a cell-by-cell basis. They are less suited to traditional biochemical approaches because the quantity of material obtainable from these cultures usually is limited, although modern molecular techniques can compensate for this limitation to some degree. For example, now it is possible to analyze the populations of RNAs present in individual cells, even in individual dendrites or growth cones (Miyashiro et al., 1994; Crino and Eberwine, 1996).

Another inherent limitation of primary cultures is that they often contain a heterogeneous population of cells. In specific cases, cultures can be prepared whose cellular composition is much simpler than that of the tissues from which they derive. For example, principal sympathetic neurons can be obtained in culture essentially free of contamination by small, intensely fluorescent cells, fibroblasts, Schwann, and satellite cells (see chapter 11) and biochemical studies of such preparations have yielded considerable information concerning neurotransmitter choice during the development of sympathetic neurons (Patterson, 1978). More commonly, cultures are as complex as the tissue from which they originate.

The issue of heterogeneity also complicates studies using morphological and physiological techniques, because consistent results require the identification of specific cell populations. Developing approaches to deal with the heterogeneity of cell types is integral to the successful use of primary cultures. Such considerations begin with the choice of tissue to culture. Some regions of the nervous system are simply more complicated than others. One important reason for the use of dissociated cultures of autonomic and sensory ganglia in so many studies is that they contain a single predominant cell population (although even in sensory ganglia, there are subpopulations of cells that can be distinguished by neurotransmitter phenotype and neurotrophin dependence; see chapter 10).

In the CNS, the hippocampus and cerebellar cortex both contain a single dominant cell type, pyramidal cells and granule cells, respectively. In more complicated systems, it is important that markers be available to identify the cell type of interest after it has been introduced into culture. Finally, it may also be possible to simplify the cellular composition of the cell cultures. For example, if the cells of interest can be labeled in the living state, either by retrograde transport of a fluorescent dye in situ or with an antibody directed against a cell surface constituent applied after dissociation, they can be purified before being placed into culture (Assouline et al., 1983; O'Brien and Fischbach, 1986a; DiPorzio et al., 1987; see chapters 16 and 18). Alternatively, unwanted cells may be killed, either by specific cytotoxins or by complement-mediated lysis using antibodies against the cell surface (Brockes et al., 1979; Vogel and Weston, 1988; see chapter 19).

One final drawback of working with primary cultures: Success is not automatic. In the preceding discussion, we have emphasized what can be accomplished by using dissociated cell cultures. However, finding the conditions that permit good neuronal maturation, getting cultures to grow reproducibly, and documenting that you have accomplished all of this entails plenty of hard work. Some of these aspects of using dissociated cell cultures are covered in the next three chapters.

Explant or Organotypic Cultures

Culture of intact fragments of tissue—the kinds of cultures that Harrison developed—now would be termed *explant cultures*. Making explant cultures can be quite simple. Thin slices of the tissue of interest are allowed to attach to an appropriate substrate and are cultured in a rich medium, usually one containing serum. As with dissociated cell cultures, immature tissue grows best, and explants generally are prepared from embryonic or neonatal tissue. The need for nutrients and oxygen to diffuse to the center of the tissue limits their thickness to approximately a millimeter (Lumsden, 1968). In experienced hands, explant cultures can be maintained for months, and cells within the explant continue their development appropriately, extending processes and forming synapses with one another (Wolf and Dubois-Dalcq, 1970; Crain, 1976; Hendelman et al., 1977; Hendelman and Marshall, 1980). Non-

neuronal cells migrate out from the explant, and long neurites grow out from the nerve cell bodies within the explant.

Though this general approach continues to be used profitably, the last decade has seen the elaboration of this methodology in two different directions, one focused on maintaining the organotypic organization within the explant, the other on analysis of the neurites that grow out from the explants. Organotypic slice cultures, pioneered by Beat Gahwiler et al. (1981 a,b; 1984a), were developed with the aim of preserving tissue structure in thin slices that are more accessible to observation and experimental manipulation than are conventional explants (see chapter 17). Slices approximately 0.4 mm thick are cut on a tissue chopper and cultured in a plasma clot on glass coverslips. The coverslips are maintained in tubes that are rotated slowly so that the tissue alternately is submerged within the medium and exposed to the atmosphere (see also Hild and Tasaki, 1962; Hild, 1977). More recently, it has become possible to grow slice cultures on membrane filters (Stopini et al., 1991), eliminating the need for roller tubes and the vagaries of chicken plasma and putting this technique well within the realm of expertise of most laboratories.

Compared to the conventional explant technique, slice cultures "thin out" to as little as 15 μm in thickness during the first few weeks of culture, greatly improving the ability to visualize cells within the explants and making them much more accessible for physiological study. This approach has proved particularly fruitful for study of cortical structures such as the hippocampus, in which salient features of the normal organization of the tissue can be captured in a two-dimensional culture.

Explant cultures are of interest also because of the extensive fiber outgrowth that often occurs (see figure 2.6). Indeed, the remarkable halo of fibers that can be induced to form from explanted sympathetic ganglia still serves as the basis for the standard bioassay of Nerve Growth Factor activity. Thin strips of tissue that give rise to axons aligned in parallel (Bonhoefer and Huf, 1980, 1985; Halfter et al., 1983) also can be used (figure 2.7). By choice of appropriate substrates and use of antimitotic agents, it is possible to eliminate nonneuronal cells from the outgrowth zone, leaving a pure population of nerve fibers (Wood, 1976). Such preparations have been used to investigate the response of axonal growth cones to putative neurotropic substances (Heffner et al., 1990) or to contact with other fibers and tissues (Verna, 1985; Kapfhammer and Raper,

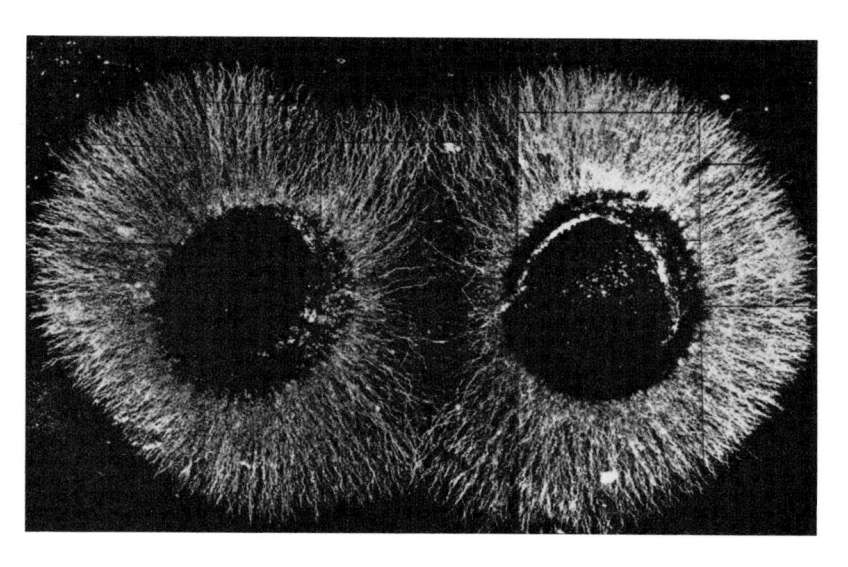

Figure 2.6 Explant cultures. Two dorsal root ganglia (from chick embryos) cultured together in a plasma clot. (From G. A. Dunn, Mutual contact inhibition of extension of chick sensory nerve fibres in vitro. J. Comp. Neurol. 143:491. © 1971.)

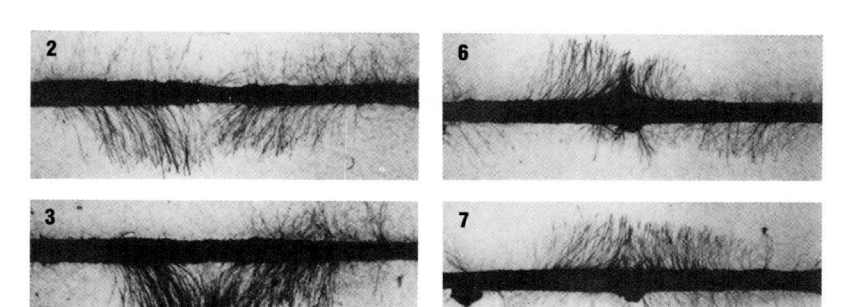

Figure 2.7 Fiber outgrowth from thin strips of embryonic chick retina explanted into culture. The tissue was placed on a filter so that it could be cut into strips of defined orientation. The principal direction of growth in culture reproduces that observed in situ. Outgrowth from strips 2 and 3, taken from superior retina, emerges largely from the inferior edge (toward the optic nerve head); outgrowth from strips of inferior retina (6, 7) is from the superior edge. Scale bar: 1 mm. (From Halfter et al., 1983, with permission.)

1987; Raper and Kapfhammer, 1990); for studies of the interactions of axons with myelinating Schwann cells or oligodendroglia (Wood and Bunge, 1975, 1986; see chapter 19); and to harvest populations of axons, free from somata and dendrites, for biochemical study (Black and Smith, 1988). By preparing explant cultures in collagen gels it is possible to establish gradients of soluble guidance molecules and examine the response of axons to these factors (Lumsden and Davies, 1986; Tessier-Lavigne et al., 1988; Sato et al., 1994). This approach has led to the isolation and characterization of the first molecularly identified chemotropic agents that guide growing axons (Kennedy and Tessier-Lavigne, 1995). Finally, placing two explants side by side allows fibers emerging from one explant to enter and innervate cells in the other (Crain, 1976; Gähwiler and Brown, 1985a; Distler and Robertson, 1993).

Reaggregate Cultures

Dissociated cells kept in suspension rather than allowed to settle on and attach to a solid substrate tend to reaggregate into small balls. This process can be encouraged by culturing cells in flasks maintained on a gyrotory shaker. Such reaggregate cultures originally were developed to study the process of cell association and "histotypic reaggregation" (Garber and Moscona, 1972; Garber, 1977), following from the classic experiments of Moscona's group on nonneuronal tissues (Moscona, 1965). It soon became apparent that reaggregate cultures offered a favorable environment for neuronal maturation, and several laboratories have adopted this procedure as their principal technique for culturing neurons. As in dissociated cell and explant cultures, cells in reaggregates extend processes, form synapses, synthesize transmitters; and express appropriate receptors (Seeds, 1983; Honegger, 1985; Hsiang et al., 1988). Moreover, reaggregate cultures permit cells to develop in three dimensions and, by combining cell populations dissociated from different brain regions, they allow a novel approach to study the interactions between afferents and target cells (Adler et al., 1976; Hsiange et al., 1987; Choi et al., 1993; Vidal et al., 1995). The conditions within small reaggregate cultures also appear to be favorable for the division of neural precursors, which do not proliferate well in dissociated cell cultures (Gao et al., 1991; Gage, Coates, et al., 1995). This approach has been exploited very

effectively by Gao et al. (1991, 1992) to elucidate the cell interactions that regulate neurogenesis and neuronal differentiation in
the cerebellum.

The price of culturing cells in reaggregates is lack of access.
Microscopy must be performed on fixed, sectioned preparations,
and physiological analyses are difficult.

Tumor Cell Lines

Although widely used, primary cultures are not ideal for many
purposes. The amount of material that can be obtained limits biochemical analysis and, because most primary cultures contain a
heterogeneous population of cell types, interpretation of such experiments can be ambiguous. Moreover, most genetic techniques
simply are not applicable to primary neuronal cultures. Because
neurons in primary cultures do not divide, mutant cells cannot be
propagated, and foreign genes cannot be stably integrated into the
genome (for further discussion, see chapter 4).

Since the pioneering work of Augusti-Tocco and Sato (1969) and
Schubert et al. (1969), cell lines derived from neural tumors have
provided an alternative approach that overcomes some of these
disadvantages. In contrast to primary cultures, nerve cell lines are
relatively easy to grow. In many cases, it is simply a matter of
thawing a vial of frozen cells, plating them into standard tissue
culture dishes or flasks, and subculturing them until the desired
number of cells is obtained. Then they can be induced to "differentiate" by any of a variety of factors, ceasing division, extending
processes, and increasing their expression of some neural-specific
genes (for review, see Kimhi, 1981; Schubert, 1984). Cells from
some clonal lines are electrically active, synthesize transmitters or
peptides, and express certain transmitter receptors. Moreover, the
cell population is clonally derived and therefore, to a first approxi-
mation, is genetically homogeneous.

These advantages must be weighed against the fact that many
important aspects of neuronal differentiation are not expressed by
tumor cell lines. Among the lines studied to date, none gives rise to
cells that develop definitive axons or dendrites, form synapses with
one another, or elicit the formation of myelin by appropriate glial
cells. Although cell lines express some generic properties of neurons or glia, for the most part the cell lines presently available do
not express the particular subset of neuronal properties that char-

acterize specific neuronal populations, say, cerebellar Purkinje cells or spinal motoneurons—and that set them apart from other types of neurons. Thus, tumor cell lines are one further step removed from "real" neurons than are primary cultures

Among the most commonly used of the neural clonal cell lines is the rat pheochromocytoma line PC12, which was derived from a tumor of the adrenal medulla that arose following x-irradiation (Greene and Tischler, 1976). PC12 cells represent an exception to the rule that cell lines do not express subsets of neuronal properties characteristic of specific cell types. Under routine culture conditions, PC12 cells exhibit many of the properties of adrenal chromaffin cells. As with adrenal chromaffin cells (Unsicker et al., 1978; Aloe and Levi-Montalcini, 1979; Doupe Landis, et al., 1985a; Anderson and Axel, 1986), when PC12 cells are exposed to nerve growth factor, they stop dividing and develop properties similar to sympathetic neurons. They extend long processes, become electrically excitable, synthesize catecholamines and release them in a calcium-dependent fashion (Guroff, 1985). PC12 cells synthesize acetylcholine as well, but this is true also of some populations of sympathetic neurons in situ. Although PC12 cells induce tumors when injected into animals, they differ from most other transformed cells lines in their near diploid number of chromosomes and their relatively slow growth. Methods for culturing PC12 cells are described in chapter 6.

Other commonly used cell lines derive from the C-1300 neuroblastoma, a tumor that arose spontaneously in the body cavity of a mouse, apparently from peripheral neural tissue. Hundreds of clonal lines, which differ markedly in their phenotype, have been derived from this tumor. This diversity reflects in part the unstable karyotype of these cells. Clones with average chromosome numbers varying between 60 and nearly 200 have been isolated, and even after subcloning, the number of chromosomes is unstable (Kimhi, 1981). To increase further the diversity of phenotypes expressed, clonal cell lines have been derived from hybrids of neuroblastoma cells fused to glioma or fibroblast cell lines (Hamprecht, 1977; Hamprecht et al., 1985). Other such cells express properties not found in either parent line. In addition, other neuroblastoma cell lines have been developed, including some from human tumors and some from tumors induced in rats by treatment with carcinogens (for review, see Schubert, 1984). Another human cell line that exhibits some neuronal features in culture was derived from a

patient with megalencephaly (Ronnett et al., 1990, 1994; Poltorak et al., 1992).

A recent approach to developing tumor cell lines uses transgenic technology to express immortalizing oncogenes under the control of cell-type specific promoters. For example, the GT-1 cell line was derived from a hypothalamic tumor induced by expressing the SV40 large T antigen under the control of the gonadotropin-releasing hormone promoter (Mellon et al., 1990). These cells, which express several neuron-specific markers, have been used extensively to study the expression and secretion of GnRH (Maggi et al., 1995; Belsham et al., 1996; Voight et al., 1996). A similar approach has been used to derive catecholaminergic cell lines from brain and adrenal gland (Suri et al., 1993) and cell lines from the retina (Hammang et al., 1990) and from neural progenitors in the olfactory epithelium (Largent et al., 1993).

Another, very different approach begins with continuous cell lines derived not from neural tissue but from multipotential cells with features of early embryonic tissues. When grown under appropriate conditions and treated with appropriate factors, such as retinoic acid, the cells develop a neuronlike phenotype.

This approach is typified by the studies of P19 cells initiated by McBurney and colleagues (McBurney and Rogers, 1982; McBurney et al., 1982; MacPherson and McBurney, 1995). P19 Cells derive from a mouse tumor induced when a mouse embryo was implanted into the testicular capsule of an adult mouse. The cells, which have a normal karyotype and divide rapidly, have a broad developmental potential, as evidenced by the tissue types to which they give rise following transplantation to an embryo or when differentiated in culture. In the last few years, several laboratories have developed strategies for inducing efficient neuronal differentiation of P19 cells and have begun to explore the value of such cultures as models for CNS neurons (Bain et al., 1993; Staines et al., 1994; Finley et al., 1996; see chapter 7). The cultures obtained by this strategy are not homogeneous, but the neuronlike cells they contain exhibit many desirable features not typical of conventional neural cell lines. They synthesize and release glutamate, GABA, and glycine and express receptors for these neurotransmitters, including glutamate receptors of both AMPA and NMDA subtypes. And like neurons in primary cultures, they become polarized and make real synapses, as confirmed by both morphological and physiological methods.

Like mouse P19 cells, the human teratocarcinoma cell line N-Tera 2 can be induced to differentiate as neurons in culture following treatment with retinoic acid, replating on appropriate substrates, and exposure to mitotic inhibitors (Pleasure et al., 1992). Under optimal conditions, nearly homogeneous cultures of cells that exhibit many of the structural and cytoskeletal features of polarized neurons can be obtained. They express a variety of receptors, including glutamate receptors of the AMPA and NMDA subtypes, and exhibit glutamate-induced excitotoxicity (Hardy et al., 1994; Munir et al., 1996). The procedures required to induce neuronal differentiation in N-Tera 2 cells require many weeks, but terminally differentiated N-Tera 2 cells can be purchased commercially (Stratagene, La Jolla, CA).

More recently, it has been shown that embryonic stem (ES) cells, the totipotent embryonic mouse cell line used in creating mice with targeted disruptions in endogenous genes, can also be induced to differentiate into neuronlike cells in culture exhibiting many of the same features (Bain et al., 1995; Fraichard et al., 1995; Strubing et al., 1995; Finley et al., 1996; see chapter 7). This offers many exciting possibilities, because the well-established techniques for homologous recombination in ES cells allow knocking out genes and introducing genes downstream of native regulatory elements. Such manipulations could be studied in neuronal cells in culture as well as in transgenic mice. Moreover, unlike tumor-derived cell lines, ES cells are genetically normal.

Alternative Strategies for Generating Nerve Cell Lines

The many potentially important uses of nerve cell lines, together with the limitations exhibited by those presently available, has stimulated the development of new strategies for creating neural cell lines. A particularly important impetus for such work comes from the possibility of using genetically engineered neural cell lines as a source of tissue for transplantation—a situation in which tumorigenic cells lines would be particularly undesirable. Might this approach also provide new cell lines that more closely resemble differentiated neurons in culture? As yet, the new lines that have been generated do not exhibit the well-developed neuronal properties routinely found in primary neuronal cultures, but they offer many features that complement tumor cell lines.

One advantage common to these new methods is that they allow cell lines to be derived from cells in specific regions of the nervous system. One strategy that has been used to accomplish this is to form somatic cell hybrids between embryonic cells dissociated from the brain region of interest and continuous cell lines. Hybrid clones can be isolated by choosing cell lines that are deficient in hypoxanthine phosphoribosyltransferase and that, therefore, cannot multiply in medium containing hypoxanthine, aminopterin, and thymidine (the same selection procedure used in preparing monoclonal antibodies). This approach was applied first by Greene et al. (1975), who obtained a catecholamine-producing hybrid cell line from fusion of mouse sympathetic neurons with a neuroblastoma cell line that did not synthesize catecholamines. Similar results were obtained from fusions of rat dorsal root ganglion cells with neuroblastoma cells (Platika et al., 1985).

Beginning in 1986, Wainer and his colleagues have applied this approach systematically to develop hybrid lines from discrete regions of the CNS, including the striatum, hippocampus, septal area, and mesencephalon (Hammond et al., 1986; Eves et al., 1992; Blusztajn et al., 1992; Choi et al., 1992). Similar approaches have been used to develop hybrids expressing properties of spinal motoneurons (Cashman et al., 1992) and mesencephalic dopaminergic cells (Crawford et al., 1992). In general, such cells appear to exhibit more features characteristic of the mature neuronal phenotype than typical neural tumor cell lines. For example, often they express a neurotransmitter phenotype appropriate to the region from which they were derived, but they do not become polarized or establish synapses.

One serious limitation in this technique concerns the neuroblastoma cell lines currently used as fusion partners. For example, N18TG2 cells exhibit chromosome numbers ranging from 59 to 120, compared with the normal mouse complement of 42 (Crawford et al., 1992). These chromosomal abnormalities carry over to the hybrid cell lines. For example, dorsal root ganglion–neuroblastoma hybrids contained on average 140 mouse chromosomes (from the neuroblastoma cell line) but only 10 rat chromosomes (Platika et al., 1985).

A second approach is based on infecting cells with oncogene-containing retroviruses (for review, see Gage et al., 1995a; Whittemore and Snyder, 1996). The viral oncogenes, which are capable of immortalizing cells, are inserted into the host genome, copied

along with host DNA, and transmitted to progeny. An important limitation of this procedure is that the incorporation of viral DNA requires a round of DNA synthesis. Thus, cell lines can be made only from cells that retain the capacity to divide, not from post-mitotic neurons. An important advantage, particularly compared to the hybrid lines, is that only a single gene is added to the genome of the cell type of interest, and none of the cell's genes are lost. Temperature-sensitive mutants of oncogenes also are available, so that in principle, cells might be propagated indefinitely at the permissive temperature that allows the oncogene to be expressed, then induced to stop dividing and exhibit the properties of more differentiated cells by transfer to the nonpermissive temperature.

Sympathoadrenal precursor cells, isolated by fluorescence-activated cell sorting, have been immortalized successfully by using a retrovirus containing v-*myc* (Birren and Anderson, 1990; Sommer et al., 1995). Exposure of the cells first to fibroblast growth factor, then to nerve growth factor; causes some to acquire a sympathetic phenotype. More than a dozen cell lines have been derived in this way from various regions of the CNS, including the cerebellum, hippocampus, striatum, olfactory bulb, mesencephalon, and medullary raphe; most have used v-*myc* or the SV40 large T antigen (Whittemore and Snyder, 1996). Nearly all are multipotential, capable of generating cells with both neuronal and glial properties. When transplanted into the brain, cells from many of these cell lines acquire a highly differentiated neuronal phenotype. Cells transplanted to the hippocampus closely resemble dentate granule neurons, those transplanted to the cerebellum appropriate cerebellar cell types, and so on. Remarkably, this capacity need not depend on the region from which the cell line was derived (Renfranz et al., 1991; Vicario-Abejon et al., 1995a; Cunningham et al., 1995). For example, a cell line derived from the medullary raphe can, when transplanted to the hippocampus, give rise to neurons that look remarkably like hippocampal pyramidal neurons; when transplanted to the cerebral cortex, derivatives include both pyramidal and stellate neurons (Whittemore and White, 1993; Shihabuddin et al., 1996). Though study of these cell lines offers a promising means to examine the epigenetic signals that regulate neural differentiation, too little is presently known to induce them to acquire such mature neuronal phenotypes in culture.

One limitation in understanding the control of proliferation and lineage in the CNS has been the difficulty of culturing the progeni-

tor cells that give rise to neurons. The last few years have seen remarkable progress in this area (for reviews, see Gage, Goates, et al., 1995; Kilpatrick et al., 1995; Temple and Qian, 1995), progress that certainly will improve the prospects of exploiting retrovirally derived cell lines as culture models.

Glial Cells in Culture

Cell culture is a particularly valuable approach for studying glial development and function. Because of the inherent heterogeneity of nervous tissue, it has been difficult to investigate the function of glia in situ. In culture; it is relatively easy to obtain pure preparations of astroglia, oligodendroglia, and Schwann cells, free of contaminating neurons. As discussed in chapter 18, this process has become the method of choice for many studies.

Astrocytes (more correctly astroglial precursor cells) are particularly hardy and grow readily in primary cultures (see chapter 18). Typically, cell suspensions are prepared from neonatal brain and are plated into tissue culture flasks or dishes. The cells divide relatively rapidly, forming a confluent monolayer of astroglia within a week or two. Conditions are chosen to preclude the survival of neurons but, in some cases, additional steps are needed to remove other nonneuronal contaminants. Using this approach, one can produce amounts of cells suitable for biochemical as well as morphological or physiological analysis (Federoff and Vernadakis, 1986; Kimelberg, 1988). Some caution is required in interpreting observations made in these preparations, because it is not clear yet to what extent the cultured cells exhibit the properties of mature astrocytes as opposed to developing astrocytes or astroglial precursors. Obviously, some aspects of astroglial maturation may require interaction with other cell types or constituents not available in culture.

Culturing oligodendrocytes and Schwann cells is somewhat more difficult. The elegant studies of Raff and colleagues have demonstrated that oligodendrocytes and a subpopulation of astrocytes develop from a common precursor cell, the O-2A cell (reviewed by Raff, 1989; see chapter 18). They also have defined the conditions that control the differentiation of these cells in culture. Most approaches for culturing oligodendroglia involve first allowing the proliferation of this precursor cell in neonatal brain cultures, then separating it from contaminating cell types and manipulating cul-

ture conditions to induce the differentiation of oligodendroglia (see chapter 18). Schwann cell cultures commonly are prepared from neonatal peripheral nerve (Brockes et al., 1979); alternatively, they can be obtained from explant cultures of spinal ganglia (Wood, 1976; see chapter 19). Culture conditions must be chosen to enhance the proliferation of the rather slow-growing Schwann cells, and contaminating fibroblasts must be killed selectively; either with antimitotic agents or by immune lysis. The oligodendrocytes and Schwann cells prepared by these methods can be induced to form myelin sheaths when cocultured with an appropriate population of nerve cells. Such cultures have facilitated studies of the properties of oligodendrocytes and Schwann cells grown in the absence of neurons. They have also served to define the cell interactions that occur during myelination: the stimulation of Schwann cell pro-liferation by contact with axons, the events that lead to axonal en-sheathment, and the role of extracellular matrix in this process (reviewed in chapter 19).

Primary cell cultures also are used widely for the study of micro-glia, the population of macrophages resident in the CNS. Microglia, which often appear as loosely attached cells atop monolayers of type I astrocytes, can be harvested by shaking and can be obtained in quite pure preparations (Giulian and Baker, 1986; Gebicke-Haertner et al., 1989). This approach has been instrumental in elu-cidating the functional properties of microglia, which secrete many cytotoxic substances and have been implicated in the destruction of neurons that occurs in several neural diseases (Giulian et al., 1993, 1995; Chao et al., 1995; Gehrmann et al., 1995).

Although many cell lines derived from glial tumors have been developed, they are used less commonly than are primary cell cul-tures. Considerable disappointment resulted when investigation of cell lines thought to resemble oligodendrocytes revealed that none was competent to form myelin (Pfeiffer et al., 1977). There are astrocytic lines that can be used to advantage, particularly when results can be confirmed with other approaches (Martin et al., 1989; Shain et al., 1989). But because primary cultures of glia can be propagated easily, can be grown so readily in primary culture, and relatively large quantities can be obtained, there has been little need for such cell lines. With the development of molecular biol-ogy, and the possibility of developing stably transfected lines, there may be a renewed interest in glial cell lines.

3 *Primary Dissociated Cell Cultures*

Dennis Higgins and Gary Banker

Regardless of the type of cells to be grown—neuronal or glial, peripheral or central, vertebrate or invertebrate—all methods for preparing dissociated-cell cultures share several features: a source of tissue containing the cells of interest must be obtained, the tissue must be dissociated without damaging these cells, and the dissociated cells must be cultured on a suitable substrate and in an appropriate medium. Careful attention to each of these features provides the foundation for the successful culturing of nerve cells. Each is considered in some detail in this chapter.

Working with cell lines and organotypic cultures involves many of the same considerations as those that apply to primary cultures, particularly regarding the choice of medium and substrate. Methods that pertain specifically to cell lines, such as passaging cells and obtaining and storing cell stocks, are described in chapters devoted to culturing PC12 cells (chapter 6) and to P19 and ES cells (chapter 7). Additional information regarding these subjects can be found in standard textbooks of cell culture. Similarly, methods for preparation and maintenance of organotypic cultures are described by Gähwiler et al. in chapter 17.

Before beginning to grow nerve cells, you will also need to be familiar with more general methods of tissue culture, the most fundamental of which is sterile technique. Microorganisms reproduce so rapidly that if even only a few "bugs" are introduced into culture along with your neurons, they will soon win out. This means that every component involved in preparing cultures must be sterilized, and its sterility must be maintained. Fifty years ago, the sterile technique needed to culture cells required heroic endeavors. Fortunately, in this era of laminar flow hoods and membrane filters, the necessary techniques are easy to learn and to apply. In addition, you will need access to, and experience in using, standard cell culture equipment: autoclaves, incubators, hoods, and inverted microscopes. For those not familiar with these basics, they are described thoroughly in general textbooks devoted to cell and tissue culture (Doyle and Griffiths, 1993; Freshney, 1994).

Source of Tissue

Species

Among mammals, rats and mice are the species used most commonly as a source of tissue for neuronal cultures. They share several generic advantages, such as genetic consistency and modest cost. The ready availability of pregnant female rats and mice of defined gestational age ("timed-pregnant" females) is also important because most neural cultures are prepared from embryonic or neonatal tissue. The preponderance of culture experiments that have used rats and mice is itself advantageous because of the database that has been accumulated, but there is no inherent reason for avoiding other species as long as animals of an appropriate age are routinely available.

When compared with rats, mice offer additional advantages. First, a large variety of neurological mutants has been catalogued. Nerve cell cultures from these mutants provide a valuable opportunity for analyzing the effects of specific genes on neural development and function (Messer and Smith, 1977; Bartlett, et al., 1989; Kofuji et al., 1996; Liesi and Wright, 1996; see chapter 16). The rapid development of transgenic and knockout technology has expanded such opportunities immensely. This approach has been combined already with a cell culture analysis to study means to reduce the susceptibility of neurons to neurotoxic damage (Farlie et al., 1995; Dawson et al., 1996), to explore the role of specific genes in the response to neurotrophins (Bar-Peled et al., 1996; Dawson et al., 1996; Lawrence et al., 1996), and to evaluate the role of certain cytoskeletal proteins in axonal outgrowth (Harada et al., 1994) Finally, transgenic mice that constitutively express marker genes such as lacZ (Friedrich and Soriano, 1991) could serve as a useful source of labeled cells for certain types of coculture experiments. One limitation in this approach must be kept in mind: If mutations or gene deletions are sufficiently deleterious that the mouse lines are maintained by mating heterozygotes, the cells from each littermate must be cultured separately, and their genotype must be determined after the fact.

Techniques similar to those developed for culturing neurons from rodents have been applied with considerable success to cultures of human fetal neurons, permitting a unique approach to

studies of neurological disorders that cannot be studied in animal models. Successful dissociated cell cultures have been obtained from spinal and sympathetic ganglia (Scott et al., 1982; Zeevalk et al., 1982; Kim et al., 1984; Nieminen et al., 1988; Yong et al., 1988) as well as from spinal cord (Kato et al., 1985), dopaminergic brainstem nuclei (Dong et al., 1993; Levallois et al., 1995; Othberg et al., 1995; Spenger et al., 1995), cerebral cortex (Louis et al., 1983; Mattson et al., 1992), and retina (Osborne and Beaton, 1985). These cultures typically have used tissue from therapeutic abortions performed. Recently, several groups have had success in culturing and propagating human Schwann cells (Morrissey et al., 1995; Rutkowski et al., 1995a; Li et al., 1996) and oligodendroglia (Scolding et al., 1994) from adult tissues. Cultures of neuronal cells from adult brain biopsies also have been described (Kirschenbaum et al., 1994).

Among nonmammalian vertebrates, two species have proved particularly valuable as a source of tissue for neuronal culture and have been used extensively for developmental studies: the domestic chicken, *Gallus*, and the exotic clawed toad, *Xenopus*. By comparison with mammals, both offer a welcome simplicity. Fertilized chicken eggs are inexpensive and readily available, and *Xenopus* can be reared easily in the laboratory. Both species can be staged accurately, and neither requires elaborate animal care facilities.

Embryonic chicks frequently are used as a source of tissue for culture studies of sensory and autonomic ganglia (Nishi, 1996; see chapter 10 and references therein) and of spinal cord and nerve-muscle interactions (Falls et al., 1993; Hory-Lee and Franks, 1996). Cultures from chick brain (Sensenbrenner et al., 1978; Davenport et al., 1996; Dyatlov et al., 1996) have received comparatively little attention, perhaps because many aspects of the anatomy of the avian brain are quite different from those of mammals.

Although less widely used than are chicks, cultures from *Xenopus* have proved particularly valuable for studies of muscle innervation (Kuromi et al., 1985; Buchanan et al., 1989; Hirano and Kidokoro, 1989; see chapter 9). *Xenopus* embryos are accessible for observation and experimentation from the time of fertilization, making it possible to inject cells within the blastomere with fluorescent tracers that persist in all the progeny after they are placed in culture (Sanes and Poo, 1989). Likewise, one can inject proteins (Vallorta et al, 1995), antibodies (Lin and Szaro, 1995), or vectors

that direct the expression of specific proteins (Alder et al., 1995), then test their effects on neuronal development in culture. Cultures of *Xenopus* spinal neurons have become a favorite preparation for analysis of the role of calcium currents in neural development (Spitzer et al., 1995) and for study of the properties of growth cones and the synapses they make on muscle cells (Zheng et al., 1994, 1996; Dai and Peng, 1995; Dan et al., 1995; Fu et al., 1995).

Finally, invertebrates. Successful neuronal cultures have been obtained from a variety of invertebrates, particularly molluscs, annelids, and arthropods (for reviews, see Thomas et al., 1987; Townsel and Thomas, 1987; Beadle et al., 1988). Most attention has focused on cultures from the now-famous sea slug *Aplysia* (Camardo et al., 1983; Katz and Levitan, 1993; Eliot et al., 1994; Fisher et al., 1994; Murphy and Glanzman, 1996; see chapter 8), on the land snail *Helisoma* (Kater and Mattson, 1988; Davenport et al., 1993; Guthrie et al., 1994; Williams and Cohan 1995; figure 3.1), on the leech *Hirudo* (Chiquet and Nicholls, 1987; Szczupak et al., 1993; Neely and Gesemann, 1994; Bruns and Jahn, 1995; Fernandez-de-Miguel and Drapeau, 1995), and on the moth *Manduca* (Levine and Weeks, 1996)—primarily because of the large body of neurobiogical work on these species. The advantages that these preparations offer for studies in situ—their ability to identify individual cells from animal to animal and the large size of their somata—have proved to be of equal value for studies undertaken in cell culture. Such cultures typically are prepared from juvenile animals, so that the growth observed in culture reflects regenerative events in cells that are relatively mature, compared with those taken from embryonic vertebrates.

A very different motivation underlies the development of cultures of nervous tissue from *Drosophila* (Seecof et al., 1971; Wu et al, 1983; Salvaterra et al., 1987), whose neurons are among the smallest known. Following from the advances that have derived from the combination of classical genetics and molecular biology, cell cultures of *Drosophila* neurons offer a remarkable opportunity to investigate the functions of specific genes in development. This approach has been applied most extensively to analyze the regulation of ion channel expression (O'Dowd and Aldrich, 1988; O'Dowd et al., 1995; Wright and Zhong, 1995) and the mechanisms of neurite outgrowth (Kim and Wu, 1987; Broughton et al., 1996). The use of molecular genetic methods for "marking" specific cell types in culture (Zhang et al., 1994) and the formulation of an

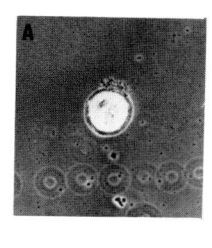
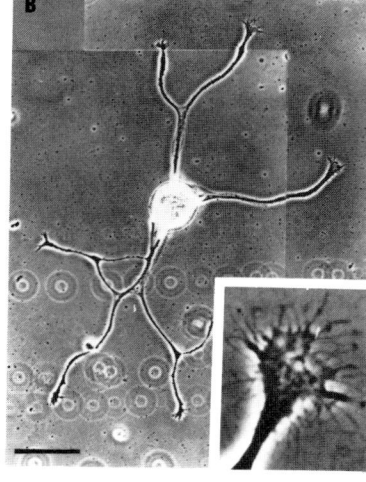
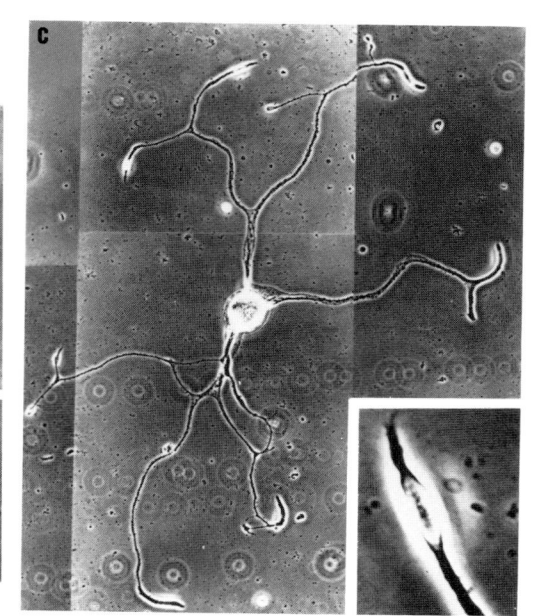

Figure 3.1 Snail neurons are among the many invertebrate types that have been cultured. Illustrated here is neuron 5 from the buccal ganglion of *Helisoma*. Outgrowth usually begins during the first day in culture (*A*) and progresses at a rapid pace for the next 2 days (*B*). Growth ceases after 3 days and the cell acquires a stable morphology (*C*). During active outgrowth the processes exhibit typical growth cones (*B*, inset), while in the stable state they are tipped by slender, elongated, phase bright structures (*C*, inset). Different identified neurons consistently exhibit different morphologies in culture. Scale bar: 100 μm; 20 μm for insets. (From Hadley et al., 1985, with permission.)

appropriate serum-free medium for *Drosophila* cultures (O'Dowd, 1995) should facilitate this work.

Age

Traditionally, neuronal and glial cultures have been prepared from embryonic or early postnatal animals. There are several reasons for this preference. Neurons are much less susceptible to damage during dissociation if prepared while their somata are still small and before they have developed extensive axonal and dendritic arbors and have become highly innervated. They also may be less dependent on their target cells for trophic support at early stages in their development. Glial cultures, which derive predominantly from populations of progenitor cells, are prepared most easily when the number of these progenitors is near its peak, during the early

postnatal period. On a more prosaic level, meninges and connective tissue sheaths are easier to remove cleanly at these earlier stages of development.

Obviously, the appropriate developmental age for preparing cultures will be determined by the time at which the cells of interest are generated. Detailed information about the birthdates of cells throughout the central and peripheral nervous system is available regarding most commonly used animals, based on labeling with ^{3}H-thymidine. For example, in the rat, cerebellar Purkinje cells are generated well before birth, whereas most granule cells arise during the first 2 weeks after birth. Thus, cultures enriched for Purkinje cells are best prepared from embryonic animals, whereas granule cells can be cultured only from postnatal animals (for details, see chapter 16).

The relationship between the stage of a cell's development in situ and its growth in culture can be studied quite precisely. For example, by administering ^{3}H-thymidine to animals at different stages of gestation, it is possible to label neurons generated at different times, so that subsequently they can be identified in culture by using autoradiography (Banker and Cowan, 1977; Ahmed and Fellows, 1987; Krushel et al., 1989). In studies of hippocampal cultures, we found that the cells generated 24 to 48 h before dissociation, which were in the process of migration at the time they were introduced into culture, survived somewhat better than did either cells that were generated earlier and had completed migration and had begun to elaborate dendrites or cells that had just completed mitosis (Banker and Cowan, 1977). The culture conditions used in these early experiments were admittedly Spartan, and we have found since that the age-related differences in ability to survive in culture can be overcome to some extent by improvements in culture conditions (Fletcher and Banker, 1989). Nevertheless, these results show how rather small differences in a cell's age can affect its survival in culture. Other studies, using similar approaches, have shown that differences in cell age can influence other parameters of neuronal development in culture, including dendritic growth and the rate of axonal elongation (Argiro et al., 1984; Bruckenstein et al., 1989).

Recent advances, particularly the development of gentler, more reproducible methods of cell dissociation, have made it possible to obtain cultures from progressively older animals. Dorsal root and sympathetic neurons from adult rats and mice are cultured readily,

although the recovery of cells may be substantially less than that from neonates (Scott, 1982; Johnson, and Argiro, 1983; Orr and Smith, 1988; Delree et al., 1989; Acheson et al., 1995; Edstrom et al., 1996). Even neurons from adult human ganglia have been maintained in culture (Scott et al., 1979). Though it is not routinely possible to obtain dissociated cell cultures of neurons from the adult central nervous system (CNS), considerable success has been achieved in preparing cultures from rats and mice during the first few postnatal weeks (Huettner and Baughman, 1986; see chapter 12). At these ages, nerve cells already exhibit many of their mature properties, and anatomically defined regions may be recognized precisely and dissected cleanly .

The ability to prepare cultures from postnatal rather than from embryonic animals also has practical advantages. For instance, it is possible to sacrifice only one postnatal animal at a time, saving the rest of the litter for later use. This is clearly impossible with embryonic animals. Also, when embryonic rats or mice must be used, their true stage of development can be determined only after the pregnant mother has been killed, a fact that can lead to occasional, unhappy surprises. The promising results of Magistretti et al. (1996), who have obtained successful cultures from adult guinea pig cortex, raise the possibility that it even may become routinely possible to break the 2 week barrier. Unlike most neurons from the adult CNS, magnocellular neurons from the hypothalamus can be maintained in long-term culture (Erickson and Watkins, 1981; Weiss and Cobbett, 1992). Perhaps this ability is related to the fact that these cells do not synapse on other neurons but instead project to the hypophyseal portal system. Culture of adult retinal neurons also has been possible with the envelopment of appropriate substrates (O'Malley and MacLeish, 1993).

Preparation of Cells

Balanced Salt Solutions and pH Control

At all stages, tissues and cells must be maintained in an osmotically balanced solution at physiological pH. A *balanced salt solution* (BSS) consists of a simple mixture of salts, including Na, K, Mg, Ca, Cl, PO_4, and HCO_3 at concentrations approximating those of extracellular fluid, together with glucose. They are intended for

short-term use, such as for collecting or dissociating tissue. *Media* contain, in addition, the nutrients needed for long-term growth of cells: amino acids, vitamins, and other ingredients. (Details concerning the composition of media are discussed in a later section).

There are several variations of balanced salt solutions that differ primarily in the buffers they contain. Some balanced salt solutions, such as Earle's salts, are buffered with bicarbonate and require equilibration with an atmosphere containing 5% to 10% CO_2 to maintain pH (whereas ambient atmosphere contains 0.03%). Earle's BSS is used as the basis for many of the media most commonly used for culturing cells (see below). Balanced salt solutions buffered with bicarbonate are unsatisfactory for use in an ambient atmosphere because they rapidly become basic, reaching pH levels above 8.0. For equilibration in air, other buffers must be used. These include a combination of low concentrations of $NaHCO_3$ and PO_4 (as in Hank's BSS) or "Good" buffers such as HEPES (Good et al., 1966). Buffers commonly used in biochemical studies, such as phosphate or TRIS at high concentration, are toxic to cells when used for long periods of time. For collecting and dissociating tissues, many laboratories use BSS that they prepare themselves according to formulae that vary slightly depending on their intended use (for examples, see chapters 8, 10, and 19); alternatively, Hank's BSS, sometimes supplemented with HEPES, also is widely used.

Because pH control is so important for cell survival, the pH indicator phenol red is included routinely in BSS and medium. With experience, one can gauge the pH of phenol red-containing solutions to within 0.2 units simply on the basis of the color, which ranges from yellow (pH $\sim$6) to red (pH $\sim$7.3) to purple (pH $\sim$8.0). To become familiar with the color changes that phenol red exhibits, it is useful to titrate a container of medium while measuring pH with a meter or to prepare a series of standard solutions of phenol red at known pH values (Freshney, 1994). Despite the widespread use of phenol red, a bit of caution is needed. Phenol red interacts with estrogen and prostaglandin receptors (Berthois et al., 1986; Hubert et al., 1986; Greenberg et al., 1994), and a common impurity in phenol red affects some ion transporters (Hop and Bunker, 1993). Toxic products also may be generated on exposure to intense light, as can occur during microscopy for long periods or with intense light sources.

Dissecting the Desired Tissue

The first step in the preparation of any primary culture is the dissection. Obviously, the tissue must be obtained aseptically, and the dissection itself usually is performed in a laminar flow hood. At all stages, the tissue must be kept moist and, once obtained, usually it is placed in BSS until all the needed material has been collected. It is customary to work at room temperature, although in some cases, tissue is maintained on ice after it has been collected. If the specific area of interest is too small to be obtained by dissection, methods have been developed for obtaining cells from discrete regions of tissue slices (Turner et al., 1995).

In cell culture work, it is seldom necessary to oxygenate the solutions used during tissue preparation. This finding may seem surprising in view of the importance of proper oxygenation for in vitro physiological studies using ganglia or tissue slices. It reflects, in part, the predominant use of embryonic and neonatal tissue for culture, when metabolism still is largely anaerobic. Once the tissue has been dissociated, the levels of dissolved O_2 in solutions exposed to air are more than adequate to achieve the O_2 tensions necessary for optimal growth. In fact, the level of dissolved O_2 in culture medium is significantly higher than it is in the intact brain and, in some cases, it may be beneficial to maintain nerve cell culture in an atmosphere containing less O_2 than air (Kaplan et al, 1986; Brewer and Cotman, 1989). In contrast, in tissue slices or in organ culture, diffusion of O_2 to the center of the tissue often is limiting.

Dissociation

After the dissection, the tissue obtained must be dissociated to give a suspension of single cells. The stronger the cell-cell associations and the greater the number of synapses, the more difficult it is to dissociate tissue. Dissociation is difficult when there are strong intercellular associations, such as synaptic junctions. Synapses frequently remain intact even when tissue is homogenized, pulling with them fragments of membrane of the pre- and postsynaptic cells. Presumably, this is why mature tissue is difficult to dissociate without damage to its constituent cells.

Dissociation is facilitated by removal of divalent cations, which are required for some classes of cell-cell adhesion (Takeichi, 1988).

Thus, it is common to collect and dissociate tissue in calcium- and magnesium-free balanced salt solutions. In some cases, this will weaken cell associations sufficiently to allow dissociation, but frequently protease treatment is also necessary. As enzymes are large molecules that do not enter cells, protease treatment can remove externally exposed cell surface proteins and proteins of the extracellular matrix (including components involved in cell association) without significant damage to the cell. During this process, other cell surface components also may be attacked. For example, trypsin treatment preferentially destroys some classes of transmitter receptors, which reappear only after a day or so in culture (Fischbach and Nelson, 1977; Allen et al., 1988).

Typically, the tissue to be dissociated is cut into small fragments and is incubated with protease at 37°C for periods ranging from 10 min to an hour or more. Obviously, the protease cannot be used in the presence of serum or other protein-containing solutions, which would competitively inhibit protease activity. A variety of enzyme preparations have been used to dissociate tissues for culture. The most commonly used is trypsin 1:250 (so called because it will hydrolyze 250 times its weight of casein in 10 min, under the standard conditions of assay). In fact, this preparation, which is prepared from hog pancreas, contains a mixture of other enzymes, including chymotrypsin and elastase, in addition to trypsin. For many purposes, the use of a mixture of proteases is desirable, and this crude preparation gives quite satisfactory results. It is important, however, that the preparation be screened for viruses and mycoplasma.

If more careful control of the dissociation procedure is important, as when dissociating tissue from postnatal animals, it may be advantageous to use a purified protease. In addition to purified trypsin, other commonly employed proteases include the neutral protease from *Bacillus polymyxa* ("Dispase"), pronase (Johnson and Argiro, 1983), or papain (see chapter 12). Collagenase also may be beneficial when a significant amount of connective tissue is present, as in peripheral ganglia from older animals (Johnson and Argiro, 1983).

Careful control of pH during enzyme treatment is important, because some proteolytic enzymes have narrow pH optima. Trypsin, for example, is almost completely inactive below pH 7.0. If substantial cell lysis occurs, the released strands of DNA can form a sticky, viscous "goop" that interferes with dissociation. Some pro-

tocols include DNAse in the dissociation step to hydrolyze released DNA.

After enzyme treatment, protease activity must be stopped. This is accomplished by rinsing the tissue after fragments have settled out or after centrifugation to pellet the cells. Enzyme activity can also be inhibited by the addition of serum or of a specific inhibitor, such as soybean trypsin inhibitor (chapter 12). The tissue fragments then are dissociated mechanically. Usually, this process is accomplished by repeated passage through a Pasteur pipette, a process termed *trituration*. The mechanical shearing force that this action produces disaggregates the tissue; the fragments become smaller and smaller, and the medium turns cloudy, owing to light scattering by the suspended cells. To increase the effectiveness of dissociation, the tip diameter of the Pasteur pipette may be decreased by flaming in a Bunsen burner. This also increases the possibility of damaging the cells. The larger the cells, the more susceptible they are to shearing damage. Thus, it may be desirable to allow the undissociated fragments to settle out periodically, so that the supernatant containing dissociated cells can be removed. Fresh BSS then is added, and the trituration process is resumed. It is important to avoid frothing during trituration, as cells at an air-liquid interface can be lysed. In expelling the tissue fragments from the pipette, its tip should be above the surface of the liquid and directed toward the wall of the container. In some preparations, clumps of tissue will remain undissociated after this procedure, and these can be removed by sieving: passing the cell suspension through a sheet of nylon bolting cloth of the desired mesh size (see chapters 8 and 13).

Purifying Specific Cell Populations

Once the tissue has been dissociated, it is possible to enrich the population for a desired cell type or to eliminate an unwanted one. One of the simplest methods for separating cell populations prior to plating is based on differential adhesion. Neurons and some classes of glial cells adhere poorly to untreated glass or plastic surfaces, whereas nonneuronal cells, particularly fibroblasts, adhere rapidly. If a mixed cell suspension is plated into untreated dishes and left for a short time, unattached cells (including nearly all neurons) can be removed and replated on an appropriate substrate (McCarthy and Partlow, 1976; see chapter 10). A similar principle forms the

basis for one standard method of obtaining purified glial populations (McCarthy and DeVellis, 1980). In mixed glial cultures
from the CNS, type 1 astrocytes adhere tightly to the tissue culture
dish, whereas type 2 astrocytes and oligodendrocytes develop on
top of the monolayer formed by type 1 astrocytes. The less tightly
attached oligodendrocytes and type 2 astrocytes can be removed by
vigorous shaking, leaving type 1 astrocytes attached to the substrate.

Other methods for cell separation, such as density gradient centrifugation, also have been useful for obtaining neural cell populations enriched in a particular cell type. For example, centrifugation
on Percoll gradients can be used to separate cerebellar cell suspensions into a small cell fraction consisting principally of granule
neurons and a large cell fraction containing astroglia and larger
neurons (Hatten, 1985; this approach is described in detail by
Hatten and her colleagues in chapter 16). Centrifugation on gradients of metrizamide (G. M. Smith et al., 1986; Martinou et al.,
1989, 1992) has permitted 4- to 12-fold enrichment of motoneurons
in cell suspensions prepared from the embryonic spinal cord.

These methods are relatively fast and do not require complicated
equipment but, because they are based on differences in physical
properties such as cell size, they seldom will yield pure populations of neurons from a tissue as heterogeneous as the CNS. Indeed,
this can be a formidable problem, considering that some much-
studied classes of neurons account for only a small percentage of
the cells present in the region in which they reside (Barres et al.,
1988; Martinou et al., 1989). Two general approaches have been
developed that permit cell separation with this degree of selectivity: immunoselection techniques and fluorescence-activated cell
sorting. The first requires antibodies that recognize surface constituents on the cell type of interest; the second requires a means of
labeling the cells selectively with a fluorescent marker.

If an antibody directed against a specific surface antigen on the
cells of interest is available, any of several immunoselection methods can be used to purify cells that express it (Sharpe, 1988;
Fleischer and Fleischer, 1989). Of these, "cell panning" is probably
the method of choice; the application of cell panning to purification of cerebellar neurons and glial progenitor cells is described
in detail in subsequent chapters. In this approach, antibodies are
adsorbed to plastic Petri dishes to create a surface that permits
the rapid and selective attachment of the desired cell population.
A two-step antibody procedure, analogous to that used in indirect

immunofluorescence, commonly is used. Antibodies directed against immunoglobulins from the species used to prepare the cell-specific antibody are adsorbed to the panning dish. Then the cell-specific antibody may be applied to the dish as a second layer, and the mixed cell suspension can be added. Alternatively, the cell suspension can be incubated with the cell-specific antibody and added to the dish. After allowing time for cell attachment, unbound cells are removed by washing, and bound cells are collected, often by trypsinization. Cell panning is comparatively simple, inexpensive, and rapid. Suspensions containing more than 10^8 cells can be applied to one 100-mm Petri dish, and adsorbtion usually is complete is less than an hour.

This approach has been used widely to prepare purified populations of both glia and neurons (Assouline et al., 1983; Barres et al., 1988b; Gard and Pfeiffer, 1989). Often two or more steps are used: a negative-selection step to remove an unwanted cell type and a positive-selection step to obtain the cell type of interest. For example, to obtain purified populations of Purkinje cells, Hatten et al. (chapter 16) first remove glia and immature neurons by immunopanning with an antiganglioside antibody, then they harvest Purkinje cells by immunopanning with antibodies directed against the Purkinje cell–specific antigen Thy-1. Immunopanning also can be combined with gradient centrifugation, as in the protocols for preparing spinal motorneurons developed by Henderson and colleagues (Camu and Henderson, 1992; Mettling et al., 1995). These methods can yield remarkably pure cell populations. For example, Barres et al. (1988b) report obtaining ganglion cell preparations more than 99% pure with yields of 25% to 50%, impressive figures considering the ganglion cells account for less that 1% of the cells in the retina.

Antibodies directed against cell surface constituents also can be used to remove an unwanted cell type by complement-mediated lysis. This approach was introduced by Brockes et al. (1979) to remove fibroblasts, which express the cell surface glycoprotein Thy 1, from cultures of Schwann cells, which are Thy 1–negative (for details, see chapter 19). A similar method can be used to remove O-2A progenitor cells from astroglial cultures (see chapter 18). Cells first are incubated in the specific antibody, then rinsed and incubated with complement. Once triggered by interaction with the membrane-bound antibody, the cascade of complement reactions ultimately produces pores in the cell membrane, leading

to osmotic lysis. The procedure can be applied to cells in suspension or attached to a substrate (Vogel and Weston, 1988).

Cells that have been labeled with a fluorescent dye can be separated from unlabeled cells by using a fluorescence activated cell sorter (FACS). In this device, individual cells travel in single file through a laser beam, and their fluorescence is measured. Then, depending on their fluorescence intensity, they are sorted into two populations. Cells can be sorted at enormous speeds (2000–3000 per sec), but because each is sorted individually and because it may be necessary to sort 3 to 4×10^7 cells to collect 500,000 viable, labeled cells, several hours often are required. FACS is an extremely valuable tool because it offers a means of isolating specific populations of cells that have been labeled by retrograde transport. For example, motorneurons from the spinal cord have been purified following injection of fluorescently labeled wheat germ agglutinin (Calof and Reichardt, 1984; Schaffner et al., 1987) or carbocyanine dyes (Martinou et al., 1989, 1992; St. John, 1990) into the muscles to which they project. Preganglionic sympathetic neurons from the spinal cord (Clendenning and Hume, 1990) and nigrostriatal neurons from the brain (Lopez Lozano et al., 1989; Kerr et al., 1994) also have been purified successfully by this approach. Alternatively, antibodies against cell surface components can be used to label cells for FACS (Abney et al., 1983; Maxwell et al., 1988; Barald, 1989). Clearly, FACS is a powerful tool, but its successful use requires dedication. A considerable investment of time is needed to work out the parameters necessary to isolate specific cell populations, yields can be low, and the necessary equipment is complicated and expensive.

A similar device, the anchored cell analysis system, can be used to purify cells attached to a substratum (Schindler et al., 1985; Barald, 1989). Using a microscope equipped with stage control motors to scan a culture dish and a laser beam to measure the fluorescence intensity of individual cells, unlabeled cells are killed by a high-energy laser pulse.

Cell Counting and Assays of Viability

To control the number of cells plated, it is necessary to determine the cell density. This is accomplished most easily using a hemacytometer, a specially designed slide with a counting chamber 0.1 mm deep and ruled in a grid pattern (figure 3.2). It is also frequently

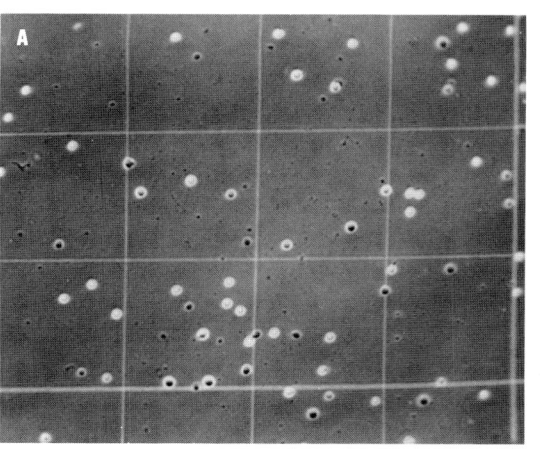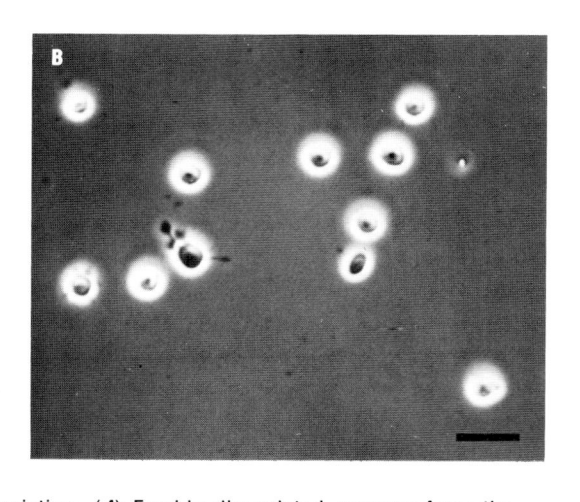

Figure 3.2 Neurons immediately after dissociation. (*A*) Freshly dissociated neurons from the embryonic rat hippocampus on a hemacytometer slide used for determining cell density. The squares in this section of the hemacytometer measure 0.25 mm on a side. (The aberration present in some low-magnification objectives is also apparent.) (*B*) Cells from the same preparation shortly after attachment to a polylysine-treated substrate. Scale bar: 25 µm.

desirable to estimate the proportion of cells that have been damaged by dissociation. This can be done by using any of several dyes (e.q., trypan blue, erythrosin, or nigrosin) that are excluded from "viable" cells whose membranes are intact but are taken up by damaged cells (Phillips, 1973; Patterson, 1979). Following one standard protocol, a drop of cell suspension is mixed with an equal volume of 0.08% trypan blue dissolved in BSS. After 4 min, the cells suspended in the dye solution are examined and are counted in a hemacytometer. Serum interferes with this assay by binding dye (Phillips, 1973). Of course, these are crude measures of cell viability, and there is no guarantee that cells that exclude dye are healthy enough to grow in culture. Nevertheless, they offer a useful approach for monitoring the adequacy and consistency of tissue dissociation.

Other methods for assessing cell viability can be applied to cells growing in culture as well as to cells in suspension. For example, fluorescein diacetate (Rotman and Papermaster, 1966; Novelli et al., 1988; Paramore et al., 1992; Petroski and Geller, 1994) is a compound that crosses intact cell membranes readily but, once inside a cell, it is hydrolysed rapidly to the impermeable and brightly fluorescent dye, fluorescein. Thus, fluorescein is trapped and accumulates in intact cells but not in cells whose membranes have been

damaged. In recent years, a variety of fluorescent dyes have been developed for assessing cell viability, including some available in kit form that stain living cells one color and dead cells another (Molecular Probes). Tetrazolium dyes, which enter living cells and are converted enzymatically to a colored, insoluble product, are also popular for quantifying cell viability in culture (Mosmann, 1983). For example, MTT (3-[4,5-dimethylthiazol-zy]-2,5-dipheryltetra-zolium bromide), which is converted to a blue reaction product within mitochondria, is widely used to assay neuronal cell death and to test the efficacy of possible neuroprotectants. The reaction, which requires several hours, can be quantified spectrophoto-metrically via a plate reader (Manthorpe et al., 1986). In chapter 18, Noble and Mayer-Pröschel provide a detailed protocol for the use of MTT to assess the effects of growth factors and antioxidants on the survival of oligodendroglia.

Freezing Cells

It has long been known that cells from continuous lines can be frozen, stored at low temperature, and regenerated successfully. Cells can be kept at −80° for a month or two and can survive indefinitely when stored in liquid nitrogen. More recently, it has been shown that primary cells can be frozen successfully in the same manner and, when thawed, will give rise to cultures that are in many respects comparable to those obtained with control cells placed directly into culture (Kawamoto and Barrett, 1986; Scott and Lew, 1986; Petite and Calvet, 1995). This method has been applied successfully to cells from many regions of the peripheral and CNS (Mattson and Kater, 1989; Collier et al., 1993), and to both human and rodent cells (Mattson and Rychlik, 1990; Frodl et al., 1994). Thus, for some purposes, it may be possible to start primary cultures from the freezer rather than from the animal.

To maintain maximum viability, cells usually are frozen in a medium containing serum or serum proteins and a cryoprotectant, usually 5% to 10% dimethylsulfoxide; suitable freezing media also are available commercially from suppliers of reagents for cell culture. Optimal conditions vary somewhat among different cell types (see references cited earlier). Cells must be frozen slowly to minimize the formation of ice crystals and must be thawed rapidly. For further details, see chapters 6 and 13.

Media

A complete medium for culturing cells consists of a basal medium, such as minimum essential medium (MEM), supplemented either with serum or, in the case of serum-free medium, with a defined set of hormones and growth factors. These mixtures often are modified further, depending on the particular use intended, and antibiotic and antimitotic agents also may be included. Each of these components will be considered in turn.

Basal Media

Most media are based on balanced salt solutions to which are added amino acids, vitamins, and other nutrients at concentrations roughly similar to those found in serum. The composition of the media commonly used in cell culture is provided in standard texts (Freshney, 1994) and in catalogs from companies that sell supplies for tissue culture. The most commonly used media range in complexity from Eagle's MEM, which contains only 13 essential amino acids and 8 vitamins, to Ham's F-12, which also includes non-essential amino acids, and a wider array of vitamins, minerals, and additional metabolites (such as nucleosides). MEM/F-12, a half-and-half mixture of the two, also is popular. Dulbecco's modification of MEM (D-MEM), developed for use with rapidly growing cells, contains largely the same nutrients as does MEM but at two to four times higher concentrations. In choosing a medium, it's worth reading the fine print in the catalog and remembering that more is not always better. For example, some media include glutamate among their amino acids. Although this makes sense for most uses outside neurobiology, it might not be the best choice for neurons that are susceptible to excitotoxic damage, especially if they are to be cultured in the absence of glia. Ferrous sulphate, which is included in F-12, also has been reported to have neurotoxic effects (Brewer et al., 1993).

In all these media, glutamine is present at much higher concentrations than are other amino acids, reflecting its instability and its use as a carbon source by many cells in culture (Reitzer et al., 1979). For neuronal cultures, it is common to increase the concentration of glucose to the range of 0.6% (Murray, 1965) and to add pyruvate to basal media that do not contain it (Selak et al., 1985b; O'Donnell-Tormey et al., 1987). Both MEM and F-12 are intended for equilibration in an atmosphere containing 5% CO_2; D-MEM,

which contains a higher concentration of $NaHCO_3$, was intended to be equilibrated at 10% CO_2, although lower levels sometimes are used.

The formulation of these basal media was based on studies of the growth of various cell lines, but generally they have proved satisfactory for use with primary cultures. Recently, Brewer et al. (1993) reexamined the formulation of basal media with primary neuronal cultures in mind. The medium they developed, Neurobasal, was derived from D-MEM, but has a much reduced osmolarity and contains some nonessential amino acids and vitamin B_{12}; it has been tested on several types of central neurons (Brewer et al., 1995). The addition of serine but not other nonessential amino acids enhances neurite outgrowth of chick sensory and retinal neurons (Savoca et al., 1995).

In principle, a buffer such as HEPES could be substituted for bicarbonate, eliminating the need for incubation in a CO_2-enriched atmosphere. In practice, it is not this simple. Apparently, dissolved CO_2 or bicarbonate are important for good cell growth. Leibovitz's L15 medium, which was designed to permit the growth of cells in an ambient atmosphere, is formulated quite differently from other basal media. It contains high concentrations of amino acids, which provide buffering capacity, and uses galactose rather than glucose as a carbon source to prevent the build-up of lactic acid in the medium. Small amounts of dissolved CO_2 are generated by the metabolism of pyruvate, which is present at a high concentration. The advantages of such a medium are obvious, especially for studies wherein maintaining a CO_2-enriched atmosphere is inconvenient, such as during long-term microscopic or physiological studies. L15 has been used with reasonable success for the culture of peripheral neurons (Hawrot and Patterson, 1979; see chapters 9–11), but its ability to support the development of central neurons has not been investigated thoroughly.

Serum

Cells cannot live by basal medium alone. To provide the trace nutrients and growth factors necessary for growth and maintenance of specific cell types in culture, basal media frequently are supplemented by the addition of serum, usually at a final concentration of 5% to 20%. The most appropriate source of serum for a particular application must be determined empirically. Both horse serum

and fetal calf serum are used widely and readily available from commercial sources. Fetal calf serum, which is rich in mitogenic factors, usually is the preferred serum for proliferating cells, cell lines or primary cultures of glia; for culturing postmitotic neurons, horse serum commonly is used. However, many investigators use fetal calf serum for neuronal cultures, and some (including ourselves) use horse serum for culturing glia. Some investigators, particularly those who prepare neuronal cultures from rats, have found it preferable to use homotypic serum (Dichter, 1978; Hawrot and Patterson, 1979; Huettner and Baughman, 1986; see chapter 12). Finally, human placental serum, which long has been used for organotypic culture of neural tissue, remains the serum of choice for some specific applications (see chapter 19).

Not surprisingly, serum varies considerably in composition from batch to batch, and most investigators find it necessary to test the suitability of individual lots of serum before use. Most commercial suppliers will provide samples, and once a satisfactory lot has been identified, it is common to purchase a sufficient amount to permit its use for up to 12 months. Serum sold commercially often is heated in a water bath to a temperature of 56° for 30 min, which destroys complement (a process called *heat inactivation*). Recently, there has been some controversy over the relative benefits of heat inactivation, as some desirable serum constituents also may be affected.

Serum-Free Media

An important advance in nerve cell culture occurred in 1979, with the introduction of chemically defined media that support the survival of neural cells without the need for supplementation with serum (Bottenstein and Sato, 1979a,b; see also Honegger et al., 1979; Snyder and Kim, 1979). This advance developed from a broad effort to define the role of serum in culture medium and to develop suitable combinations of hormones, nutrients, and attachment factors to replace it, an effort whose remarkable success has changed the entire field of cell culture. The medium termed N_2, developed by Bottenstein and Sato in 1979, has been particularly useful for culturing nerve cells. It was developed initially for use with B104 rat neuroblastoma cells in culture, using their rate of proliferation as an index for formulating its specific composition. As originally formulated, it consists of a 1:1 mixture of D-MEM and

Ham's F-12, supplemented with insulin, transferring, progesterone, putrescine, and selenium. Insulin and insulinlike growth factors are important for the growth and survival of a broad variety of cell types, as is transferrin, an iron-transport protein (Barnes and Sato, 1980; see also Oh and Markelonis, 1982). Putrescine is a precursor for the synthesis of polyamines, which are thought to play an important role in cell growth in general and in brain maturation in particular (Seiler, 1981; Seiler et al., 1984). Selenium, a cofactor in glutathione production, may assist in the breakdown of peroxides and superoxides (McKeehan et al., 1976). It has been reported also to protect cells against light-induced damage (Boder et al., 1983). Additional formulations (N_1, N_3), which contain lower concentrations of transferrin, followed (for review, see Bottenstein, 1985).

Somewhat unexpectedly, considering that they were formulated to support the rapid proliferation of neuroblastoma cell lines, the media developed by Bottenstein and Sato have been able to support the growth of a variety of neurons in *primary* culture and have supplanted the use of serum-containing media in many laboratories. In some protocols, cells are plated directly into serum-free medium. In others, cells are plated into serum-containing medium, which facilitates cell attachment, then are transferred to serum-free medium. Such media eliminate the variability inherent in the use of serum. More important still, they permit examination of the growth factors and other agents that improve neuronal growth and survival or protect neurons from environmental toxins, a rapidly growing areas of neuroscience. The neuronal media developed by Bottenstein and Sato have the added advantage of reducing the rate of proliferation of nonneuronal cells under some circumstances, resulting in a purer population of neurons. On the other hand, serum-free media formulated for the cultivation of glial cells also have been developed (see chapters 18 and 19).

Many workers have obtained adequate results by using the original Bottenstein and Sato formulations. Others have attempted to optimize serum-free media specifically for use in primary nerve cell cultures (Bottenstein, 1985; Huck, 1983; see also Barnes and Sato, 1980). The extensive studies of Romijn and colleagues (Romijn et al., 1984; Romijn, 1988) and Brewer and Cotman (1989), which have served as a starting point for several subsequent studies (Brewer et al., 1993; Brewer, 1995; Martin and Wiley, 1995), illustrate some of the important considerations and complexities in developing chemically defined media for a specific neuronal popu-

lation. Nearly all these investigations concur on the importance of including insulin, transferrin, and selenium; many include thyroid hormone. Romijn's formulation is enriched with vitamins and fatty acids not included in, say, MEM and contains reduced concentrations of some hormones.

It seems probable that the optimal composition of a defined medium will depend critically on other variables in the culture protocol: the type of neuron to be cultured, cell density, substrate, and the specific growth factors included. From a practical standpoint, it is much easier to begin by testing a few commercially available media than to embark on a systematic study.

Components present in serum, such as serum albumin, can act as scavengers of metabolic toxins that can accumulate in media. In their absence, neurons growing in serum-free medium, especially in low-density cultures, are particularly vulnerable to peroxides and free radicals. This has been noted by many workers. Catalase and superoxide dismutase, which prevent the buildup of peroxides and superoxides in the medium, have been reported to enhance cell survival in low-density cultures (Walicke et al., 1986a; Saez et al., 1987). Brewer and Cotman (1989) found that cell survival could be increased at reduced O_2 tensions. Often, formulations of serum-free media contain agents that act as antioxidants. For example, vitamin E often is included, as is pyruvate, which also acts as a scavenger of peroxides (O'Donnell-Tormey et al., 1987). These concerns become less important in high-density cultures, especially when neurons are cocultured with glia, which can take up and metabolize neurotoxins such as glutamate (Sugiyama et al., 1989).

Finally, it should be emphasized that although serum-free medium initially is defined chemically, its composition changes during culture, as original components are depleted, and products secreted by the cells accumulate. Indeed, conditioned medium—medium that has been used for culturing cells—frequently enhances neuronal and glial development (see next section)

Growth Factors

Most embryonic mammalian neurons are fastidious in their trophic requirements, and failure to provide the appropriate growth factor or combination of factors typically causes most neurons to die within the first few days in vitro. Therefore, one of the most

important steps in establishing a culture system is the identification of an adequate means of providing trophic support for the cell type of interest.

There are two basic approaches to this problem: to allow the cultured cells to produce their own trophic factors or to add purified growth factors to the medium. The rationale behind the first approach is straightforward. Most types of glia cells, and many types of neurons, secrete trophic factors in vitro. Therefore, if appropriate mixtures of cells are grown at high density, significant amounts of the needed trophic factors will accumulate, especially if the medium is changed infrequently. This process is obviously the method of choice for growing cells whose trophic requirements are poorly defined, and it also has the advantage of being economical. However, the self-conditioning approach suffers from several disadvantages. Often, it is difficult to generate reproducibly the same mixed cell populations in the proper proportions, and the growth conditions are defined poorly. Moreover, this approach tends to work only with very-high-density cultures, because the conditioning of the medium becomes less effective at lower density. In some cases, however, low-density cultures of purified neuronal populations can be supported by using medium that has been conditioned by high-density cultures or by growing the neurons in apposition to glial monolayers (see chapter 13).

The second way to satisfy the trophic requirements of neurons is to add growth factors to the medium. For several decades, the only factor that was available for routine use in tissue culture was nerve growth factor (NGF) and, consequently, only the few types of cells that responded to this protein could be grown in this manner. During the last 10 years, however, a significant number of new growth factors have become widely available at modest cost. Owing to these advances, there also has been significant progress in defining the growth requirements for the major classes of neurons. It is, therefore, becoming an increasingly common practice to grow purified neuronal populations under low-density conditions in at least the relative absence of nonneural cells.

Of the various classes of growth factors, the neurotrophins have been the most extensively used in neural cell culture. The neurotrophin family has four members—NGF, brain-derived neurotrophic factor (BDNF), NT3, and NT4/5—and receptors for these molecules are distributed widely, with one or more subtypes found in most regions of the embryonic brain (Eide et al., 1993; Snider,

Table 3.1 Neuronal Selectivities of Neurotrophin Growth Factors

	RESPONSIVE NEURONS	
NEUROTROPHIN	PNS	CNS
NGF	Sympathetic neurons Neural crest sensory neurons	Basal forebrain cholinergic neurons Striatal cholinergic neurons Cerebellar Purkinje cells
BDNF	Placode-derived sensory neurons Neural crest sensory neurons Nodose ganglion neurons	Basal forebrain cholinergic neurons Proprioceptive trigeminal neurons Substantia nigra dopaminergic neurons Retinal ganglion neurons Facial motoneurons
NT-3	Sympathetic neurons Sensory neurons	Basal forebrain cholinergic neurons Locus coeruleus neurons
NT-4/5	Sympathetic neurons Dorsal root ganglion neurons Nodose ganglion neurons	Basal forebrain cholinergic neurons Locus coeruleus neurons

PNS, peripheral nerve system; CNS, central nervous system; NGF, nerve growth factor; BDNF, brain-derived neurotrophic factor.
After Eide et al., 1993.

1994; Ip and Yancopoulos, 1996). Moreover, the various family members can regulate the survival or differentiation of many types of neurons from the central and peripheral nervous systems (table 3.1). Thus, in establishing growth conditions for new culture systems, exploration of the effects of neurotrophins represents a reasonable starting point. A sampler kit, containing small amounts of each of the four members of the neurotrophin family, is available for this purpose (Pepro Tech, Inc., Rocky Hill, NJ), and recommended methods for handling these molecules are described in box 3.1. However, it is also important to note that there is compelling evidence that many other types of growth factors are involved in regulating the survival and differentiation of neurons in vivo, including members of the following families: neuropoietic cytokines, such as ciliary neurotrophic factor and leukemia inhibiting factor (Patterson and Nawa, 1993; Ip and Yancopoulos, 1996); fibroblast

Box 3.1   Suggestions for the Handling of Growth Factors

1. Use a carrier for making all stock solutions. Many growth factors avidly bind to glass and also exhibit significant adsorption to plastic surfaces. Losses during transfer and dilution can be minimized by using a carrier, such as 2 mg/ml of high-quality BSA (nuclease and protease-free). BSA has the added advantage that it may serve as an antioxidant (Halliwell, 1988), thus perserving critical disulfide bonds.
2. Do not filter dilute protein solutions. Even with the use of nominally low-protein binding filters (0.22 μm), large adsorptive losses are incurred when the protein concentration in the filtrate is below 20 to 50 μg/ml.
3. Do not subject stock solutions to repeated freeze-thaw cycles. In this respect, it is important to note that activity can be lost by storage in −20°C frost-free freezers. Some growth factors, such as the basic fibroblast growth factors, become more resistant to freezing and thawing when complexed with specific stabilizing agents, such as heparin.
4. The interaction of serum with the factor of interest needs to be considered. For example, serum stabilizes NGF but inactivates TGF-β.
5. The interaction of the medium with the factor of interest also needs to be considered. For example, the high concentration of cysteine in F12 medium causes the rapid inactivation of insulin ($T\frac{1}{2} < 30$ min) (Barnes and Sato, 1980). Therefore, the use of a large proportion of this medium may be contraindicated with molecules that have critical disulfide bonds, especially in the absence of serum. To avoid inactivation of growth factors under low serum conditions, many laboratories find it useful to freeze freshly prepared media in small aliquots (10–20 ml, −80°C) and to thaw them immediately before use.

growth factors (Eckenstein et al., 1994); transforming growth factor β (Krieglstein et al., 1995) and the related bone morphogenetic proteins (Lein et al., 1996); interleukins (Mehler et al., 1995; Merrill and Jonakait, 1995); epidermal growth factor and transforming growth factor–α (Sensenbrenner et al., 1994); platelet-derived growth factors (Yeh et al., 1993); stem cell factor (Carnahan et al., 1994); vasoactive intestinal peptide (Pincus et al., 1990); insulin-like growth factors (Zackenfels et al., 1995); and the neuregulins (Carraway and Burden, 1995).

Many types of peripheral nervous system (PNS) neurons exhibit simple trophic requirements in vitro; often, provision of a single trophic factor is adequate to allow long-term survival. For example, rat sympathetic neurons require only NGF for their survival and, in its presence, these neurons can be grown for several months under rigorously defined conditions (i.e., in a serum-free medium, in the absence of glia, and on a chemically defined substrate; Iacovitti et

al., 1982). Moreover, there is substantial evidence that NGF is one of the physiological regulators of the survival of sympathetic neurons in situ (Snider, 1994). However, despite the obvious appeal of such a system, there are also reasons to be cautious. Sympathetic neurons also respond to glial cell line-derived neurotrophic factor (GDNF), NT3, LIF, and CNTF, and their survival is impaired in animals which do not produce GDNF (Moore et al., 1996) or NT3 (Zhou and Rush, 1995). The differences between trophic requirements in vitro and in situ may be explicable in terms of the amounts of NGF available under the various circumstances: saturating amounts of NGF are provided in culture, whereas limiting amounts probably are available at most stages in situ. Nonetheless, these observations suggest that one must be very careful in making extrapolations from cell culture to the intact animal. They point out also the importance of using growth factors at appropriate concentrations. Although it is customary to use maximally effective amounts of trophic factors in most experiments, synergistic effects are seen more easily with suboptimal doses. In addition, high concentrations of trophic factors may render cells more resistant to toxins and other stresses (Levi-Montalcini, 1982). Accordingly, lower amounts may be preferable in examining phenomena such as the response to free radicals or toxic concentrations of excitatory amino acids (Cheng and Mattson, 1995; Mattson et al., 1995).

There are many other PNS culture systems in which a single trophic factor is adequate to maintain a substantial proportion of the cells. Two of the most popular are chick ciliary parasympathetic neurons and rat dorsal root sensory neurons. However, there are also limitations to these models. In the case of the ciliary ganglion, up to 90% of the neurons survive for extended periods when cells are exposed to CNTF; however, CNTF does not appear to be the endogenous target-derived trophic factor and there is controversy as to whether a related molecule, GPA, fulfills this role (Nishi, 1994b). Rat dorsal root ganglia contain several cell populations. The small cell population, which includes nocioceptive cells, is responsive to NGF, but other neurons, such as the large cell population involved in proprioception, respond to different neurotrophins (Snider, 1994). Thus, cultures grown under the most commonly used conditions do not mirror faithfully all the characteristics of the parental population. The problem of cell selection is likely to be especially problematic in CNS cell cultures, because means for identifying all the various neuronal subtypes are much more limited.

Current evidence suggests that the trophic requirements of CNS neurons are more complex than those of PNS neurons. Studies of spinal motorneurons and retinal ganglion cells indicate that these neurons respond to a much wider variety of trophic factors than do most PNS neurons. For example, at least 15 different molecules have been found to increase the survival of motorneurons in vitro (Oppenheim, 1996). Moreover, it has been observed that the survival response of retinal and motorneurons to any individual trophic factor tends to be less complete than that typically observed with PNS neurons (Nishi, 1994a; Meyer-Franke et al., 1995; Oppenheim, 1996). Thus, most of the trophic factors affecting motoneurons and retinal ganglion cells support only a subpopulation of the neurons, and optimal survival requires a combination of factors. In the case of retinal ganglion cells, the optimal combination of factors (BNDF, CNTF, IGF1, bFGF) includes representatives from several different growth factor families (Meyer-Franke et al., 1995). The generality of this observation has not yet been assessed fully but is consistent with the finding that targeted deletions of the individual neurotrophin genes do not appear to affect greatly the survival of most classes of CNS neurons (Snider, 1994). Moreover, it is known that the long-term survival of oligodendrocytes also requires multiple trophic interactions (Barres et al., 1993).

Depolarization

Depolarization induced by either high potassium or other agents can alter profoundly the neuronal response to growth factors. At least three different types of interactions have been observed. In a few systems, responsiveness to growth factors is observed only after depolarization or indirect activation of intracellular kinase cascades (Cohen-Cory et al., 1991; Birren et al., 1992; Meyer-Franke et al., 1995; see figure 3.3). In contrast, in many other systems, depolarization can act as a substitute for one or more growth factors, allowing the growth and differentiation of neurons in their absence (Scott and Fisher, 1970; Lasher and Zagon, 1972; Chalazonitis and Fischbach, 1980; Nishi and Berg, 1981; Wakade and Thoenen, 1984). The latter type of response to depolarization has been observed most frequently in the case of peripheral neurons, and it is thought to be mediated by an influx of calcium ions (Franklin and Johnson, 1994). Finally, there is also evidence that depolarization

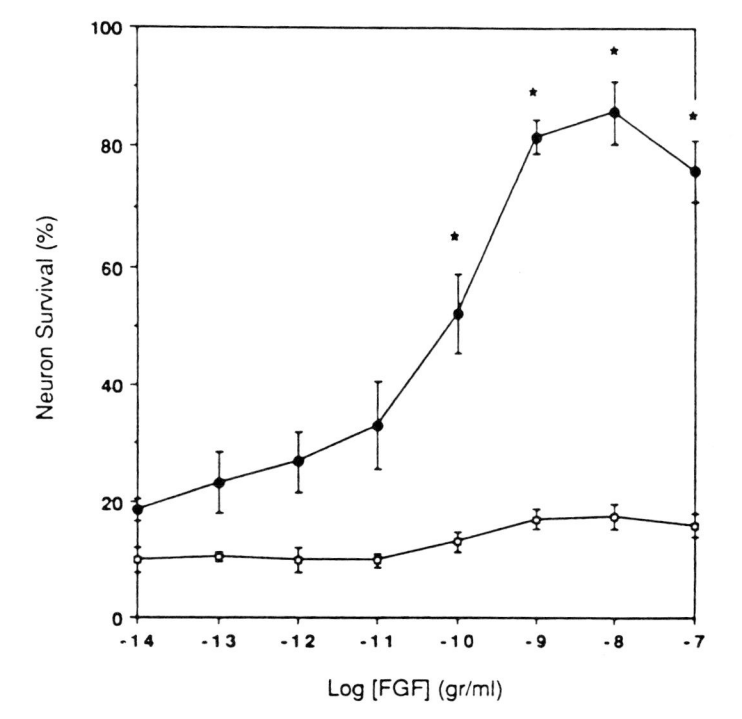

Figure 3.3 Synergistic interaction between bFGF and depolarization. Under control conditions (open squares), ciliary neurons are unresponsive to bFGF. In the presence of 20 mM potassium, bFGF markedly enhances neuronal survival. (From Schmidt and Kater, 1993, with permission.

may increase the synthesis and release of some neurotrophic factors from cultured glia and neurons (Lu et al., 1991; Patterson et al., 1992; Ghosh et al., 1994). Typically, depolarization is induced by increasing the concentration of potassium ions in the culture medium to 20 to 50 mM.

Antibiotics

The antibiotics used most commonly in cell culture are penicillin (usual concentration, 25–100 units/ml) and streptomycin (25–100 µg/ml), which often are used together; in some laboratories, they are added routinely to all culture medium. Gentamicin (10–100 µg/ml), which is effective against a broader range of microorganisms and is more stable over time, is also used, particularly when low levels of contamination are detected. These agents are not effective against molds and yeasts.

Although antibiotics often are added to media used for culturing cell lines (which are carried continuously), there are several reasons for avoiding their routine use in primary culture. First, provided the cells can be obtained aseptically, bacterial infection of primary cultures is relatively rare. Moreover, even if a culture preparation becomes contaminated, relatively little damage results, as individual cultures are not carried indefinitely. Although most cells appear to tolerate them well, antibiotics are not without effect on neuronal metabolism (Amonn et al., 1978). Whether or not you choose to use antibiotics, it is important to learn to recognize the principal types of contamination—bacteria, mold, or yeast—as discussed in chapter 19 (see also Freshney, 1987). The type of contamination usually suggests the source of the problem.

Antimitotics

Certain inhibitors of DNA synthesis are toxic to dividing cells but have relatively little effect on cells that are not undergoing DNA synthesis. As neurons ordinarily are incapable of DNA synthesis and hence are unaffected by antimitotics, such agents are used frequently in neuronal culture to eliminate or reduce the population of nonneuronal cells. If it is desirable to kill all nonneuronal cells, proliferation usually is stimulated by the addition of serum or of growth factors to ensure that the highest possible number of nonneuronal cells are synthesizing DNA when the antimitoics are added (Patel et al., 1988; see chapter 19). Even so, some cells will be at stages of the cell cycle when they are insensitive. Therefore, repeated rounds of stimulation of proliferation followed by antimitotic treatment may be necessary. In culturing CNS neurons, antimitotics also are added frequently after a confluent monolayer of astroglial cells has formed. Because at this stage the glial cells are inhibited from further division by cell-cell contact, they are not killed by antimitotic treatment, but further proliferation, especially of fibroblasts, is prevented so that the cultures do not become overgrown.

Two antimitotic agents commonly are employed in neuronal cultures. Fluorodeoxyuridine, a suicide inhibitor of thymidylate synthetase, commonly is employed at concentrations of $\sim 10\,\mu M$. Uridine ($10\,\mu M$) usually is included as well, to prevent inhibition of RNA synthesis in nondividing cells. Cytosine arabinoside (arabinofuranosylcytosine; araC) also is commonly employed, typically

at concentrations of 5 to 50 µM. In any use of antimitotics, the possibility of toxic effects on neurons must be considered; use of the lowest possible effective concentration is recommended. AraC, even at low concentrations, is cytotoxic to some populations of neurons, apparently because it triggers apoptotic cell death (Martin et al., 1989; Wallace and Johnson, 1989; Dessi et al., 1995; Enokido et al., 1996; Ishitani and Chuang, 1996). Other antimitotic drugs do not exhibit this toxicity (Martin et al., 1990).

Maintenance of Cultures

Typically, cultures are maintained in an incubator that is perfused automatically with a mixture of air and CO_2, the latter at the level appropriate to the medium being used. The O_2 concentration in air is considerably higher than that in blood or cerebrospinal fluid, and the growth of some cells, including neurons, may be enhanced at reduced levels of O_2 (Kaplan et al., 1986; Brewer and Cotman, 1989). Incubators that permit use of reduced O_2 levels are available, but they are not used widely.

High humidity is necessary to minimize evaporation from the culture dishes. Humidity usually is maintained by placing a large dish of water in the bottom of the incubator. It is essential that this water be changed frequently and the container sterilized to prevent the buildup of mold. Once an incubator becomes heavily contaminated with mold spores, it can be next to impossible to decontaminate it. When cultures must be kept for long periods or in a small volume of medium, evaporation can be eliminated further by cultures in sealed containers, such as dessicators flushed with the appropriate gas mixture (see chapter 19).

The accuracy of temperature regulation should be checked periodically. Incubator temperature sometimes is set a degree or so below 37°C (Holtzman et al., 1982). Cells tolerate considerable periods at reduced temperatures but die after even a few hours at temperatures above 39°C.

The optimal schedule for feeding cultures varied. For culturing glial cells, frequent feeding is necessary to maintain maximal rates of proliferation (see chapters 18 and 19). In contrast, some populations of neurons require surprisingly infrequent feedings and benefit from the conditioning that occurs between feedings. Cultures of cerebral cortex have been maintained for up to a month without any feeding (Yavin and Yavin, 1980; see also Bartlett and

Banker, 1984). On the other hand, cells such as hippocampal neurons, which depend on a conditioning of the medium, rapidly degenerate if the medium is replaced completely (see also Rosenberg and Dichter, 1989). In such situations, a reasonable compromise may be to exchange only a fraction of the medium at each feeding (see chapters 13 and 18).

Dishes and Substrate

Dishes

A variety of plastic culture dishes are commercially available. These include traditional Petri dishes (35-mm, 60-mm, and 100-mm diameters), multiwell plates with wells ranging in size from 6 to 35 mm, and flasks with surface areas ranging from 25 to 150 cm^2. All are available "ready to use," without the need for cleaning or sterilization. All are prepared from "tissue-culture-grade" plastic, a polystyrene that has been treated during manufacturing to decrease its hydrophobicity. Untreated, microbiological-grade plastic dishes do not provide an adequate substrate for cell attachment and growth.

Despite their convenience, plastic dishes are not suitable for all purposes, particularly for uses involving microscopy. Their bottoms are too thick to allow use of high-magnification objectives, and they are incompatible with such techniques as differential interference microscopy, because plastic is birefringent. For microscopy of cells after fixation and staining, it may be most convenient to grow cells on glass coverslips placed inside Petri dishes or multiwell plates. The coverslips then can be removed, stained, and mounted on glass slides in the usual way. Coverslips that have been etched with a grid pattern make it possible to study individual cells in living cultures and relocate them following staining (available from Bellco; see chapter 10). Tissue culture chamber slides (Lab-tek Division, Miles Laboratories Elkart, IN) provide an alternate approach. These consist of standard glass microscope slides with plastic wells attached to their surface with a silicone gasket. After fixation, the wells and gasket can be removed, and the slide can be processed using standard histological techniques. Dishes designed for microscopy of living cultures are described in chapter 5.

If glass coverslips are used, first they must be cleaned and sterilized. Most commonly, they are cleaned by immersion in concentrated nitric or sulfuric acid (see chapters 6, 8, 9, 13, and 17); for some purposes, immersion in ethanol is satisfactory. Chromate-dichromate-based cleaning solutions usually are not used for cell culture work, as they contain toxic heavy metals. Coverlips may be sterilized by dry heat (at least 160°C for at least 1 h) or may be autoclaved.

It is worth remembering that coverslips are not intended by their manufacturers for use in cell culture; thus, you may encounter batches that are not suitable for this use. Some glass may release toxic elements slowly into the medium. Other glass may be treated chemically during manufacturing in a way that alters its ability to adsorb substrates, such as polylysine. Having recently suffered through a series of bad cultures that were ultimately attributable to just this cause—brought about when one of the leading US companies that fabricates coverslips for scientific distributors changed its glass supplier—we can attest to the importance of this variable (see chapter 13 for details). If you suspect this problem, you will find certain manufacturers and importers of coverslips are aware of this issue and are willing to help (Erie Scientific Co, Portsmouth, NH, 1-800-258-0834; Carolina Biological, Burlington, NC, 1-800-334-5551).

Substrate

The adhesion of cells in situ involves cell-cell and cell-matrix interactions mediated by specific cell surface receptors, which are rapidly being identified and characterized (Venstrom and Reichardt, 1993; Letourneau et al., 1994; Brummendorf and Rathjen, 1995). The nature of the cell attachment that occurs in culture is less certain. When known extracellular matrix molecules or cell adhesion molecules are used as the substrate, cell adhesion well may involve the same mechanisms that operate in situ. On other substrates, such as tissue culture plastic or polylysine, adhesion may involve the adsorption of biological molecules present in the serum or released from the cultured cells. For example, the binding of some cells to a glass surface requires the serum component vitronectin, which adsorbs to glass and binds to an integrin on the cell surface.

Untreated Glass or Tissue-Culture Plastic

Most types of glial cells are undemanding in their substrate requirements; they grow well on tissue-culture plastic and somewhat less
well on untreated glass surfaces. To some extent, this tendency
may be related to their ability to secrete molecules that then form
the surface to which they adhere. Neurons, in contrast, are quite
"finicky" with regard to substrate; obtaining successful neuronal
cultures depends strongly on finding an appropriate substrate. For
specific, short-term studies, some neurons can be cultured on plain
glass or plastic substrates (Bray, 1991), but this technique is not
suitable for long-term cultures. For most purposes, the glass or
plastic surface must be treated to improve its adhesive properties,
usually by the adsorption of macromolecules. This approach is
used widely and is quite successful (see next section). Its one
potential drawback is that the process of adsorption is slowly
reversible, so that with time, neurons may detach from the substrate, or their processes may become highly fasciculated. An
alternative approach meriting further attention involves chemical
modification of the glass surface. For example, incorporation of
aminosilane derivatives provides a surface chemically similar to
that produced by adsorbed polylysine (Kleinfeld et al., 1988), and
the attached amino groups also can serve as sites for coupling
to proteins via a cross-linking agent such as glutaraldehyde
(Matsuzawa et al., 1996).

Polylysine and Polyornithine

Surfaces prepared by treating glass or plastic with polymers of
basic amino acids (Yavin and Yavin, 1974; Letourneau, 1975a)
presently are the substrate of choice for culturing many different
types of neurons, particularly those from the CNS. They may be less
suitable for culturing PNS neurons. Surfaces treated with polylysine or polyornithine appear to be strongly adhesive (Letourneau,
1975a; Zheng et al., 1994). Nearly all types of cells adhere to them,
though not all grow well. They were introduced first with the intent
of promoting cell adhesion by altering the surface charge on the
substrate. One of the reasons for thinking that glass is a poor substrate is that it is charged negatively and the net charge on cell
surfaces also is negative. This is certainly one factor in the adhesion of cells to polylysine (Lein et al., 1991) but, in practice, the
situation often is more complicated. Most laboratories plate cells

onto polylysine- or polyornithine-treated surfaces in media that contain serum, and components from the serum that are adsorbed to the treated surface may contribute to the improvement of cell attachment and growth. In fact, surfaces are often pretreated with polylysine for the purpose of enhancing the adsorption of other substrate proteins, such as extracellular matrix constituents or lectins.

Polylysine or polyornithine is dissolved in sterile water or in borate buffer, and the surface being treated is covered completely by this solution. Although polymers of the L-isomers of these amino acids are adequate for most applications, the D-isomers may be preferred because they are not subject to breakdown by proteases, which are released by cells in culture. If glass coverslips are being used, they must be cleaned first, as described earlier. All sterilization procedures should be completed before this treatment, as heat, ultraviolet irradiation, and ethanol may disrupt the substrate. After the polylysine or polyornithine solution is removed, the substrate is rinsed with water, BSS, or medium to remove the unbound material. Polybasic amino acids commonly are used at concentrations ranging from 5 µg to 1 mg/ml and are applied for times ranging form 15 min to 24 h, the amount of adsorbed polylysine being dependent on these variables. At low concentrations signs of poor adhesion—clumping of neuronal cell bodies and fasciculation of processes—may become evident, whereas high concentrations may be toxic to some cell types. The wide range of concentrations commonly used reflects the different requirements of individual culture paradigms. For example, high concentrations usually are necessary to ensure rapid, long-lasting attachment of neurons directly to the substrate. In many protocols, an underlying monolayer of glial cells forms the true substrate for neuronal attachment. Under such conditions, lower concentrations may be sufficient to enhance neuronal attachment.

Nitrocellulose

Nitrocellulose is used widely in protein blotting techniques as a substrate for the rapid, noncovalent adsorption of proteins. This polymer does not support the growth of most neural cells. However, Lagenaur and Lemon (1987) found that many cell adhesion molecules exhibit greater neurite activity when they are bound to this substrate than when they are adsorbed to either plastic or

polylysine. Nitrocellulose, therefore, has been used extensively in studies of the cadherins and of adhesion molecules belonging to the immunoglobulin superfamily. Nitrocellulose also has been used in studies of extracellular matrix molecules. Its advantages in this respect are not as clear-cut, because many matrix molecules exhibit significant binding to both plastic and polylysine. In fact, the concentrations of laminin required to obtain maximal effects on nitrocellulose-coated dishes (100–1 000 µg/ml) typically are much greater than those that elicit maximal effects on other substrata (∼10 µg/ml).

Nitrocellulose most commonly has been applied to plastic dishes (Lagenaur and Lemmon, 1987), although a variant method allowing adsorption to glass coverslips has been described (Hankin and Lagenaur, 1993). The procedure for coating plastic is simple and fast (∼10 min). A disc of nitrocellulose is dissolved in methanol, and aliquots are rapidly spread onto the plastic. After the solvent has evaporated, test protein samples are applied for ∼60 s. Subsequently, the samples are aspirated, and the plates are washed with a solution containing a blocking agent, such as bovine serum albumin (BSA). If large amounts of nitrocellulose are applied, the culture dishes will be opaque. Proper titration of the concentration and volume yields a clear surface.

Extracellular Matrix Constituents

The extracellular matrix (ECM) contains a complex set of large molecules, including 14 types of collagens, at least 25 noncollagenous glycoproteins, and numerous proteoglycans (Reichardt and Tomaselli, 1991; Letourneau et al., 1994). Neurons are exposed to a rich mixture of these molecules during development. For example, cells in the spinal cord are in contact with at least 10 different matrix components (Letourneau et al., 1994). Moreover, the exposure is dynamic, differing complements of molecules appearing at different developmental stages. Tissue culture techniques have been used extensively to analyze the effects of various individual ECM molecules on the development of neurons and glial cells, to identify particular amino acid sequences within the large ECM molecules that mediate these effects, and to characterize the membrane receptors that mediate these responses (Venstrom and Reichardt, 1993; Letourneau et al., 1994).

Functional studies of individual ECM molecules indicate that they can profoundly affect the behavior of neurons and glial cells. For example, particular ECM molecules have been found to regulate such critical processes as cell division, survival, adhesion, differentiation, myelination, process outgrowth, cell polarity, cell migration, and synapse formation (Bunge et al., 1985; Venstrom and Reichardt, 1993; Letourneau et al., 1994; Noakes et al., 1995). Such activities obviously are relevant to the establishment of culture models. Three of the most prominent and important ECM constituents—laminin, fibronectin, and collagen—are available commercially (Collaborative Research, Indianapolis, IN; Boehringer Mannheim; Gibco/BRL, Gaithersburg, MD; and Calbiochem, San Diego, CA). Unfortunately, many other ECM reagents are difficult to prepare and are still available only in limited quantity.

The ECM molecule that has been used most frequently in neural cell culture is mouse laminin prepared from the Engelbreth-Hoth-Swarm tumor; this protein recently was renamed *laminin-1* to distinguish it from related isoforms in the laminin family of proteins (Burgeson et al., 1994). Laminin-1 is a large molecule (M_r $\sim 900,000$ Da) that is retained by 0.22 µm filters. Therefore, usually it is sterilized by dialysis against chloroform during the purification procedure (Timpl et al., 1979). Concentrated laminin stocks (>1 mg/ml) need to be thawed slowly at 4°C to avoid the formation of gels. Thereafter, the material is diluted in saline with 50 mM TRIS (pH 7.6) or tissue culture media to a concentration (~ 1–100 µg/ml) appropriate for coating untreated plastic or polylysine-coated dishes. Optimal adsorption typically requires 4 to 8 h, then plates are rinsed extensively.

Coating dishes with laminin-1 enhances the adhesion of most types of neurons and glia. In contrast, fibroblasts appear to lack laminin receptors and thus do not bind as well to this substrate. Consequently, laminin-1 usually produces an increase in the number of adherent neural cells and a slight alteration in the composition of the population. However, it is important to note that laminin, like many other ECM molecules, also has anti-adhesive effects on certain types of neurons and may interfere with their attachment (Gotz et al., 1996). A second effect of the adsorption of laminin is a marked stimulation of process formation. Virtually all types of CNS and PNS cells exhibit this response, which usually includes both a decrease in the time to initial process extension

and an increase in the total length of the processes extended. The effects of laminin on neuritic growth appear to be specific for axons, whereas dendritic elongation is not enhanced on this substrate (Lein and Higgins, 1989; Lein et al., 1992). A third effect of laminin is that frequently it alters the cell's response to trophic factors. In some cases, a laminin substrate allows survival in the absence of growth factors (Ernsberger et al., 1989a) but, more commonly, laminin acts synergistically (Edgar et al., 1984; Schmidt and Kater, 1993), increasing both the sensitivity to and the efficacy of trophic factors. Finally, laminin and other ECM components have been shown to regulate the differentiation of neurons, precursor cells, and also glia (reviewed by Reichardt and Tomaselli, 1991). For example, laminin-1 specifically increases the activity of certain enzymes involved in norepinephrine biosynthesis (Acheson et al., 1986) and plays an important role in regulating myelination by Schwann cells (Bunge et al., 1985).

Fibronectins are glycoprotein multimers that exist in several forms and are produced by the alternative splicing of a single gene (Letourneau et al., 1994). They provide a favorable substrate for the adhesion, spreading, and locomotion of neural crest cells, which may interact with fibronectin during some phases of their migration. Like laminin, fibronectin stimulates both cellular adhesion and neurite outgrowth in cultures of many types of PNS neurons. However, the response of CNS neurons to fibronectin is much weaker, with only a few types of neurons forming processes on this substrate (Rogers et al., 1989).

Type I collagen was introduced as a substrate for neuronal cell culture by Bornstein in 1958. As collagen is not found in brain, it was known at the time that collagen was not a physiological substrate for CNS neurons, but it offered many advantages over the substrates then available. Methods for preparing collagen and for forming collagen monolayers are described in chapter 19.

Although the use of type I collagen seems to be declining, it still offers certain advantages: It is easy to use, is readily obtainable, and can form stable three-dimensional matrices. In addition, when a high concentration of collagen is polymerized rapidly, a thick gel is formed, which restricts protein diffusion and allows gradients to be established. By using this technique, Lumsden and Davies (1986) were able to demonstrate a chemotropic effect of a target epithelium on the developing sensory neurons. Subsequently, others used this approach to study chemotropic phenomena in the spinal

cord (Tessier-Lavigne et al., 1988) and to isolate and clone the first family of chemotropic factors, the netrins (Serafini et al., 1994).

Other Substrate Molecules

Cell adhesion molecules (CAMs) are an obvious choice for use as substrates for cultured neurons, given the important roles they are thought to play in controlling neurite outgrowth in situ (Kreis and Vale, 1993; Brummendorf and Rathjen, 1995). As one might expect, a variety of CAMs permit vigorous neurite outgrowth in culture. Among those most studied are N-CAM and L1 from the Ig super-family (Lagenaur and Lemmon, 1987; Chuang and Lagenaur, 1990) and N-cadherin from the cadherin family of calcium-dependent adhesion molecules. To test their effects, the desired CAM can be adsorbed to the plastic substrate or to a precoating of nitrocellulose (Lagenauer and Lemmon, 1987; Ignelzi et al., 1994; see previous discussion). Alternatively, fibroblast cell lines whose endogenous surface molecules support neurite outgrowth only poorly can be engineered to express the CAM of interest (Doherty et al., 1991; Beggs et al., 1994). The cell culture approach has played a key role in refining our understanding of the function of CAMs in neural development. From such studies, it has become clear that CAMS play instructive roles in guiding fiber outgrowth that are indepen-dent of their adhesive properties (Lemmon et al., 1992), and it has been possible to elucidate many of the intracellular signaling path-ways that mediate these actions (Schuch et al., 1989; Williams et al., 1992, 1994a,b; Bixby et al., 1994).

Unfortunately, CAMs are not available in the quantities needed for routine use as cell culture substrates. Nevertheless, they can be valuable in specific circumstances. For example, when combined with techniques for patterning the culture substrate, they provide a means for regulating the signals that impinge on growth cone out-growth in a geometrically precise way (see following section). This ability has permitted a high-resolution analysis of temporal changes in growth cone behavior that occur when contact first is established with a given CAM (Burden et al., 1995). Simultaneous exposure of individual cells to different CAMs has rendered it pos-sible to control which of a cell's initial neurites becomes specified as its axon (Esch, 1995).

Still another possibility, based on the same idea as cell pan-ning, is to prepare substrates derivatized by adsorption of anti-

bodies directed against surface antigens on the cell type of interest (MacLeish et al., 1983). One potential advantage of such an approach is that substrates can be tailored to facilitate the growth of only a single cell type from within a heterogeneous cell population. For example, substrates derivatized with anti-Thy 1.1 preferentially enhance adhesion and process outgrowth by retinal ganglion cells in culture (Leifer et al., 1984; see also Messer et al., 1984). This approach has allowed culture of adult primate retinal neurons, which do not adhere well to substrates appropriate for young cells (O'Malley and MacLeish, 1993).

Growth of Neurons on Monolayers of Nonneuronal Cells: Mass Cultures and Microislands

When plated onto a nonadhesive substrate, such as untreated glass or plastic, neurons will adhere to and grow on the surface of any nonneuronal cells present. Even when treated substrates are used, neurons may prefer to grow on glia rather than directly on the substrate. In addition to providing a good substrate for neuronal growth, glial cells are thought to be the source of trophic substances that enhance the survival of neurons in culture. Further, in the CNS, there is evidence that glial processes are the normal substrate for neuronal migration and neurite outgrowth. Thus, there are compelling reasons to think that glial monolayers could form an attractive substrate for neuronal growth in culture.

This approach has proved to offer a relatively simple and reliable method for preparing cultures from many regions of the nervous system (Dichter, 1978; Huettner and Baughman, 1986; Yamada et al., 1989; see chapter 12). It is particularly appropriate for physiological studies, where long-term survival is important and where fine neuronal processes (obscured by the underlying cell monolayer) can be examined by intracellular injection of fluorescent tracers.

Preparing small patches of nonneuronal cells, now called *microislands*, it is possible to culture individual neurons in isolation from other cells for extended periords. This idea was pioneered by Furshpan and colleagues (Furshpan et al., 1976; 1986 a, b), who grew single sympathetic neurons on heart cells, and followed changes in the physiological makeup of individual cells over the course of weeks in culture. Using glial cells as substrate, this approach has been extended to prepare microisland cultures of CNS neurons (Huettner and Baughman, 1988; Segal and Furshpan, 1990;

Mennerick et al, 1995). Often, cells in microisland cultures form numerous synapses on themselves, sometimes exhibiting levels of spontaneous electrical activity that are seizurelike (Segal and Furshpan, 1990; Segal, 1994). Methods for establishing microislands cultures are described in chapter 12.

In using nonneuronal cells as a substrate for growth, it is important to characterize the population of cells present. For example, astroglia provide an excellent substrate for neuronal development, but fibroblasts and meningeal cells, which sometimes contaminate astroglial cultures, do not (Sensenbrenner and Mandel, 1974; Noble et al., 1984; Fallon, 1985; Schwab and Caroni, 1988). In addition, the region of the brain from which the glial cells are derived also may be important. For example, mesencephalic neurons develop dendritic arbors when cultured with mesencephalic, but not with striatal glia (Rousselet et al., 1988).

Patterned Substrates, Campenot Chambers, and More

Several approaches have been developed to confine or orient the growth of neurites developing in culture. These methods depend on creating local variations in the adhesiveness of the substrate, so that fibers extend on regions that are suitably adhesive and avoid regions to which they cannot adhere. The possibility of patterning neurite outgrowth in dissociated-cell cultures was explored first by Letourneau (1975). By using vacuum evaporation to apply a thin layer of palladium to a polyornithine-treated coverslip while shielding the coverslip with an electron microscope grid to prevent palladium deposition beneath its bars, he created a gridlike pattern of adhesive stripes and nonadhesive, palladium-coated squares. Neurite growth was restricted to the stripes. In a variant of this approach, a grid is laid onto a coverslip that has been treated with an ECM molecule, then is exposed to intense ultraviolet light (Rauvala et al., 1994). Neurites avoid the regions of substrate that have been denatured by the light, remaining confined to the stripes.

This approach subsequently has been refined through the use of photolithography to create more precise patterns (Kleinfeld et al., 1988). For example, by derivatizing a silicon substrate in a pattern of alternating stripes using alkyl-trichlorosilane (nonadhesive) or amino trihydoxysilane (adhesive)—cells can be confined to grow on lines only 10 μm wide and to maintain this pattern of growth for 12 days. Additional photolithographic techniques for creating pat-

terns of chemically derived substrates have been developed with resolutions approaching 1 to 2 μm (Britland et al., 1992; Matsuzawa et al., 1993; Schaffner et al., 1995; St. John et al., 1997). It has also been possible to use this approach to generate patterns of biological substrates, either by creating patterns that permit selective protein adsorption (Clark et al., 1993; Lom et al., 1993) or by chemical cross-linking of synthetic peptides that correspond to neurite-promoting domains of matrix molecules (Matsuzawa et al., 1996).

Bonhoeffer and colleagues (Walter et al., 1987; Vielmetter et al., 1990) have developed a silicone matrix device containing a series of 50 μm-wide channels that enables formation of substrates in a pattern of alternating stripes. The goal of this work is not to create patterned neurite outgrowth but to present fibers with a choice of two different substrates. Striped substrates can be prepared either from membrane fractions obtained from different cell populations or by adsorbtion of two different soluble molecules (figure 3.4). This assay has been used to identify molecules that guide differentially axons from different regions of the retina (Drescher et al., 1995) and to observe the moment-by-moment changes that occur when a growth cone contacts a new substrate (Burden-Gulley et al., 1995). The matrices required to prepare these substrates are available commercially (Juergen Jung, Max-Planck Institut für Entwicklungsbiologies, Spemannstrasse 35, Tubingen, Germany).

Finally, it is possible to examine the interaction of growing neurites with a complex tissue by culturing them on the surface of cryostat sections (Carbonetto et al., 1987; Covault et al., 1987; Anton et al., 1995). For visualization of the dissociated cells, usually they are labeled first with a long-lasting dye, such as diI. In an elegant variant of this approach, Hotary and Tosney (1996) have developed methods for maintaining cross-sections of chick embryos in slice culture. This process has allowed analysis of the responses of sensory and motor axons to several tissues that they would encounter normally as they grow within the embryo (Hotary and Tosney, 1996). One also can capture a cellular imprint of a fresh tissue section by touching it to anitrocellulose-coated coverslip. This approach has been used to obtain glial cells for physiological recordings (Barres et al., 1990) or as a substrate to observe the migration of fluorescently labeled neurons (Komuro and Rakic, 1996).

Certain experiments depend on the ability to control independently the chemical environment surrounding nerve cell bodies

P ▌A ▌P ▌A ▌P ▌A ▌P ▌A

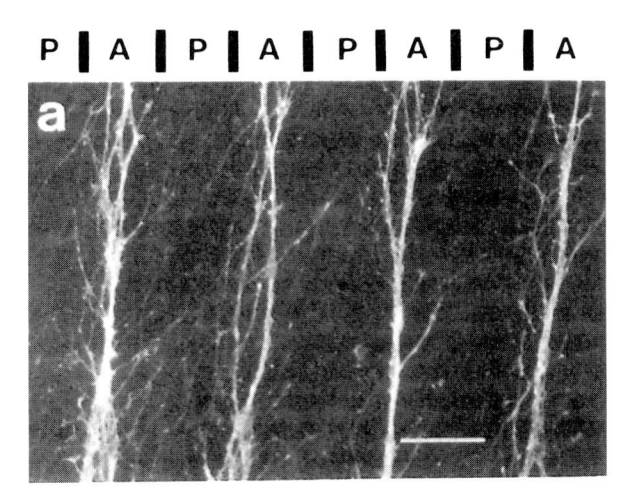

P ▌A ▌P ▌A ▌P ▌A ▌P ▌A

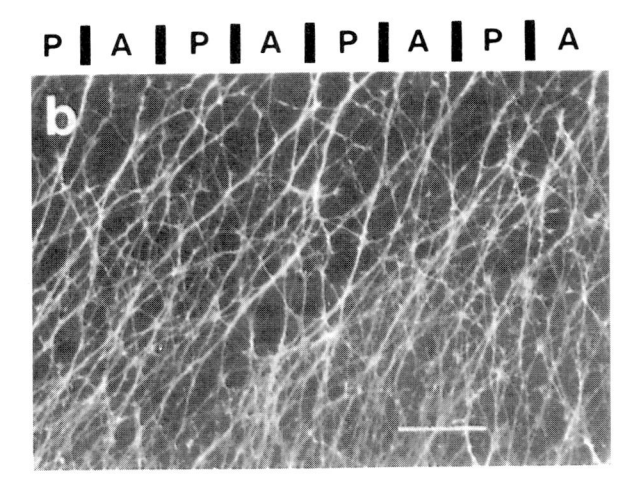

Figure 3.4 The stripe assay of axonal guidance. (*A*) Under control conditions, axons from an explant of temporal retina avoid stripes composed of membrane fractions from the posterior tectum and are guided onto stripes containing membranes from the anterior tectum. (*B*) Guidance is abolished when membrane fractions are treated with an antibody against tectal membrane. (From Stahl et al., 1990, with permission. Copyright 1990 Cell Press.)

and their processes. For this purpose Campenot developed special, three-well chambers (Campenot, 1977). Cells are plated into the central chamber, and their processes extend under grease seals and enter chambers on either side, a distance of a few millimeters. Using these chambers, Campenot (1977, 1982a,b) demonstrated that the survival of sympathetic neurons was not dependent on exposing their cell bodies to NGF directly as long as their neurites extended into a region where NGF was present. Independent of cell survival, individual branches of sympathetic fibers were maintained only if NGF was present in their local environment (Campenot, 1994). This approach has since proved useful for a variety of purposes: to follow the anterograde and retrograde transport of growth factors and neuroactive viruses (Bergstrom et al., 1992; Penfold et al., 1994; Ure and Campenot, 1994), to study the biosynthetic capacity of isolated axons (Posse de Chavis et al., 1995), to monitor simultaneously two populations of axons as they interact with common target cells (Davenport et al., 1996), and to enable selective stimulation of a subpopulation of afferents converging on a single postsynaptic cell (Fields et al, 1991; Nelson et al., 1993). The components for preparing these chambers are available commercially (Tyler Instruments, Edmonton, Alberta, Canada).

4 Transfecting Cultured Neurons

Ann Marie Craig

Neurons are difficult to transfect because they are postmitotic cells; thus, methods that allow entry of DNA into the cytoplasm are not sufficient. In dividing cells, if one can get the DNA into the cytoplasm, it will enter the nucleus during breakdown of the nuclear envelope during mitosis. Standard, physical methods for transfecting dividing cells can be used to transfect neurons but at low efficiencies, generally ≤1%. These standard methods include calcium phosphate coprecipitation, lipid or DEAE-dextran (diethylaminoethyl-dextran) mediated transfection, and electroporation. Calcium phosphate and lipid-mediated methods have been used successfully for neuronal transfection by several labs and are are discussed further in following sections. I know of no success stories with DEAE-dextran or electroporation of neurons, even at low efficiency. Other physical methods that have been used for transfecting neurons include microinjection and biolistics. A novel transfection method using a complex of plasmid DNA, transferrin, polylysine, and inactivated adenovirus (Cotten et al., 1992; Wagner et al., 1992) leads to very high efficiency transfection of cell lines, presumably by a combination of receptor-mediated endocytosis and adenovirus-mediated disruption of endosomes. It remains to be seen whether this method will be enough to overcome that last hurdle of nuclear entry of the DNA in postmitotic neurons. The cationic polymer polyethyleneimine was used to facilitate oligonucleotide delivery to the nuclei of hypothalamic neurons in culture and may also prove to be a general (and inexpensive) agent for transfecting neurons (Boussif et al., 1995).

To overcome the limitations in efficiency with physical methods, many neuroscientists have turned to viral methods. These methods make use of the natural means viruses have evolved for ensuring that their DNA reaches the nucleus of infected neurons, while in most cases debilitating the virus so it will not undergo a full lytic cycle. The most commonly used viral vectors are derived from herpes simplex virus 1 (HSV) or adenovirus, although adeno-associated virus, vaccinia virus, and semliki forest virus (SFV) also

have been adapted as neuron transfection vectors. An advantage of viral vectors is that they can be used to transfect neurons in vivo with fairly high efficiency, and in fact most have been developed by labs interested in potential applications in gene therapy. All these viral vectors can induce very-high-efficiency transfection of neurons in culture (90% and higher). Their limitations are threefold and vary in severity among particular viral vectors: potential toxicity to the neurons, potential safety hazard to lab personnel, and effort and time for constructing each viral vector.

Thus, there is no perfect way to transfect a neuron. One has to compromise on something, either transfection efficiency, or longevity, or effort required. The method you choose will depend on which of these factors is most important. We switch between several methods depending on the experiment: calcium phosphate transfection for low-efficiency, long-term, low-effort perturbation studies; defective HSV amplicon-based herpesvirus vectors for high-efficiency, short-term, moderate-effort targeting experiments; and recombinant adenovirus for high-efficiency, long-term, high-effort expression (actually, high-effort for the labs kind enough to pass on their adenovirus vectors to us). Figure 4.1 illustrates some of the differing features of calcium phosphate versus adenovirus-mediated transfection of a membrane-associated green fluorescent protein in low-density hippocampal cultures.

Physical Methods

Calcium Phosphate Coprecipitation

Calcium phosphate–mediated transfection seems to have been the most successful of the "fast and easy" transfection methods for neurons. It has been possible to obtain transfection efficiencies up to 20% and consistently in the range of 0.5 to 3% and to use this method to do more than just produce blue cells. Neurons that have been transfected by the calcium phosphate method include cultured chick or rat cortical, hippocampal, spinal cord, dorsal root ganglion, and retinal neurons (Werner et al., 1990; Gabellini et al., 1992; Kanai and Hirokawa, 1995; Watson et al., 1995; Xia et al., 1996). In particular, this method has been used to study targeting and microtubule-binding properties of MAP2 and tau (Kanai and Hirokawa, 1995) and analysis of transcriptional induction through

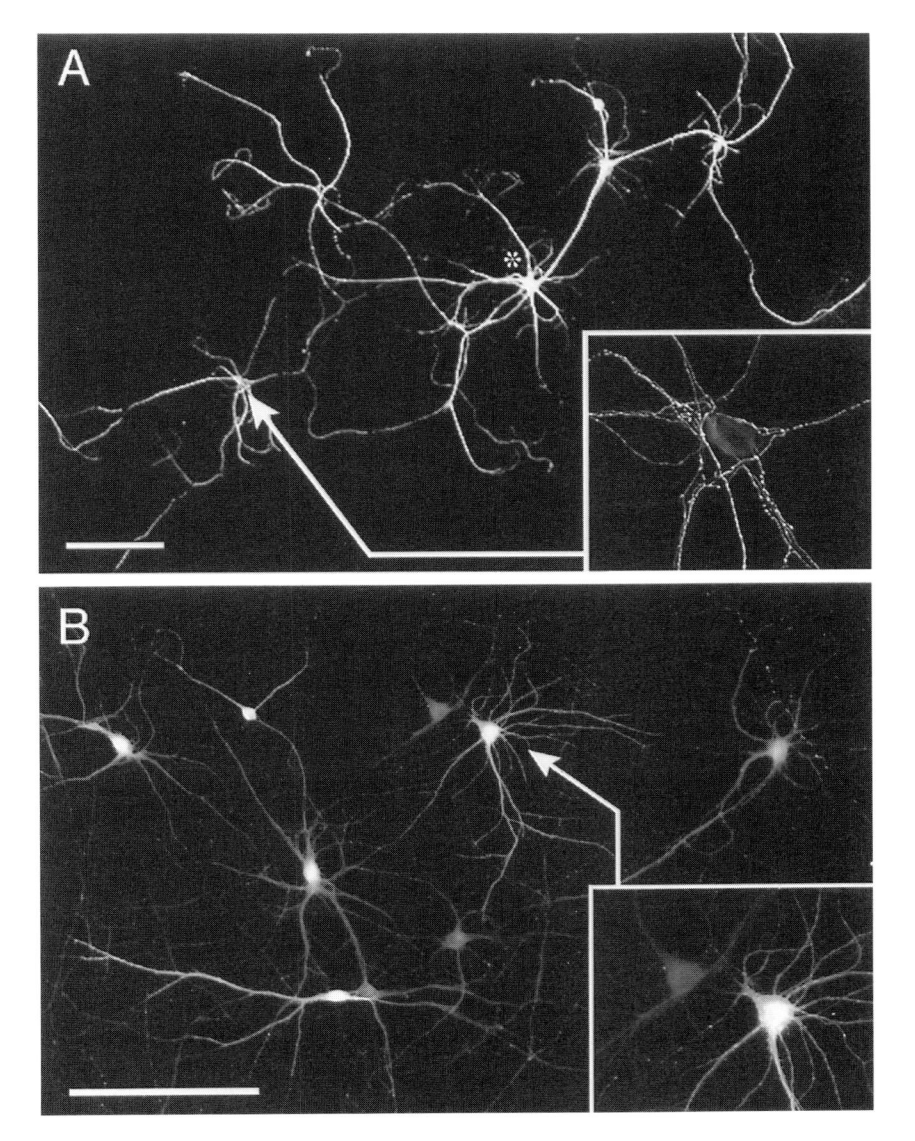

Figure 4.1 Transfection of rat hippocampal neurons in low-density culture for membrane-associated green fluorescent protein. (*A*) The calcium phosphate coprecipitation method using pCA-GAP-GFP (S65A). (*B*) An adenovirus vector AdV-CA-GFP (S65A)-Ras (using vectors generously provided by Moriyoshi et al., 1996). Neurons were transfected at 8–13 days in culture and were imaged 3–6 days later. By the calcium phosphate method (*A*), few neurons are transfected and brightly labeled. In panel (*A*), the labeled axon from the single transfected neuron (asterisk) surrounds other nearby cells, as shown at higher magnification in the inset. With the adenovirus vector (*B*), many neurons are labeled at low to moderate levels. Some individual arbors of the most brightly labeled neurons can be distinguished from the more moderately expressing cells. Scale bars: 200 μm. (Courtesy of D. W. Allison, J. N. Stowell, F. T. Crump, and A. M. Craig, University of Illinois.)

the serum response element of the c-fos promoter (Xia et al., 1996). In a very encouraging series of experiments, Nikolic et al. (1996) used calcium phosphate–mediated transfection of cultured cortical neurons with both dominant negative and antisense constructs against the cdk5/p35 kinase to show its essential function in neurite outgrowth (figure 4.2). The transfected neurons were identified and neurite length was determined by coexpression of β-galactosidase. A nice control included the rescue of antisense effects by coexpression of wild-type p35.

A detailed protocol for calcium phosphate transfection of neurons is given in box 4.1. The method is similar to the original protocol of Graham and van der Eb (1973). The method was discovered empirically, and its basis still is not clear. It is believed that the DNA–calcium phosphate coprecipitate enters the cytoplasm by endocytosis and that some DNA makes its way to the nucleus (more, alas, in dividing cells, where the nuclear envelope breaks down). Practically speaking, the goal is to incubate the neurons in a "fine sandy" precipitate of DNA-calcium phosphate prepared by mixing DNA–calcium chloride with HEPES buffered saline. The pH of the buffer is critical; it is advisable to prepare several batches of buffer, varying slightly in pH between 7.05 and 7.15, to test which works best, and to store it frozen in aliquots. Alternatively, the Stratagene (La Jolla, CA) kit buffers work well for preparing precipitates for neurons. Another critical parameter is the quality of the plasmid DNA. Plasmid DNA prepared by using Qiagen kits does not work as consistently as the method of equilibrium centrifugation in CsCl–ethidium bromide density gradients (see Sambrook et al., 1989, for protocol).

The maturity of the neurons is also a factor. Surprisingly, transfection by this method only works after 2 days in culture, and we routinely transfect at 4 to 9 days in culture. Older neurons also will transfect but generally are more sensitive to any manipulations. Expression is detectable by 2 days after transfection, increases in level over the next couple of days, and persists for at least a couple of weeks (and probably for as long as the neurons survive). As for all the transfection methods, addition of kynurenate and $MgCl_2$ to block glutamate receptor ion channels can enhance neuronal health and survival. Xia et al. (1996) also found that a 2% dimethyl sulfoxide shock at the end of the transfection protocol helped to reduce variability, and a 5% glycerol shock increased transfection efficiency for cortical and hippocampal neurons. Depending on the

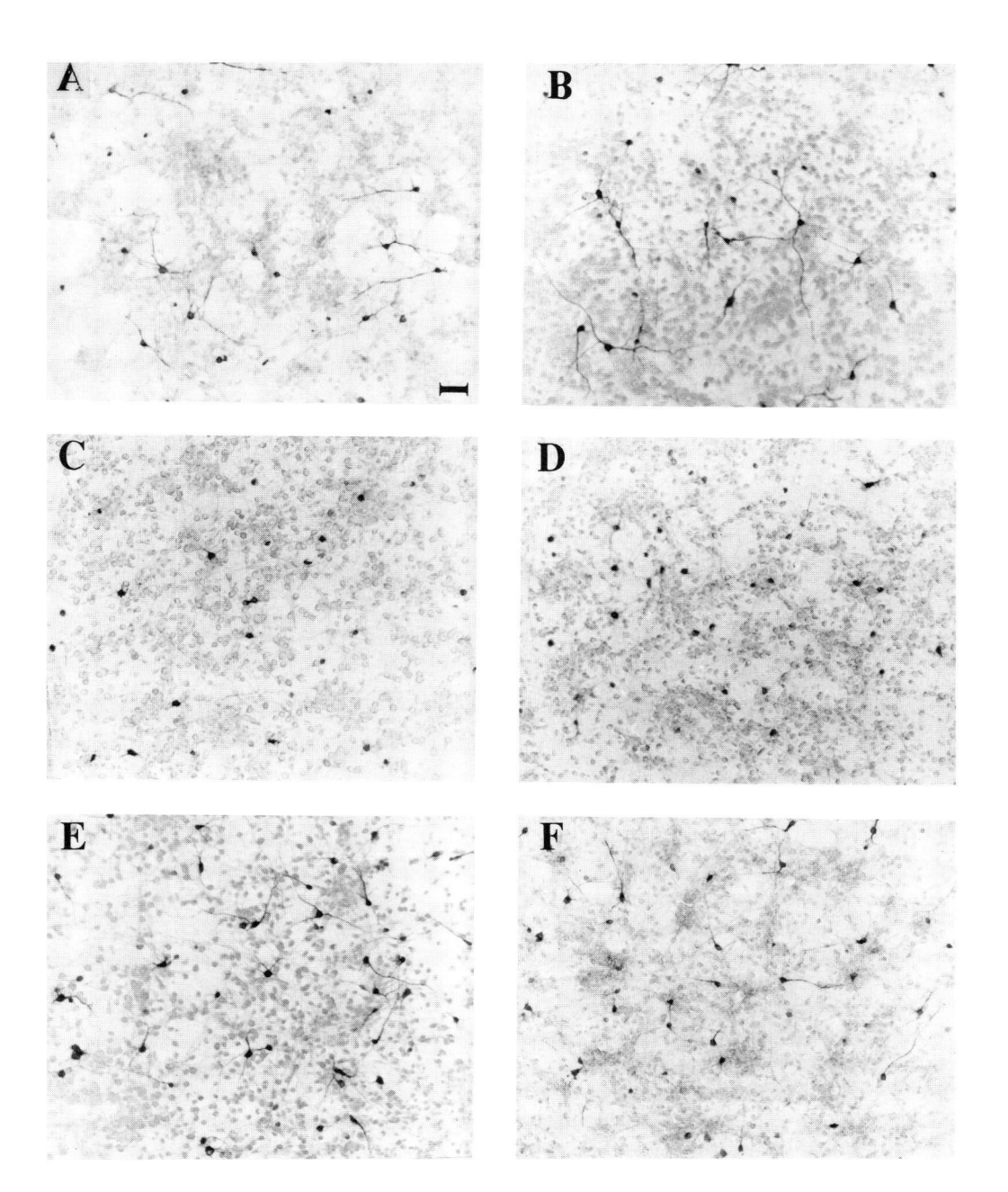

Figure 4.2 Use of calcium phosphate–mediated cotransfection to demonstrate the role of the cyclin-dependent kinase cdk5 and its activator, p35, in neurite outgrowth. Cultured rat cortical neurons were cotransfected with CMV-β-gal and the following expression vectors: (*A*) CMV-β-gal alone; (*B*) CMV-p35; (*C*) CMV-cdk5N[144]; (*D*) CMV-cdk5T[33]; (*E*) equal amounts of CMV-cdk5N[144] and CMV-cdk5; or (*F*) equal amounts of CMV-cdk5N[144] and CMV-p35. The figure shows immunostaining for β-galactosidase, which identifies the transfected neurons. Expression of β-galactosidase alone or coexpression of p35 did not affect neuron morphology (*A, B*). Expression of two different dominant-negative forms of cdk5 (cdk5N[144] of cdk5T[33]) inhibited neurite outgrowth (*C, D*), and this effect was rescued by coexpression of wild-type cdk5 or p35 (*E, F*). (From Nikolic et al., 1996, with permission.)

Box 4.1 Calcium Phosphate-Mediated Transfection

Method

1. Mix sterile reagents in hood: 15 μl 2.5 M $CaCl_2$
                                              5–20 μg DNA
                                              dH_2O to 150 μl
   These volumes will make enough precipitate to transfect two to three 60-mm dishes. The amount of DNA is determined best experimentally, as different amounts have been found to be optimal by different investigators. A mixture of plasmid vectors can be used for coexpression of multiple proteins. Expression level per cell can be regulated by using a constant amount of DNA consisting of differing ratios of expression vector to an inert plasmid, such as pUC19.

2. Place 150 μl 2×HeBS in another tube. To this, add the DNA/$CaCl_2$ mix dropwise with a pipetman, swirling the tube between drops. Bubbling in air through a plugged Pasteur pipette while adding drops also can aid in mixing. We use the mixture immediately, although some investigators have found that incubation for up to 20 min enhances precipitate formation.

3. Choose neurons to be transfected at 3–10 days in culture. Transfer neuron coverslips with cell side up to a new 60-mm dish containing 3 ml of transfection medium. Save the original glial dish or conditioned media in the incubator.

4. Drip 80–160 μl of the DNA/$CaCl_2$/HeBS mix per dish in small drops evenly over the neuron coverslips and incubate for 15–75 min. Check periodically on a microscope and stop when there is a moderate to heavy layer of fine precipitate. This is the most critical step of the procedure. Too much precipitate will lead to toxicity, whereas too little precipitate will result in very low transfection efficiency. For a new set of experiments, it is best to do a pilot transfection, testing different amounts of the DNA/$CaCl_2$/HeBS mix per dish and stopping the transfection at 15, 30, and 60 min to determine the optimal conditions.

5. To stop the transfection, rinse the coverslips once in fresh transfection media and transfer them back to their original culture dishes. For hippocampal and cortical cultures, addition of 100 μM APV (to block NMDA receptor-mediated toxicity) can aid in survival.

6. Assay for transfection at ≥1 day later.

Reagents

DNA
Prepare by banding through CsCl gradients (Qiagen kits do not work as well).

2×HeBS

NaCl	274 mM final	3.2 g	Baker no. 3642-05; Mallinckrodt
KCl	10 mM	142 mg	Mallinckrodt no. 6858
$Na_2HPO_4 \cdot 7H_2O$	1.4 mM	76 mg	Mallinckrodt no. 7914
D-glucose	15 mM	540 mg	Baker no. 1916-01; Mallinckrodt
HEPES (free acid)	42 mM	2 g	Calbiochem no. 391338

Box 4.1 (continued)

Add dH_2O to 200 ml. Adjust pH with 10 N NaOH to pH 7.05–7.15. It is best to prepare several batches with slightly different pH, test which works best for transfection (generally whichever gives the finest precipitate), and store in aliquots at −20°C.

Alternatively, we have found that the Stratagene Transfection Kit 2×BBS works fairly well.

TRANSFECTION MEDIA

1. DMEM Gibco/BRL no. 11960 (bicarbonate-buffered; incubate in CO_2 incubator)

or

2. MEM Gibco/BRL no. 12370 and bring to pH 7.7–7.85 with NaOH (HEPES-buffered: incubate in air during precipitate formation).

We prefer transfection in DMEM, which can be the most efficient, although its pH is more difficult to control. If using MEM for better consistency, the pH must be raised for efficient precipitate formation (pH 7.85 is best if tolerated by the neurons).

Optional: For hippocampal and cortical neurons, addition of 1 mM kynurenic acid and 10 mM $MgCl_2$ to the transfection media can aid survival by inhibiting glutamate-induced toxicity.

type of neuron, it may be possible to use harsher methods, and Watson et al. (1995) found that the presence of 10 μg/ml poly-ornithine throughout and a 30% dimethyl sulfoxide shock at the end increased transfection efficiency of dorsal root ganglion cultures. Finally, a useful feature of calcium phosphate–mediated transfection is the ability to cotransfect two or more plasmids. Nearly 100% cotransfection can be obtained by mixing plasmids prior to precipitate formation, although with varying ratios of expression. Cotransfection can be useful for decreasing the expression level of a particular construct by mixing it with an inert DNA such as pUC19 to keep the amount of DNA constant for precipitate formation.

Lipid-Mediated Transfection

Lipid-mediated transfection of cultured neurons also has proved successful as a fast and easy method not only for expression of reporter genes but also for studying the targeting of a neuromodulin

fusion protein and of transferrin receptor (Liu et al., 1991; Kaech et al., 1996). Unlike the calcium phosphate method, lipid-mediated transfection works best at the time of plating and thus may be particularly useful for studying early stages of development. There are a number of commercially available cationic lipids that interact with DNA to form a complex that is taken up by cells (first described by Felgner et al., 1987). The DNA is not encapsidated in a liposome but rather is coated with the lipids and thus is neutralized. When the lipids fuse with the plasma membrane, the DNA presumably is endocytosed, with some of the DNA eventually reaching the nucleus (more so in dividing cells). Kaech et al. (1996) optimized the conditions for transfection of hippocampal neurons in low-density culture and provided the protocol in box 1.2. They found that DOTAP (Boehringer Mannheim, Indianapolis, IN) works better than does Transfectam or Lipofectamine and that sequential incubation of the neuronal cell suspensions with DOTAP and then the plasmid DNA prior to plating is optimal, yielding efficiencies of 0.5% to 3%. As for the calcium phosphate method, if the neurons survive the initial onslaught and begin to express a transfected gene product, they will continue to express it throughout their lifetime. Cotransfection of two or more plasmids also occurs with very high efficiency using the DOTAP method.

Microinjection

Transfection by microinjection has been used widely for invertebrate neurons and for some mammalian neurons, primarily cultured sympathetic neurons. Transfection can be achieved either by injection of plasmid DNA into the nucleus (Martinou et al., 1995) or by injection of cRNA into the cytoplasm (Ikeda et al., 1995). A particularly effective use of this method was the expression of Bcl-2 or of a dominant negative form of c-Jun containing the DNA binding and dimerization domains but lacking the transactivation region of c-Jun (Garcia et al., 1992; Ham et al., 1995). Expression of Bcl-2 or of this dominant negative c-Jun protected the cultured sympathetic neurons from programmed cell death induced by nerve growth factor (NGF) withdrawal.

Microinjection obviously works on a cell-by-cell basis, so it is inherently inefficient, but one can inject hundreds of cells per day with practice, particularly with an automated micromanipulator and pressure microinjector (Eppendorf makes a good one). A very

Box 4.2 Lipid-Mediated Transfection

Method

1. Dissect, trypsinize, and triturate hippocampi from E18 rat embryos in Ca, Mg-free Hank's BSS with 10 mM HEPES pH 7.2 as described in chapter 13.
2. To remove debris, pellet the cells by gentle centrifugation and resuspend in MEM. Determine the cell count and adjust the density to 5×10^5 cells/ml.
3. For each construct to be transfected, aliquot 6 μl DOTAP into a polystyrene tube and mix with 1 ml MEM. To this, add 1 ml of the cell suspension (i.e., 5×10^5 cells) and incubate at 37°C in a water bath for 10 min.
4. Dilute 1 μg of DNA in 100 μl MEM, add to the preincubated cells, and gently mix by inversion. Continue incubation at 37°C for an additional 30–40 min.
5. Transfer the contents of the tube to a 60-mm dish containing polylysine-treated coverslips in MEM with 10% horse serum. After 4 h in the incubator, flip coverslips with neurons attached onto glial feeder layers in N2.1 as described in chapter 13.
6. Depending on the sensitivity of the assay, transgene expression can be detected as early as 16 h after plating.

Reagents

DOTAP is available from Boehringer (no. 1811177 or no. 1202375). As suggested by the manufacturer, use a sterile plastic or glass syringe to remove DOTAP from the vial.
MEM: We supplement MEM from Life Technologies (no. 41090-028) with 0.6% glucose (Sigma G-7021, St. Louis, MO).
DNA: We prepare our plasmids routinely using Qiagen kits, preferably Endo-Free Plasmid Maxi Kit no. 12362.

good pipette puller also is required to produce sharp and reproducible pipettes on the order of 60 MΩ resistance. All cultured neurons potentially are amenable to microinjection, but cells such as hippocampal neurons are smaller and flatter than are sympathetic neurons and thus much more difficult to microinject.

Biolistics

A potentially promising new method is biolistics which uses a "gene gun" and involves bombarding cells at high velocity with micron-size gold particles coated with plasmid DNA. Biolistics has been used to generate beautiful transfected neurons in both

dissociated culture and slice culture (Jiao et al., 1993; Lo et al., 1994; McAllister et al., 1995). The method is conceptually simple and relatively straightforward if one has access to a biolistic device that uses high-pressure helium (e.g., the Bio-Rad PDS-1000), although it may require optimization of conditions for particular cultures (as is true for all the physical methods). Lo et al. (1994) optimized parameters to obtain 50 to 200 transfected neurons per cultured cortical slice and found that transfection correlated with the presence of a gold particle in the nucleus. More recent experiments that used a hand-held accelerator have improved on this efficiency 10-fold (D.C. Lo, personal communication). McAllister et al. (1995) used biolistics to label a subpopulation of neurons in slice cultures of ferret visual cortex to determine the effects of neurotrophins on dendritic morphology (figure 4.3 and color plate 1).

Viral Methods

Molecular neuroscientists took notice when Geller and Breakefield (1988) reported the first high-efficiency, virally mediated transfection of a foreign gene into neurons. They used a defective HSV vector, a natural choice as neurons are a normal host for HSV. Instead of a recombinant vector, they used a helper-mediated plasmid amplicon-based HSV vector, an ingenious and fast method first proposed by Spaete and Frenkel (1982). More recently, the discovery that adenovirus vectors can infect neurons with reasonable efficiency (Akli et al., 1993; Davidson et al., 1993; La Salle et al., 1993) even though neurons are not a natural host led to another wave of virally mediated neuron transfections. These two methods, HSV amplicons and recombinant adenoviruses, have been the leaders over the last few years in terms of productive use for transfection of neurons both in culture and in vivo.

Other lesser-used viral vectors for neurons include recombinant HSV, adeno-associated virus, vaccinia virus, and SFV. A comparison of these viral vectors is given in table 4.1 Commonly used for other cell types, retroviruses do not transfect postmitotic neurons (with the exception of a novel human immunodeficiency virus–based vector described by Naldini et al., 1996). Excellent chapters including detailed methods for most of these viral vector systems can be found in Roth (1994); a shorter overview is provided by Slack and Miller (1996).

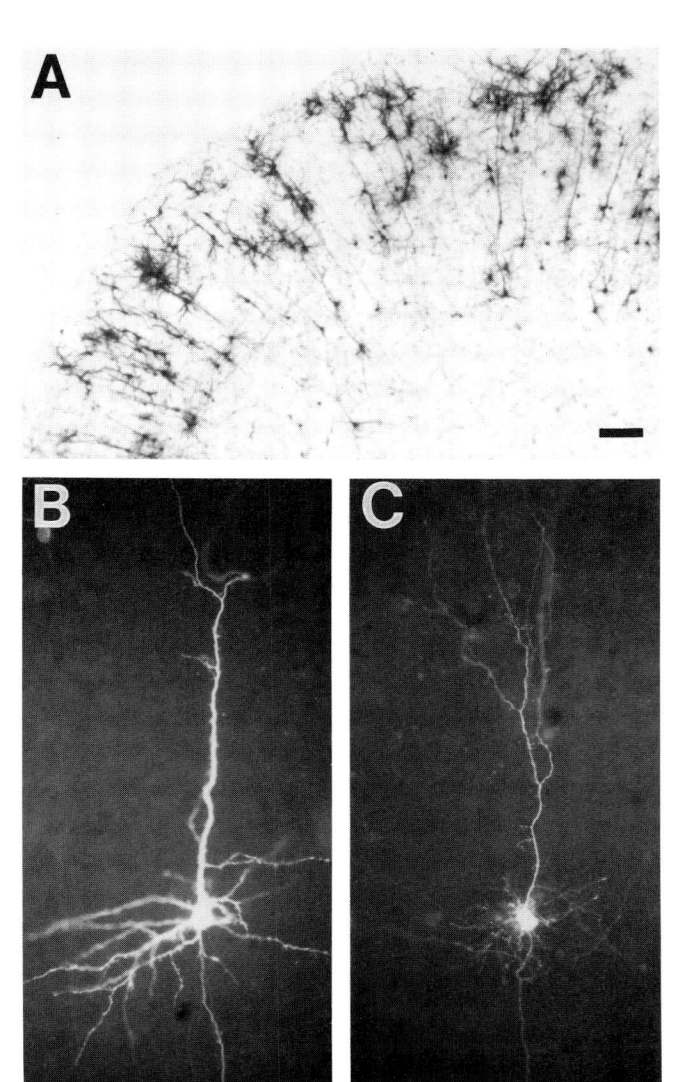

Figure 4.3 Transfection of pyramidal neurons in ferret organotypic slice cultures by biolistics. (*A*) Field of the slice culture after bombarding with the gold particles coated with a lacZ expression plasmid and staining with X-gal. (*B*) Layer 5 pyramidal neuron from a transfected slice treated with BDNF and immunostained for β-galactosidase. (*C*) Layer 5 pyramidal neuron from a transfected slice treated with NT-4 and immunostained for β-galactosidase. Note the halo of neurites extending from the cell body owing to the effects of NT-4 on increasing the number of basal dendrites. (From McAllister et al., 1995, with permission.) See color version in plate 1.

Table 4.1 Viral Vectors for Neuron Transfection

VIRAL VECTOR	DEFECTIVE	HELPER REQUIRED	GENOME	MAXIMUM INSERT	TITERS[a] (pfu/ml)	EXPRESSION TIME	CONSTRUCTION TIME
Recombinant herpes simplex virus (HSV)	Yes	No	150 kb DNA episomal	≥30 kb	$\sim 10^8$	$\sim$12 h to weeks[b]	1–2 months
Amplicon-based HSV	Yes	Yes (nonseparable)	$\sim$15 kb plasmid (+ helper HSV)	15 kb	$\sim 10^6$	$\sim$12–48 h (then toxicity)[c]	$\sim$2 weeks
Recombinant adenovirus	Yes	No	36 kb DNA episomal	7.8 kb	$\sim 10^{11}$	$\sim$12 h to weeks	1–2 months
Adeno-associated virus	Yes	Yes (separable)	4.7 kb DNA integrating	4.7 kb	$\sim 10^4$	$\sim$12 h to weeks	$\sim$2 weeks
Recombinant vaccinia virus	No	No	190 kb DNA cytoplasmic rep.	≥30 kb	$\sim 10^9$	6–16 h (then toxicity)	1–2 months
Semliki forest virus	Yes	Yes (not packaged)	11 kb (+) RNA cytoplasmic rep.	3 kb optimal	$\sim 10^9$	5–8 h. (then toxicity)	<1 week

[a] Titers can vary easily 10-fold from estimates here for crude cell extracts and almost all can be increased 10- to 100-fold by further purification.
[b] We have observed survival for weeks, but many other laboratories have reported toxicity within a couple of days.
[c] There have been reports of longer survival times but, in our experience with a variety of amplicon-based vectors, the neurons always have exhibited signs of toxicity within 2 days and death within 6 days.

There are some advantages and disadvantages that apply to all these viral vectors. All can give transfection efficiencies up to 90% in cultured neurons (except perhaps adeno-associated virus). Of course, this is the maximal efficiency, and one usually can use less virus if the goal is to transfect only a subpopulation of neurons. Another advantage is that all seem to be capable of transfecting neurons at any age in culture. For example, we have performed HSV and adenovirus-mediated transfections anywhere between day 1 and day 25 in hippocampal cultures. Some toxicity is associated with all the viral vectors, more so at higher multiplicities of infection. Of the commonly used vectors, adenovirus is least toxic, then recombinant HSV, and then amplicon-based HSV vectors. Finally, safety to lab personnel is a consideration for all the viral vectors. Although there are no reported incidences of infec-

tion in laboratory personnel to date and none of these viruses are airborne, it is necessary to follow National Institutes of Health biosafety level 2 guidelines. Wild-type adenovirus induces a mild infection, and HSV can induce life-threatening encephalitis. Even though most of these vector systems use replication-defective viruses, recombination can produce infectious virus at low frequency. Moreover, recombination theoretically could produce an infectious virus expressing the gene of interest. Thus, generally it is necessary to monitor stocks for the presence of nondefective viruses by testing for plaque formation on a cell line that does not complement the defect in the parent virus. One of the current aims is to generate packaging systems wherein recombination cannot easily generate an infectious virus. Practically, biosafety level 2 is not too difficult to achieve. It requires awareness by lab personnel and the use of a class II biosafety cabinet, protective clothing, and autoclaving or bleach treatment of all waste.

Recombinant HSV

Recombinant HSV vectors have been used to express reporter genes in neurons in culture and in vivo (Ho and Mocarski, 1988; Chiocca et al., 1990; Dobson et al., 1990; Fink et al., 1992; Johnson et al., 1992b). They have also been used to study targeting of glycosyl-phosphatidylinositol (GPI)-anchored proteins and to enhance neuron survival by expression of a kinase (Buckmaster and Tolkovsky, 1994; Lowenstein et al., 1994b), but such functional studies have not been abundant. The likely reason is that recombinant HSV vectors are much more difficult and time-consuming to construct than are the amplicon-based HSV vectors and are somewhat more difficult than recombinant adenoviruses, owing to the larger 150-kb genome. The usual method is to cotransfect viral DNA (which itself can be finicky to purify intact) and a plasmid containing the expression cassette flanked by viral sequences corresponding to the desired site of insertion. The resultant virus stock then must be screened for in vivo recombinants, which are plaque-purified and confirmed by Southern blotting. A commonly used insertion site is the thymidine kinase locus; growth in acyclovir then can be used as an initial selection for recombinants. The efficiency of recombination may also be enhanced by addition of loxP sites from bacteriophage P1 to the viral genome and shuttle vector and incubation with the Cre recombinase prior to transfection (Gage et al., 1992).

For both recombinant and amplicon-based HSV vectors, it is desirable to begin with a parent virus that is defective in replication. Temperature-sensitive mutants or mutants in accessory genes have been used, but the best (least toxic) appear to be deletion mutants lacking genes essential for HSV replication. Deletion mutants and packaging cell lines that express the deleted gene have been developed for the essential gene IE3 (also known as ICP4, α4, and Vmw 175), which encodes the major transcriptional activator: N. A. Deluca, University of Pittsburgh, virus d120 and cell line E5 (DeLuca et al., 1985); R. D. Everett, MRC Virology Unit, Glasgow, Scotland, virus D30EBA (Paterson and Everett, 1990); P. A. Johnson, Dept. of Pediatrics, UCSD, RR1 cell line (Johnson, et al., 1992a). Using an IE3 mutant (from Dobson et al., 1990), we have obtained β-galactosidase expression for at least 2 weeks in cultured hippocampal neurons, but other labs (Johnson et al., 1992b) have found considerable toxicity within a few days with similar IE3 deletion mutant recombinant HSV vectors. A recent improvement is the generation of viruses with deletions in multiple genes and a consequent reduction in toxicity of the viral vector (Johnson et al., 1994; Marconi et al., 1996). Additional information about recombinant HSV vectors can be found in Johnson and Friedmann (1994) and Fink et al. (1996).

Amplicon-Based HSV

HSV amplicon vectors have been used widely for neuron transfection in dissociated cultures, slice cultures, acute slices, and in vivo (Geller and Breakefield, 1988; Kaplitt et al., 1991; Casaccia-Bonnefil et al., 1993; Bahr et al., 1994). Experiments keyed toward enhancing neuron survival include expression of NGF, p75 NGF receptor, trkA NGF receptor, the glucose transporter, and the apoptosis inhibitory protein Bcl-2 (Battleman et al., 1993; Geschwind et al., 1994; Ho et al., 1993; Xu et al., 1994; Lawrence et al., 1996a). In a study of excitotoxicity, amplicon-mediated expression of GluR6 in a small number of neurons led to transsynaptic neuronal loss (Bergold et al., 1993). Enhanced neurotransmitter production has been reported by expression of a constitutively active adenylate cyclase or by expression of tyrosine hydroxylase, in the latter case leading to behavioral recovery in a Parkinsonian model (Geller et al., 1993; During et al., 1994). Amplicon vectors have been used also in cell biological studies to show addition of membrane pro-

teins to axonal growth cones and to study protein targeting to axonal versus somatodendritic domains (Craig et al., 1995; figure 4.4).

An HSV amplicon is a plasmid cloning-amplifying vector that contains an HSV origin of replication, HSV packaging signals, and an expression cassette for the foreign gene of interest (figure 4.5). First, the gene of interest is cloned into the amplicon vector, generally an easy step, as the amplicons are in the range of 6 to 15 kb, and many have been designed with multiple cloning sites. Then, the amplicon is transfected into a packaging cell line by standard methods, such as lipid-mediated transfection. Finally, the transfected cells are superinfected with helper virus to provide HSV replication and packaging functions in *trans*. DNA replication occurs from the HSV origin on the amplicon and generates a large DNA containing head-to-tail repeats of the plasmid. This DNA is cleaved at the nearest packaging site to generate a $\sim$150-kb genome-sized DNA that is packaged into virions. The result is the production of new virus particles, some corresponding to more helper virus and some corresponding to virions containing head-to-tail copies of amplicon DNA but no other HSV DNA. Ideally, the next step would be to separate physically amplicon-containing virions from helper virions, but that goal has not yet been achieved. Thus, as for recombinant HSV vectors, it is necessary to use a defective helper virus with the deleted gene, generally IE3, supplied by the packaging cell line. In addition, because it is necessary to expose neurons to both amplicon-containing vector and helper virus, one tries to achieve a good ratio (roughly 1:1) of vector to helper. This is done by passaging the viral stock two to three more times. As the vector has approximately 15 copies of the HSV origin of replication (e.g., for a 10-kb amplicon) versus 3 origins in the helper virus, the amplicon vector will multiply selectively, at least up to a point at which the needed helper virus has diminished. Usually, it is possible to obtain viral stocks suitable for neuron transfection after approximately three passages. The titer of helper virus can be determined by plaque formation on the packaging cell line, whereas the titer of amplicon vector can be determined by protein expression in another cell line. Transfection of neurons with these mixed stocks results in expression of protein from cells that have taken up amplicon DNA regardless of whether they also have taken up helper virus DNA (Lowenstein et al., 1994a). Partial purification of the final vector-helper mix by centrifugation or microfiltration can help to concentrate the viral stock and to reduce toxicity to

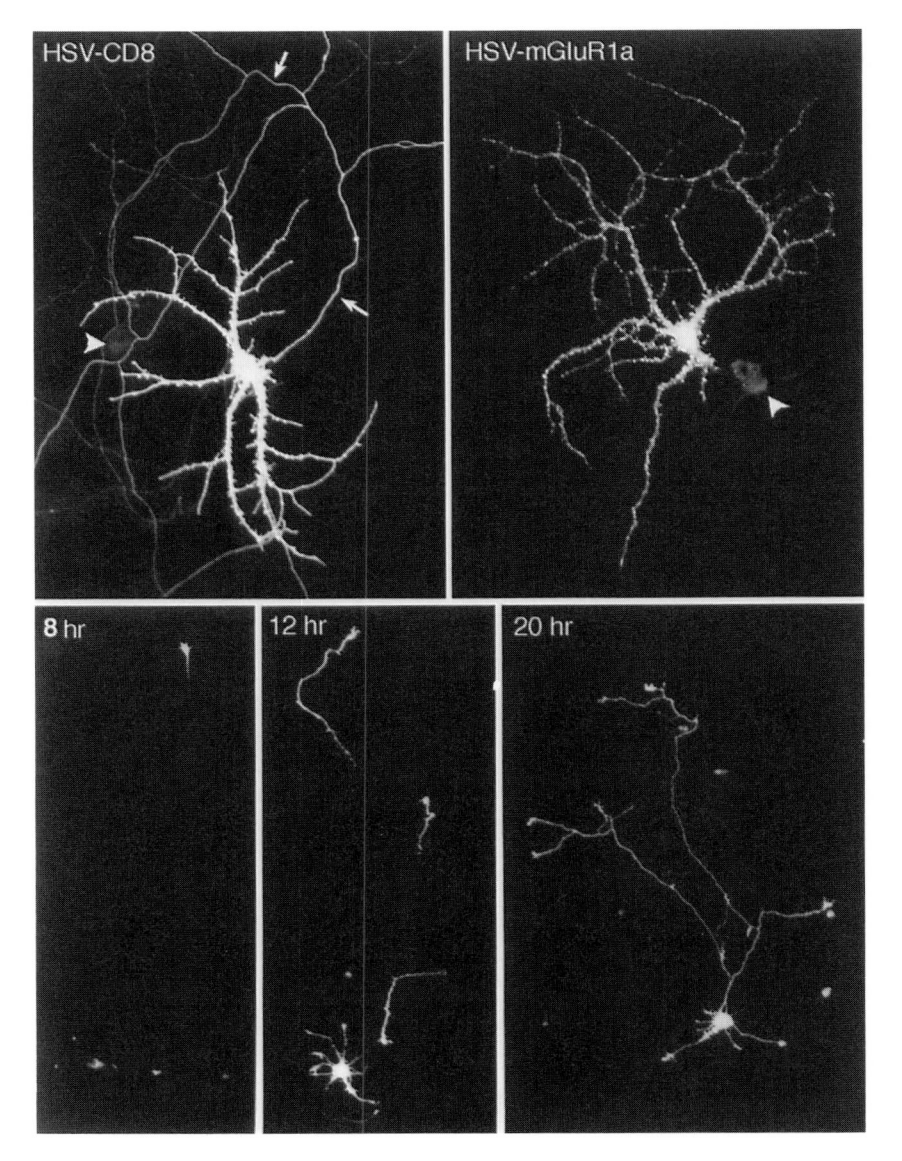

Figure 4.4 Use of herpes simplex virus amplicon-based vectors to study membrane protein targeting in rat hippocampal cultures. (Top row) Hippocampal neurons were exposed to HSV amplicon-based vectors expressing the lymphocyte protein CD8α or the metabotropic glutamate receptor mGluR1α at 3 weeks in culture and were immunolabeled 1 day later for the expressed proteins. CD8α is targeted to the entire plasma membrane surface, including the axon, whereas mGluR1α is excluded from the axon and restricted to the somatodendritic domain. (Bottom row) Neurons were exposed to the HSV-CD8α vector at 2 days in culture, fixed between 6 and 24 h later, and immunolabeled for surface CD8α. At the earliest time at which the expressed CD8α could detected on the cell surface (8 h), it was detected only at the growth cones, indicating specific sites of addition to the plasma membrane. By 18–24 h, the expressed protein reached a more uniform steady-state distribution. (Bottom row from Craig et al., 1995, with permission.)

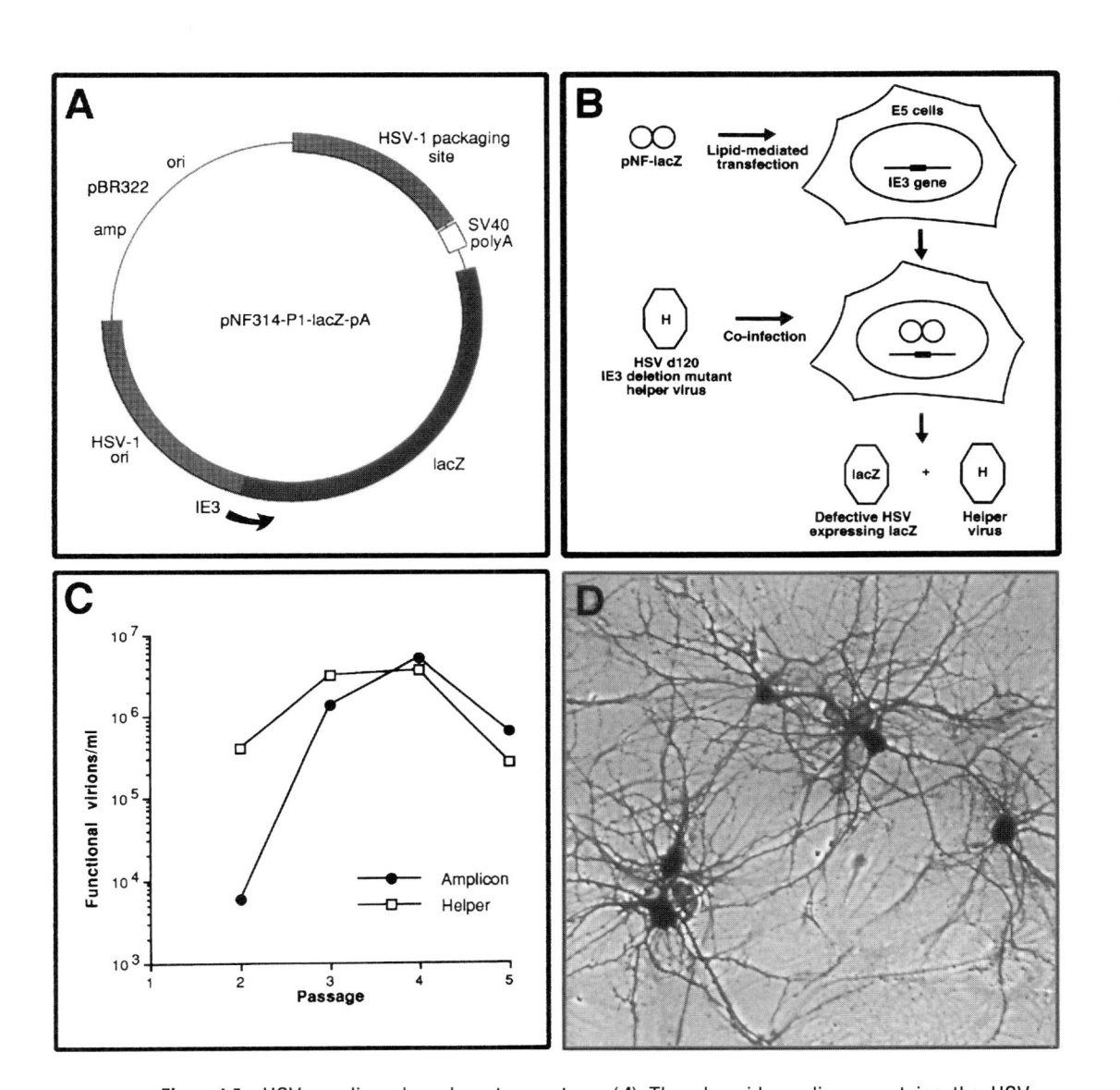

Figure 4.5 HSV amplicon-based vector system. (*A*) The plasmid amplicon contains the HSV origin of replication and packaging site and the expression cassette, in this case lacZ driven by the HSV IE3 promoter and followed by the SV40 polyadenylation signal. (*B*) The packaging method involves transfection of the plasmid amplicon into the E5 cell line that carries the HSV IE3 gene and then coinfection with the d120 IE3 deletion mutant helper virus. This leads to production of a mixed viral stock containing more d120 helper virus and virions containing head-to-tail repeats of the plasmid amplicon DNA. (*C*) The initial ratio of packaged amplicon to helper virus is low. The amplicon-containing virions are replicated preferentially on subsequent passages, owing to their numerous origins of replication but, after a few passages, the helper virus titer drops off, so all replication is decreased. (*D*) Hippocampal neurons in low-density culture were exposed to an amplicon-based HSV-lacZ vector (passage 3, purified by centrifugation through a sucrose cushion) and stained with X-gal 1 day later.

mature neurons. Crude cell lysates, even those lacking virus, can induce neuron toxicity, in part via activation of glutamate receptors (Ho et al., 1995).

In summary, three components are needed to make amplicon-based vectors: amplicon plasmid DNA; defective helper virus, preferably a deletion mutant of IE3; and a packaging cell line expressing the defective gene. No company is marketing these products, so it is necessary to obtain components from individual laboratories. The amplicon plasmid should be easy to obtain from any of the many laboratories referenced earlier. IE3 defective virus and packaging cell lines have been produced by a few groups (listed under Recombinant HSV). Detailed methods for amplicon-based vector production are given in box 4.3. Also, there is an excellent methods chapter on the amplicon vector system by Ho (1994) and a report on optimizing packaging efficiency by Wu et al. (1995).

An advantage of this vector system over recombinant viruses is the rapidity of constructing each vector. For most of us, this is a very strong advantage. Another advantage is that each virion contains multiple copies of the expression cassette, so that there is no problem in obtaining high-level expression. However, there are two major disadvantages. The vector stock cannot be propagated indefinitely because each replication cycle leads to varying ratios of amplicon vector to helper virus, and there are reports of difficulties in obtaining good ratios. We have not found this to be a serious disadvantage and always have been able to obtain sufficient usable vector, sometimes by redoing a single passage from frozen stocks and, rarely, by starting the protocol over from the first transfection. The other, major disadvantage for us is the toxicity, which appears after a few days and prevents the use of amplicon-based vectors for long-term functional studies. This toxicity is apparent with partially purified stocks regardless of the protein being expressed. The cause of the toxicity still is not clear; it is not mimicked by the same amount of helper virus alone. One theory is that it is an unavoidable consequence of the packaging method. The amplicon vector is in a sense a defective interfering particle, a virion with a defective genome, and so optimization of amplicon vector production necessarily leads to high-level production of other defective interfering particles that themselves may be toxic and cannot at present be separated physically. It is surprising that some of the functional studies reported earlier were possible, given this level of toxicity in

Box 4.3 Production of HSV Amplicon-Based Viral Vectors

All steps must be performed in a certified biosafety cabinet according to National Institutes of Health biosafety level 2 standards.

Packaging

Day 1
Seed two T-25 flasks with 8×10^5 E5 cells each. E5 cells are derived from the VERO monkey kidney cell line and express the HSV IE3 gene (DeLuca et al., 1985). We grow the E5 cells in DMEM + 10% FCS + Pen/Strep + 125 mg/ml active G418, and passage with trypsin-EDTA. Many other kinds of media will work, but the G418 is required to select for the antibiotic resistance gene that was originally cotransfected with the HSV IE3 gene in generating the cell line. The cells must be used within the first 15–20 passages, as later passages eventually become resistant to propagation of d120 virus, even with continued G418 selection (presumably through loss of the HSV IE3 gene). RR1 cells, a line derived from BHK cells that also expresses the IE3 gene, also can be used. They are reported to transfect more efficiently (Johnson and Friedmann, 1994).

DAY 2

1. Prepare:
   A. 14 µl Lipofectamine (GIBCO/BRL) in 280 µl Opti-MEM I medium (GIBCO/BRL)
   B. 4 µg amplicon DNA in 280 µl Opti-MEM I medium (plasmids prepared with Qiagen kits work fine)
   Mix A and B and leave at room temperature for 30 min.
2. At the end of the incubation, rinse a flask of E5 cells plated on day 1 with Opti-MEM I.
3. Add 2.2 ml Opti-MEM I to the DNA-lipofectamine complex and add to the cells.
4. Incubate 6 h, then add 2.7 ml DMEM with 20% FCS.
5. Incubate 18–24 h.

In setting up the system, cells can be fixed and stained at this point to test transfection efficiency. Maximal transfection efficiency (ideally 30%–40%) is important to optimize the subsequent ratio of packaged amplicon to helper virus.

DAY 3

1. Remove the medium from the flask of transfected E5 cells and add the HSV IE3 deletion mutant helper virus (d120 or D30EBA) at a multiplicity of infection of two in a final volume of 1.5 ml medium. Replace the flask in the incubator and allow the virus to adsorb 90 min, shaking periodically.
   Some laboratories use a multiplicity of infection of 0.1 here and collect virus after several days when cytopathic effects are widespread, in a sense combining the multiple passages in a single step. Sometimes, this has worked for us as well but has yielded variable results in our hands.

Box 4.3 (continued)

2. Remove the virus-containing medium from the flask and add 4 ml of fresh medium containing 8×10^5 E5 cells obtained by trypsinizing the extra flask of E5 cells seeded on day 1. The purpose of overlaying cells with each passage is to allow virus, released from the bottom cell layer, to infect the top cell layer and, in a sense, induce two rounds of infection in the same flask.
3. Incubate for approximately 40–48 h until most cells exhibit cytopathic effects. Ideally, all the cells should be rounded but with few detached, as the virus inactivates quickly in the medium.

DAY 4
Seed two T-75 flasks with 3×10^6 E5 cells each.

DAY 5

1. Assuming widespread cytopathic effects have developed, freeze the cells by laying the flask flat in a $-80°C$ freezer for 5 min. Thaw, tapping the flask vigorously so the ice will scrape off any remaining cells attached to the substrate. Collect the cells and medium in a screw-cap tube.
2. Freeze the cell suspension again rapidly in a dry ice-ethanol bath. Thaw rapidly at 37°C with agitation; leave at 37°C only long enough to thaw.
3. Repeat step 2. These freeze-thaw cycles will disrupt the cells, releasing the virus. Alternatively, the virus can be released by sonicating the mixture on ice.
4. Centrifuge the suspension at 2000 rpm for 10 min at 4°C to remove cell debris.
5. Freeze 2 ml of this viral stock of passage 1 (P1) on dry ice-ethanol and store at $-80°C$.
6. Use 2 ml of the P1 stock to start P2. Remove the medium from a flask of E5 cells seeded on day 4, add 2 ml P1, and incubate 90 min.
7. Remove the virus-containing medium and add 10 ml of fresh medium containing 3×10^6 E5 cells obtained by trypsinizing the extra flask of E5 cells seeded on day 4.
8. Incubate for approximately 40–48 h until most cells exhibit cytopathic effects.

DAY 6
Seed two T-75 flasks with 3×10^6 E5 cells each.

DAY 7
Harvest P2 and start P3 as for day 5; as volume now is 10 ml, freeze 8 ml and use 2 ml to start P3. The frozen stocks can be used later to make more virus simply by repeating a single step (e.g., P2 to P3).

DAY 9
Harvest P3 as for day 5, freezing all of it.
   If desired, one more passage could be performed to obtain P4 stocks. Initially, we determined the titers of helper virus and packaged amplicon in all

Box 4.3 (continued)

viral stocks (see further for methods). Now, we tend to go ahead and use the P3 or P4 stocks for neuron transfection and only determine titers if there is a problem. P3 or P4 stocks usually are optimum for neuron transfection, with titers of 10^5–10^6/ml (before concentration) and approximately equal ratios of packaged amplicon to helper virus. Further passaging tends to decrease titers without improving the ratio of packaged amplicon to helper virus.

We usually perform a crude purification of the virus stocks before using them for neuron transfection. This last step serves both to concentrate the viral stock up to 50-fold and to remove components of the crude cell lysate that are toxic to neurons (probably mainly glutamate). We layer the viral stock onto a cushion of 25% sucrose in PBS and centrifuge at 27,000 rpm overnight to pellet the virus. Viruses also can be concentrated by centrifuging at lower speeds in buffer or by using a microfiltration device.

Titering Helper Virus
Helper virus d120 can be titered by plaque formation on E5 cells as follows.

1. Plate E5 cells in six-well dishes, 2×10^5 cells per well, and incubate overnight.
2. Prepare a series of 10-fold dilutions of the virus in media. Remove media from the cell wells and add 250 µl per well of virus dilutions 10^{-2}–10^{-7}.
3. Incubate for 1 h, occasionally rocking the dish.
4. Remove virus and add 3 ml per well of media supplemented with 0.5 mg/ml human immune γ-globulin (Armour Pharmacentical, Fort Washington, PA). This mixture contains antibodies against HSV that will prevent spreading of the virus from individual plaques.
5. Incubate for 3 days to allow plaques to develop. Plaques will appear as clear areas of dead cells on a lawn of live cells (much like bacteriophage λ plaques on a lawn of *E. coli*). Cells can be fixed and stained with cresyl violet to help to visualize plaques. Count plaques and calculate the titer.

Titering Amplicon-Based Vector
The titer of virions containing packaged amplicon is determined by detecting expression of the exogenous protein in a cell line that is nonpermissive for d120 replication, such as VERO cells (the parent line for E5; available from American Type Culture Collection, Rockville, MD).

1. Plate VERO cells in six-well dishes, 2×10^5 cells per well, and incubate overnight.
2. Prepare a series of 10-fold dilutions of the virus in medium. Remove medium from the cell wells and add 250 µl per well of virus dilutions 10^{-2}–10^{-7}.
3. Incubate for 1 h, occasionally rocking dish.
4. Remove virus and add 3 ml per well of medium.
5. Incubate for approximately 24 h. Fix and stain with antibody against the expressed protein or with Xgal if expressing β-galactosidase. Count the number of individual expressing cells and calculate the titer (sometimes termed *bfu* for blue-forming units).

Box 4.3 (continued)

6. Also check for the absence of plaques on VERO cells to ensure the absence of recombinant infectious virus.

Preparing Helper Virus
Stocks of the d120 helper virus usually last us for more than a year if we prepare them from several flasks as follows.

1. Seed 5–10 T-75 flasks with 1.2×10^6 early passage E5 cells. Grow approximately 40 h until 70–80% confluent.
2. Remove medium and add d120 virus at a multiplicity of infection of 0.01–0.05 in a final volume of 2.5 ml medium per flask. (A higher MOI would allow too much replication of defective virus.) Incubate for 90 min, shaking occasionally.
3. Add an extra 7.5 ml medium per flask and incubate for approximately 2 days until most cells have become rounded.
4. Harvest virus. Freeze flask at −80°C and shake off cells while thawing.
5. Centrifuge cells plus medium at 3000 rpm at 4°C for 10 min. Save both pellet and supernatant.
6. Centrifuge the supernatant at 10,000 rpm at 4°C for 2 h and save this pellet.
7. Resuspend the pellet from step 5 in 2 ml of medium. Perform three freeze-thaw cycles in dry ice-ethanol at 37°C, then centrifuge at 4000 rpm at 4°C for 10 min to remove cell debris, saving the supernatant.
8. Use the supernatant from step 7 to resuspend the pellet from step 6. Freeze in aliquots. The titer should be 10^7–10^8 pfu/ml.

our low-density culture system; it seems that high-density cultures or tissue can absorb the toxic effects better.

The amplicon vector system is relatively new and certainly is open for improvement. Ideally, one would like a packaging cell line that obviates the need for any helper virus. This development seems unlikely in the near future, given the complexity of HSV replication and the toxicity of many viral gene products when constitutively expressed in mammalian cells. An exciting new method that approaches this ideal is to cotransfect amplicon DNA together with a set of five HSV-derived cosmids that lack packaging signals but can support *trans* replication and packaging of the amplicon (Fraefel et al., 1996). This method resulted in the production of helper virus–free amplicon vectors that could induce high-level expression of β-galactosidase with little toxicity even at 8 days after transfection. Vector titers were lower than those with helper-mediated packaging, and the actual packaging step was

somewhat finicky but also very fast, only a couple of days. This method sounds ideal for our lab, and I have my request in for the cosmid set.

Recombinant Adenovirus

Although the first reports of neuron transfection in vivo by defective adenoviral vectors came only a few years ago (Akli et al., 1993; Davidson et al., 1993; La Salle et al., 1993), adenovirus vectors have already come into widespread use. Cultured neurons that have been transfected include those from the superior cervical ganglion, dorsal root ganglion, retina, cortex, and hippocampus (both dissociated and slice cultures) (Caillaud et al., 1993; La Salle et al., 1993; Jomary et al., 1994; Moriyoshi et al., 1996; Vogt et al., 1996; Wilkemeyer et al., 1996; figure 4.6 and color plate 2). A number of interesting experiments have been performed by adenovirus-mediated transfection of cultured neurons. Expression of p53 induced apoptosis, whereas expression of superoxide dismutase protected neurons against glutamate toxicity (Slack and Miller, 1996; Slack et al., 1996). Cell biological questions have been studied by expression of peptide-processing enzymes and axonal cell adhesion molecules (Paquet et al., 1996; Vogt et al., 1996). Calbindin expression suppressed posttetanic potentiation (Chard et al., 1995) and, in a particularly elegant experiment, expression of brain-derived neurotrophic factor (BDNF) partially rescued the defect in long-term potentiation (LTP) in hippocampal slices from BDNF-deficient mice (Korte et al., 1996; figure 4.7). An adenovirus expressing a membrane-targeted green fluorescent protein (GFP) (Moriyoshi et al., 1996; see also figure 4.1) will no doubt see widespread use as a means of labeling neuron profiles in culture and in vivo.

Adenoviral vectors are most often constructed by in vivo recombination in a packaging cell line. One method developed in Frank Graham's laboratory (McGrory et al., 1988; Bett et al., 1994; see also Becker et al., 1994) uses a shuttle plasmid together with another large plasmid (originally pJM17) containing the entire adenovirus genome but with an insert in the E1 region such that it is too large to be packaged (figure 4.8A). Recombination between pJM17 and the shuttle plasmid generates viral DNA that meets the size requirements for packaging and that now contains the gene of interest. Another method selects for recombination between a linearized shuttle plasmid containing the expression cassette flanked by

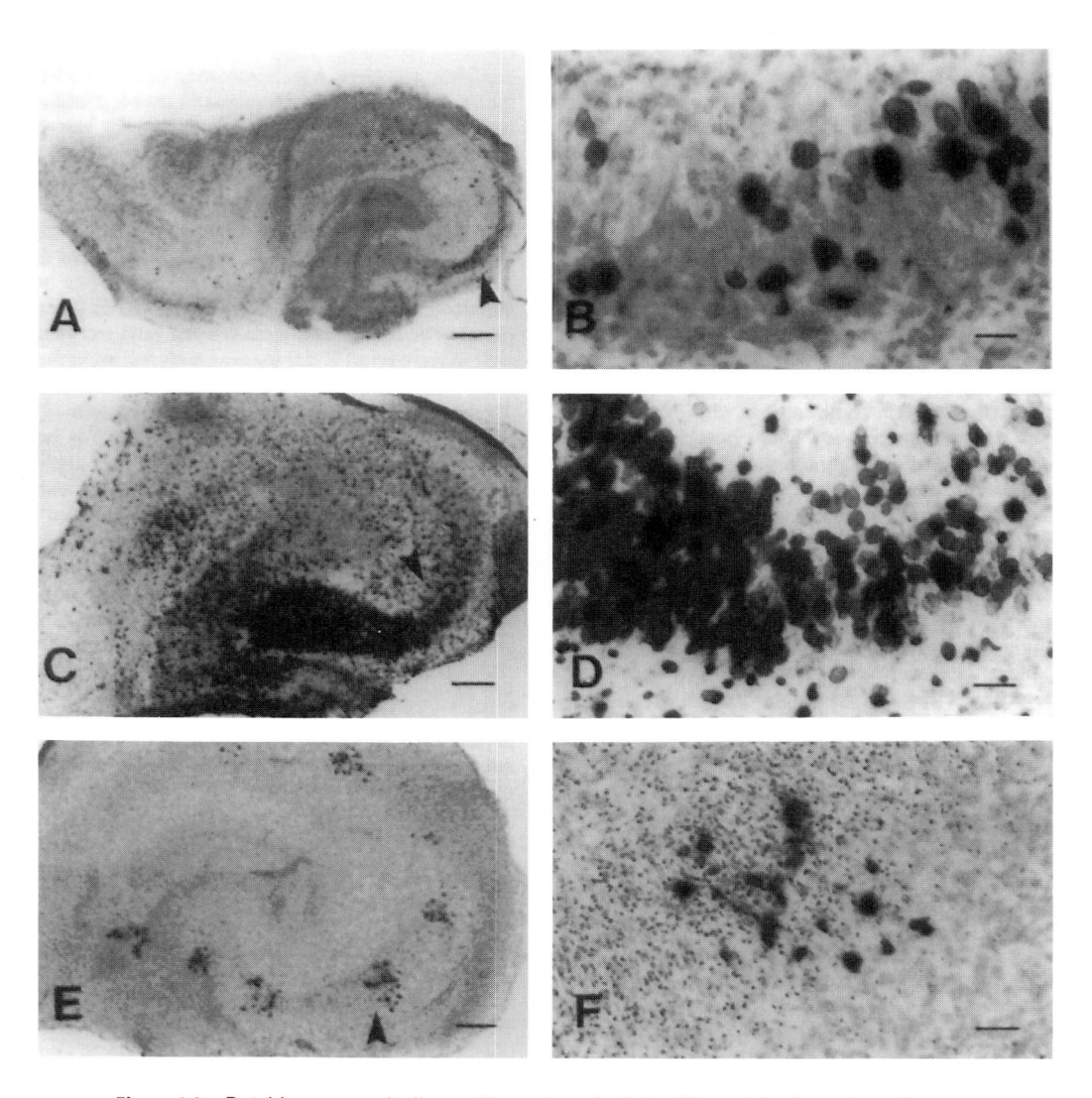

Figure 4.6 Rat hippocampal slice cultures transfected with a defective adenovirus vector expressing β-galactosidase with a nuclear localization signal (Adv/RSVβ-gal). After 1–3 days in explant culture, the slices were exposed to Adv/RSVβ-gal by application of a droplet to the surface (*A–D*) or by pressure injection (*E, F*). At 2 weeks in culture, the slices were stained with X-gal to detect β-galactosidase and were counterstained lightly with Nissl. The extent of transfection varied with application of different amounts of the viral vector: *A, B,* 5×10^7 pfu; *C, D,* 5×10^8 pfu; *E, F,* 1×10^4 pfu per injection site. (From Wilkemeyer et al., 1996, with permission.) See color version in plate 2.

viral DNA and a large fragment of adenoviral DNA restricted to remove 5' packaging and E1 sequences (Stow, 1981; figure 4.8B). Thus, with both methods there is a selection for recombinants, and both generate viruses with deletions in the E1 region and, thus, are defective for replication. The packaging must be performed and vectors must be propagated in the 293 cell line that supplies E1 gene products in *trans*. Of course, it still is necessary to plaque-purify potential recombinants and to check the viral DNA directly for the presence of the gene of interest. The original vectors had insert size limits of 4.8 kb, but newer variations of these methods use vectors that have deletions in the non-essential E3 region as well as in E1 and can accommodate insertions of up to 8.3 kb (Bett et al., 1994).

Shuttle plasmids and plasmid pJM17 and derivatives are commercially available singly or in a kit (Microbix Biosystems, Toronto, Canada), as Dr. Graham, who has been making plasmids available for years, recently has been overwhelmed with requests. The 293 cells are available from Microbix and also from American Type Culture Collection (Rockville, MD); for recombination, early passage 293 cells are preferable. I know of no commercial source for the shuttle plasmids and virus DNA for the linear recombination method, but these components are used widely and usually are available from individual laboratories on request. Detailed methods for generating recombinant adenovirus are not reproduced here but can be found in Becker et al. (1994) and Hitt et al. (1994). If you can obtain a little of your desired recombinant virus from another lab, you can easily prepare a large supply by propagation on 293 cells. You start with a subconfluent layer of 293 cells, add the virus (1–10 plaque-forming units/cell) in a minimal volume of medium and allow to adsorb for 1 hr, then add more medium and incubate until cells are mostly rounded but not yet detached (generally 2 days). Harvest the virus by scraping the cells, collect the cells plus media, freeze-thaw three times to release virus, spin out cell debris at low speed, and freeze the viral stock in aliquots. This crude stock often is on the order of 10^9 pfu/ml and is adequate for use on neurons.

Advantages of defective adenovirus vectors for transfection of cultured neurons include lower toxicity than HSV vectors, relative ease of construction compared with other recombinant vectors (because there are selection techniques), and the ability to propagate to high titers. The lower toxicity also is a very big advantage.

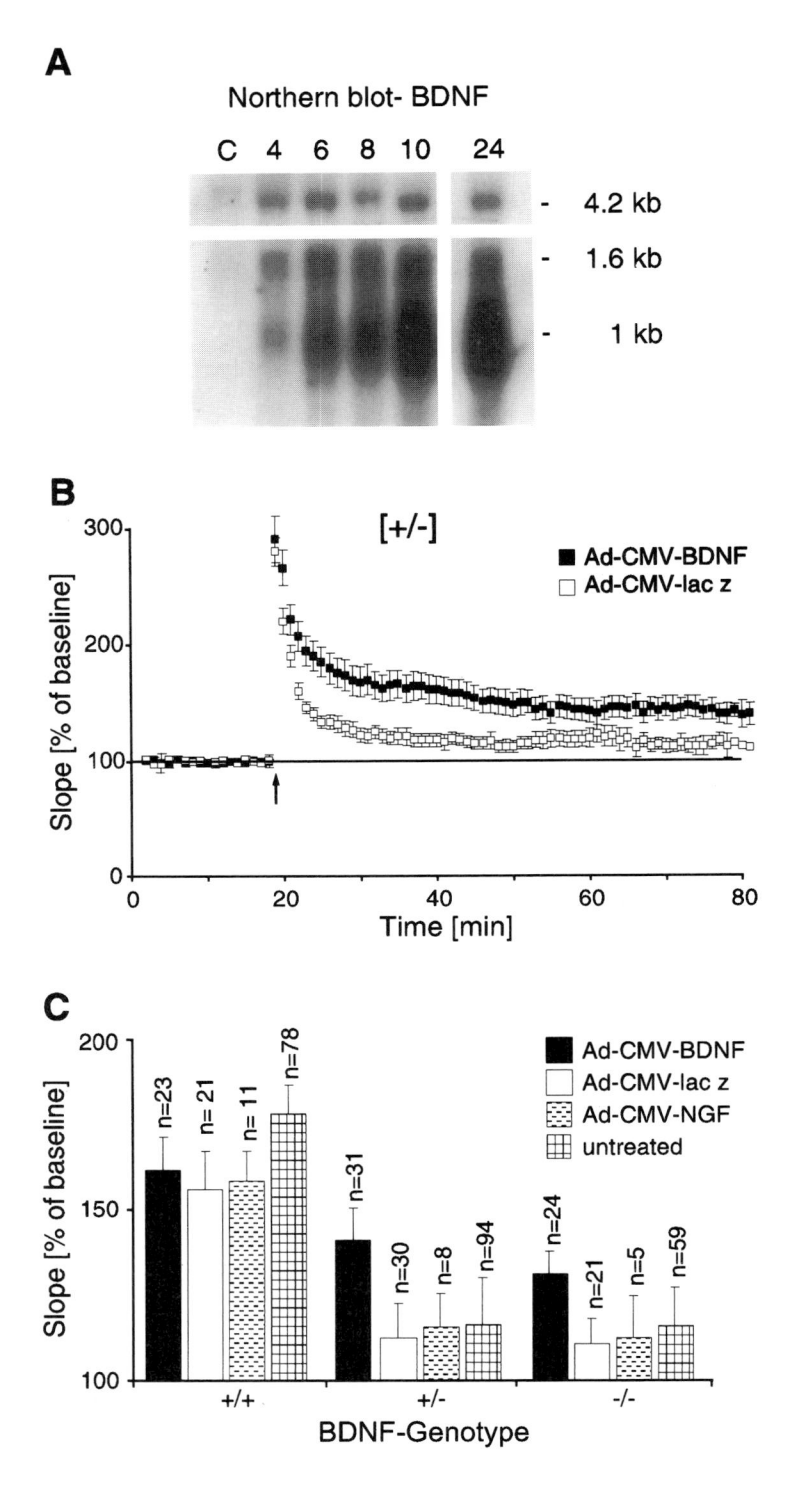

A

Northern blot- BDNF

C 4 6 8 10 24

- 4.2 kb

- 1.6 kb

- 1 kb

B

[+/-]

■ Ad-CMV-BDNF
□ Ad-CMV-lac z

C

■ Ad-CMV-BDNF
□ Ad-CMV-lac z
▨ Ad-CMV-NGF
▦ untreated

However, there are some potential drawbacks. Whereas HSV vectors yield high transfection efficiencies at a multiplicity of infection (MOI) of 1, adenovirus vectors can require an MOI of 10 to 100 for efficient transfection of neurons, perhaps because neurons are not a natural host for adenoviruses. Still, even with such high MOI, a range usually can be found wherein toxicity is not a problem. Slack and Miller (1996) found that a MOI of 10 was sufficient to induce expression in 80% of cultured sympathetic neurons with no effect on cell survival, electrophysiological function, or cytoarchitecture, whereas a MOI of 100 was toxic. In another very thorough study, Wilkemeyer et al. (1996) infected cultured hippocampal neurons with adenovirus at a MOI of 1, 10, or 100. The MOI of 1 did not affect survival and gave 30 to 70% transfection efficiency, whereas the MOIs of 10 or 100 resulted in toxicity after 10 or 5 days, respectively. Others have reported optimal transfection efficiencies at a MOI of 100 (Caillaud et al., 1993) or even 500 (Chard et al., 1995). It is not clear why the reported optimal MOIs vary so greatly, perhaps it depends on the promoter and expression level. The expression levels appear to be lower for recombinant viral vectors than for methods that introduce multiple copies of an expression cassette. We have found that infection by multiple defective adenoviruses is required to obtain detectable expression of membrane-associated GFP (from Moriyoshi et al., 1996), whereas calcium phosphate transfection of the corresponding plasmid can lead to high-level expression in individual cells (see figure 1). Another consideration is that optimal expression, in terms of protein levels, occurs only a few days after transfection. Finally, though most of the available transfection methods are more effective on glia cells than on neurons, this difference is particularly pronounced for adenovirus vectors and can lead to difficulties in transfecting neurons in mixed cultures.

Figure 4.7 Use of an adenovirus-BDNF vector to restore long-term potentiation (LTP) in slices from BDNF knockout mice. Hippocampal slices were exposed to the Ad-CMV-BDNF vector immediately after their isolation from BDNF-mutant mice, then were tested for their ability to undergo LTP 6–14 h later. (*A*) Time course of expression of the BDNF RNA in injected wild-type slices. The 1-kb BDNF RNA expressed from the viral vector was detectable by 4 h after injection and increased steadily to 24 h reaching much higher levels than the endogenous BDNF transcripts at 4.2 and 1.6 kb. (*B*) Expression of BDNF in a slice from a heterozygote increased the amount of LTP by 2.6-fold compared with expression of lacZ from a similar adenovirus vector. (*C*) Summary graph for all genotypes with different treatments. (From Korte et al., 1996, with permission.)

A
CMV
lacZ
0 mu
ΔE1 (0.9-9.8 mu)
pΔE1sp1-lacZ
Shuttle plasmid
15.8 mu
+
4.3 kb pBRX
insert at 3.7 mu
0/100 mu
pJM17
Plasmid carrying
Ad5 genome with insert
Co-transfect into 293 cells
Recombination event
CMV
lacZ
Recombinant adenovirus vector
(ΔE1; expresses lacZ; 36 kb genome)
Pick single plaques,
re-infect 293 cells,
prepare lysates and viral DNA,
check by Southern blotting,
prepare high titer purified stocks...
B
CMV
lacZ
0-1 mu
9.4-15.5 mu
Linearized shuttle plasmid
+
9.4 mu
100 mu
Right end of Ad5 DNA
(left end packaging site and E1 region removed
using unique restriction site at 9.4 mu)
Co-transfect into 293 cells
Recombination event
CMV
lacZ
Recombinant adenovirus vector
(ΔE1; expresses lacZ; 36 kb genome)
Pick single plaques,
re-infect 293 cells,
prepare lysates and viral DNA,
check by Southern blotting,
prepare high titer purified stocks...

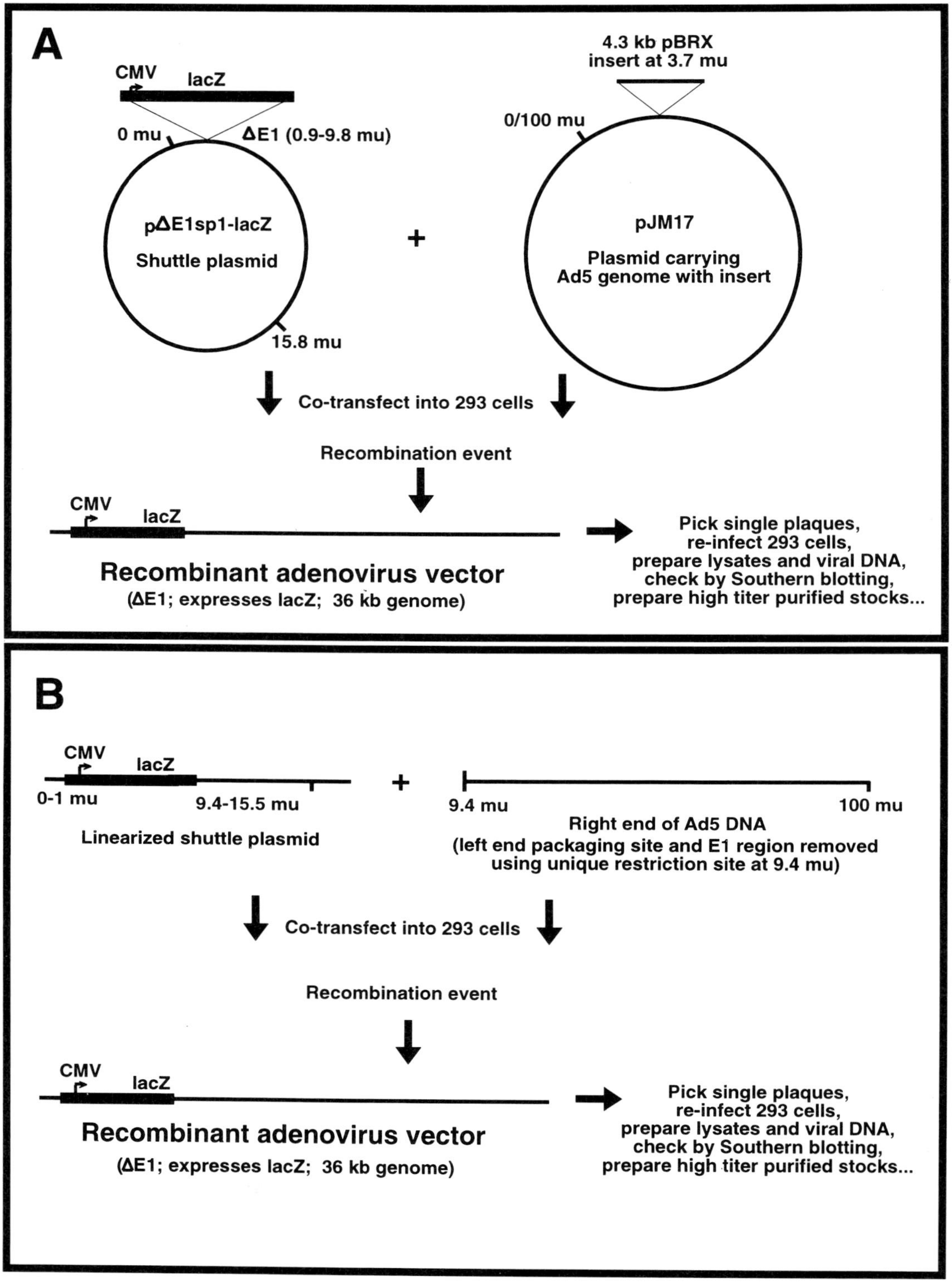

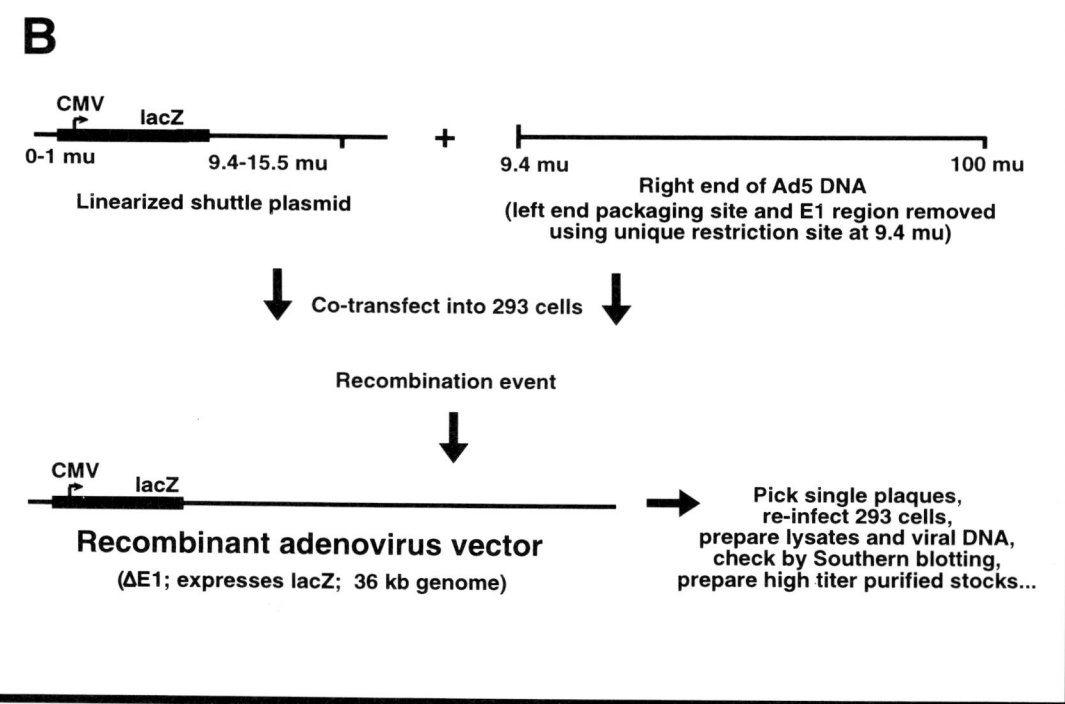

Considering all factors, defective adenovirus vectors still are one of the most promising methods for neuron transfection. More recent improvements in adenovirus vector construction include the generation of adenoviruses defective in both E1 and E4 and a complementing packaging cell line (Yeh et al., 1996). This may reduce further the toxicity of adenovirus vectors. A novel method that is not quite efficient enough for routine use but that seems promising is the production of recombinant adenovirus deleted of all viral genes that are propagated in the presence of an E1-deleted helper virus (Fisher et al., 1996). In some ways, this technique is analogous to the HSV amplicon method, except that the vector does not have a growth advantage over the helper, although they physically can be separated at least partially. One would think that direct cloning might offer the easiest method of all. The adenovirus genome is only 36 kb, much smaller than the other recombinant viral vectors described in this chapter. By use of 8-bp restriction enzyme recognition sites, it should be possible to design a vector for direct cloning in *E. coli* that would also lack E1, E3, E4, and possibly other viral genes and that could be propagated in a complementing cell line.

Adeno-Associated Virus

Adeno-associated viruses (AAVs) have a number of advantages as potential gene therapy agents: they are nonpathogenic, they require

Figure 4.8   Methods for production of recombinant adenovirus vectors. The two commonly used methods for producing recombinant adenovirus vectors involve cotransfection and selection for in vivo recombination between a shuttle plasmid and a partial or oversized Ad5 genome. The vectors are defective, owing to a deletion in the E1 region and thus are propagated in the 293 cell line, which expresses the E1 gene products. (*A*) The shuttle plasmid contains the expression cassette (in this case, CMV-lacZ) inserted in the deleted E1 region and contains flanking viral DNA on both sides. It is cotransfected with pJM17, which contains a full Ad5 genome but with an insert in the E1 region so that it is too large to be packaged. Recombination leads to replacement of the large pBRX insert and complete E1 region with the smaller expression cassette and deleted E1 region. (*B*) Alternatively, the right end of the Ad5 genome can be used instead of pJM17 as a substrate for the in vivo recombination. This viral DNA, obtained by cleavage at a unique restriction site, cannot be packaged because it lacks the left end packaging site. This is restored by recombination with a linearized shuttle plasmid that contains the left end packaging site followed by the expression cassette replacing the E1 region and then flanking viral DNA. With both methods, the resulant viral stocks are plaque-purified and tested by viral DNA isolation and Southern blotting for the presence of the gene of interest.

a helper virus for replication and can be separated physically from that helper virus, and they have the potential for site-specific integration (Muzyczka, 1992; Kaplitt et al., 1994b; Zolotukhin et al., 1996). Thus, they are the least toxic of viral vectors. The method of construction involves cotransfection of a plasmid containing *cis*-acting replication sequences and the expression cassette with a nonpackaging complementing AAV plasmid and then superinfection with a helper adenovirus. The resultant AAV vectors (which do not require recombination for production) then can be separated from helper adenovirus on CsCl gradients or by heat inactivation. However, their limitations make AAV much less than ideal as a choice of vector for transfection of neuron cultures at present. They have a maximal insert size of 4.7 kb and, more seriously, are finicky to propagate, yield very low titers (on the order of 10^4/ml) and, thus, do not yield high efficiency transfection readily. However, improvements in packaging efficiency already are being reported (Tamayose et al., 1996).

Recombinant Vaccinia Virus

Vaccinia virus vectors are generated by homologous recombination between a plasmid and a virus in a cell line, as for the other recombinant viral vectors. Insertion of the expression cassette usually is engineered into the nonessential viral thymidine kinase gene to allow for selection of recombinants (Weisz and Machamer, 1994). Vaccinia virus vectors can be slightly more difficult to construct because they undergo a cytoplasmic replication cycle and use viral rather than cellular transcriptional control signals. Two consequences are that inserts cannot accomodate introns and that the sequence TTTTTNT is recognized as a transcription termination signal and must be removed by silent mutagenesis from any gene of interest prior to expression. The other main difference from other viral systems is that these vaccinia vectors are not defective. These viruses are cytopathic to most mammalian cells by 6 to 8 h after infection, exhibited by cell rounding and inhibition of host protein synthesis.

Nonetheless, rat neurons in hippocampal slices have been transfected with vaccinia virus vectors, resulting in foreign protein expression at 6 to 16 h postinfection, with no detrimental effect on synaptic transmission or LTP, at least at the earlier times of expression (Ozaki et al., 1993; Pettit et al., 1995). Only postnatal, not

adult, slices could be transfected. Expression of active CaMKII resulted in potentiated transmission and prevention of further LTP in the hippocampal slices (Pettit et al., 1994). Although vaccinia vectors may not be ideal for dissociated cultures owing to their complicated transcriptional control and toxicity, they do have the advantage of extremely high-efficiency transfection of neurons in slice cultures. Their effectiveness is not limited to rat neurons. Vaccinia viruses also have been useful for transfecting frog neurons where, perhaps owing to the lower temperature, expression occurred over a much slower timecourse of 1.5 to 6 days (Wu et al., 1995).

Semliki Forest Virus

SFV is an RNA-based virus that encodes its own enzyme for cytoplasmic replication. The SFV expression vector system involves cotransfection of two types of in vitro transcribed RNA: one containing RNA replication and packaging signals and the gene of interest under control of an SFV transcription initiation site, and the other a helper RNA that encodes viral structural proteins but lacks replication and packaging signals (Liljestrom and Garoff, 1991; Olkkonen et al., 1994). The products of this cotransfection are SFV particles containing only the expression cassette RNA and flanking sequences. However, although these vectors are defective in the sense that they cannot produce new virus, they still are toxic to cells within approximately 8 h because they shut off host protein synthesis. In spite of the narrow window of expression (at approximately 5–8 h), SFV vectors have been used extensively by the Dotti laboratory to study intracellular protein trafficking in cultured hippocampal neurons (Ikonen et al., 1993; de Hoop et al., 1994; Simons et al., 1995). These studies included the first report of transcytosis in neurons and expression of a dominant-negative Rab5a with subsequent disruption of endocytosis.

Promoters

A large number of promoters have been used successfully for expression in neurons. The most popular have been strong constitutive viral promoters: cytomegalovirus (CMV) immediate-early promoter, Rous sarcoma virus LTR, Moloney murine leukemia virus LTR, SV40 early promoter, and the HSV1 IE3, IE4/5, and gC

promoters. The CMV promoter is a good first choice for high-level expression in most neurons. Cellular promoters that have been used include globin, β-actin, elongation factor 1α, and phosphoglycerate kinase. The level of expression from many promoters, including the most commonly used viral promoters such as the CMV and SV40 early promoters and the Rous sarcoma virus LTR, generally can be increased many-fold by exposure to 1 to 10 mM sodium butyrate (Gorman and Howard, 1983; Tanaka et al., 1991).

Of particular interest are the potentially neuron-specific promoters for neuron-specific enolase, neurofilament, and sodium channel. However, expression from any promoter can be affected by its insertion site in the recombinant viral vectors and, for example, expression from a neuron-specific enolase promoter in a recombinant HSV vector was not neuron-specific (Johnson and Friedmann, 1994). Preliminary studies with HSV amplicon-based vectors have also found that these three promoters are not neuron-specific. A greater degree of specificity has been found with tyrosine hydroxylase and preproenkephalin promoters (C. Fraefel, personal communication; Kaplitt et al., 1994a). Also of particular interest are the inducible promoters. The metallothionein promoter in an HSV vector gave only a two-fold induction by zinc in superior cervical ganglion neurons (Buckmaster and Tolkovsky, 1994). An HSV amplicon-based vector with a glucocorticoid-inducible promoter gave up to 50-fold induction in hepatocytes (Lu and Federoff, 1995), but its efficacy in neurons was not reported. Ho et al. (1996) obtained an impressive 50-fold controlled range of gene expression in neurons using the tetracycline-responsive promoter system. In this system, tetracycline is used to maintain repression and is removed for induction (derepression) of gene expression. This system requires the incorporation of a tet operator in the promoter controlling the gene of interest and expression of a tet transactivator from another promoter; still, it is the most promising of the inducible promoter systems.

Expression of multiple genes in a single neuron from viral vectors can be achieved in a few ways. Transfection with mixed viral stocks will yield some neurons expressing both products and some expressing only one or the other; the number of doubly expressing cells actually appears to be higher than that expected by chance. Two expression cassettes can be packaged into a single vector. Although this technique also can lead to unequal expression, usually it is very effective (Lawrence et al., 1996). Another interesting way

around this problem is through the use of an internal ribosome entry site to induce translation initiation of a second gene product on a single mRNA (Dirks et al., 1993). This method has been used, for example, to add humanized GFP as a coexpressed marker in AAV vectors (Zolotukhin et al., 1996).

Concluding Remarks

The notorius difficulty in transfecting neurons has held back the field of neuronal cell and molecular biology for some time. However, progress has been extremely rapid over the last 5 years, and it seems likely that some enterprising young company soon will be marketing a safe, fast, and user-friendly viral packaging method for constructing high-efficiency vectors for neuron transfection. Some of the novel defective HSV amplicon or adenovirus vectors now are approaching this stage.

Acknowledgments

I am very grateful to Henryk Dudek and Michael E. Greenberg (Harvard University), and Jason Chang, Laura Greenlund, and Eugene M. Johnson (Washington University) for much advice concerning calcium phosphate mediated transfection and HSV amplicon-based vectors, respectively. I also wish to thank members of the lab, particularly Daniel W. Allison, F. Thomas Crump, and Julia N. Stowell, for their contributions.

Work in the author's laboratory was supported by National Institutes of Health Grant NS33184, the Lucille P. Markey Charitable Trust, and the Pew Charitable Trust.

5 Characterizing and Studying Neuronal Cultures

Ginger S. Withers and Gary Banker

We should say at the outset that we seriously considered not including this chapter at all. There were many reasons why we hesitated. First, because almost every method used by neurobiologists has been applied to characterizing cells in culture, it would be an overwhelming task to attempt to describe each one. Moreover, the relevancy of these methods depends, to a great extent, on the particular cell type chosen for study and the specific problems being addressed, and only a few are likely to be of interest to any one reader. And our experience with many of these techniques is quite limited. Most important, it would have been one less chapter to write.

As you see, we have gone ahead with it anyway. With regard to the first part of the chapter, which concerns characterizing neuronal cultures, specific approaches may differ, but the general issues that must be addressed are similar: What cell types are present, how can they be recognized, and how accurately do the cell populations present in culture represent those in situ? Moreover, some of the methods used to answer these questions, such as immunostaining to localize cell-specific markers, are used so widely that we hardly could avoid discussing them. The second half of the chapter, which concerns some of the practical details of studying neurons in culture, focuses almost exclusively on microscopic methods. This is not because we believe that this is the only approach for studying cells in culture. Rather, this approach is what we know best, and most labs will, on occasion, find some need to use this approach. Nevertheless, we do not claim to be experts, and we have made no attempt to treat these topics exhaustively. Instead, we have emphasized aspects of these methods that are specifically relevant to cells grown in culture, including some "tricks of the trade" that we have acquired through years of experience and mistakes. The protocols provided are not intended to be definitive—they simply illustrate the standard approach used in our lab. As they have worked reliably for us, they may offer a reasonable starting point for others.

Bookkeeping

An important, sometimes overlooked, approach for characterizing neuronal cultures involves nothing more than bookkeeping:
determining the yield of cells obtained after dissociation and
quantifying cell attachment and survival over time in culture.
These data are simple to collect, and can reassure you that your
cultures are on the right track or alert you to serious defects in
culture technique.

The yield of cells obtained after dissociation, and the proportion
of these cells that are viable, can be determined readily by counting
in a hemacytometer, as described in chapter 3. To interpret these
counts, the number of cells present in the tissue before dissociation
must be known. Counts of neuronal number have been performed
for most regions of the nervous system, at least in rats and mice.
Usually, such counts are performed in adult animals, where the
histological identification of neurons is most certain, so it may be
necessary to adjust the expected yield, either because the tissue
was obtained before neurogenesis is complete or because a period
of naturally occurring cell death occurs at a stage after the cultures are prepared. Nevertheless, it should be possible to confirm
that the yield of cells is consistent with that expected, at least to
within a factor of two or so.

The number of cells that attach and that survive can be assessed
in a similar fashion, by counting the cells in randomly selected
regions of the culture, using a grid inserted into the microscope
eyepiece to define the dimensions of the area counted and extra-
polating this measurement to the total surface area of the culture.
The area of the grid can be determined from the magnification
(being careful to include factors due to intermediate lenses between
objective and ocular) or by using a stage micrometer, a slide
embossed with a line ruled in hundredths and tenths of a millimeter (available from most microscope suppliers).

Usually, cell attachment is complete within a few hours of
plating (perhaps longer when collagen is used as the substrate), and
can be assessed by tapping the microscope stage (attached cells
don't move) or by rinsing away unattached cells. The majority of
viable cells should attach; if not, the dissociation procedure may
have left them unhealthy (though viable by conventional assays),
or the substrate or serum may be unsatisfactory. Once attached,
the number of surviving neurons should remain constant for an
extended period, with loss of (at most) a small percentage of the

cells per week. This slow attrition is not of serious concern if the remainder of the cells are healthy. At some point, when the culture's time has come, cell loss of a different sort begins. Neurons throughout the entire culture begin to degenerate, usually with a fairly rapid time course, and this process continues until only nonneuronal cells remain. Often, this process will have a patchy distribution at first, then will involve the entire culture. Thus, in monitoring neuronal survival, sampling from many regions of the culture is important. Early signs of degeneration, such as cell body swelling and beading of processes, often can be recognized before overt cell death.

Whenever significant cell loss occurs, during dissociation, plating, or culturing, it raises the concern that the loss will affect some classes of cells preferentially, skewing the population available for study in culture. From the data presently available, it is not known how common differential cell loss is, but it certainly can occur. For example, interneurons seldom survive in cultures of sympathetic ganglia (see chapter 11), whereas in some cultures of hippocampal neurons, they represent a disproportionately large fraction of the neurons (Hoch and Dingledine, 1986). Obviously, the more homogeneous the starting cell population and the fewer the cells lost, the less one must be concerned. However, in most cases, unless the extent of differential cell loss can be assessed directly, its effect on experimental observations must be considered.

Telling Neurons from Glia

One of the most important steps in getting to know your cultures is learning to identify the different cell types that are present, particularly to distinguish neurons from glial cells. This is not always as simple as it may seem. Admittedly, the morphology of mature neurons in culture usually is quite distinctive. As in situ, they have a large, clear nucleus with a prominent nucleolus. And of course, the ability to extend long processes is one of the distinctive characteristics of nerve cells. Moreover, independent of their length, neuronal processes tend to have a recognizable contour: Axons usually are quite constant in diameter, dendrites taper continuously with distance from the cell body, and both are distinctly cylindrical in shape. But early in development—when their somata are small and their processes short—neurons are more difficult to identify positively. The morphology of glial cells is much more variable (see

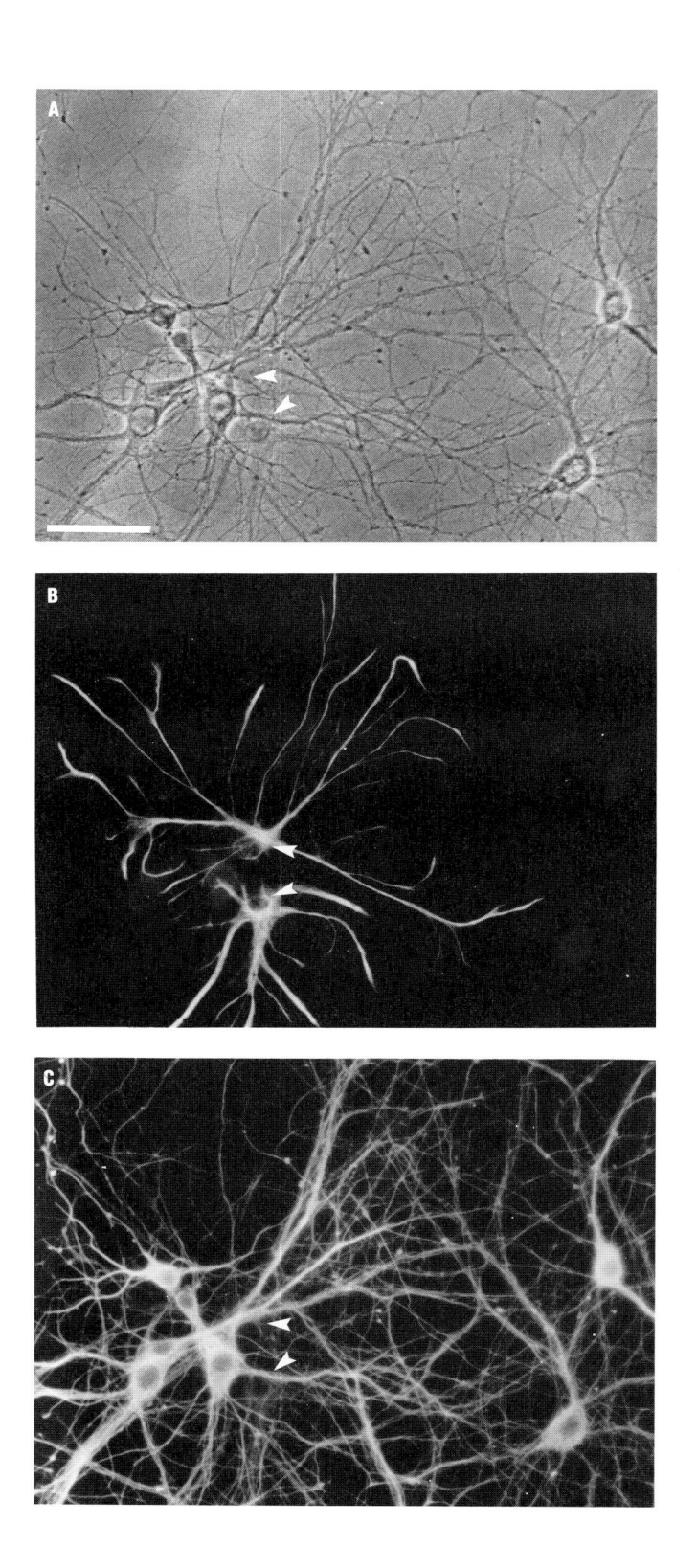

chapter 18). In some cases, they are flattened and polygonal, much like epithelial cells in culture. In other cases, they may give rise to many, highly branched, radially symmetrical processes or to one or two processes that can be quite long. High cell density makes it that much more difficult to identify individual cells, as the length of their processes may be obscured. And glial cells are easy to overlook when they lie within a dense network.

For all these reasons, the development of immunostaining methods for identification of neurons and glial cells has been of exceptional value (figure 5.1). Neuron- and glia–specific markers offer an independent means to confirm a cell's identity. Of course, physiological recordings or electron microscopy can be used as well, but both of these approaches must be applied on a cell-by-cell basis and can be remarkably tedious. The most commonly used markers for identifying cell types in cultures from the central nervous system (CNS) are outlined in table 5.1 (Fields, 1979, 1985; Raff et al., 1979; Loffner et al., 1986).

Ideally, a cell type–specific marker should be expressed in all cells of the class and in no other cells. Moreover, it should be present at high levels so that it can be detected easily, should appear early in development, and should be distributed throughout the cell. It is hardly surprising that no such marker has been identified. Most antigens that have been proposed as neural cell–type–specific markers have turned up in unexpected places: A2B5 in islet cells, class III β-tubulin in various tumors. Several proteins used as neuronal markers—proteins such as GAP-43, microtubule-associated proteins, and ion channels that once were thought to have uniquely neuronal functions—since have been identified in certain types of glial cells, where they undoubtedly have equally important functions (Vitkovic, 1992). A second problem is developmental. Some proteins that are excellent markers of mature cells are not expressed at the early stages when cells are taken for culture; to complicate things further, this restriction may vary from one type of neuron to another. For example, antineurofilament antibodies usually give excellent staining in early cultures of spinal cord and

Figure 5.1 Identification of neurons and astroglia in a culture of rat hippocampal neurons. (*A*) Phase-contrast microscopy reveals all cells and their processes. (*B*) Astroglia are stained with antibodies against glial fibrillary acidic protein. (*C*) Antibodies against class III β-tubulin reveal neurons and their processes. Cultures were maintained for 2 weeks without addition of antimitotic agents. Arrowheads indicate the location of glial nuclei. Scale bar: 50 μm.

Table 5.1   Selected Markers for Distinguishing Cell Types in Central Nervous System Cultures

MARKER	CELL TYPE	LOCALIZATION
Class III β-tubulin	Neurons	Cytoskeletal protein (neuron-specific isoform of β-tubulin)
Neurofilament proteins	Neurons	Cytoskeletal protein (68, 105, 135-kD type IV intermed. fil. subunits)
Neuron-specific enolase	Neurons	Cytoplasmic protein (gamma-gamma isoform of glycolytic enzyme)
Tetanus toxin receptor	Neurons, O-2A progenitors, and type II astrocytes	Cell-surface gangliosides
A2B5 (monoclonal antibody)	Neurons, O-2A progenitors, and type II astrocytes	Cell-surface gangliosides
Glial fibrillary acidic protein	Astrocytes (both type I and type II)	Cytoskeletal protein (51-kD type III intermediate filament subunit)
Galactose cerebroside	Oligodendrocytes	Cell-surface glycolipid
Vimentin	Astrocytes and fibroblasts	Cytoskeletal protein (53-kD type III intermediate filament subunit)
OX42 (monoclonal antibody)	Microglia (macrophages)	Cell-surface protein (complement type 3 receptor)
PGP9.5	Neurons	Cytoplasmic protein (ubiqutin carboxyl-terminal hydrolase)
O4	Oligodendrocytes and their precursors	Sulfatide (and perhaps another determinant)

peripheral ganglia but work less well in cultures from other regions of the CNS. Conversely, neurons express the nonneuronal form of enolase early in development (Marangos and Schmechel, 1987), and both immature neurons and astrocytes express vimentin, a fibroblast intermediate filament protein, before expressing neurofilament subunits or glial fibrillary acidic protein (GFAP). All this is simply to say that caution and common sense are necessary in using markers to analyze the cell types present in culture. Whenever possible, use two or three different markers to be certain that a consistent pattern emerges. Double-staining also can be used to verify that two different neuronal markers stain identical cell populations or to confirm that cells that fail to express one marker do stain with another.

For staining fixed cultures, antibodies against cytoskeletal proteins are particularly useful because they are expressed in large amounts and often are distributed throughout the cell. One isotype of tubulin, class III beta-tubulin, is expressed by neurons and by some tumor cells but not by glial or most other nonneuronal cells (Sullivan et al., 1986; Burgoyne et al., 1988; Lee et al., 1990). Because this isotype is expressed shortly after terminal mitosis and extends throughout the neurites, antibodies that selectively recognize it have proved to be extremely useful for identifying neurons in culture (figure 5.1). Antibodies against neurofilaments are another commonly used neuronal marker. Certain microtubule-associated proteins also can be useful markers, with the previously discussed caveats.

Some applications require markers that can be visualized in living cells. Polypeptide toxins, such as tetanus or cholera toxin (Dimpfel et al., 1977; Mirsky et al., 1978), or monoclonal antibodies (Eisenbarth et al., 1979) commonly are used to label living neurons. Fluorescently labeled toxin fragments that bind to the cell surface but lack the components that mediate toxicity are commercially available. And of course, the usual caveats about testing their specificity apply.

In characterizing neuronal cultures, usually it is desirable to identify the population of nonneuronal cells present, using appropriate markers. The most common nonneuronal "contaminants" in cultures prepared from the CNS are astrocytes and fibroblasts. Astrocytes (both type 1 and type 2) can be identified by their content of GFAP. Fibroblasts and meningeal cells probably are identified best by the presence of vimentin and the absence of glial or

neuronal markers. Fibronectin, which is secreted but retained on the cell surface, also can be used to identify these cells. Astrocytes secrete a form of fibronectin that does not bind to the cell surface, so they appear fibronectin-negative on immunostaining (Price and Hynes, 1985). Oligodendrocytes most frequently are distinguished by using antibodies against galactose cerebroside, a cell-surface glycolipid. Microglia, the macrophages of the CNS, express receptors for immunoglobulins and complement. If glial cells rather than neurons are the cells of interest, many additional markers are available for their rigorous characterization. They are discussed in chapters 18 and 19.

Domain-Specific Markers

Dissociated cell cultures can be very useful for studying the subcellular localization of neuronal proteins. For this purpose, it can be helpful to compare the localization of the antigen in question with that of known markers that selectively label axons or dendrites, presynaptic terminals or postsynaptic specializations. In using this approach, the usual caution applies: In every case, there are instances where these markers do not exhibit the expected distribution.

Probably the most widely used dendritic marker is microtubule-associated protein 2 (MAP2), which is present in the somata and dendrites of most neurons but virtually absent from most axons. Antibodies against MAP2 have been used effectively to identify dendrites in cultures from many regions of the nervous system (Caceres et al., 1984; Matus et al., 1986; Higgins et al., 1988). When visualized by use of peroxidase immunocytochemistry, the morphological detail rivals that in a Golgi preparation, so that MAP2 staining can be used to quantify dendritic development and to investigate factors that influence dendritic morphology (Banker and Waxman, 1988; Lein and Higgins, 1989; Withers et al., 1995). Other markers for dendrites are discussed by Craig and Banker (1994).

None of the markers for axons is as broadly applicable as is MAP2. Antibodies against the microtubule-associated protein tau, especially the antibody called tau-1, which recognizes a specific dephosphoepitope, often are used to stain axons (for references, see Mandell and Banker, 1996). Certain phosphorylated forms of MAP1b also are distributed preferentially in axons (Gordon-Weeks

et al., 1993; Ulloa et al., 1994; Boyne et al., 1995). Antibodies against the phosphorylated form of the high-molecular-weight neurofilament subunits selectively label the axons of cultured sympathetic neurons, whereas unphosphorylated forms of these proteins are confined largely to cell bodies and dendrites (Higgins et al., 1991). In the case of hippocampal cultures, with which we have direct experience, useful axonal markers include the cell adhesion molecule L-1, the membrane-associated protein GAP-43, and tau, but all have limitations as well (see chapter 13). Immunostaining methods for identifying growth cones in neuronal cultures also have been described (Devoto and Barnstable, 1989; Goslin et al., 1989; figure 5.2).

In a similar manner, antibodies against synaptic vesicle proteins can be used to identify sites of vesicle aggregation. In some cases (e.g., in cultures of hippocampal neurons), concentrations of synaptic vesicles are restricted largely to presynaptic specializations, so that immunolocalization affords a light microscopic means to identify synapses (Bekkers and Stevens, 1989; Fletcher et al., 1991, 1994). In other situations, such as in cultures of cerebellar granule cells or sympathetic neurons, synaptic vesicle antigens appear to be much more broadly distributed throughout the axonal network (Higgins et al., 1991; T. Fletcher and G. Banker, unpublished observation). Postsynaptic sites can be identifed by the clustering of neurotransmitter receptors (Craig et al., 1993, 1994a,b; Eshhar et al., 1993; figure 5.3 and color plate 3) or of other postsynaptic proteins (Kornau et al., 1995; Apperson et al., 1996; Craig et al., 1996). Antibodies against glutamate receptors also can be used to visualize dendritic spines (Craig et al., 1993).

Identifying Specific Types of Neurons in Culture

Once cells are dissociated, most of the anatomical cues that allow one to identify specific populations of neurons in situ are lost. Some fundamental characteristics of cell shape are maintained in culture—including cell body size and rudimentary aspects of dendritic morphology but these features often are too variable to serve as reliable criteria for distinguishing one type of neuron from another. Thus, the development of independent methods that allow individual cell types to be identified is of key importance for the study of dissociated neuronal cultures. The region of the nervous system from which cultures are taken, and the particular features of

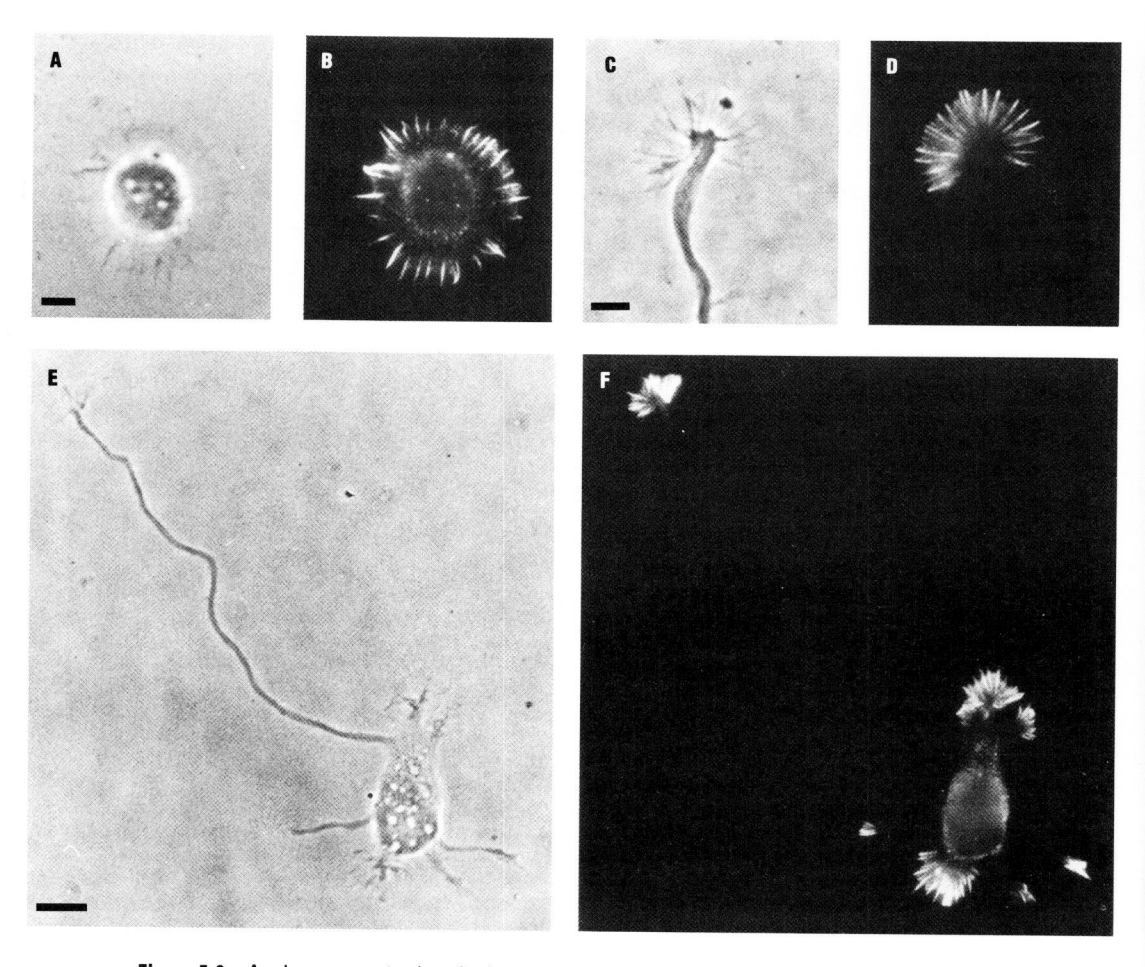

Figure 5.2 An immunocytochemical marker for growth cones. A monoclonal antibody, 13H9, preferentially labels lamellipodia and growth cones of cultured hippocampal neurons (Goslin et al., 1989). The antibody, prepared by Birgbauer and Solomon (1989), labels an isotype of ezrin, a protein that appears to interact with both actin and microtubules. Scale bars: *A* and *C*, 5 μm; *E*, 10 μm. (Reproduced with permission from Birgbauer and Solomon, *J. Cell Biol.* 1989, 109: 1609–1620. Copyright 1989 the Rockefeller University Press.)

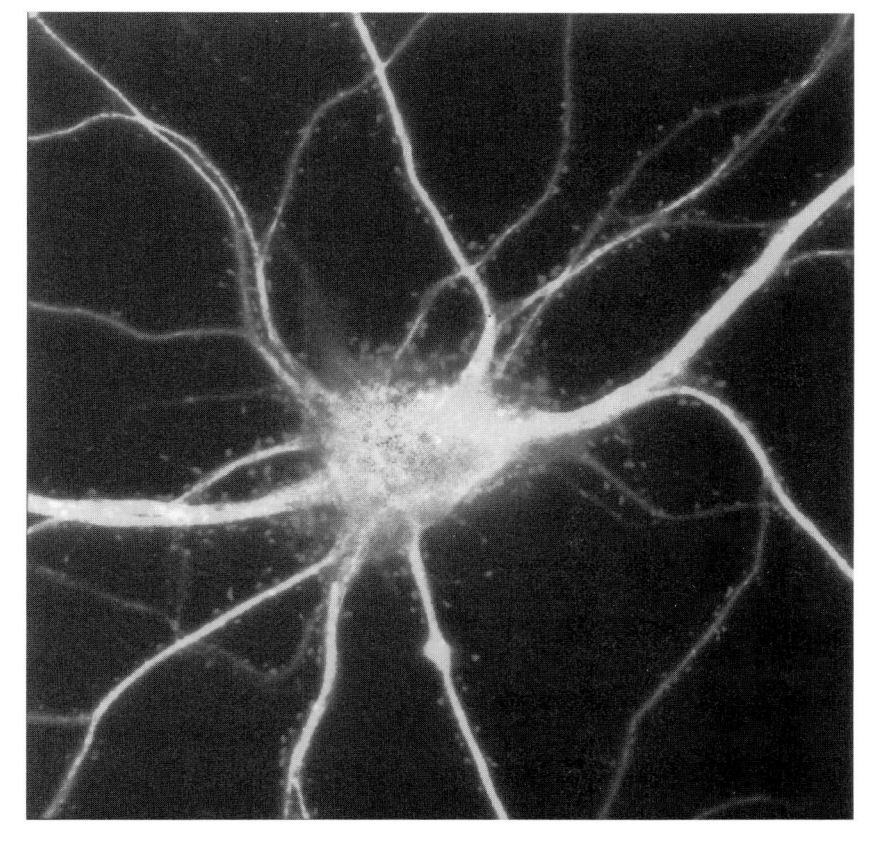

Figure 5.3 Double-label immunofluorescence microscopy shows the clustering of the AMPA-type glutamate receptor subunit GluR1 on dendritic spines of a cultured hippocampal neuron. Neurons were fixed at 3 weeks in culture and stained for the dendritic protein MAP2 (red) and for GluR1 (green). GluR1 is segregated to the somatodendritic domain and is concentrated in dendritic spines. (Courtesy of A. Rao, A. Gelfand, and A. M. Craig, University of Illinois.) See plate 3 for color version.

the cell types it contains, dictate the particulars of the approaches that can be taken. Nevertheless, some generalities do apply.

Because the transmitter phenotype of neurons in many regions of the nervous system is known, one common approach is to identify cell types in culture on the basis of their neurotransmitters. This can be done by using physiological methods, but often it is more convenient to immunostain cultures with antibodies directed against the neurotransmitter itself or against its biosynthetic enzymes. For example, spinal motorneurons have been identified by their content of choline acetyltransferase (Martinou et al., 1989), inhibitory interneurons by their content of GABA or of glutamic acid decarboxylase (Neale et al., 1983; Hoch and Dingledine, 1986; Benson et al., 1994), and dopaminergic neurons by their content of tyrosine hydroxylase (Won et al., 1989). Neurons that contain particular peptides can be identified in a similar fashion (Huettner and Baughman, 1986). Similarly, neurons with high-affinity uptake systems for specific transmitters can be localized in dissociated cell cultures, either by incubation with radiolabeled transmitter followed by autoradiography (White et al., 1980; Neale et al., 1983; Denis-Donini et al., 1984) or by immunostaining with antibodies against the appropriate neurotransmitter transporter (Johnson, 1994).

Virtually any immunogen that is restricted to a specific cell type in a given brain region may be used to identify such cells in culture, but some classes of proteins have proved particularly valuable for this purpose. They include calcium-binding proteins, cell adhesion molecules, and neurotrophin receptors. For example, spinal motoneurons can be identified by immunostaining with antibodies against SC1, a cell adhesion molecule, islet 1, a homeobox domain protein, and the p75 nerve growth factor (NGF) receptor (Mettling et al., 1995). Antibodies against Thy-1, a member of the immunoglobulin superfamily, selectively mark ganglion cells in the retina (Barres et al., 1988b; Taschenberger and Grantyn, 1995). Cerebellar Purkinje cells can be recognized by their content of the cyclic guanosine monophosphate–dependent protein kinase, the calcium-binding protein calbindin, and a peptide antigen termed PEP-19 (Hockberger et al., 1989). Although the reasons for these proteins' restriction to Purkinje cells are not understood completely, all these proteins have proved to be useful markers for confirming the identity of Purkinje cells in culture (figure 5.4).

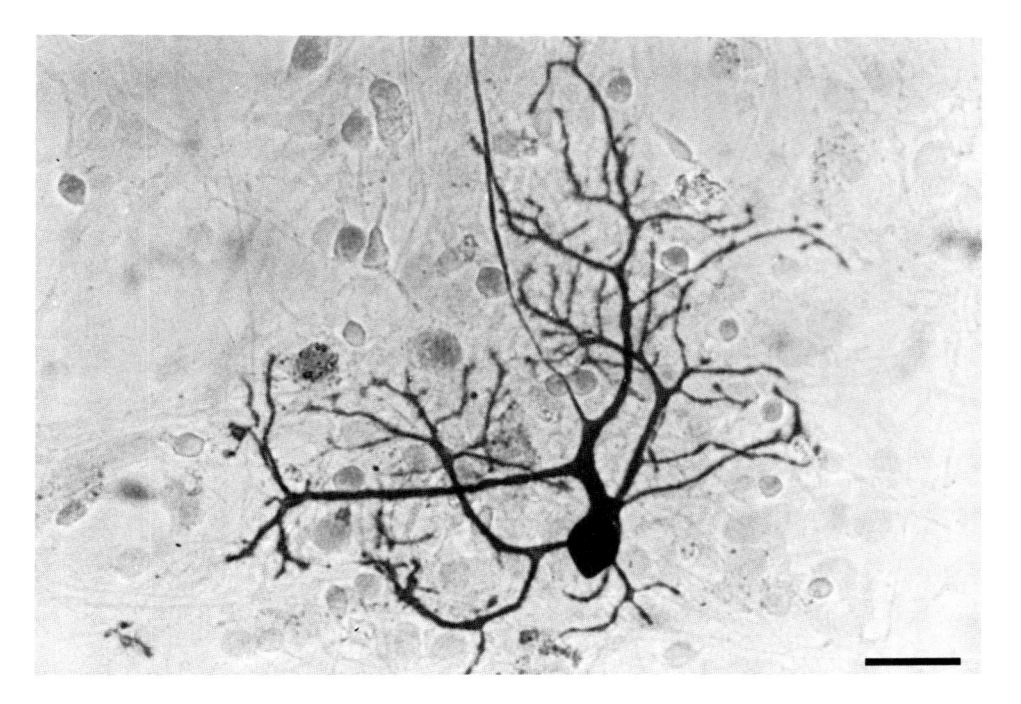

Figure 5.4 Identification of a cultured Purkinje cell using antibodies directed against polypetide PEP-19, a specific marker (see Hockberger et al., 1989). This cell's dendrites bear the unmistakable features of Purkinje cells in situ. Its axon, which passes out of the field at the top of the picture, could be followed for several hundred micrometers. Cultures were prepared from the cerebella of embryonic rats at E16 and maintained for 34 days. Scale bar: 40 μm. (Courtesy of Drs. Karl Schilling and John Connors.)

A very different approach for recognizing specific cell types in culture is based on the use of retrograde tracer techniques, originally developed for investigating the connectivity of cells in situ. When labeled tracer is injected into the vicinity of a cell's terminals, it is taken up and transported retrograde to the cell body, allowing that specific class of projection neurons to be identified. The label is retained after dissociation, so that labeled cells subsequently can be identified in culture. This approach initially was used to identify cells with peripheral targets, such as somatic and autonomic motoneurons (Okun, 1981; Honig and Hume, 1986; O'Brien and Fischbach, 1986a; Martinou et al., 1992; Tuttle and Steers, 1992) and specific populations of sensory neurons (Honig and Kueter, 1995; Honig and Zou, 1995). Subsequently, it has been applied to intrinsic neurons of the CNS, including cortical, hippocampal, and septal projection neurons (Huettner and Baughman, 1986; Yang et al., 1993; Webb et al., 1995), cells of origin of the

nigrostriatal pathway (Lopez Lozano et al., 1989; Kerr et al., 1994), and retinal ganglion cells (McCaffery et al., 1984; Johnson et al., 1986b). Fluorescent latex microspheres and the carbocyanine dyes diI and diO have proven particularly useful as tracers because they can be detected in cell bodies of neurons even after several weeks in culture. Some cell types appear to be more susceptible to damage from labeling with diI than with other dyes in this family (St. John, 1991). Viruses that drive the expression of green fluorescent protein could be used in a similar fashion, with the added advantage that the label extends throughout the neurites that develop in culture (Moriyoshi et al., 1996)

Microscopy of Neuronal Cultures

Light Microscopy of Fixed Cultures

Cell cultures are ideal for the lazy microscopist, because the cell layer is so thin that sectioning is unnecessary. This also allows rapid penetration of solutions; procedures that may take days when applied to sections can be finished in a few hours in monolayer cultures. Microscopic techniques are most successful and convenient when cells are cultured on glass coverslips or on chamber slides rather than in culture dishes (see chapter 3).

Fixing cultures so that they can be examined and analyzed at a later date or can be maintained as permanent documentation of specific experiments is straightforward. In general, glutaraldehyde gives the best preservation of structure, although fixation in formaldehyde also works well (box 5.1). Cultures may be fixed in buffered fixative solution as for immunostaining or electron microscopy (see following discussion) but, for routine purposes, usually it is satisfactory simply to add sufficient concentrated glutaraldehyde (25–70%) directly to the culture medium to give a final concentration of 1% or 2%. After 15 to 30 min, cultures are rinsed in phosphate-buffered saline (PBS), and are mounted on slides. Phase-contrast and differential interference–contrast microscopy depend on differences in the optical properties of the cultured cells and on their surrounding medium. We have yet to find mounting media that give images quite as good as those obtained from living cells, but several acceptable preparations are available (box 5.2).

Box 5.1 Fixation in Formaldehyde for Light Microscopy

Recipes

PBS
Composition: 140 mM Nacl, 15 mM phosphate buffer, pH 7.3. To prepare 10× stock solution, dissolve NaCl (82 g), sodium phosphate monobasic (NaH$_2$PO$_4$2H$_2$O, 4.3 g), and sodium phosphate dibasic (Na$_2$HPO$_4$, 17.4 g) in a final volume of 1L. Crystals form during storage at 4°C; they can be redissolved by heating. Check pH after dilution to 1× concentration.

FIXATIVE
The fixative consists of 4% formaldehyde (prepared from paraformaldehyde) in PBS containing 4% sucrose. Heat ∼60 ml H$_2$O to 60°C. Working in a fume-hood, add 4 g paraformaldehyde, 1 or 2 drops of 1 N NaOH, and stir or swirl. Within a minute or so, the initially milky mixture will turn clear as the para-formaldehyde is hydrolysed to formaldehyde and dissolves. Then, add 10 ml 10× PBS, 4 g sucrose (or 20 ml of a 20% stock solution), and H$_2$O to 100 ml. Any residual cloudiness can be removed by filtration. Check pH. For critical applications (including electron microscopy), prepare the formaldehye imme-diately before use.

USE
Bring fixative to 37°C and fix cultures for 15–30 min.

Cell cultures also can be stained by the methods traditionally used for neural tissue: Nissl stains to reveal RNA within the cell body, silver stains for processes, even Golgi impregnation (Wolf and Dubois-Dalcq, 1970; Toran-Allerand, 1976). These methods are most useful for staining explant cultures, which resemble tissue sections in their thickness. For dissociated cell cultures, these classical methods have largely been supplanted by immunostaining techniques. For example, peroxidase cytochemistry using anti-bodies against tubulin gives a picture of neuronal processes that is every bit as beautiful as traditional silver stains but is easier and more reliable.

Immunostaining

If you plan to culture nerve cells, immunostaining may well become one of the techniques that you rely on most. The theory and practice of immunofluorescence and immunocytochemistry have been discussed extensively by others (Osborn and Weber,

Box 5.2 Mounting Media

Gurr's Fluoromount (Immiscible with Water)
A proprietary product from Gurr Microscopy Materials, BDH Ltd. Available in the United States from Biomedical Specialties, Santa Monica, CA.

USE

Dehydrate cultures grown on glass coverslips or slides (25%, 50%, 70%, 95%, 100% ethanols, 2 min each; xylene, 5 min). Remove from xylene and, while still wet, attach coverslip to slide with a drop of fluoromount. Hardens overnight.

COMMENTS

Preparations do not deteriorate over time; gives an adequate phase-contrast image. Comparable mountants (Permount, DPX) render the processes of cultured cells nearly invisible by phase contrast. For specimens involving peroxidase localization using the diaminobenzidine reaction and for routine observation by phase-contrast microscopy.

Polyvinyl Alcohol (Aqueous Base)

RECIPE

Add 8 g polyvinyl alcohol (also known as *Gelvatol*, *Mowiol*, or *Elvanol*) to 40 ml 0.2 M TRIS-HCl, pH 8.5. Dissolve by heating to 50°C–60°C with occasional stirring. After cooling, add 20 ml glycerol. For use with fluorescence microscopy, add 1%–2.5% DABCO (1,4 diazoabicyclo[2,2,2]octane) to reduce photobleaching. Centrifuge at 5000 rpm for 15 min and store in aliquots at −20°C.

USE

After thawing, mount coverslip in a drop of mounting medium. Medium hardens within a few hours. To view the specimen immediately, "tack" the coverslip onto the slide with a bit of nail polish. Store the mounted specimens in the dark at 4°C.

COMMENTS

Good phase-contrast image. Our standard mount for immunofluorescence, it is also useful for routine preservation of specimens to be examined by phase contrast. Reported to preserve fluorescence for months to years.

1982; Cuello, 1983; Harris, 1986; Sternberger, 1986; Harlow and Lane, 1988). Typical protocols are presented in box 5.3.

For most purposes, we prefer immunofluorescence localization (where a labeled antibody is visualized directly from its emitted fluorescence) rather than immunocytochemistry (where an antibody coupled to an enzyme is visualized by deposition of a colored reaction product). Fluorescence microscopy readily permits simultaneous identification of two or three antigens, using antibodies labeled with different fluorochromes and, in our experience, gives a more precise localization and a more accurate picture of relative antigen concentration. However, immunocytochemical techniques, such as the peroxidase-antiperoxidase method, also offer advantages: Preparations can be examined indefinitely without concerns about photobleaching, and the method can be adapted easily to electron microscopy.

For immunostaining, the method of fixation matters: Cells must be fixed well enough to immobilize the antigen but not so well that the antigen's ability to react with antibody is impaired. Further, the pattern of staining observed with some antibodies depends on the type of fixation used. For example, the staining with tubulin antibodies has a more filamentous appearance in cells fixed in methanol than in those fixed with formaldehyde. Although we do not know precisely why this is, we interpret such differences as being due to the nature of the fixation process. Because methanol is a coagulative fixative and permeabilizes the cell membrane, soluble proteins may be at least partially extracted from the cytoplasm, whereas those bound to the cytoskeleton may remain. Such cross-linking fixatives as formaldehyde and glutaraldehyde, which convert the cytoplasm into a gel, may better retain soluble proteins that might be extracted during methanol fixation. In practice, it simply is important to determine to what extent the pattern of staining observed depends on the conditions of fixation.

The most commonly used fixative for light microscopic immunostaining of cultured cells is 4% formaldehyde, prepared from paraformaldehyde (see box 5.1). Generally, it is agreed that this fixative should be "freshly prepared," but there is no agreement on what this means. Usually, we store this fixative for a week or so at 4°C but, for critical applications (including electron microscopy), it may be safest to make it immediately before use. We routinely prepare this fixative in PBS containing 4% sucrose, which seems to improve cell preservation (see Luduena, 1973); others use isotonic

Box 5.3 Immunostaining

Fixation and Permeabilization

Fix cultures in 4% formaldehyde, 4% formaldehyde plus 0.25% gluta-raldehyde, or cold methanol.
Rinse in PBS (2×1 min).
Permeabilize with Triton X-100 (0.25% in PBS) for 5–10 minutes, then return to PBS; alternatively, dehydrate in graded ethanols, leave in 100% ethanol for 30 min, and rehydrate to PBS.

Application of Primary Antibody

Block in 10% BSA or 10% serum in PBS for 30 min.
Incubate in primary antibody, diluted in 2–3% BSA or serum in PBS, for 2 h at room temperature or 37°C or overnight at 4°C.
Rinse 3×5 min in PBS.

Detection of Primary Antibody

A. IMMUNOFLUORESCENCE

Incubate in fluorochrome-conjugated antibody directed against immuno-globulins from the species used to prepare the primary antibody. For example, to localize monoclonal antibodies prepared in mice, incubate in fluorescein- or rhodamine-conjugated goat anti-mouse IgG (1:400, Boehringer Mannheim, Indianapolis, IN) for 1 h at 37°C.
Rinse 3×5 min in PBS.
Rinse 1 min in dH_2O.
Mount on slides in polyvinyl alcohol–based mountant.

B. AVIDIN-BIOTIN IMMUNOFLUORESCENCE

Incubate in biotinylated antibody directed against immunoglobulins from the species used to prepare the primary antibody. For example, to detect mono-clonal antibodies prepared in mice, incubate with biotinylated horse anti-mouse IgG (1:700, Vector Laboratories, Burlingame, CA) 1 h at 37°C.
Rinse 3×5 in PBS.
Incubate in either avidin-fluorescein or avidin-rhodamine (Vector Laboratories, 1:700), 1 h at 37°C.
Rinse 3×5 min in PBS.
Rinse 1 min in dH_2O.
Mount on slide in polyvinyl alcohol–based mountant.

C. AVIDIN-BIOTIN IMMUNOPEROXIDASE

Incubate in biotinylated antibody directed against immunoglobulins from the species used to prepare the primary antibody. For example, to detect mono-clonal antibodies prepared in mice, incubate in biotinylated rabbit anti-mouse immunoglobulins diluted in PBS with 3% BSA for 1 h at 37°C.

Box 5.3 (continued)

Rinse 3 × 5 min in PBS.
Incubate in avidin-biotinylated horseradish peroxidase complex (1:50 solution A, 1:50 solution B in PBS with 3% BSA, Vectasatin Elite ABC kit, Vector), 45 min at 37°C.
Rinse 3 × 5 min in PBS.
Prepare reaction mixture consisting of 0.05% diaminobenzidine tetrahydrochloride in 10 mM imidazole-50 mM TRIS-HCl, pH 7.4. Then add 0.03% H_2O_2. Observe the reaction via an inverted microscope. After the desired intensity is reached, usually within 1–2 min, stop the reaction by transfer to PBS.
Dehydrate in graded EtOH to 100%, 2 min per step.
Transfer to xylene for 5 min.
Mount on slides in Gurr's Fluoromount.

or hypertonic buffers, usually phosphate buffer. Cultures fixed in formaldehyde are not completely stable. For example, they remain osmotically active; treatment with hypotonic solutions or simply storage overnight in PBS can result in extensive blebbing of processes, particularly of young cells. The permeabilization step required to allow penetration of antibodies into the cell also eliminates the danger of further osmotic damage, so we permeabilize cells immediately after formaldehyde fixation by treatment with detergent (0.05–0.3% Triton X-100 in PBS) or by dehydration in graded ethanols. Following permeabilization, we sometimes store cultures in PBS at 4°C for a week or more before immunostaining (usually adding 0.01% sodium azide to prevent bacterial growth). However, the advisability of this practice is likely to depend on the antigen to be localized; cross-links formed by formaldehyde are slowly reversible, so that soluble proteins can be lost during storage.

Fixation in formaldehyde alone sometimes is inadequate. Glutaraldehyde consistently gives better preservation but frequently reduces antigenicity, increases autofluorescence, and may increase nonspecific staining because unreacted aldehyde groups nonspecifically cross-link antibodies. Often, the addition of a low concentration of glutaraldehyde (0.1–0.25%) to formaldehyde fixatives improves preservation sufficiently without impairing immunostaining. When glutaraldehyde fixation increases background staining to unacceptable levels, reaction with sodium borohydride (0.5 mg/ml in PBS for 5 min, repeated up to three times) commonly is used to quench unreacted aldehydes (Osborn and Weber, 1982).

Another common fixation method that simultaneously permeabilizes cells uses either methanol or acetone. This is simple, quick, and often gives surprisingly good results, especially for immunolocalization of cytoskeletal antigens. Cultures first are rinsed in PBS (to prevent precipitation of proteins from the culture medium), then are immersed for 5 to 10 min in either reagent, usually at $-20°C$.

A common problem with chemical fixatives is that they act relatively slowly (Heuser et al., 1979), allowing time for proteins to move from their natural distribution and associate artifactually with other structures (Smith and Reese, 1980; Landis et al., 1987; Tatsuoka and Reese, 1989). Rapid freezing is an alternative method that can overcome many of these problems. In many ways, monolayer cultures are ideally suited to this approach. Ice-crystal demage, the principal limitation to the rapid-freezing approach, is a significant problem only at tissue depths of more than 10 to 15 µm below the surface, thicker than the average monolayer. This method yields excellent preservation and, when combined with freeze substitution, is suitable for both light and electron microscopic immunocytochemistry (Landis and Reese, 1981; Rees and Reese, 1981; Bridgman and Reese, 1984; Bridgman et al., 1986; Moreira et al., 1996). Though rapid freezing usually is done with a slam-freezing device—not something every laboratory would have—cells grown on coverslips can be fixed by immersion in a mixture of isopentane and butane with quite satisfactory results (Robards and Sletyr, 1985).

Aside from fixation, the most important variable in an immunostaining protocol is the concentration of the primary antibody. In working with a new antibody, appropriate concentrations must be established empirically. Usually, there is a fairly broad range of acceptable concentrations but, obviously, concentrations that are too high lead to nonspecific staining, and those that are too low reduce specific staining. Controls are needed to assess nonspecific staining (see Osborn and Weber, 1982; Harlow and Lane, 1988). If a polyclonal antiserum is being used, preimmune serum or normal serum from the same species gives a reasonable estimate of the nonspecific staining. For monoclonal antibodies, it is common to omit the primary antibody from control samples. This control is worthwhile but tends to underestimate the background because it measures only the contribution due to nonspecific binding of the

secondary antibody. It does not take into account nonspecific binding of the primary antibody, which will be detected and amplified by the secondary antibody. For antibodies generated against a synthetic peptide, the optimal control for specificity is to use an excess of the peptide to compete against binding sites in the tissue. The antibody is diluted in blocking buffer, and a 10-fold excess concentration of the peptide is added and left overnight at 4°C or for several hours at room temperature. This solution then is used in place of the primary antibody. Finally, if specific cell types in the culture lack the antigen, they can serve as internal controls for nonspecific binding.

To reduce nonspecific binding, antibody solutions always should be prepared in buffers that contain additional protein, either normal serum or albumin. Also, it is important to centrifuge antibody solutions to remove any precipitates that may have formed during storage (we centrifuge at 10,000 rpm for 10 min in a microfuge). Fine precipitates, either in the primary antibody solution or in labeled antibodies, adhere tenaciously to the surfaces of cultured cells, producing a generalized staining that obscures any specific signal. To conserve reagents, we place coverslips face up on a strip of dental wax (available from suppliers of products for electron microscopy), whose extreme hydrophobicity ensures that the antibody solution does not run off the coverslip, and apply only a small volume of antibody solution (50–100 μl for an 18-mm coverslip). Others place a drop of antibody on a hydrophobic surface such as parafilm and invert coverslips onto it. During staining, the coverslips are placed in a "humidified chamber," a large Petri dish containing moistened filter paper, which minimizes evaporation of the antibody.

Commonly used protocols apply primary antibodies for times ranging from 30 min to 2 h at room temperature or 37°C to overnight or longer at 4°C. Short incubations have obvious advantages. Sometimes, overnight incubations are convenient to schedule and may allow use of lower antibody concentrations; in principle, long incubations increase the probability that both antibody-combining sites bind to the antigen, greatly reducing the chance of dissociation (Sternberger, 1986). Rinse volumes and times must be adequate not only to remove antibody by dilution but also to allow unbound antibody within the cytoplasm and nuclear matrix to diffuse back out into the rinse solutions. We do three, 5-min rinses in a large volume of PBS, but others simply aspirate the antibody solution

and apply PBS directly to the coverslip ($\sim 200\,\mu$l PBS for an 18-mm coverslip) for 2 min, repeating this process six times.

For most purposes, acceptable immunostaining can be obtained by using fluorochrome-labeled secondary antibodies directed against immunoglobulins from the species used to prepare the primary antibody. If greater signal amplification is needed, avidin-biotin techniques or other multistep procedures are available. After staining, coverslips are mounted on slides with an appropriate mounting medium. The pH of this medium is particularly important when fluorescein conjugates are used; maximal fluorescence occurs only at pH 8.5 or higher. We use a polyvinyl alcohol-based mountant that hardens over time and forms a relatively permanent preparation (Harris, 1986; see box 5.2), and we include 1,4-diaza bicyclo(2.2.2) octane as an antibleaching agent (Langanger et al., 1983).

By comparison with immunofluorescence methods, immuno-cytochemistry is unsurpassed in one regard: Preparations are stable indefinitely. This is particularly important when cells must be examined for a long period, as for morphometry or camera lucida drawing, or when permanent preparations are important for documentation. For such purposes, we use the biotin-avidin method (Vectastain Elite ABC kit, Vector Laboratories; see box 5.3), although many other equally sensitive procedures have been developed. We detect the ABC reagent (avidin-biotinylated horseradish peroxidase complex) by reaction with diaminobenzidine. Addition of imidazole (Straus, 1982; Trojanowski et al., 1983) or cobalt (Adams, 1981) greatly increases the intensity of the staining.

Light-Microscopic Autoradiography

Because of their accessibility, cells in culture are ideal also for autoradiographic studies. Historically, autoradiography has been used to identify sites of protein synthesis and posttranslational processing, to trace the subsequent redistribution of the labeled macromolecules within the cell, and to label populations of neurons and glial cells with high-affinity uptake systems or receptors for particular neurotransmitters. More recently, in conjunction with in situ hybridization, autoradiography has been used to identify cell populations that express specific mRNAs. Unfortunately, the autoradiographic method requires patience—it can mean waiting for a week (and sometimes several weeks) to obtain adequate

exposure. For many purposes, autoradiography has been supplanted by faster methods, but it still has its place (box 5.4).

The autoradiographic procedure itself is similar to photography (for details, see Rogers, 1979). Fixed cultures are coated with a layer of emulsion containing crystals of a silver halide that is sensitive to nuclear emissions, are left for a time, then are treated with a photographic developer to convert silver halide crystals that have been sensitized by radiation exposure to insoluble, metallic silver. Small black grains appear in the emulsion overlying regions of the culture that contain radioactivity. Low-energy beta emitters—^{3}H, ^{35}S, and ^{125}I—are the isotopes of choice for light-microscopic autoradiography. These isotopes give *both* the highest resolution and the highest efficiency of grain production (Rogers, 1979), an important truth that will seem counterintuitive to those who work with other methods for detecting isotopes. Compounds labeled to the highest possible specific activity are used to keep exposure times as short as possible. For metabolic labeling, it is important that the medium not contain unlabeled precursor. Modified media, lacking a specified amino acid, are commercially available for studies of protein synthesis.

After metabolic labeling or exposure to radioactive ligands, tissue may be fixed as for light microscopy. Formaldehyde often is used in metabolic labeling studies because it does not cross-link most commonly used precursors. Glutaraldehyde is preferred if it is desirable to cross-link diffusible or reversibly bound label, as in studies of neurotransmitter uptake or radioligand binding.

In general, the same autoradiographic procedures can be used regardless of the method of labeling, as long as the incorporated isotope is bound irreversibly to the tissue (see box 5.4). Different, and more demanding, procedures are required for localization of reversibly bound or diffusible molecules (Rogers, 1979). Coating with emulsion and subsequent developing must be carried out in a darkroom. The safelights usually recommended for working with nuclear track emulsions do not provide much light; thus, dipping is rather tedious. We prefer a sodium safelight (such as a Duplex Super Safelight, available from suppliers of photgraphic equipment, and used with vanes closed), which is much brighter and, under most circumstances, does not increase background significantly. Cells are coated by dipping the slides in emulsion (such as Kodak NTB-2) that has been melted in a water bath at 41°C. Many workers dilute the emulsion 1:1 with water. Though this is satisfactory for

Box 5.4   Autoradiography

Fixation and Mounting

Fix cultures in 4% formaldehyde in PBS-sucrose or alternative, depending on radioactive compounds used.
Rinse in PBS to remove fixative.
Dehydrate in ethanols (2 min each in 25%, 50%, 70%, 95%, and 100%).
Place coverslips cell-side-up on filter paper and allow to dry.
Attach coverslips to clean glass microscope slides, cell-side-up, using a drop of Permount or Fluoromount. Position coverslip 5–10 mm from one end of the slide (to conserve emulsion during dipping). Allow to dry completely (several hours to overnight).

Coating with Emulsion (perform the following steps in a darkroom)

Scoop emulsion into a container just large enough to accommodate a slide and place the container in a water bath at 41°C until the emulsion is melted (approximately 30 min). Glass containers designed for staining single slides (Pelco cat. no. 22500) or plastic slide mailers (e.g., Thomas cat. no. 6707-M25) are handy containers and minimize the volume of emulsion needed.
Dip test slides to ensure that the emulsion is free of bubbles and to check its depth. The layer of emulsion should extend approximately 1 cm higher on the slide than the upper edge of the coverslip.
Dip each slide in emulsion, removing it with a steady motion to ensure even coating. Wipe excess emulsion off back and bottom and place in a test-tube rack for a few hours to gel and dry.
Load slides into black plastic slide boxes (Clay Adams no. 3843) and include a small container of silica gel dessicant. Place this box in a light-tight storage box (such as those supplied with EM film) or wrap in aluminum foil. Store in a refrigerator at 4°C for the period of exposure.

Developing and Mounting

Working in a darkroom, remove slides from boxes and transfer to glass staining racks. Check the color of the dessicant; it should not have become saturated.
Develop in Kodak D-19, 3 min at 15°C.
Rinse in 1% acetic acid (30 s).
Fix in Kodak Fixer, 4 min. Subsequent steps can be performed under normal lighting.
Rinse in gently running H_2O for 20 min.
Mount in polyvinyl alcohol mountant. Place large drop of mounting medium onto the coverslip and cover with a second, slightly larger coverslip.

coating sections or cultures of flat cells, it may give incomplete coverage of neuronal cell bodies, which protrude above the substrate.

Appropriate exposure time obviously depends on the amount of radioactivity incorporated and must be determined empirically. In our experience, studies of amino acid or uridine incorporation typically require exposures of a week or less, whereas receptor labeling or in situ hybridization may require significantly longer exposure. After exposure, slides are developed very much like photographic film. We mount the autoradiograms under a second coverslip with a gelatin-based mountant.

In Situ Hybridization

Cell cultures are ideal preparations for in situ hybridization to detect specific messenger RNAs. This approach can indicate which cells express a given message and how its level of expression changes under different conditions (Figure 5.5). In comparison to immunostaining, in situ hybridization has the advantage that it does not require production of an additional reagent. If you have a cDNA or know the sequence, you can perform in situ hybridization.

In general, the method involves fixing the cultured cells to immobilize their mRNAs, followed by incubation with labeled nucleotide probes that contain sequences complementary to the RNA to be localized. Typically, cells in culture are fixed for 15 to 30 min in 4% formaldehyde, rinsed in PBS, dehydrated, and stored in 70% ethanol at 4°C (see Lawrence and Singer, 1985; Singer et al., 1986). Many methods for in situ hybridization with DNA, RNA, and oligonucleotide probes have been described, and their advantages and disadvantages have been discussed at length (Valentino et al., 1987). This goes well beyond the scope of this chapter (and the expertise of its authors). We focus instead on our admittedly limited experience with cultured hippocampal neurons (Kleiman et al., 1993b). Though DNA and oligonucleotide probes can be used, we prefer to use riboprobes (500–1000 bases in length) because they bind at high stringency and because unbound (single-stranded) probe can be removed by treatment with RNase, thus reducing background. We have used radioactive probes labeled with either ^{35}S-UTP or ^{3}H-UTP, followed by autoradiography (as described in box 5.4). Each has its advantages and disadvantages. ^{35}S-labeled probes have a much higher specific activity, so often

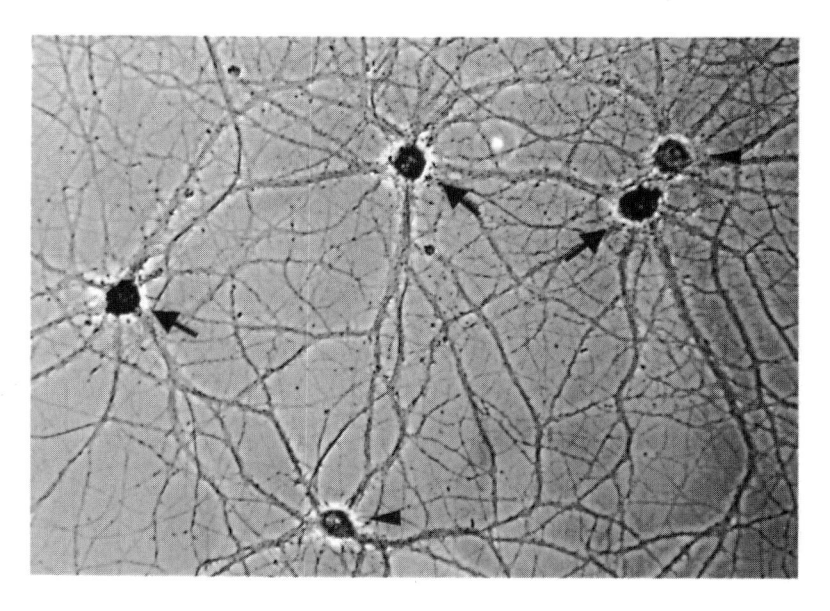

Figure 5.5 Nonradioactive in situ hybridization using a probe for the immediate early gene NGFI-A (Milbrandt, 1987). Hippocampal neurons (28 days in vitro) were stimulated for 45 min with the calcium channel agonist BAY K 8644 (1 μm) and then were fixed and prepared for in situ hybridization as described in box 5.5. Under these conditions, approximately half the neurons respond with elevated levels of NGFI-A mRNA over their cell bodies (arrows). Arrowheads indicate neurons that do not contain detectable NGFI-A mRNA. (Courtesy of G. Withers and C. Wallace, Oregon Health Sciences University.) See plate 4 for color version.

they can be detected after exposures of only a week or two. ^{3}H-labeled probes require much longer exposure times but offer better resolution and a clearer view of the distribution of mRNAs that extend into dendrites (Kleiman et al., 1993b).

In comparison with radioactive probes, probes labeled with digoxygenin (a compound isolated from *digitalis* plants) offer several advantages. The labeling reagents are less expensive than are most isotopes, and their use and disposal are not subject to stringent regulations. Most important, there is no need to wait for autoradiograms to expose; the entire procedure can be performed in 3 days. Our current protocol for in situ hybridization with digoygenin-labeled probes is shown in box 5.5. This protocol largely follows the methods for in situ hybridization on cultured nerve cells developed by Stefanie Kaech and Evelyn Ralston, who were kind enough to share their results prior to publication. Details of the hybridization conditions must be adjusted for each probe, but the protocol provided may serve as a reasonable starting point. For cul-

Box 5.5   Nonisotopic In Situ Hybridization

Probe Preparation

Nonradioactive cRNA probes are synthesized by using the Ambion maxiscript in vitro transcription kit in the presence of digoxygenin-11-uridine-5'-triphosphate (Boehringer Mannheim, cat no. 1209256). Concentration of RNA can be determined by comparing the probe against a dilution series of digoxygenin-labeled RNA of known concentration (Boehringer Mannhiem, cat no. 1585746) using dot-blot hybridization performed according to manufacturer's instructions. Approximately 0.2–0.5 μg of cRNA probe is added to each coverslip.

Culture Preparation

Fix cultures grown on coverslips for 15–20 min in 4% formaldehyde in PBS-sucrose. Rinse in DEPC-treated PBS and store at 4°C in DEPC-treated 70% ethanol.

Hybridization

The volumes given here are for 18-mm round coverslips; they can be adjusted for other preparations. For rinses, four coverslips are placed in a 60-mm culture dish with 8–10 ml of rinse solution. All solutions except TRIS buffers are treated with DEPC.

1. Rehydrate coverslips in 5 mM $MgCl_2$ in PBS for 10 min at room temperature.
2. Rinse with 0.1 M glycine in 0.2 M TRIS (pH 7.4) for 10 min.
3. Place in prehybridization buffer for 1 h at 42°C. Prehybridization buffer consists of 50% deionized formamide, 2× SSC, 0.5% Denhardt's reagent, 5% dextran sulfate (Sigma, cat. no. D-7037), 0.25 mg/ml *E. coli* tRNA (Sigma, cat. no. R-1753), 0.125 mg/ml salmon sperm DNA (Sigma, cat. no. D-7656), 0.25 mg/ml heparin (Sigma, cat. no. H-3393) in DEPC-treated water).
4. For each coverslip, place 180 μl of hybridization buffer (50% deionized formamide, 2× SSC, 1% Denhardts reagent, 10% dextran sulfate, 0.5 mg/ml *E. coli* tRNA, 0.25 mg/ml salmon sperm DNA (Sigma, cat. No. D-7656), 0.5 mg/ml heparin in DEPC-treated water) in a 35-mm culture dish. To this drop, add 20 μl of probe mixture (0.2–0.5 μg cRNA diluted to a final volume of 20 μl in DEPC-treated H_2O). Remove the coverslip from the prehybridization dish, place it cell-side-down onto the droplet of hybridization mix, close the Petri dish, and place in a humidified chamber in a 55°C oven overnight.
5. Rinse with 50% formamide-2× SSC for 30 min at 55°C. This solution can be made the night before and stored overnight in the oven so it will be at the correct temperature first thing in the morning.
6. Treat with RNase A (20 μg/ml, Sigma, cat. no. R-5503) in 0.5 M NaCl, 10 mM TRIS, pH 8.0 for 30 min at 37°C.
7. Rinse with 50% formamide-1× SSC for 30 min at 55°C.
8. Rinse with 1× SSC for 30 min at room temperature.

Box 5.5 (continued)

Antibody Labeling

For the remaining steps, we recommend preparing solutions in glass-distilled water to reduce the amount of precipitate that forms during the colorization reaction. We detect digoxygenin-labeled probes by using the Genius Kit (Boehringer Mannheim).

1. Rinse coverslips 3× for 5 min in TRIS-buffered saline (TBS).
2. Block with 10% BSA (or serum) in TBS for 30 min at room temperature in a humid chamber.
3. Incubate coverslips in alkaline phosphatase–conjugated antidigoxigenin FAb fragments (Boehringer Mannheim, cat no. 1093274) diluted 1:1000 in TBS plus 10% BSA for 1 h at 37°C in a humid chamber.
4. Rinse 2× for 10 min each with TBS, then for 10 min with NMT (see following recipe).
5. Immerse in colorization solution overnight at 4°C in the dark. To avoid accumulation of precipitate on coverslips, we use staining racks to keep the coverslips oriented vertically. The volume of solution needed will depend on the staining rack used: For 10 ml, add 45 µl NBT reagent (nitroblue tetrazolium chloride, 100 mg/ml; Boehringer Mannheim, cat no. 1383213) and 35 µl X-phosphate reagent (5-bromo-4-chloro-3-indolyl phosphate, 50 mg/ml; Boehringer Mannheim, cat no. 1383221) to 10 ml NBT. The colorization solution is light- and temperature-sensitive. Immediately after preparation, filter through Whatman no. 1 paper into a foil-wrapped container on ice.
6. Rinse 3× for 10 min in 1 mM EDTA, 0.1 M TRIS, pH 8.5 to quench the alkaline phosphatase reaction.
7. Rinse with H_2O and mount coverslips in an aqueous mounting medium, such as Elvanol.

Solutions

Denhardt's Reagent: 1 g ficoll, 1 g polyvinylpyrrolidone, 1 g BSA in 50 ml DEPC-treated water; aliquot and store at −20°C.
20× SSC: 3 M NaCl, 0.3 M sodium citrate; DEPC-treat, then autoclave.
TRIS-buffered saline: 25 ml 1 M TRIS, 7.5 ml 5 M NaCl, fill to 250 ml with dH_2O.
NMT: 0.1 M NaCl, 0.05 M $MgCl_2$, 0.1 M TRIS, pH 9.5

tured cells, usually it is unnecessary and undesirable to pretreat with detergents or proteinases, as is usual for in situ hybridization on tissue sections.

One final practical matter must be addressed. As the goal of in situ hybridization is to detect mRNA, it is essential to avoid RNAse contamination. RNases are lurking everywhere: in the water, on glassware, on your own person. Precautions are necessary. We use plastic dishes from unopened packages whenever possible; bake spatulas, forceps, and glassware at 250°C for 4 h; and wear gloves. Diethylpyrocarbonate (DEPC) is used to treat all buffer solutions, and other solutions are prepared in DEPC-treated water (Sambrook et al., 1989): Add DEPC at 1 part per 1000, shake vigously to mix, allow to stand for several hours, then autoclave. We DEPC-treat all solutions listed in box 5.5 except buffers containing TRIS (which inactivates DEPC; these are prepared in DEPC-treated water and are sterile-filtered).

Microscopy of Living Cells

An obvious advantage of tissue culture is that it renders observing living cells easy. Well, it can be easy, depending on just what you want to observe. What is observed can range from monitoring cell growth over a period of hours by phase contrast microscopy—an experiment almost any laboratory could afford to undertake—to imaging the calcium content within individual dendritic spines with a time resolution of tens of milliseconds; entire laboratories are devoted to such problems as this. Each application will require a somewhat different approach, but some issues will have to be faced regardless of the specifics of the experiment. We concentrate here on these issues.

MAINTAINING CELLS ON THE MICROSCOPE STAGE
Looking at living cells on a microscope, even for the simplest of experiments, presents two immediate problems. You must have a means of getting the cells close enough to the microscope objective so that they can be brought into focus, and you must keep them alive long enough to see something interesting. Both concerns require some modification to the methods ordinarily used for cell culture. Obviously, inverted microscopes help to solve some of these problems, as they are designed to enable observation of cells growing in dishes that are too deep to be observed from above. But

if you intend to make observations at higher magnifications, say at 40× or above, you will find that the bottom of an ordinary culture dish is simply too thick. The working distance of high-resolution objectives (i.e., the clearance between the front of the objective and the specimen focal plane) is barely more than the thickness of a glass coverslip (typically 0.17 mm). Moreover, the optical qualities of most plastics are inferior to those of glass, and plastic's birefringence makes it incompatible with techniques such as differential interference contrast microscopy, which use polarized light. And unless you plan to put your microscope in an incubator, you will have to make some arrangements to keep the cells warm, moist, and in an atmosphere that provides the requisite pH buffering.

There are two basic approaches to the problem of working distance. One approach is to grow the cells in culture dishes modified with microscopy in mind. This typically is accomplished by cutting a hole in the bottom of an ordinary culture dish and attaching a glass coverslip over this hole from the outside (see chapters 8 and 12). This alteration forms a shallow well into which the cells are plated. The coverslip can be attached with a 3 : 1 mixture of paraffin and Vaseline (which is a little messy to apply but will allow the coverslip to be pried off at the end of the experiment) or with silastic. Such dishes are relatively easy to make, or they can be purchased from commercial sources. An alternative approach is to grow the cells on coverslips placed in culture dishes or in multiwell plates, mounting the coverslips in a specially designed chamber when the time comes to observe them in the microscope. A typical design uses a teflon or silicone rubber spacer coated with silicone grease to seal the cell-bearing coverslip to a second coverslip, with room for a bit of medium in between (Forscher et al., 1987; Ryan et al., 1993; see chapter 10). In one design, the resulting sandwich is held between two aluminum plates screwed together to form a frame. These chambers can be left open at opposite ends to enable perfusion of medium, or they can be sealed completely. Many investigators have simple chambers made in local machine shops to meet their particular requirements; more sophisticated (and more expensive) chambers are commercially available (McKenna and Wang, 1989).

High-resolution DIC microscopy, the method that has produced such stunning views of intracellular organelle transport and growth cone motility (Smith, 1994a; Dai and Sheetz, 1995; Lin et al., 1996; see chapter 8 and 10), is more demanding still. This technique re-

quires that the surface of the condensor lens be positioned only a millimeter above the cells, which means that the entire chamber can be only 1 mm thick. This is not an issue for phase contrast microscopy, because long-working-distance condensors are available.

To observe cells for any length of time, it is important to control temperature, osmolarity, and pH. Using a sealed chamber eliminates problems of evaporation and pH control, as long as the medium is equlibrated to the correct pH before the chamber is sealed and no air bubbles are allowed to enter. Temperature can be controlled by a stage heater, by incorporating heating elements within the chamber itself, or by blowing a current of warm air onto the specimen. Commercial units designed for this purpose are available, but some labs simply use a hair drier and a temperature controller.

Open chambers are required for many applications, such as micromanipulation, local application of drugs, physiological recording, or stimulation. Usually, this means using a medium that will maintain its pH in air rather than in 5% CO_2, either by replacing bicarbonate with HEPES or by using a medium such as L-15 that is formulated for use in air. Evaporation can be reduced by constant perfusion or by adding a few drops of silicone oil onto the surface of the medium. Alternatively, chambers have been designed to blow a gentle current of a defined, humidified gas mixture across the surface of the medium.

PHOTOTOXICITY

Cells are damaged by exposure to light, a definite drawback for light microscopy. For many purposes, this problem can be circumvented simply by lowering the level of light that reaches the cells. In some cases, this only requires turning down the light source or inserting neutral-density filters into the light path. Even inexpensive video cameras can produce good images at relatively low light levels. More sophisticated approaches are helpful for such microscopic techniques as high-resolution DIC or fluorescence microscopy, which require exposing the cells to intense light. Image-processing software can enhance greatly the signal in a dim image, and a computer-controlled shutter makes it possible to limit light exposure to the period actually needed to record an image. Photodamage is especially problematic in fluorescence microscopy, because the light-induced decomposition of fluorescent dyes (that causes the photobleaching so familiar to all who use fluorescence microscopy) also produces free radicals that are highly

toxic to living cells. Photodecomposition involves reaction of the excited dye with oxygen in the medium. Thus, in addition to taking advantage of all the means available to reduce light exposure, many laboratories eliminate oxygen from the culture medium or include antioxidants when performing fluorescence microscopy (Taylor and Salmon, 1989; Waggoner et al., 1989; Tanaka and Kirschner, 1991). We use a cocktail of *N*-acetyl-cysteine (50 μM, Sigma, St. Louis, MO) and Trolox (10 μM, Aldrich, Milwaukee, WI). We also use medium without phenol red, as this pH indicator has been reported to undergo photodegradation and can contribute to autofluorescence.

CAMERAS AND RECORDING DEVICES

A serious discussion of the equipment available for imaging living cells is beyond the scope of this chapter—far beyond. There are many good sources that can provide an introduction to the basic ideas (Herman and Lemasters, 1993; Shotten, 1993; Inouyé and Spring, 1997). Because this field is changing very rapidly as new technology emerges, you might also consider one of the many courses devoted to this topic, where you can see the latest equipment and get advice from real experts. We will attempt to say just enough to give the novice a sense of the kinds of approaches available (and perhaps to whet your appetite a bit).

At some time or another, everyone who works with cultured cells wants to view their movements or growth by time-lapse recording. This can require nothing more than an inexpensive video camera and a video cassette recorder to record images on videotape, equipment that is likely to be available in a nearby lab or can be purchased for a few thousand dollars. Even for such straightforward applications, however, there are real advantages to including a computer in the system to control image acquisition and to perform some simple image processing. With the appropriate software, you can collect images at whatever interval you prefer; you can greatly improve the quality of the images by averaging to reduce camera noise, enhancing the contrast, and subtracting out those annoying bits of dirt that appear on optical surfaces; and you can store the images on a device that allows their immediate recall, either in digital form on a hard disk or CD-ROM or in analog form on an optical magnetic disk recorder. If you've ever spent time playing through minutes or hours of videotape looking for particular images, you can understand how valuable that can be. For those who must do extensive time-lapse recording, addition of a

motorized stage and focus controls can be a great boon. By using software that steps the microscope from one cell to the next and automatically corrects the focus at each position, it is possible to obtain many hours of recordings from 5 or 10 different cells, all from the comfort of home.

More sophisticated cameras—such as those capable of low-light-level imaging—come in two basic forms: One generates a video (analog) signal, the other produces a digital signal. There are advantages and disadvantages to each. Video cameras, such as silicon-intensified-tube (SIT) cameras and intensified charge-coupled device (CCD) cameras, acquire images "at video rates" (30 images per second), an important consideration if, say, you're interested in recording rapid changes in intracellular calcium. Digital cameras (such as slow-scan, chilled CCD cameras) offer somewhat higher resolution and an output that is linear over a much greater range of signal intensities but can acquire a new image only once every second or so. There are inexpensive boards for personal computers that enable conversion between the two formats, so that analog images can be enhanced digitally and stored in a digital format. If your application requires investment in a sophisticated camera you certainly will also want to invest in image-processing software.

FLUORESCENT PROBES

One of the remarkable advances in the last decade has been the development of a vast armamentarium of fluorescent probes suitable for live cell imaging. Among the first probes to be applied widely in neurobiology were diI and diO, lipophilic dyes that partition into the cell membrane and diffuse over the entire cell surface, permitting individual cells to be viewed in their entirety. As cultures mature and the density of processes becomes so heavy that individual cells can no longer be distinguished, labeling with diI or diO can allow visualization of the arbor of a single cell at a resolution sufficient to follow the movements of individual filopodia or dendritic spines (Papa and Segal, 1996; Ziv and Smith, 1996). Expression of appropriate constructs of green flourescent protein (GFP) also works well to label individual cells (Moriyoshi et al., 1996). Construction of additional GFP/protein chimeras should be useful for following the targeting of specific proteins in living cells (Kain et al., 1995; Gerdes and Kaether, 1996; McKiernan et al., 1996), as has been done with the N-methyl-D-aspartate receptor (Marshall et al., 1995).

Other fluorescent compounds label specific cellular compartments (Wang and Taylor, 1989; Molecular Probes Catalog). Such probes include fluorescent derivatives of ceramide that label the Golgi apparatus and Golgi-derived vesicles (Pagano, 1989); fluorescent markers of the endoplasmic reticulum (Terasaki et al., 1984); mitochondrial dyes, such as rhodamine 123 and Mitotracker; and such RNA stains as the Syto dyes (Knowles et al., 1996). The lipophilic dye FM1-43, which becomes incorporated into the plasma membrane, can be used to label recycling synaptic vesicles (Betz and Bewick, 1992), an approach that has allowed optical monitoring of vesicle dynamics in dissociated cell cultures (Ryan and Smith, 1995).

Finally, a number of indicator dyes enable monitoring of spatial and temporal changes in ion concentrations or pH. The calcium dyes have been used extensively in neurobiology, but probes for hydrogen, sodium, potassium, magnesium, and chloride also are available. Many of these dyes are available in ester forms that enter the cytoplasm of living cells, eliminating the need for intracellular injection.

Electron Microscopy of Cultured Neurons

Methods for preparing cultured cells for electron microscopy are very similar to those routinely used for preparing tissue specimens. Usually, cultures are fixed by immersion in glutaraldehyde (1%–4%), then are rinsed and postfixed in osmium tetroxide (1–4%). Traditionally, these fixatives are added in isotonic or hypertonic buffer solutions, most laboratories having developed specific recipes that they prefer. Our approach is slightly different (box 5.6); we simply add glutaraldehyde to an aliquot of the culture medium. For some purposes, simultaneous fixation in glutaraldehyde and osmium, rather than sequential fixation, may be preferred because it gives improved preservation of such labile structures as growth cones (Hasty and Hay, 1978; Ruthel and Banker, 1998). After osmication, the entire culture is stained en bloc with uranyl acetate. This step is important; cultured cells are notoriously low in contrast when observed by electron microscopy, and staining of sections alone usually is insufficient.

Specimens cultured on glass coverslips can be dehydrated and embedded by any of the procedures used for processing tissue blocks. If cells are grown in culture dishes, dehydrating agents

Box 5.6   Fixation and Embedding for Transmission Electron Microscopy

> Remove one-third of the medium from the dish to be fixed; add sufficient 70% glutaraldehyde (EM grade) to make the aliquot 10.5%, warm to 37° in a water bath, then gently add it back to the culture. Reaction with the glutaraldehyde lowers the pH of the medium, but this is not deleterious to the fixation.
> Rinse in 0.125 M phosphate buffer (3 × 2 min).
> Add 1% OsO_4 for 30 min.
> Rinse in 3.6% NaCl to remove excess OsO_4 (2 × 2 min).
> Rinse in dH_2O (2 × 2 min).
> Stain in 5% aqueous uranyl acetate (1 h in the dark).
> Rinse in dH_2O (2 × 2 min).
> Dehydrate in methanol and acetone: 25%, 50% methanol (2 min each), 70%, 95% methanol (5 min each), 100% methanol (2 × 10 min); 100% acetone (10 min).
> Infiltrate overnight with 1:1 mixture of resin and acetone.
> Embed in resin (see text).

and resins that attack polystyrene must be avoided. These include acetone, propylene oxide, and Spurr's resin. Complete penetration of the resin is important—otherwise, cell processes that lie at the interface with the substrate tend to pull out of the polymerized resin when the coverslip is pulled away or when the block is sectioned. Usually, we leave the cultures overnight in a mixture of acetone and resin (1:1) before transferring them to the complete resin mixture for final embedding. For embedding coverslips, we have fabricated molds from silicone rubber that are 3 mm deep and just slightly smaller in diameter than the coverslips. The mold is filled with resin, the coverslip is inverted over it, and the entire assembly is placed in an oven to polymerize the resin. After polymerization the resin, with coverslip attached, can be popped out of the mold.

One of the trickiest aspects of the electron microscopy of cell cultures is separating the polymerized resin containing the embedded cells, from the substrate, and doing this in such a way that the entire resin block remains intact, allowing the cells of interest to be relocated and examined by electron microscopy. The resins used for embedding form an extremely tight bond to glass and to plastic culture dishes. The method we prefer involves dipping the embedded culture alternately into boiling water for 2 min, then into liquid nitrogen for 2 min. The differential rates of expansion and contraction of the resin and glass cause the coverslip

to shatter and to detach from the resin, which remains intact (well, usually). Glass fragments can be wiped away or picked off with a forceps. This technique also can be used for specimens in tissue culture dishes. A different approach favored by some laboratories involves dissolving the glass substrate with hydrofluoric acid (Buchanan et al., 1989). This technique requires great care in rinsing away residual acid, as microscope objectives can be hopelessly damaged by hydrofluoric acid vapors from such specimens.

An alternative approach to the problem of separating resin from substrate involves using a substrate that is more hydrophobic than glass or tissue-culture plastic, so that the resin adheres less tightly. For example, cells can be cultured on coverslips or minidishes prepared from Aclar 33C, a plastic film that can be readily peeled away from the resin after polymerization (see chapter 19). Evaporating a layer of carbon onto glass coverslips or treating glass coverslips with dicholoro-dimethylsilane (1% in benzene; see Deitch and Banker, 1993) also simplifies separating coverslip from resin. Coverslips prepared by any of these methods can be treated with polylysine or extracellular matrix constituents in the usual way, and most cells adhere to them quite well. However, in our studies of hippocampal cultures, we have found that dendrites develop less consistently on these substrates than on conventionally prepared glass coverslips (see chapter 13). Some plastic films suitable as a culture substrate can themselves be sectioned, so that separation of the polymerized resin is unnecessary.

Although osmium causes tissue to turn black, monolayer cultures are so thin that the cell layer remains invisible after osmication. Embedded cultures can be examined by phase-contrast microscopy. Alternatively, because the cells lie immediately at the surface of the resin, they can be stained by the same methods used for staining thick plastic sections. For example, we immerse the embedded cultures in toluidine blue (1.0% in 0.1% borax) at 60°C for 5 to 15 min. This makes it easy to choose areas to be sectioned and makes it possible to visualize individual cells during trimming and sectioning. After the areas to be examined by electron microscopy are marked, they can be sawn or punched out of the resin and cemented onto a suitable stub in the orientation desired for sectioning.

Cutting sections perpendicular to the substrate, so that neuronal processes may be viewed in cross-section, is quite straightforward. However, it is often more desirable to cut sections parallel to the

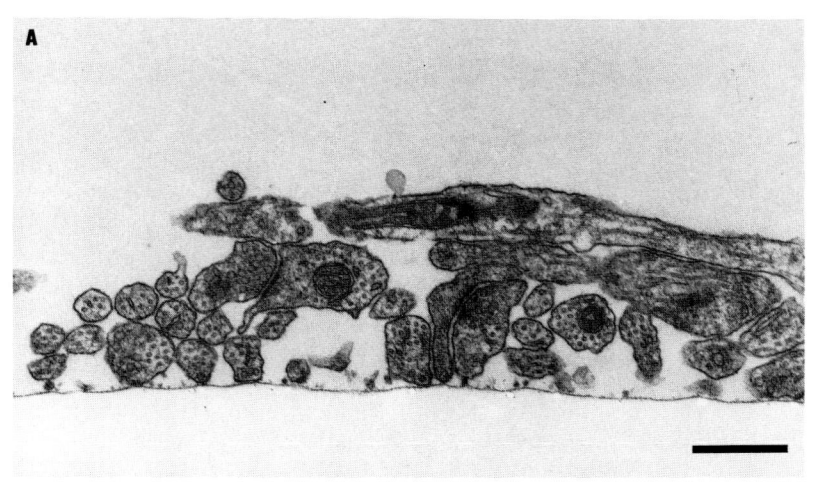

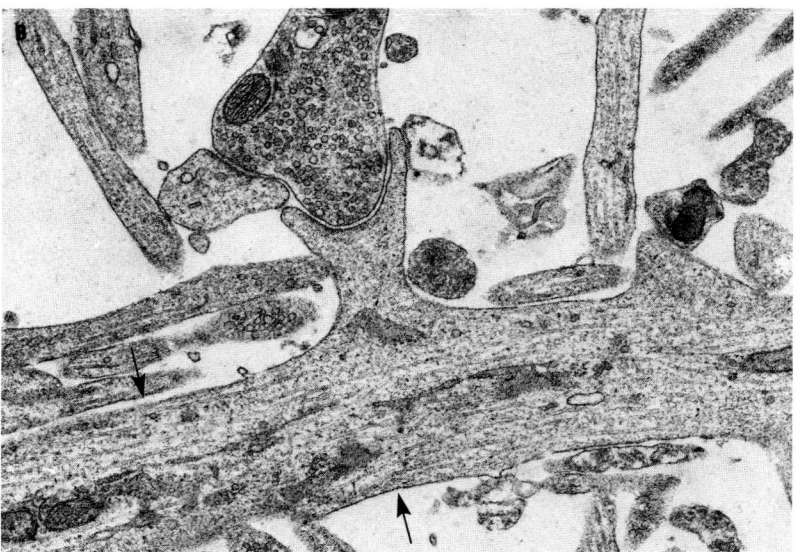

Figure 5.6 Electron micrographs of neuropil regions from hippocampal cultures that had been maintained for 3 weeks. (*A*) A culture sectioned perpendicular to the substrate. Processes lie within a micrometer or two of the culture surface, thus forming a narrow band that runs across the section. (*B*) A comparable culture that has been sectioned parallel to the substrate. Individual processes, such as the dendrite indicated (arrows), often can be followed for some distance. Note synapse on dendritic spine. Scale bar: 0.5 μm. (Courtesy of O. Steward and P. Falk, University of Virginia.)

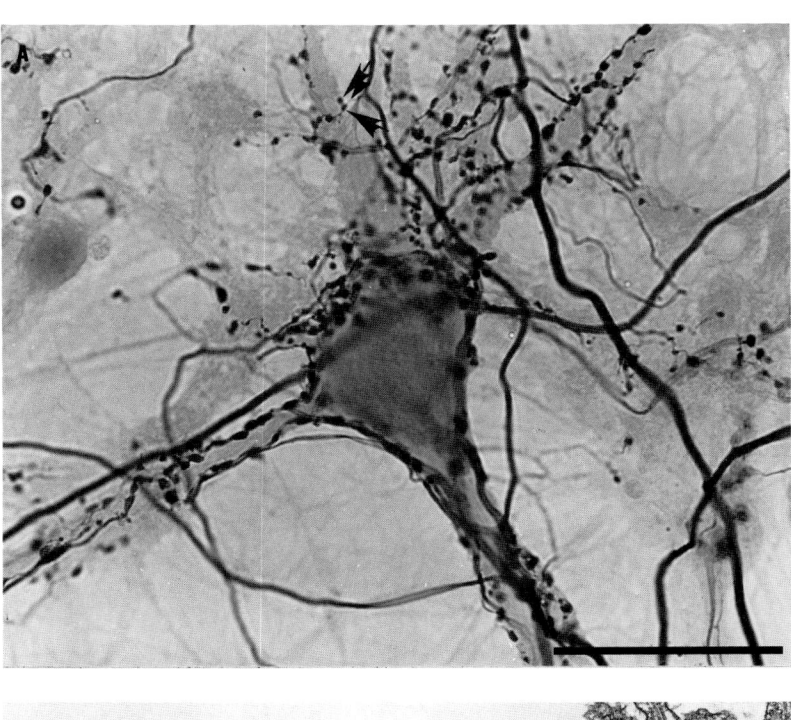

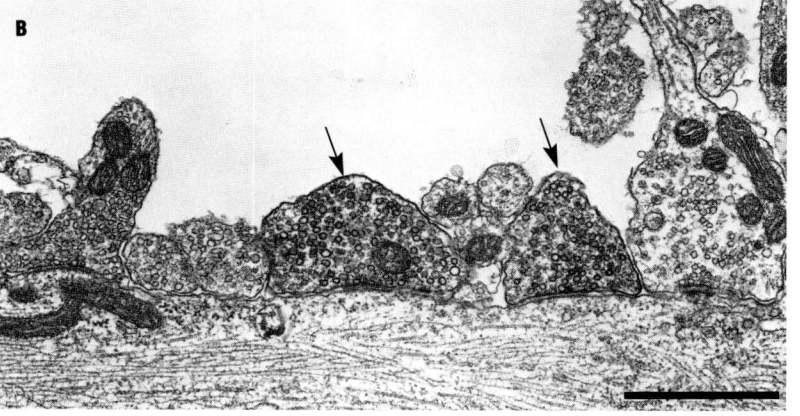

Figure 5.7 Use of intracellular injection of horseradish peroxidase for correlated light- and electron-microscopical investigation of cultured neurons. (*A*) The peroxidase-labeled axon from a spinal cord neuron as it forms varicosities (arrows) along the cell body of an unlabeled cell. Electron microscopy of this same preparation (*B*) reveals that the two peroxidase-labeled varicosities denoted by arrows in *A* are, in fact, synaptic boutons (arrows). Scale bars: *A*, 50 μm; *B*, 1 μm. (From Neale et al., 1978, with permission.)

substrate, as this allows visualization of much larger areas of the culture in a single section (figure 5.6). This approach is technically demanding, because neuronal processes are so thin that interesting features may be contained entirely within the first few sections. Proper alignment of the block face requires a microtome that has good lighting and allows easy, precise orientation of the block in all three dimensions; practice and patience also help. However, the information that can be gained by this approach, which permits correlation with light micrographs to relocate specific cells, processes, or even synapses, can more than make up for these frustrations (figure 5.7).

Choosing the Right System

The chapters that follow illustrate the diversity of techniques presently available for preparing cultures of nervous tissue. They range from the simple to the complex, from methods that are easy enough to use as teaching exercises for students to those that are demanding even for the most experienced. All the chapters include the protocols and recipes you will need to grow these cells successfully. Equally important, the authors discuss the specific experimental issues that motivate their work and the rationale behind their approaches so that you can get a sense of how these recipes evolved.

We begin with two chapters devoted to cell lines that exhibit neuronal properties. In chapter 6, Greene et al. describe their work on PC12 cells. The PC12 pheochromocytoma cell line derives from a rat adrenomedullary tumor and, as do normal adrenal chromaffin cells, PC12 cells acquire many characteristics of sympathetic neurons when exposed to nerve growth factor. The most widely used cell line of interest to neurobiologists, PC12 cells have been particularly valuable for studies of the mechanism of action of nerve growth factor and of the regulation of gene expression associated with differentiation to a neuronal phenotype. Green et al. describe the practical considerations necessary for successful culture of PC12 cells, emphasizing the importance of standardizing culture conditions to prevent development of variant cell lines. One particular advantage of cell lines is that they permit development of lines that express foreign genes. Greene et al. provide extensive protocols for transient and stable transfection of PC12s.

The approach of Bain and colleagues in chapter 7 is very different. They begin with embryonic stem cells and P19 cells, two continuous lines whose cells resemble those of the primitive ectoderm in that they have an extremely broad developmental potential. When grown under appropriate conditions and treated with appropriate factors, the cells develop a neuronlike phenotype. The differentiated cultures are not homogeneous—they contain cells with glial characteristics and their population of neuronal cells is itself heterogeneous. The compensation for this is that, unlike

conventional neural cell lines, the neuronlike cells exhibit many of the differentiated properties of central nervous system (CNS) neurons: They synthesize and release glutamate, γ-aminobertyric acid, and glycine; they express receptors for these neurotransmitters, including glutamate receptors of both AMPA and NMDA subtypes; they become polarized into axonal and dendritic domains; and they make synapses, as assessed by physiological and morphological methods.

We next turn to primary cell cultures from "simple" systems. As described by Goldberg and Schacher (chapter 8), cultures of Aplysia neurons represent the ultimate in a defined system, allowing for the culture of individual, identified neurons. The large size of the cell bodies of these neurons makes them ideal candidates for electrophysiology and for microinjection experiments. These large cells also have large growth cones, which have become a favorite object for analysis by high-resolution video microscopy. Cultures of Aplysia neurons are also widely used for analysis of synaptic specificity and synaptic plasticity.

Tabti, Alder, and Poo (chapter 9) take an equally simple approach to the culture of neurons from the spinal cord of Xenopus embryos. In addition to lending themselves to studies of process outgrowth and neuronal differentiation, such cultures are particularly useful for examining the formation of synapses with muscle cells. Early events in the development of synapses can be studied at sites of contact between single, identified growth cones and individual myoblasts, using both physiological and morphological methods. These cultures also offer other, unique experimental opportunities. Because Xenopus embryos are relatively large and accessible, fluorescent markers, antibodies or expression vectors containing foreign genes can be injected into individual cells at the blastomere stage. The injected materials persist through many rounds of division and are still present when cells are placed in culture, thus, specific populations of cells can be identified in culture, and the developmental effects of altering the function of specific genes and proteins can be assessed in the cultured neurons.

The next two chapters concern cultures of peripheral neurons and adrenal chromaffin cells. In chapter 10, Smith describes methods for preparing cultures of sympathetic and dorsal root ganglia from chick embryos. Cultures from chick ganglia have a unique place in neuroscience history. Explant cultures of chick sympathetic ganglia served as the assay system for isolation of

the first neurotrophic factor, and the first successful dissociated neuronal cultures were prepared from chick ganglia. The methods involved in preparing these cultures are easy, convenient, and inexpensive: Even the embryos come prepackaged in individual, sterile containers that need not be housed in expensive animal facilities. Yet, as Smith makes clear, these cultures continue to offer a remarkably useful preparation for analysis of trophic factors and for elucidating the cell biology of growth cones and neurite outgrowth.

In chapter 11, Mahanthappa and Patterson describe their methods for preparing cultures of sympathetic neurons from the rat superior cervical ganglion, cultures that have played a key role in studies of the control of neuronal differentiation. Such cultures are the envy of those of us who have chosen to work with other cell types. Compared to most regions of the nervous system, sympathetic ganglia contain a relatively homogeneous population of neurons. Furthermore, because their natural trophic factor is known, these cells can be cultured more or less indefinitely in the absence of nonneuronal cells. Sympathetic cultures have become a standard model for investigating the influence of the environment on neuronal differentiation and for studying the control of axonal and dendritic outgrowth. Mahanthappa and Patterson also provide methods for culturing adrenal chromaffin cells, another valuable system for studying the control of cell fate.

Chapters 12 to 16 treat dissociated-cell cultures of the mammalian CNS. Together, these chapters illustrate very different approaches tailored to distinct experimental paradigms. Culture lore points to the importance of glial cells for the long-term survival of CNS neurons, and the protocol of Segal et al. follows directly from this idea (chapter 12). They first prepare monolayer cultures of astroglia, then plate cortical neurons onto this glial monolayer. Thus, the glia serve both as substrate and source of trophic support. This work is noteworthy also for refinements in cell dissociation procedures that permit the culture of neurons from postnatal animals. Finally, these authors describe the preparation of microisland cultures that allow long-term survival of single, CNS neurons.

The approach of Segal et al., based on gentle dissociation and coculture with glial cells, solves many of the problems inherent in obtaining good CNS cultures. With minimal modification, it has been used successfully to culture neurons from hippocampus,

striatum, spinal cord, and basal forebrain. Assuming it is compatible with the experiments you plan, the coculture approach appears to be among the simplest and most reliable methods for culturing CNS neurons.

Unfortunately, such cocultures cannot be used for the experiments of Goslin et al., which require that hippocampal neurons be grown at low density and in the absence of direct glial contact. As described in chapter 13, our approach has been to prepare separate monolayer cultures of neurons (on coverslips) and glial cells (in dishes), then to culture the two together to foster trophic interactions. The coverslips themselves contain a reasonably pure population of neurons and can be removed from the dishes to be used for experiments. The access this system offers has allowed experiments that would otherwise be extremely difficult: transection of individual axons at defined distances from the cell body or immunocytochemical and electron-microscopic study of single cells whose developmental histories are known.

The next two chapters describe methods for preparing dissociated-cell cultures from two other regions of the cerebrum, the striatum and the habenula. Both chapters represent relatively recent excursions into CNS cell culture by laboratories best known for discoveries based on tissue culture of the peripheral nervous system. Over and above their intrinsic interest, these chapters are instructive for the view they provide of how experienced laboratories approach the task of developing protocols to culture new cell types.

Chaper 14, by Ventimiglia and Lindsay, concerns cell cultures from the striatum, a portion of the brain best known for its involvement in human motor disease. The goal of the authors' work is to define the response of striatal neurons to soluble growth factors, and the specifics of the culture system they describe follow directly. Cells are grown at low density so that the number of surviving cells can be counted accurately, in serum-free medium so that no undefined factors are included, and with minimal contamination by glial cells, as glia also are a source of growth factors. Finally, the authors have developed simple immunocytochemical methods to identify the different cell types present in order to define their distinct trophic requirements.

Why culture neurons from the habenula, you ask? As Krauss and Fischbach explain in chapter 15, the medial habenular nucleus contains a very well-defined, homogeneous population of neurons that receive cholinergic inputs and that themselves use acetylcho-

line as neurotrasmitter. Thus, it provides an ideal system for analyzing the role of cell-cell interactions and of known growth factors
in the regulation of cholinergic differentiation in the CNS. As glia
are not undesirable for the experiments these authors have in
mind, their approach uses a serum-containing medium to stimulate the proliferation of glial cells, which form a feeder layer that
helps support long-tem neuronal survival. Their approach permits
growth at low cell density, which is optimal for microscopy and
physiology, and at the high cell density needed for molecular
studies.

In chapter 16, Hatten and colleagues take the cerebellum apart
and put it back together again—literally. To study the cell-cell
interactions that produce the exquisite architecture of the cerebellar cortex, they have developed elegant methods for purifying
each of the major cell populations—granule neurons, Purkinje
cells, and astroglia—so that they can be studied in isolation and so
that their interactions with other defined cell types can be analyzed
in a controlled environment. They also describe methods for preparing explant cultures from some of the regions that innervate the
cerebellum and for studying their interaction with specific populations of cerebellar neurons.

Chapter 17, by Gahwiler and colleagues, describes the methods
that they have pioneered for preparing organotypic slice cultures,
an elegant approach that "updates" the classic techniques of explant culture to make them compatible with current morphological
and physiological methods. Thin slices of neonatal tissue are prepared with a tissue chopper and cultured in plasma clots or on
membrane filters under conditions that foster their thinning still
further. The result truly is remarkable: an organized culture that
faithfully reproduces many features of the architecture and the
pattern of neuronal connections characteristic of the intact nervous
system but that provides accessibility approaching that found in
dissociated-cell cultures.

Finally, glia. In chapter 18, Noble and Mayer-Pröschel provide
methods for culturing astrocytes, oligodendrocytes, and O-2A progenitor cells from both neonatal and adult rats. Studies of O-2A
progenitor cells, which give rise to two mature glial populations in
culture, have provided remarkable insights into the intracellular
signals that regulate the proliferation and differentiation of a precursor cell population. These authors describe the methods for cell
culture and cell purification that have permitted these advances. In

addition, they describe the use of oligodendrocyte cultures as a model for studying cytotoxin-mediated cell death, focusing particularly on the protective effects of trophins and antioxidants.

Chapter 19 by Kleitman et al. represents a tour de force, pushing present techniques for dissociated-cell culture to their limits. The goal of their work is to investigate the cell interactions involved in myelination. The authors first describe methods for preparing purified cultures of Schwann cells and of oligodendrocytes, based on the use of antimitotic agents to kill unwanted nonneuronal cells, augmented in some cases by complement-mediated lysis- or fluorescence-activated cell sorting. They also describe cultures of dorsal root ganglion neurons that give rise to an outgrowth zone consisting entirely of axons and completely free of nonneuronal cells. Finally, they describe conditions that permit the formation of myelin when purified populations of myelin-forming glial cells and axons are combined. In addition to the methods themselves, this chapter provides an excellent account of the contributions that cell culture has made to our understanding of the cell-cell interactions that regulate myelination.

6 Culture and Experimental Use of the PC12 Rat Pheochromocytoma Cell Line

Lloyd A. Greene, Stephen E. Farinelli, Matthew E. Cunningham, and David S. Park

The aims of this chapter, which is a revised version of that appearing in the previous edition of this book, remain largely the same: to provide technical guidance for those who wish to establish and exploit PC12 cell cultures in their own laboratories and to serve as a troubleshooting manual for those who already work with these cells but are experiencing difficulties. In many instances, the methodological details remain largely unchanged from the previous version, though in others we have included additional, improved, or updated information. A number of previous reviews consider the culture and use of PC12 cells (Greene and Tischler, 1982; Guroff, 1985; Greene et al., 1987; Greene and Rukenstein, 1989; Halegoua et al., 1991; Shafer, 1991; Teng and Greene, 1994), and the reader is referred to these for additional detail.

The PC12 cell line was cloned in 1976 (Greene and Tischler, 1976) from a transplantable rat pheochromocytoma (Warren and Chute, 1972). The original tumor appeared in an X-irradiated male New England Deaconess Hospital–strain rat. The characteristic features of the PC12 cell line have been reviewed (Greene and Tischler, 1982; Guroff, 1985; Shafer, 1991), but a brief account thereof underscores the reasons for the widespread experimental use of these cells.

In general, PC12 cells exhibit many of the phenotypical properties associated with pheochromocytoma cells and their nonneoplastic counterparts, adrenal chromaffin cells. For instance, they synthesize, store, release (in response to typical secretagogues and depolarizing agents), and take up considerable levels of catecholamines (Greene and Rein, 1977). Thus, they have served as a major model for elucidating the molecular mechanisms underlying each of these events. The PC12 line also manifests many features of sympathicoblasts, the cells that give rise to postmitotic sympathetic neurons. Of particular importance, PC12 cells respond to nerve growth factor (NGF) and, in its presence, undergo a dramatic change in phenotype wherein they acquire many of the properties characteristic of sympathetic neurons. Among the salient responses

to NGF are cessation of proliferation, generation of long neurites, the appearance of electrical excitability, hypertrophy, and a number of changes in composition associated with acquisition of a neuronal phenotype. These features have promoted a large number of studies dedicated, in particular, to uncovering the mechanism of action of NGF and, in general, to unraveling the molecular mechanisms by which neuroblasts differentiate into mature, postmitotic neurons (for review see Greene, 1984; Aletta et al., 1990; Halegoua et al., 1991; Levi and Alemá, 1991; Kaplan and Stephens, 1994). The revelation that NGF also may serve, as it does in the case of neurons, as a survival factor for PC12 cells in serum-free medium (Greene, 1978) has propelled further the use of the line to study mechanisms for the promotion and prevention of neuronal apoptotic cell death (Rukenstein et al., 1991; Pittman et al., 1993).

The last 20 years have seen an ever-increasing use of PC12 cells to approach a number of fundamental problems related to neuronal cell differentiation and function. This widespread utility of the line is attributable in part to its relative stability, homogeneity, high degree of differentiation and of differentiative capacity, robust response to NGF and dramatic change in phenotype brought about by this factor, fidelity to many of the features of normal neuroblasts and neurons, potential for genetic manipulation and the accrual of a large number of studies regarding its characterization. It is well beyond the scope of this chapter to review the many applications of the PC12 line. These can be ascertained from the past reviews cited earlier and by perusal of the abundant past and present literature on this subject (which now includes more than 4000 papers). Most likely, the reader has been drawn to this account with an idea already in mind for exploitation of the PC12 line and, as expressed earlier, this chapter is designed to aid in its implementation.

For those considering the PC12 cell line for their studies, it is appropriate at this point to consider some of the limitations of this system. First, PC12 cells are tumor-derived and, therefore, by definition must differ from nontransformed cells in their behavior. In this respect, it is interesting that the defects responsible for their transformed phenotype have yet to be revealed. Second, despite their attractiveness and utility for studying neuronal differentiation, PC12 cells cannot be taken as an exact model of developing neurons. In certain respects, they are less than perfect counterparts even for chromaffin cells and sympathetic neurons. For example, there is no evidence that they are capable of receiving or forming

synaptic connections or that they form dendrites. Thus, in light of these realities; it is paramount to consider that the line should be used only as a starting point for investigations and that findings made with it ultimately must be verified with primary tissues.

A third issue stems from stability and variation of the line. As do all proliferating cells, PC12 cells undergo spontaneous mutations and the consequent production of variants. This opens the potential for the population to become heterogeneous. Even more serious is the possible selection of subpopulations significantly different from the wild type. This can lead to loss of phenotypically interesting properties and to significant variation of the cells (and, therefore, of experimental observations) from one laboratory to another. Although such changes over time are inevitable, one aim of this article is to advocate adherence to a set of standardized culture practices for the line which we feel minimize variation and maximize the propagation of a stable phenotype.

Routine Culture of PC12 Cells

Culture Medium for Cell Growth

The culture medium recommended for propagating and maintaining PC12 cells consists of 85% RPMI 1640 medium (available from Gibco/BRL, Gaithersburg, MD, and many other suppliers in either powdered or liquid form), 10% horse serum (heat inactivated at 56° for 30 min), 5% fetal bovine serum, 25 units/ml penicillin, and 25 µg/ml streptomycin (Greene and Tischler, 1976). Pretesting of horse serum batches is prudent, as not all are satisfactory for optimal cell growth and maintenance. At present, consistently good results have been obtained with "donor" horse serum purchased from JRH Biosciences (Lenexa, KS). With respect to horse serum from JRH, it has come to our attention that two separate herds are maintained and that the one used to supply American laboratories west of the Mississippi is composed of geldings. This will, of course, affect the composition of the serum, especially with respect to hormone content. Therefore, it may be prudent to inquire regarding the source of supply and to request serum from unaltered animals.

If necessary, PC12 cells can be adapted to grow in Dulbecco's modified Eagle's medium (DMEM) supplemented as previously outlined. The adaptation is more successful if carried out in stages

with intermediate mixtures of the two media. Also, although the cells may be maintained for up to several weeks with medium containing horse serum alone, it has been our experience that continued propagation of the line requires supplementation with fetal bovine serum.

Although we do not routinely add an antifungal agent to the medium, PC12 cells will tolerate fungizone at 2.5 μg/ml. Also, in cases of bacterial infections that escape the penicillin and streptomycin present in the medium, treatment with 50 μg/ml of gentamycin generally has proved to be effective. However, usually it is advisable to discard infected cultures.

Culture Substrate

PC12 cells adhere poorly to tissue-culture plastic. Although it is possible to propagate these cells on such a surface, nonadherent cells are lost over time, and there is the inevitable selection of a plastic-adherent subpopulation. Cells selected in this manner may prove to be rather different from the original wild-type population. Therefore, it is recommended strongly that maintenance of stock cultures occur on an adhesive coating to which all the cells attach well. Another advantage of growing the cells on a substrate to which they adhere tightly is that monolayers can be washed repeatedly during experimental manipulations. This provides a rapid means to change culture medium and to remove extracellular material without resorting to detachment of the cells or to centrifugation.

COLLAGEN

The most useful and cost-effective coating for plastic culture dishes used for PC12 cell culture has proved to be rat tail collagen. It either may be purchased from commercial sources (e.g., Boehringer Mannheim, catalog no. 1 179 179 or Sigma Biochemicals, catalog no. C 7661) or may be prepared in the laboratory. We prefer the latter route because of cost and the advantage of preparing a large stock that, once characterized, may be used over a long period. The preparation and application of this reagent is described in box 6.1.

ALTERNATIVE COATINGS FOR PLASTIC DISHES

There are several alternative substrates that may be used to maintain PC12 cells. "Matrigel," a commercially available preparation of extracellular matrix (Collaborative Research, Inc.) provides an

Box 6.1 Preparation and Application of Collagen

A. Preparation of Rat Tail Collagen Stock

Collagen stock is prepared from adult rat tails by modifications of the procedure of Bornstein (1958). The tails (freshly collected or stored until use at −20°C) are sterilized in 70% ethanol for 20 min and are rinsed in sterile, distilled water. Starting at the tips, sections of the tails (approximately 1 inch in length each) are progressively "broken" off with the use of sterilized hemostats or needle-nose pliers. As each piece is detached from the tail, sections of tendon also are pulled free. They are cut from the tail sections, rinsed in sterile distilled water, and minced. After harvest, the tendons are transferred to a sterile vessel containing a sterile solution of 0.1% glacial acetic acid. The collagen is extracted overnight at room temperature, then for another 2–3 days at 4° with occasional swirling. The resulting solution should be somewhat viscous but pourable. The extraction volume averages 50–200 ml per tail, with adjustments made as necessary to achieve a workable viscosity. After extraction, the solution is transferred to sterile centrifuge bottles and is centrifuged at approximately $12,000 \times g$ for 1 h at 4° to remove insoluble material. The supernatant is collected (with care to avoid admixing particulate material present in the viscous pellet) and is stored at −20° in aliquots. Once thawed, the stock collagen solutions are refrigerated and stored for up to several months. Care is taken at all stages to maintain sterility; hence, no further sterilization procedures are required. Once prepared, the collagen stock solution is too viscous to be filtered. Moreover, we find that sterilization of collagen-coated dishes by ultraviolet irradiation is inadvisable, as the cells do not show satisfactory adherence to the substrate after such treatment.

B. Coating of Plastic Tissue-Culture Dishes with Collagen

Because of the need to coat the surface of culture vessels, for routine purposes, PC12 cells are grown in plastic cell-culture dishes. There are several means of applying the collagen to these dishes. One is to dilute the collagen stock into sterile water or into sterile 30% ethanol, to add the mixture to the dishes, and to allow it to air-dry overnight within the open dishes in a tissue-culture hood. The volumes used are 0.5 ml per well in 24-well dishes, 1 ml per 35-mm dish, 5 ml per 100-mm dish, and 10 ml per 150-mm dish. The 30% ethanol hastens drying. Alternatively, the collagen (freshly diluted into sterile water) can be added in more concentrated form and in a smaller volume (100 µl per well in 24-well dishes, 200 µl per 35-mm dish, 1 ml per 100-mm dish, and 2 ml per 150-mm dish) and can be used to coat the bottom of the dish by means of a spreader. The latter can be prepared by sealing the nozzle of a Pasteur pipette and bending it into an L shape within 1–3 cm from the tip. Collagen applied in this manner is permitted to air-dry in a culture hood. Generally, this procedure requires 1–2 h. For either procedure, it is important to control the amount of collagen applied, as both adhesion and neurite outgrowth by PC12 cells are influenced by the collagen concentration on the dish. With insufficient collagen, attachment of both cell bodies and neurites is poor. With too much collagen, proliferation is slowed, and neurite outgrowth in response to NGF is retarded and sparse. Therefore, it is necessary to pretest stock collagen batches by applying various dilutions (differing by factors of 2) to the dishes as described earlier, then seeding cells and monitoring them for

Box 6.1 (continued)

satisfactory behavior (i.e., growth and NGF-promoted neurite outgrowth). Typically, on the basis of using the preparation volumes suggested, a 1:50 dilution of stock solution suffices for the overnight procedure, and a 1:10 dilution suffices for the "quick" procedure. For rat tail collagen from commercial sources, a final concentration of 1–10 µg/cm² is a good range at which to start testing. Once prepared, the collagen-coated dishes are stored closed for up to approximately 1 week. Beyond this time, the adhesive properties of the substrate appear to diminish progressively.

excellent substrate for proliferation and neurite outgrowth. The material provided by the supplier can be applied as follows. The stock solution (stored at 4°) is diluted with ice-cold, sterile distilled water at 1:50, and the chilled diluant is added to culture dishes (1 ml per 35-mm dish or 5 ml per 100-mm dish). The dishes are incubated at room temperature for at least 2 h, after which time the Matrigel solution is removed and discarded. The coated dishes then may be used for culture without further manipulation. Despite its excellent qualities, there are two disadvantages for the routine use of Matrigel to culture PC12 cells. The first, at least for laboratories using large numbers of cultures, is the high cost of this material. The second is that the matrix itself appears to have effects on PC12 cells. For instance, when cells that have been pretreated (or primed) with NGF are replated on this substrate, they undergo NGF-independent neurite regeneration.

PC12 cells also attach well to substrates coated with polylysine or polyornithine. Tissue-culture dishes can be coated by treatment for 4 h with a 1 mg/ml solution of filter-sterilized poly-L-ornithine hydrobromide (mol wt., 30,000–70,000) or poly-L-lysine hydrobromide (mol. wt. 150,000–300,000) prepared in 150 mM sodium borate buffer, pH 8.4 (Yavin and Yavin, 1974). Then the solution is removed, and the dishes are washed four times with sterile water and are permitted to dry in a sterile hood. Dishes coated in this manner are useful for short-term experiments. However, beginning at approximately 3 days, the cells show decreased adhesion to the plates and eventually detach. This release does not appear to be due to degradation of the substrate, as comparable results occur with the presumably stable D-isomer forms. A more likely cause appears to be the slow, equilibrium-driven loss of the polyornithine and polylysine from the plastic.

COATINGS FOR GLASS

For certain experimental purposes (e.g., immunohistochemistry), it is desirable to maintain PC12 cells on glass rather than on plastic substrates. However, PC12 cells to not attach to glass; therefore, a coating is necessary. Dried collagen tends to peel from glass and, thus, generally is unsuitable in this instance. Alternatives include the use of collagen gels (prepared by coating the glass with a concentrated solution of collagen followed by exposure to ammonium vapor), of Matrigel (applied as described earlier), and of polylysine. The latter is applied by exposing the glass for 1 h to an aqueous, membrane-sterilized solution of poly-L-lysine hydrobromide (50 µg/ml). The glass then is washed four times with sterile water and is air-dried in a culture hood. These coatings permit excellent adherence of PC12 cells and do not interfere with immunofluorescence; however, they also have a drawback of tending to peel from the glass after periods of culture beyond 3–5 days, especially when used with neurite-bearing cells. Therefore, often it is advantageous to pretreat the cells with NGF on a coated plastic substrate, then to passage them onto coated glass whereon they regenerate long neurites rapidly.

General Maintenance of Cultures

The doubling time of PC12 cells is quite long: 2.5 to 4 days. Thus, every effort must be made to encourage their growth but, at the same time, not to introduce conditions that would favor selection of a subpopulation. Cultures are maintained with the complete medium described earlier. Because the cells are grown on a collagen-coated substrate and are removed mechanically from the dishes for subculture (see later), growth is achieved routinely in culture dishes rather than in T-flasks. Optimal proliferation is obtained by feeding the cultures every 2 to 3 days. Only about two-thirds of the medium is exchanged so as to leave a portion of "conditioned" medium to facilitate growth. In adding fresh medium, care should be taken to avoid damaging or tearing the substrate. As noted later, especially in the case of NGF-treated cells, damage to the substrate can lead to its detachment along with the cell monolayer. For these reasons, it is best to add medium along the side of culture dishes rather than directly onto the culture surface. Cultures are maintained at 36 to 37° in a water-saturated atmosphere containing 7.5%

CO_2. Growth also appears to be adequate in atmospheres containing 5 or 10% CO_2.

When the cultures reach confluency, they are subcultured at a ratio of 1:3 to 1:4. This relatively low split ratio reflects the fact that the cells do not proliferate well at low density. Under these conditions, subculturing is carried out every 7 to 10 days. For subculturing, the cells are detached from the substrate by forceful aspiration of the medium (which is not exchanged prior to passage) through a Pasteur or tissue culture pipette. Repeated trituration of the cells before replating decreases the formation of clumps. Despite even vigorous trituration, the cells will tend to adhere to one another and to settle down and grow in clusters or small clumps. Techniques to produce suspensions that are composed mainly of single PC12 cells have been described previously (Green et al., 1986, 1987).

Although they are a relatively stable line, like all dividing cells, PC12 cells undergo spontaneous mutations. For instance, as in other systems, spontaneous mutations in the PC12 cell HGPRTase (hypoxanthine-guanine phosphoribosyl transferase) gene occur at a frequency of approximately 1 in 10^6 (Green et al., 1986). Other naturally occurring variants that have been reported include cells that have a defective protein kinase A activity (Van Buskirk et al., 1985), cells that respond to NGF purely as a mitogen (Burstein and Greene, 1982), and a number of relatively undifferentiated cells with a "flat" phenotype that adhere well to tissue-culture plastic (Leonard et al., 1987). Therefore, it is prudent to take certain precautions to insure the stability and homogeneity of the cell population. For instance, it is very important to avoid any culture conditions that might favor the selective growth of any altered subpopulation. As noted earlier, the cells should be grown on a substrate such as collagen so as not to select for a variant subpopulation that is more adherent to tissue-culture plastic than are the wild-type cells. It is recommended also that the other culture conditions previously described (medium and serum types and concentrations, feeding schedule, subculture routine, etc.) be followed as closely as possible to standardize the phenotypical properties of PC12 cell cultures from laboratory to laboratory. Finally, although no systematic changes have been noted in the population after extended subculturing (i.e., approximately 100 passages), it is suggested that frozen stocks be maintained of cells at the earliest passages available and that these be used to replace ongoing cul-

tures that have been carried beyond 50 to 60 passages. In our laboratory, most experiments are carried out with cultures of passage numbers 20 to 50.

Availability of PC12 Cell Stock Cultures

PC12 cells originally were distributed by the Greene and Tischler laboratories, and these remain sources for obtaining starter cultures. The cells now are dispersed widely and are cultured routinely in many laboratories that are, therefore, also a potential sources of new stock cultures. Because certain laboratories have altered the conditions of culture from those originally described and recommended, it is important to evaluate the properties of so called PC12 cells when received to insure that phenotypically they resemble the original population. For instance, the population should show a vigorous NGF response and should exhibit minimal morphological heterogeneity. The American *Type Culture* Collection also distributes supposed PC12 cells, but several personal communications have informed us that they vary significantly from the wild-type line. PC12 cells also are maintained and distributed by the Japanese Cell Repository Bank in Japan.

Preparation and Storage of Frozen PC12 Cells

Like many cultured lines, PC12 cells may be stored for long periods in a frozen state. The cells are detached from culture dishes, harvested by centrifugation, and suspended in complete medium supplemented with 10% dimethyl sulfoxide (DMSO). The cell suspension then is aliquoted into plastic cryovials (available from most biological supply companies) and is chilled on ice. The cells are slow-frozen to at least −60° at a rate of approximately −1° per min. This can be achieved with dedicated devices manufactured for this purpose or with special attachments to liquid nitrogen containers. Alternatively and more economically, the chilled cell-containing vials (containing approximately 1 ml of cell suspension) may be placed overnight in a freezer maintained at −70° to −80°. Though less controlled, the latter technique has yielded consistently satisfactory results. The frozen cells may be stored for up to 6 months at −70° to −80°. For long-term storage with good recovery, it is recommended that storage be in liquid nitrogen. Care must be taken that the frozen cells do not warm to above −60° during

transfer from the freezer to liquid nitrogen; therefore, this is done best by holding the cells on dry ice between transit from the freezer to liquid nitrogen. To reculture the frozen cells, they are quick-thawed at 37° in a water bath, centrifuged, resuspended in complete medium without DMSO, and plated onto collagen-coated dishes. Because PC12 cells grow best when not at too low a density, generally, they are frozen and replated after thawing at a split ratio equivalent to no less than one-third of a confluent dish.

Generation of Neurite-Bearing PC12 Cell Cultures: Treatment with NGF

Neurite Generation

For ensuring optimal production of neurite-bearing PC12 cells, several parameters merit attention. The first is cell density. At too high a density, neurite outgrowth is inhibited (Greene et al., 1982); at too low a cell density, the cells do not survive well. Empirical studies have shown a density of approximately 2.5 to 10×10^4 cells per cm^2 to be satisfactory. The second consideration is substrate. NGF treatment decreases the adherence of PC12 cells to tissue-culture plastic, and thus, a suitable coating, such as air-dried collagen, as described earlier, is quite necessary. As also previously noted, it is important to titrate the amount of coating applied to the culture plate so that the cells do not detach from the substrate and so that neurite outgrowth is not suppressed. Another related consideration is that care should be taken during feeding or manipulation of the cultures to ensure that the substrate is not damaged. Once the cells extend neurites, they appear to exert a high degree of lateral tension. As a consequence, any tear in the substrate tends to become amplified, so that in short order, the entire monolayer of cells detaches from the culture vessel. To generate neurites, PC12 cells are plated at the aforementioned density in the presence of 50 ng/ml (~ 2 nM) NGF. The latter can be prepared from male mouse submaxillary glands as described in detail by Longo et al. (1989). An alternative is to use recombinant NGF (generally the human form of which is available). Mouse or recombinant human NGF are available from a number of commercial sources (including but by no means limited to Sigma Chemical Co., Collaborative Research, Boehringer Mannheim, Upstate Biotechnology Incorporated, Chemicon). Appeals for donations also may be made to such bio-

tech firms as Genentech, which produces large amounts of recombinant hNGF for clinical trials. The NGF is stored as a stock in pH 5 sodium acetate buffer (0.1 M) at a concentration of at least 250 μg/ml and is diluted into medium just before use. Stock solutions can be stored at −80° but should not be refrozen once thawed. Alternatively, aliquots of stock NGF can be stored in polystyrene tubes for at least 6 months at 4°. However, once diluted into culture medium, NGF should be used within the same day. It should be noted also that NGF tends to stick to a variety of surfaces (particularly to glass); therefore, it is recommended that culture medium be mixed with NGF in plastic (preferably polystyrene) rather than in glass containers.

PC12 cells can be exposed to NGF in complete growth medium (containing 15% serum), in medium containing 1% horse serum, or in medium without serum. Advantages of the latter two conditions are that there is less clumping of the cells and that there is a cost saving for serum. Also, if the cultures include any cells resistant to the antiproliferative actions of NGF, the low serum retards their growth. We have not detected any effects of using 1% or no serum on the biochemical characteristics of the cells.

Under the usual conditions, PC12 cells generate neurites relatively slowly. Processes begin to appear within 1 to 2 days of NGF treatment and by only approximately a week or so do most of the cells possess neurites (Greene and Tischler, 1976; 1982). On a collagen-coated substrate, neurite elongation proceeds at an average rate of approximately 50 μm/day for at least 10 days. By 2 weeks of NGF exposure, the cultures generate a dense mat of neuritic processes. Generally, at least 90% to 95% of the cells in the cultures produce neurites. Figure 6.1 illustrates the morphology of PC12 cells before and after 10 days of exposure to NGF. The maintenance of neurites at all stages of treatment requires the continued presence of NGF. If the factor is withdrawn, the neurites either will retract or will degenerate, and within about a week, the cells will resume proliferation.

Neurite Regeneration by Primed PC12 Cells

In some instances (e.g., the bioassay of NGF; see Greene and Rukenstein, 1989 for experimental details) and for studies of neurite regeneration, it is desirable to have rapid production of processes. This process can be achieved by pretreating PC12 cells with

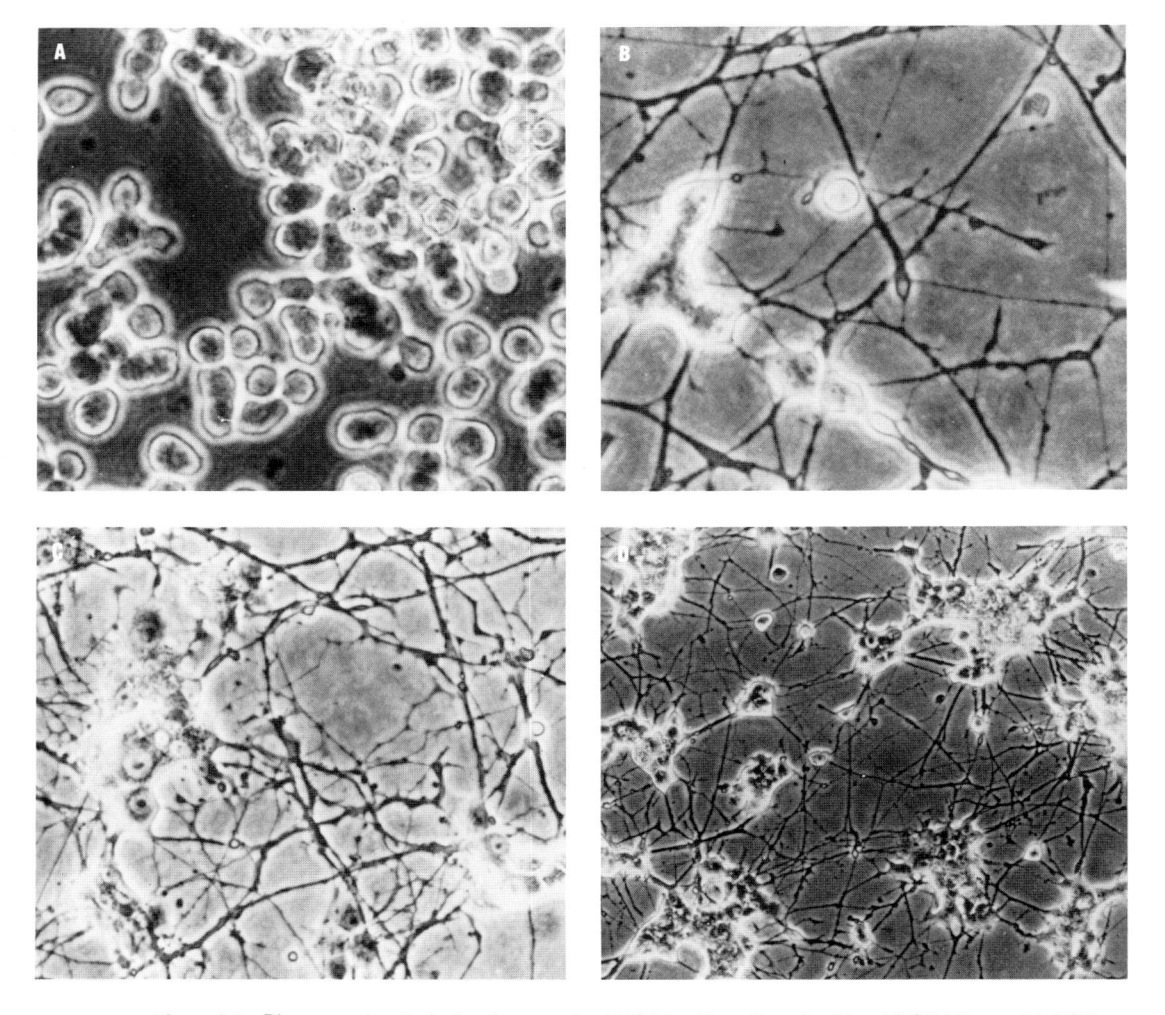

Figure 6.1 Phase-contrast photomicrograph of PC12 cells cultured without NGF (*A*) or with NGF for 9 (*B*, *D*) or 14 (*C*) days. Magnification: *A*, x625; *B* x625; *C*, x390; *D*, x195.

NGF so that they become what we have termed *primed* (Greene et al., 1982). In contrast to "naive" PC12 cells (i.e., those without NGF pretreatment), primed cells will regenerate neurites rapidly when replated. Priming and regeneration are carried out as follows. Cultures are pretreated with NGF for at least a week (i.e., primed) as described earlier. The cells are divested of their neurites and removed from the culture dish by forceful trituration of medium through a Pasteur pipette. Debris, including detached neurites, is removed by centrifuging the cells at low speed (approximately 800 rpm [ca. 125 × *g*]) in a table-top centrifuge for 5 min) and dis-

carding the supernatant. The cells are resuspended in medium with NGF and seeded onto fresh plates. Thus manipulated, the cells regrow new neurites within 4 to 16 h and, by 2 to 3 days, have produced an extensive network of processes. Under such conditions, the replated cells tend to form clumps. This formation can be minimized by triturating the cells extensively before replating. This approach is useful also for producing neurite-bearing cells for histochemical procedures. In this case, the cells are replated onto glass coverslips that have been coated with polylysine or Matrigel. PC12 cells that have been pretreated with NGF also maintain their priming in a frozen state for at least 6 months (Rukenstein and Greene, 1983). Thus, if desirable, large numbers of cells may be pretreated with NGF at one time. These may be frozen (in complete growth medium supplemented with 10% DMSO) in aliquots and, when needed, may be thawed and plated with NGF.

Washout and removal of NGF

There arise experimental situations in which it is useful to monitor the effects of NGF withdrawal on PC12 cells. Examples include studies of the effects of NGF on growth cone motility (Seeley and Greene, 1983; Aletta and Greene, 1988) and of the stability of NGF-deprived neurites (Teng and Greene, 1993). Careful removal of NGF is necessary also for bioassays using neurite regeneration by primed cells (Greene and Rukenstein, 1989). Withdrawal can be achieved by washing extensively with NGF-free growth medium. For attached cells, the medium is exchanged four to six times, then twice again after an interval of several hours. Detached cells are washed free of NGF by four repeated cycles of centrifugation and resuspension in fresh medium. Alternatively (and for more stringent removal of active NGF), the cultures can be exposed to an excess of anti-NGF antiserum. The latter can be obtained from a variety of commercial sources, such as Collaborative Research, Inc., Sigma Chemical, and Boehringer Mannheim. If anti-NGF is used, it is important to be certain that it recognizes the NGF of the species of interest. For instance, we find that the current batch of anti-mouse submaxillary NGF polyclonal antiserum sold by Sigma does not cross-react with recombinant human NGF. The foregoing measures reflect the difficulty in removing NGF from cultures, presumably because of its adherence to a variety of surfaces and to cells and because the cells themselves appear to act as reservoirs of the intact factor.

Maintenance in a Defined Medium

For certain types of experiments, it is desirable to maintain the cells in a defined medium (i.e., "defined" with respect to what is added to the cultures; no doubt the cells secrete various additional "undefined" materials into the medium). PC12 cells can be maintained for at least several weeks in RPMI 1640 medium supplemented with 1 to 3 μM insulin (Rukenstein et al., 1991). With insulin, there is some proliferation but no morphological differentiation. Maintenance in serum-free medium with insulin has proved to be particularly useful for experiments in which the presence of serum is a disadvantage. Examples include transfection with DNA and exposure to anti-sense oligonucleotides (Troy et al., 1992). Long-term cell maintenance also can be achieved with RPMI 1640 medium supplemented with NGF (Greene, 1978). Under such conditions, PC12 cells undergo neurite outgrowth. In comparison with cells exposed to NGF in the presence of serum, there is considerably less formation of clumps, and the neurites show less fasciculation. Although insulin-supplemented RPMI 1640 will sustain PC12 cells for at least several weeks, to our knowledge, conditions suitable for continuous culture of these cells in a defined medium have not been described. Defined media such as N2 contain high levels of insulin and, in our experience, maintain PC12 cells to the same degree as does insulin-supplemented RPMI 1640.

Use for Cell Death and Survival Experiments

The observations that PC12 cells rapidly die when deprived of serum and, under such circumstances, can be rescued from death by NGF has led to the use of this line for studies of the mechanisms by which trophic factors maintain neural cell survival and by which neural cells die when deprived of trophic support (Rukenstein et al., 1991; Batistatou and Greene, 1993; Pittman et al., 1993; Ferrari and Greene, 1994). It is significant that such studies can be carried out both with naive and NGF-primed PC12 cells.

A key factor in naive PC12 cell-death studies is the stringent removal of serum. This is first achieved by washing the cells five times with serum-free medium when attached to the culture dish. The cells then are removed by trituration and washed another four or five times with serum-free medium by repeated cycles of low-speed centrifugation (800 rpm on a table-top centrifuge for 5 min at

room temperature) and by resuspension. It should be noted that as the cells are brought to a serum-free state, the resultant pellet becomes progressively looser and more difficult to handle without disruption. After this extensive washing, the cells are resuspended in serum-free medium and are plated at low density. The use of low-density cultures is a key factor also in assuring rapid cell death. We find the use of collagen-coated 24-well culture dishes to be the most convenient for survival studies. In this case, the cells are plated at a density of 100,000 per well in 0.5 ml of medium. Under these circumstances, approximately 50% to 70% of the cells die within 24 h of plating, and DNA fragmentation associated with apoptosis is detectable within 3 h (Batistatou and Greene, 1993). Essentially, all the cells die by 3 days of serum-deprivation. To carry out survival studies, NGF or other agents are added at the time of plating. With NGF, essentially all cells survive for at least 7 to 10 days. A Matrigel-coated substrate is not recommended for such experiments, as cell death appears to be retarded substantially for cells plated on this material.

For studies with primed PC12 cells, the foregoing procedures are used to remove both NGF and serum. In this case, cell death is somewhat slower than that with naive cells, with 25% to 50% dead at 24 h. Otherwise, the same procedures are used.

Counting PC12 Cells

For a variety of experiments, it is necessary to have an accurate assessment of PC12 cell numbers. Because PC12 cells form clump, potentially large errors occur when one attempts to count them in the living state, even after extensive trituration. We find that there also are problems in quantification associated with the use of metabolizable chromophores such as MTT (3-[4,5-dimethylthiazol-2yl]-2,5-diphenyltetrazolium bromide). In such cases, we have noted that the amount of dye metabolized per cell may change if the cultures are stimulated with growth factors or other agents. When cells are treated with NGF, the problem is compounded, as NGF increases both overall metabolic activity and cell volume. We have found that the most accurate assessment of cell number is achieved by dissolving the cells in the detergent-containing solution described in box 6.2 and counting intact nuclei in a hemocytometer under phase-contrast optics. Under these conditions, the

Box 6.2 Assessment of Cell Number

A. Procedure for Counting Nuclei

To count attached cells, remove medium and replace with working counting solution. The amount of solution used will depend on cell number; Generally, it is useful to aim at a final cell concentration on the order of 500,000/ml. Incubate for at least 2 min at room temperature, then suspend and mix the cells by trituration. Use care to avoid excessive foaming of the detergent-containing solution. Remove an aliquot for counting in the hemocytometer. If necessary, an intermediate dilution can be made with the working counting solution. To count cells in suspension or those that have been removed from a dish, centrifuge an aliquot at low speed, resuspend in the working counting solution, and count as previously outlined. The nuclei appear to be quite stable in the counting solution and, if cell counts cannot be carried out on the same day, the solution of nuclei can be sealed to avoid evaporation of the lysis solution, refrigerated, and counted the following day.

B. Counting solutions (as described by Soto and Sonnenschein, 1985)

STOCK SOLUTION

5 g of ethylhexadecyldimethylammonium bromide (Eastman Kodak) and 0.165 g NaCl are dissolved in 80 ml of purified water. Then, 2.8 ml of glacial acetic acid is added, and the solution is brought to 100 ml and sterile-filtered. The solution may be stored at room temperature.

WORKING COUNTING SOLUTION

To prepare 100 ml, mix 10 ml of phosphate-buffered saline (PBS), 5 ml 10% Triton X-100, 200 µl 1 M $MgCl_2$, 10 ml of counting solution stock, and 74.8 ml purified water. The filter-sterilized solution may be stored for at least 6 months at room temperature.

nuclei of healthy cells show a clearly defined limiting membrane, and one or more nucleoli often are discernible. The nuclei also are homogeneous in distribution, and nearly all are unclumped.

Genetic Manipulation of PC12 Cells

One of the major potential assets of a cell line is that new genes can be introduced into it and that cells modified in this way then can be propagated as permanent lines. With the advent of new technologies and the growth in the number of genes that have been cloned, it has become routinely feasible to carry out genetic manipulation of PC12 cells. Both transient and permanently modified PC12 cells have been used for a number of studies of neuronal function. Several

examples serve to illustrate the utility and power of this approach. In one set of studies PC12 cells lacking Trk NGF receptors were transfected with a series of mutant Trk constructs. Permanent lines expressing these mutant receptors were generated and analyzed both for signaling capacities and for a variety of biological responses to NGF. In this way, it has been possible to map the domains of Trk NGF receptors responsible for activation of specific signaling pathways and to identify those pathways that are required for particular biological responses to NGF (see Greene and Kaplan, 1995 for review). A second example has been the use of both permanent and transient PC12 cell transfectants to analyze various components of the *ras* signaling pathway for their role in NGF-promoted neurite outgrowth (reviewed by Marshall, 1995). A final example involves the transient transfection of neuronally differentiated PC12 cells to demonstrate the required involvement of the Jun kinase-p38 MAP kinases in apoptosis induced by NGF withdrawal (Xia et al., 1995).

General Approaches

We have employed two general strategies to introduce new genes into PC12 cells: transfection with DNA and viral infection. The transfection approach begins with insertion of the DNA of interest into an appropriate plasmid vector and then introduction of the plasmid into cells via several possible transfection protocols. The choice of plasmids and transfection procedures appropriate for PC12 cells are discussed later. PC12 cells that take up the plasmid can express transiently the gene product of interest. Over time, most such cells lose the plasmid but, if allowed to proliferate, a small proportion of the cells randomly integrate the plasmid into their genome. By employing selectable markers that integrate along with the gene of interest, eventually one can select stable cell lines that express the inserted gene.

Presently, retroviruses are the most convenient viral vectors available for introducing new genes into PC12 cells. This approach begins with insertion of the gene of interest into a retroviral vector that then is introduced into a packaging cell line to produce infective virions. The virions are used to infect PC12 cells and, as the cells divide, the proviral DNA containing the gene of interest integrates into the host genome. By selecting cells that integrate a selectable marker also present in the proviral DNA, one can produce stable lines expressing the gene of interest.

There are certain advantages and disadvantages to each approach. The advantages of transfection include the relative ease with which plasmids may be produced. DNA, in contrast to retroviruses, also is quite stable. In addition, because the transfected DNA need not integrate into the host genome to be transcribed, transient transfections are possible both for replicating and nonreplicating (neuronally differentiated) PC12 cells. Generally, this function has not been possible with retroviruses. Although it takes considerably more time and effort to engineer and produce retroviral virions than to prepare transfection plasmids, this approach also has advantages. It has been our experience that in the production of stable PC12 cell lines, retroviral infection produces an effiency at least an order of magnitude higher and that infected cells show a higher range of expression than those obtained by transfection. Moreover, in contrast to lines obtained by transfection, at least 90% of those generated by retroviral infection express the exogenous gene of interest. Also, once the retroviruses are produced, the actual mechanics of infection are far easier than those for transfection.

Despite the experimental allure of introducing new genes into PC12 cells, it should be emphasized that the existing techniques still leave much to be desired. First, relative to results achieved with many other cell lines, present methods have a very low efficiency for both transient transfection and permanent transfection-infection. A partial solution in the near future is likely to be the development of suitable adenovirus vectors that will permit high-efficiency transient infection and gene expression in both replicating and nondividing, neuronally differentiated PC12 cells (J. Kitajewski, personal communication).

A second issue is that PC12 cells may decrease or lose expression of the transfected-infected gene over time. In our experience, the extent to which this occurs varies greatly from one line to the next. Some lines have been highly stable for many generations, whereas others may lose expression of the transgene within several passages. Thus, expression levels of the introduced gene should be monitored in each experiment.

A third issue is that it would be highly desirable to introduce genes into PC12 cells that are expressed from tightly inducible promoters. In this way, the same line could be compared before and after expression of the tranfected-infected gene. At present, the most widely used induction system in PC12 cells is the mouse mammary tumor virus promoter. Although this system certainly

has been useful (see Guerrero et al., 1986), its drawback is that there is a background level of expression in the absence of induction and that the inducing agent (dexamethasone) itself has considerable effects on PC12 cells (see Leonard et al., 1987). Although beyond the scope of this review to elaborate, several additional strategies for inducing transfected genes in PC12 cells are being evaluated in a number of laboratories, and it is anticipated that these will be widely available in the near future. One notable example is the inducible Tet-on and Tet-off systems introduced by Gossen and Bujard (1992). Suitable reagents for this approach are sold by Clontech.

In the following sections, we describe transfection and retroviral techniques that can be applied to PC12 cells. As touched on earlier' aspects of these are subject to improvement, and the reader is urged to consult the literature for the latest refinements.

Transfection of PC12 Cells

The PC12 cell line has proved to show relatively low efficiency for both transient and permanent transfection. This limitation possibly is due to their small size, limited amount of cytoplasm, and long doubling time. Nevertheless, with persistance and patience, this approach can be highly successful.

To evaluate various protocols, we have used transient transfections with a plasmid carrying the gene encoding N-*ras*. Various approaches have shown that expression of *ras* oncogenes in PC12 cells induces their morphological differentiation (Bar-Sagi and Feramisco, 1985; Noda et al., 1985). On successful transfection with the N-*ras* construct, PC12 cells extend processes that can be observed 2 days after transfection (Guerrero et al., 1986). As the average doubling time of PC12 cells is greater than this period, a reasonably accurate representation of percentage of transiently transfected cells can be achieved by scoring the cultures for proportion of process-bearing cells. Alternatively, the cells may be transfected with a plasmid containing a β-galactosidase reporter gene. The cells are fixed and developed for β-galactosidase activity (Cepko, 1992) 2 days after transfection. The percentage of blue stained cells then can be scored readily.

Although various promoters have been employed successfully to drive expression of exogenous genes in PC12 cells, we have had the most consistent results with the cytomegalovirus (CMV) promoter. A systematic evaluation of several promoters in the PC12 cell line

also found this to be the most effective of those tested (Muller et al., 1990).

Using the assays previously described, we have had very little success with transient transfections using the DEAE-dextran-mediated gene transfer procedure. We have had the most success in transfecting PC12 cells by using electroporation, lipofection, or calcium phosphate. We observe comparable efficiencies with all three transfection protocols and have used them interchangeably. Lipofection is the easiest but most costly method. The calcium phosphate method is the least costly but appears to be the most sensitive to small variations in protocol and solutions. The important factors in each of these protocols include the state of the cells to be transfected, the quality and purity of the input DNA, and variables specific to each technique. As is the case with other cell types, smaller plasmids are introduced more efficiently into PC12 cells than are larger vectors.

Cells to be transfected should not be confluent, but approximately half to three-quarters confluent. Usually, it is best to replate cells to be transfected on collagen-coated dishes the day before transfection. This technique will enhance survival by ensuring a starting population of healthy, freshly-fed PC12 cells.

Plasmid DNA to be used for transfections can be prepared by the alkaline-lysis method (Maniatis et al., 1982) with two CsCl gradient centrifugations. This ensures that no contaminating bacterial proteins (toxic to eukaryotic cells) are present. Alternatively, the DNA may be purified on a Qiagen plasmid-cosmid purification column using procedures supplied by the manufacturer (Qiagen, Inc.). We have seen no significant difference in transfection efficiency of a β-galactosidase reporter plasmid prepared by either method. Box 6.3 describes three transfection methods.

The electroporation technique results in a considerable degree of cell death. Using the foregoing procedures, we typically achieve 30% cell survival. Of the surviving cells, 2% to 5% are transfected transiently (as evaluated by the use of N-*ras*-evoked process outgrowth).

As previously noted, via the transient transfection assay with the N-*ras*-containing plasmid, an efficiency of approximately 2% to 5% is achieved with Lipofectin. Comparable levels have been achieved with a plasmid encoding the human Trk NGF receptor (Loeb et al., 1991). With Lipofectamine, we have observed a transfection efficiency of approximately 1% with a β-galactosidase reporter

Box 6.3   Transfection of PC12 Cells

A.   Transfection of PC12 Cells by Electroporation

Electroporation devices are sold by several commercial suppliers and have been used to transfect PC12 cells successfully (Andreason and Evans, 1989; Loeb et al., 1991; Loeb and Greene, 1993). We use the BRL Cell-Porator with the following procedure:

1. Triturate cells off dishes and pellet at 500 rpm in a table-top centrifuge at room temperature.
2. Remove medium and resuspend the cells in Ca^{++}, Mg^{++}-free PBS. Centrifuge again as explained earlier and repeat resuspension.
3. Count cells before final centrifugation.
4. Resuspend cells in modified PBS to a density of approximately 1×10^8/ml. This number is equivalent to the population on a confluent 150-mm culture dish. Modified PBS is PBS (containing Ca^{++} and Mg^{++}) supplemented with 1 g/L glucose.
5. Place 1 ml of cell suspension in an electroporation cuvette, add 50–100 µg DNA (in sterile buffer or water in a total volume not to exceed 100 µl), mix by inversion, and incubate on ice for 10 min.
6. Mix by inverting the cuvette gently and incubate in a room-temperature water bath for 1–2 min.
7. Mix the contents by inverting the cuvette before electroporating the cells with 450 V (1125 V/cm) at 330 µF on the low ohm resistance setting. These are the settings for the BRL electroporator device and translate to a 3.7-ms pulse time.
8. Place the cuvette on ice for 30 min to allow cells to recover.
9. Transfer the cells into two 100-mm collagenized tissue culture dishes. Rinse the cuvette with 1.5 ml of room-temperature serum-containing medium and add to the cultures. Add an additional 4 ml of room-temperature complete medium to each dish and place them in a culture incubator.

B.   Transfection of PC12 Cells via Lipofection

An alternative means to achieve transfection of PC12 cells is with Lipofectin or Lipofectamine, commercial products available from BRL. In both techniques, the DNA is bound to a lipid mixture that aids its penetration into cells (Felgner et al., 1987). Use of modifications of protocols provided by the manufacturer has made it possible to obtain transfection efficiencies comparable to those achieved by electroporation but with no significant cell death. The main potential drawback of the procedure is the cost of the lipid reagents (approximately $150 per ml; $15 per transfection of a 100-mm dish). Briefly, the procedure is as follows:

1. One day before transfection, plate approximately $2–3 \times 10^7$ PC12 cells on 100-mm collagen-coated dishes in complete growth medium. (A proportional number of cells may be used with smaller dishes).
2. In serum-free RPMI 1640 medium supplemented with 1 µM insulin, prepare the following solutions in sterile polystyrene tubes (amounts given are for one 100-mm culture dish): 2.5 ml of lipid reagent (containing 100 µg of Lipofectin or Lipofectamine) and 2.5 ml DNA (containing 50 µg

Box 6.3 (continued)

of DNA for Lipofectin; $5 \mu g$ for Lipofectamine). Increased DNA concentrations have minimal effect on the efficiency of Lipofectamine-mediated transfection. Serum-free medium is used to avoid DNAses present in serum, and insulin is used to maintain the cells without serum.

3. Mix the two solutions in a sterile polystyrene test tube and incubate for 10–15 min at room temperature.
4. Wash the cultures to be transfected three times with serum-free RPMI 1640 medium.
5. Add lipid-DNA mix to cells and incubate overnight in a 37° incubator.
6. After overnight incubation, add an equal volume of complete growth medium for experiments using Lipofectin. For those using Lipofectamine, the medium is removed and is replaced with complete growth medium.
7. On the next day, exchange the medium with complete serum-containing medium.

C. Transfection of PC12 Cells by Calcium Phosphate–Mediated Gene transfer

Schweitzer and Kelly (1985) first described the use of this approach to transfect PC12 cells successfully. We have had the best success (comparable to that achieved with Lipofectin and electroporation) with this technique based on the protocols given by Chen and Okayama (1987). The protocol is as follows:

1. Dilute the plasmid DNA (10–30 μg) in 0.5 ml of sterile 0.25 M $CaCl_2$.
2. Add to the plasmid solution 0.5 ml of sterile 2× BES-buffered saline. The latter contains 50 mM N-,N-bis(2-hydroxyethyl)-2-aminoethane-sulfonic acid (BES) at pH 6.95; 280 mM NaCl; and 1.5 mM Na_2HPO_4. Chen and Okayama (1987) stress the importance of adjusting the pH to exactly the value given earlier. If the buffer is prepared ahead of time, it should be stored in frozen aliquots so as to avoid absorption of CO_2 from the atmosphere.
3. Incubate the mixture for 10–20 min at room temperature; then add dropwise with swirling to a 100-mm dish of PC12 cells in 10 ml of complete growth medium. We have achieved no better results by replacing RPMI 1640 with DMEM.
4. Incubate the cultures overnight at 37° in an incubator containing 7.5% CO_2. In their protocol, Chen and Okayama (1987) recommend using 2–4% CO_2 but, in our experience, this does not enhance the efficiency of PC12 cell transfection.
5. The medium is removed, and the cultures are washed and refed with complete growth medium. The calcium phosphate-DNA precipitate that is formed during the procedure can be seen in the microscope and, although it coats the cells and substrate, it appears to do the cells no harm.

vector. However, the efficiency of transfection of N-*ras* with the Lipofectamine reagent has not been determined. There is no apparent toxicity of Lipofectin at the concentrations employed here. Lipofectamine can be slightly toxic to PC12 cells and, accordingly, incubations greater than 14 to 15 h are not recommended. A variety of additional Lipofection reagents have been marketed recently, but we have not systematically evaluated them.

All three methods described in box 6.3 have been used successfully to generate stable PC12 cell transfectants. For this purpose, it is necessary to use a *selectable marker*. This choice may be achieved either by including a selectable marker in the DNA construct used for transfection or by cotransfecting with a separate plasmid containing the selectable marker. As with other cell lines, neomycin resistance has proved to be a useful selectable marker for transfected PC12 cells. When challenged with G418 (a less expensive analog of neomycin) at a concentration of 500 µg/ml, nearly all wild-type PC12 cells die within a week and essentially all (survival, <1 in 10^8) die by 2 weeks. We also have found resistance to hygromycin (300 µM) to be a suitable alternative marker for selection. Before selection is begun, the transfected cultures are maintained for 5 to 7 days in complete growth medium to permit stable integration of the transfected DNA. A period of growth before selection also permits the transfected cells to undergo several divisions so that they exist as small colonies rather than as single cells. This process appears to enhance the probability of survival during the selection process, when most of the cells in the culture are undergoing death.

If neomycin resistance is to be used as the selectable marker, the cultures then are challenged with complete medium supplemented with 500 µg/ml G418 (obtainable from Boehringer-Mannheim or Sigma Chemical). The neomycin stock solution is prepared at 100× in water, sterilized by filtration, and stored at 4°. Generally, the G418 as supplied by the vendor is approximately 50 to 70% pure, and this factor should be considered when preparing the stock solution (e.g., for a final concentration of 500 µg/ml of material that is 50% pure, prepare a 100× stock at 100 mg/ml). During selection, the medium is exchanged every 2 to 3 days. Cell death will begin by the second feeding, and essentially all selection will occur by 10 to 14 days of treatment. After this time, to favor survival and growth of the transfected cells (which are neomycin-resistant), the cultures are fed only once per week and with selection medium

containing 50% fresh medium and 50% medium conditioned by confluent PC12 cultures. This medium should be passed through a 0.45-μm filter to remove any residual cells. The G418 concentration may be lowered to 250 μg/ml. Colonies should begin to appear between 3 to 8 weeks and generally are large enough to subculture by approximately 10 to 12 weeks. It is important to find and mark the locations of incipient colonies as early as possible. As the colonies increase in size, they tend to release "floaters" that form new secondary colonies elsewhere on the plate.

The marking of colonies early ensures that one is dealing with primary, independent transfectants rather than with secondary clones. Marking is achieved by visualizing the colonies at low power on the microscope and circling their locations on the bottom of the plate with a marker. To isolate and propagate the colonies, they are located under a dissection microscope using dark-field illumination and "picked" from the dishes by suction into finely-drawn Pasteur pipettes. A successful alternative technique for picking colonies is the use of a 200-μl micropipetter. The micropipetter is fitted with a sterile yellow tip, and the latter is brought into juxtaposition with the colony with the aid of a dissecting microscope. The colony is dislodged gently from the substrate with the end of the pipette tip and is drawn up with a small quantity of culture medium. The colonies are transferred to 24-well collagen-coated culture dishes. We have recovered 20 to 40 colonies per 100-mm dish by using either electroporation or lipofection.

The number of colonies, however, will vary with the type and quality of DNA introduced into the cell. When the cells become confluent in the wells, they are transferred to 35-mm dishes and, when confluent, to 100-mm dishes. We routinely have employed this approach to generate stable transfectant PC12 cell lines that express constructs of exogenous Trk NGF receptors (Loeb et al., 1994; Stephens et al., 1994). In this case, expression levels of the exogenous gene ranged from 1- to 20-fold that of the endogenous Trk gene. It should be noted that for reasons not well-understood, many of the neomycin-resistant colonies obtained in this approach do not express the gene of interest. This reaction has ranged from 30 to 90% of the isolated colonies. Thus, it is advisable to isolate and screen a number of colonies to ensure generation of the desired cell line.

In interpreting experiments based on genetically modified PC12 cells, it is important to carry out appropriate controls. That is, it is

necessary to establish that any observed changes in phenotype arise from the transfected DNA and are not merely due to the selection of spontaneous variants in the population. Also, there may be a wide variation among transfected clones in the degree to which they express the foreign gene. One control is to select and characterize a number of independent transfectants. A second control is to select and characterize clones that have been transfected independently with an "empty" construct that confers neomycin resistance but that lacks the gene of interest.

Genetic Modification of PC12 Cells by Retroviral Infection

Retroviruses represent an alternative means to produce stable lines of genetically modified PC12 cells. Various packaging systems permit the production of high-titer viral stocks that though infective, cannot replicate in normal cells (Miller and Buttimore, 1986; Miller and Rosman, 1989; Pear et al,. 1993, Pear et al., 1995). Because foreign DNA can be inserted into such viruses, they can be used for gene transfer. Transcription of the foreign gene can be driven either by the viral long-terminal repeat or by a separate promoter. Typically, the CMV promoter provides excellent constitutive expression in PC12 cells. Also, as a part of the retrovirus life cycle involves integration of its provirus form into the host genome, insertional mutagenesis can occur as a result of infection. If the provirus DNA integrates at or near a gene required for the maintenance of a given phenotype and if a means can be found to select for cells deficient in this phenotype, retroviruses can be used to create specific mutants. Further study of the mutant phenotype is facilitated particularly by the fact that the proviral DNA serves as a genetic marker for the affected gene and, therefore, provides a means for its identification during cloning. Additional information regarding the application of this approach to PC12 cells has been reviewed by Lo et al. (1988).

Our laboratory has made use of the replication-defective retroviral vector pLNCX (described by Miller and Rosman, 1989) to introduce foreign genes into PC12 cells. This vector contains a G418 resistance gene as a selectable marker.

Several packaging cell lines for production of retroviruses have been described (Mann et al., 1983; Miller and Buttimore, 1986; Pear et al., 1993). In our laboratory, we have used the Ψ2 packaging system that was produced in (and should be available from) the

Box 6.4   Ψ2 Packaging System

1. Insert the gene of interest behind the CMV promoter in the pLNCX vector.

2. Plate the Ψ2 cells on a 100-mm dish 1 day prior to transfection so that they are 60%–80% confluent on the day of transfection. Use the Ca_2PO_4 method described earlier to transfect the pLNCX vector into the packaging cell line Ψ2. Two days after transfection, select the cells with 500 μg/ml G418 for a period of 7 days. Exchange the selection medium every 2–3 days. After this initial selection period, clones may be selected individually or may be allowed to grow to confluency on the original dish. The packaging cells are maintained in 10% FCS/DMEM as described (Mann et al., 1983; Miller and Buttimore, 1986).

3. At 1–2 days before the infection, plate $1-3 \times 10^7$ of the virus-transfected Ψ2 cells on a 150-mm tissue culture dish and maintain in 11 ml of 10% FCS/DMEM. Because the retroviral vector is replication-defective, a high titer of the virus-containing medium is necessary for successful infection. This result is achieved by ensuring that the packaging cells are at their log phase of growth (usually 80% confluency) and by keeping the volume of the culture medium to a minimum.

4. On the day of infection, remove the virus-containing medium from the Ψ2 cell culture, pass through a 0.45-μm filter, and add Polybrene to a final concentration of 4 μg/ml. The Polybrene may be omitted, but this omission will decrease infection efficiency by at least severalfold. It is important to note that the virus is quite unstable at room temperature and that it should be used for infection as soon as possible after harvesting. Otherwise, the virus-containing medium should be frozen and stored in liquid nitrogen or −80°C. Freezing and thawing, however, does result in a several-fold loss of viral titer.

5. To infect PC12 cells, replace their normal culture medium with the virus-containing medium. As viral integration generally requires the host cell to undergo at least one round of replication, the PC12 cell cultures should be infected in the log, rather than in the stationary, phase of growth.

6. After 3–5 h of incubation at 37°C, supplement the PC12 cells with an equal volume of complete culture medium. Exchange the culture medium the next day with complete growth medium and maintain the cultures for 3–7 days before beginning selection.

7. Selection is carried out with complete growth medium supplemented with 500 μg/ml of G418. At this concentration, 100% cell death occurs in mock-infected cell populations within 2 weeks.

8. Under these procedures, the infection frequency for PC12 cells is approximated 1 in 10^3-10^4. However, it should be noted that a decrease in viral titer frequently is observed when the vector contains foreign genes. Also, to obtain single, isolatable colonies, it is preferable to have a considerably lower frequency of colony formation. This may be achieved by omitting Polybrene and by using diluted virus-containing medium. For instance, without Polybrene and at a dilution of 1:10, the number of colonies that form with viruses carrying a Trk gene is approximately 1 in 10^5 of the original population.

Box 6.4 (continued)

9. The surviving cells are maintained and expanded by means of the pre-viously described techniques for transfection. In contrast to the results for transfection—in which many of the G418 resistant colonies do not express the exogenous gene of interest—more than 90% of those ob-tained by retroviral infection show good expression.

10. As noted earlier for stable transfectants, it is important to select and characterize a number of independent clones of infected cells and to compare these with clones of cells derived by infection with a "blank" vector that lacks the gene of interest.

laboratory of R. C. Mulligan, Whitehead Institute, Massachusetts Institute of Technology. This packaging line requires stable inte-gration of the retroviral vector into the packaging genome and selection of clones to generate a high viral titer sufficient to infect PC12 cells. Typically, pooling of clones that result after selection produces sufficient titer to generate PC12 cell infectants. Higher titer of infectious particles, however, may require selection and evaluation of individual Ψ2 colonies. We have introduced a num-ber of different Trk mutants into PC12 cell lines by using pLNCX produced in Ψ2 cells (Cunningham et al., 1997). With the CMV promoter, we have generated lines expressing 1- to 200-fold the levels of Trk present in wild-type PC12 cells. Although we have had success with this particular packaging system (see box 6.4), the reader should be vigilant for the development of new, more efficient packaging systems that may produce viral stocks more conve-niently. One example is the Bosc system described by Pear et al. (1993, 1996). Protocols for use of the latter for PC12 cell infection have been given recently (Cunningham et al., in press).

Summary and Conclusions

The passage of nearly two decades has seen a continuing increase in use of the PC12 cell line. This chapter has addressed our current (as of Spring, 1995) procedures for culture and exploitation of the line and is intended to assist both those who have not used it previously and those who are well versed in it. As in the past, we advocate the use of standardized conditions not only to optimize the success of experiments but also to ensure the generation of comparable findings from laboratory to laboratory.

Acknowledgments

Portions of the work described here were supported in part by grants from the National Institutes of Health–NIH-NINDS and March of Dimes Birth Defects Foundation.

7 Neuronlike Cells Derived in Culture from P19 Embryonal Carcinoma and Embryonic Stem Cells

Gerard Bain, Min Yao, James E. Huettner, Michael F. A. Finley, and David I. Gottlieb

Cell lines are used widely for studying cell and molecular biology in mammals. From looking at the recent past, it is clear that many fundamental studies of cellular regulation involved cell lines and that the lines were indispensable tools of discovery. Many examples could be cited; perhaps the series of experiments leading to the identification of G proteins stands as a paragon of how creative investigations with cell lines contributed to fundamental advances (Haga et al., 1977; Ross et al., 1978; Northrup et al., 1980). Cell lines already have been instrumental in important studies of neuronal cell biology leading to fundamental advances in the neurobiology of ion channels (Catterall, 1981), trophic factors (see chapter 6), and other fields too numerous to mention. Currently, an extensive effort is underway to develop new cell lines that model an even greater range of neuronal phenotypes than do the lines already in common use. The underlying assumption of this field is that no single cell line possibly can model the diverse cellular properties of the mammalian brain. Instead, a collection of lines will be needed. This chapter focuses on two systems, P19 embryonal carcinoma cells and embryonic stem (ES) cells, in which cell lines derived from early embryonic cells are induced to differentiate into neuronlike cells in culture. Another approach for producing ES-derived cultures highly enriched in neurons and glia has recently been reported (Okabe et al., 1996). To provide a framework for these and other approaches to neuronal cell lines, it is worth considering an outline of early mammalian development and neurogenesis (reviewed in Hogan et al., 1986).

Immediately prior to implantation, the mouse embryo consists of a structure called the *inner cell mass* and several adjacent layers. One and a half days later, soon after the embryo has implanted in the uterine wall, the inner cell mass gives rise to an epithelium termed the *primitive ectoderm*. The primitive ectoderm plays a pivotal role in the future development of the embryo; it is the progenitor of the three primary embryonic layers—ectoderm, mesoderm, and endoderm—that collectively are the source of all tissues

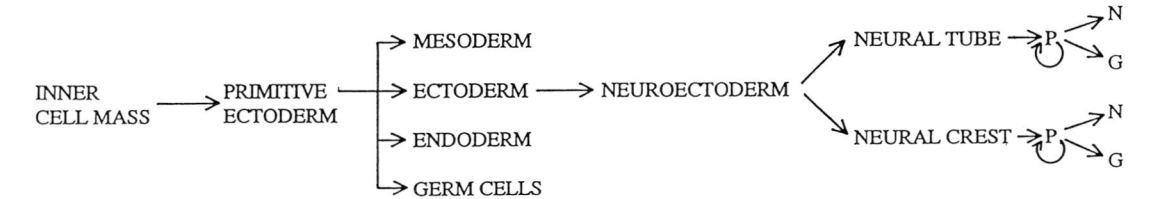

Figure 7.1 Outline of the developmental pathway from the inner cell mass to neurons and glial cells. The lineage leading to neurons and glial cells is shown in full, whereas other lineages are truncated or not shown. P, progenitor cells; N, neurons; G, glial cells. The circular arrows under P indicate that progenitors undergo replication.

of the adult body. The midline ectoderm, under the influence of adjacent mesoderm, becomes the neuroectoderm that folds to form the neural tube. The early neural tube consists predominantly of rapidly dividing progenitor cells. As development proceeds, more and more of the progenitor cells withdraw from the cell cycle and become postmitotic neurons and glia; many of the progenitor cells are multipotential in that they give rise to multiple types of neurons and also to glial cells (reviewed in Sanes, 1989; Walsh and Cepko, 1990; Wetts and Fraser, 1991). The developmental pathway from the inner cell mass to neurons is summarized figure 7.1.

Cell lines are established by isolating a single cell and allowing it to replicate so as to obtain a large number of progeny cells. Cell lines exhibit two basic characteristics that underlie their usefulness. First, the cells can be propagated for many cycles of replication (a property often termed *immortality*), making it possible to obtain large numbers of cells. This distinguishes them from most cells in the normal animal, wherein the number of cell divisions allotted is limited strictly. This limitation carries over to cells cultured directly from tissues that also are constrained to a relatively small number of replication cycles. Second, cell lines possess phenotypes characteristic of their lineage of origin. Even after many generations in culture, they express sets of genes that are strikingly similar to those expressed by the founder cells. How this "cellular memory" is encoded is mysterious. Recent discoveries showing that some transcription factors involved in specifying cell fate are autoregulatory provide an interesting hint of how stable self-perpetuating patterns of gene expression may be set up (Weintraub et al., 1991)

It is highly likely that cell lines can be established only from actively cycling progenitor cells. Establishment of useful cell lines

has two distinct requirements: First, the endogenous machinery that limits cell replication must be overcome; second, the line must express stably the phenotype of the population of progenitor from which it was derived. In the case of neural lineages, a variety of strategies have been effective for establishing cell lines. Most aim at creating lines from cycling progenitor cells in the neural tube or neural crest derivatives.

The field of neuronal cell lines is very large and is still growing; the following is intended to outline the *types* of methods used to obtain lines. (A comprehensive review of this field is beyond the scope of this work.) The simplest strategy is the isolation of naturally occurring tumors. The mouse neuroblastoma C1300 is an outstanding example of this approach (Augusti-Tocco and Sato, 1969; Schubert et al., 1969). A human cerebral cortical tumor also has been used as a source of a cell line with neuronal characteristics (Ronnett et al., 1990). Another useful strategy has been to increase the rate of tumor formation with x-rays or chemical mutagens and to establish differentiated neuronal lines from the resulting tumors. The widely used PC12 line was established from rats exposed to x-rays (Greene and Tischler, 1976). Chemical mutagenesis was used to establish a panel of neuronal and glial cell lines from the rat brain (Schubert et al., 1982). Another widely used strategy is to introduce oncogenes into a specific set of neural precursors and to establish clonal lines in which the ectopically expressed oncogene overcomes the natural limits to cell replication. Parts of the embryonic nervous system are explanted at a time when progenitor cells are still cycling and infected with a retrovirus carrying an oncogene (Geller and Dubois-Dalcq, 1988; Bartlett et al., 1989; Cepko, 1989; Birren et al., 1990; Ryder et al., 1990; Renfranz et al., 1991; Snyder et al., 1992). An advantage of this approach is that a deliberately chosen set of precursor cells can be immortalized. A variant method is to create lines of transgenic mice carrying constructs consisting of a neuronal-specific promoter driving an oncogene. By choosing a promoter used by a subset of neurons, tumors are produced selectively in the corresponding lineage; clonal cell lines then are established from the tumors. Examples of this approach include production of cell lines from the hypothalamus and retina (Mellon et al., 1990; Hammang et al., 1991). A different approach involves the use of cellular hybrids between primary neuronal cells and neural cell lines. This approach was first applied to sympathetic ganglion cells (Greene et al., 1975) and

since has been extended to central nervous system (CNS) neurons (e.g., see Choi et al., 1991). Recently, a new option has become available: clonal expansion of precursor cells from the CNS in tissue culture. This result is achieved by culturing dissociated brain cells in serum-free defined medium with epidermal growth factor. Under these conditions, precursor cells divide without limit but retain the capability of differentiating into neurons and glia (Reynolds and Weiss, 1992). A similar result has been obtained with hippocampal cells (Ray et al., 1993)

Each of these approaches has yielded useful neuronal cell lines. As a result, a set of cell lines now collectively models some of the many known neuronal phenotypes. Here we describe two additional systems in which the lines are derived, not from the developing nervous system but from extremely early embryonic cells at a stage that precedes the formation of the neuroectoderm. These systems significantly extend the range of neuronal development that can be studied with cell lines; their characteristics and potential advantages and limitations are discussed further.

The P19 System

The P19 cell line was isolated by implanting a 7-day-old mouse embryo under the testis capsule of an adult, which resulted in formation of a tumor (McBurney and Rogers, 1982). Tumor cells were grown in culture, and one clone, P19, was established as a line. Although the line's exact origin is unclear, P19 cells have a phenotype similar to cells of the primitive ectoderm (see figure 7.1). P19 cells have a normal karyotype and replicate rapidly and without apparent limit in culture; they express several early embryonic markers. When grafted into a normal early embryo, they colonize the host and join multiple cell lineages, showing that they have a broad developmental potential (Rossant and McBurney, 1982). The ability of these cells to differentiate along multiple pathways, particularly neuronal, cardiac muscle, and skeletal muscle, also is expressed in tissue culture (Jones-Villeneuve et al., 1982; McBurney et al., 1982).

P19 cells can be induced efficiently to differentiate along a neural lineage in culture (Jones-Villeneuve and McBurney, 1982; Levine and Flynn, 1986; McBurney et al., 1988; reviewed in Bain et al., 1994). To induce the neuronal pathway, stem cells are cultured in a

nonadhesive dish wherein they form aggregates; exposure of the aggregates to retinoic acid (RA) for 4 days results in a population that, when plated on an adhesive substrate, differentiates into predominantly neuronlike and glialike cells. As described further, the neuronlike cells have many basic phenotypes of normal neurons, and most studies on the P19 system refer to them as neurons. We prefer caution and refer to them as neuronlike cells (NLCs). Morphologically, NLCs have small cell bodies that give off multiple processes with a striking resemblance to the neurites seen in primary cell culture. The processes are segregated into separate axonal and dendritic compartments (Finley et al., 1995, 1996). NLCs are permanently postmitotic and electrically excitable, expressing strong inward and outward currents that generate action potentials. They express many of the marker proteins usually associated with neuronal differentiation (figure 7.2). A limitation of many widely used cell lines is that they do not express GABAergic or glutaminergic phenotypes. This limitation is crucial, because GABAergic and glutaminergic synapses are the most prevalent types in the CNS. In contrast, P19 NLCs strongly express GAD_{65} and GAD_{67}, the two genes that encode glutamic acid decarboxylase, and also have functional GABA receptors (Bain et al., 1993; Reynolds et al., 1994; Staines et al., 1994). They also express NMDA and kainate/AMPA type glutamate receptors (Turetsky et al., 1994). Synapse formation is perhaps the single most definitive property of neurons as opposed to other cell types. NLCs make synapses as demonstrated morphologically (McBurney et al., 1988) and physiologically (Finley et al., 1995, 1996). Finally, the pathway by which P19 stem cells differentiate into NLCs (reviewed in Bain et al., 1994) bears a striking resemblance to the pathway used by normal neural precursor cells in that genes are expressed roughly in the same order as that occurring in vivo.

In Vitro Differentiation of ES Cells into Neuronlike Cells

ES cells are clonal cell lines derived from the 4-day mouse embryo (Evans and Kaufman, 1981; Martin, 1981) and having biological properties similar to cells of the inner cell mass and primitive ectoderm (see figure 7.1). ES cells have three properties that, in combination, make them invaluable tools for the analysis of genetics and development. First, they replicate indefinitely in tissue culture (Suda et al., 1987). This ability is a natural property of the

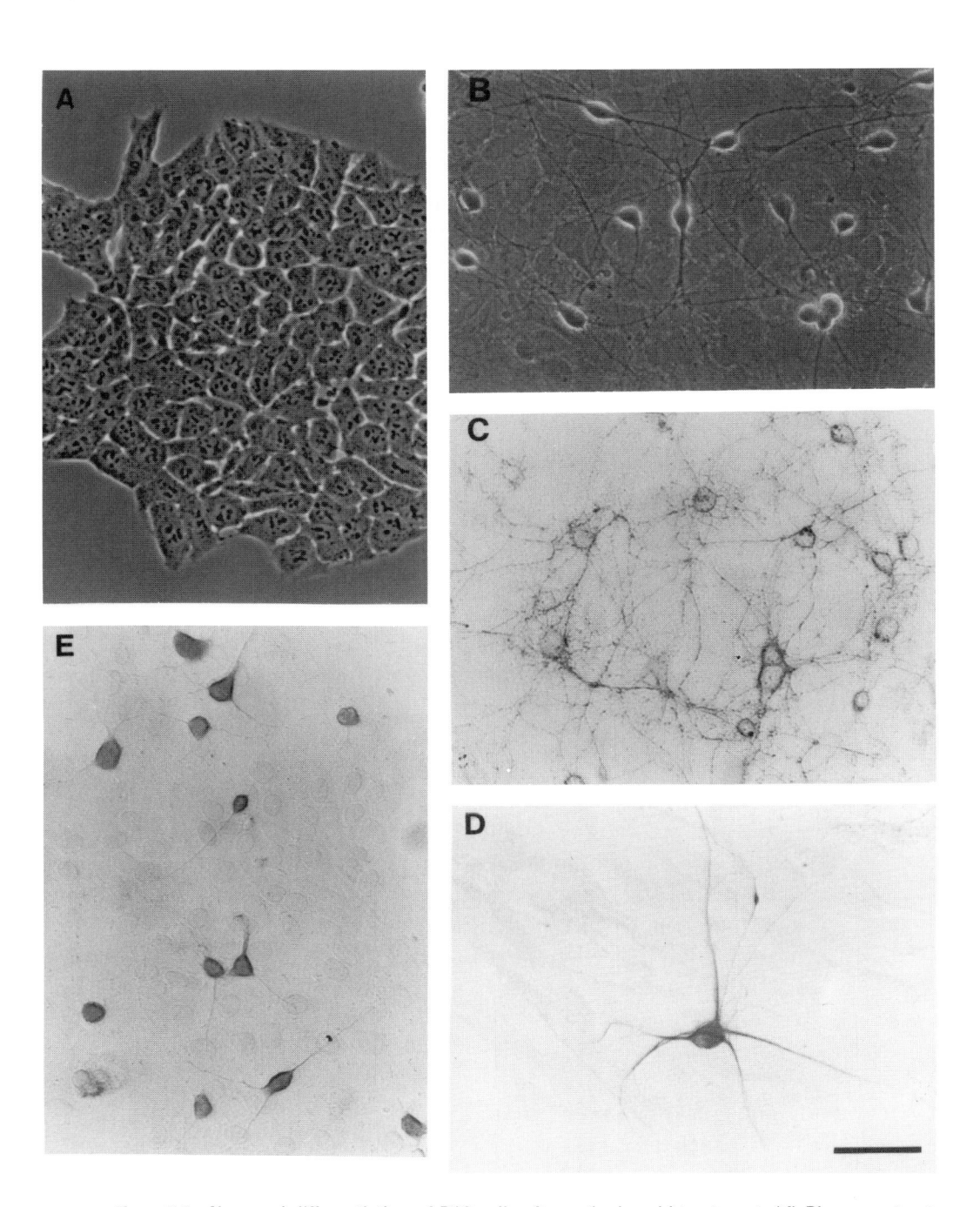

Figure 7.2 Neuronal differentiation of P19 cells after retinoic acid treatment. (*A*) Phase-contrast micrograph of undifferentiated P19 cells. (*B*) Phase-contrast micrograph of differentiated P19 cells (phase-bright, process-bearing) plated on a glial monolayer. (*C*) Immunoperoxidase staining for M6, a mouse-specific central nervous system antigen. (*D*) Immunostaining with polyclonal anti-NF 200. (*E*) Immunostaining for neuron-specific enolase. Scale bar: 50 μm (*A*, *C*, *D*, *E*) or 66 μm (*B*). (Reprinted with permission from Turetsky et al., 1993.)

cells and is not dependent on an oncogenic mutation or perturbation of the genome. In this regard, early embryonic cells are fundamentally different from cells later in development and may be thought of as "naturally immortal." The capacity for sustained replication allows the investigator to manipulate the genome of ES cells with sophisticated genetic techniques based on either homologous recombination or random integration of cloned DNA. In fact, ES cells have become the leading model for application and development of novel strategies for altering the mammalian genome.

Second, ES cells are developmentally totipotent. When introduced into the inner cell mass of a host embryo, they colonize the host and join in the formation of all tissue lineages. The resulting mouse is outwardly normal but at the cellular level is a chimera of host and ES cell contributions.

Third, in chimeric animals, ES cells give rise to germ cells with the capacity to make normal mice. This proves that the genome of ES cells is normal. These properties of ES cells are the basis for creating so-called "knock-out mice" that already have revolutionized mammalian genetics and development.

ES cells have the full potential of normal early embryonic cells to form the developing nervous system. Until recently, the only way to realize this potential was by grafting ES cells into a host embryo so as to create chimeric animals. However, we have shown that some aspects of the pathway between ES cells and neurons can be reconstituted in vitro (Bain et al., 1995). Following our report, two additional studies with similar results have appeared (Fraichard et al., 1995; Strubing et al., 1995). Our approach to inducing neuronal differentiation in ES cells was informed by the observation that P19 and ES cells share important properties. Therefore, we attempted to make ES cells differentiate into neurons with RA. Simply treating ES cells with RA either as monolayers or aggregates resulted in some neuronal differentiation but was not very efficient. Some properties of ES cells suggest that they represent a slightly earlier developmental stage than do P19 cells. Therefore we cultured ES cells as aggregates for 4 days without RA, in the hope that they would reach a stage equivalent to P19 cells, and then exposed them to RA for 4 days. This induction procedure (to which we refer as the *4−/4+ protocol*) results in very efficient neuronal differentiation. When 4−/4+ aggregates are dissociated and plated on an adhesive substrate, approximately 40% of the resulting cells have a neuronal appearance (figure 7.3). Consistent with the P19

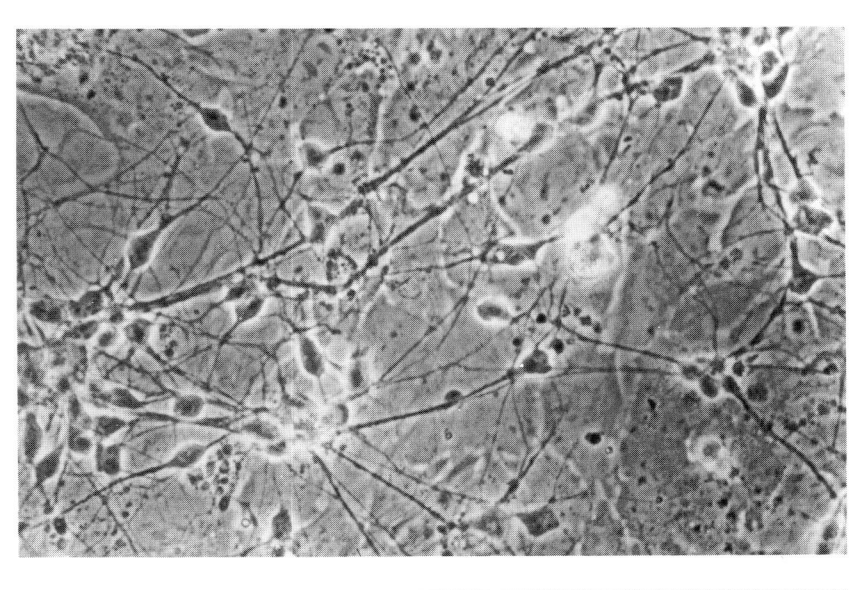

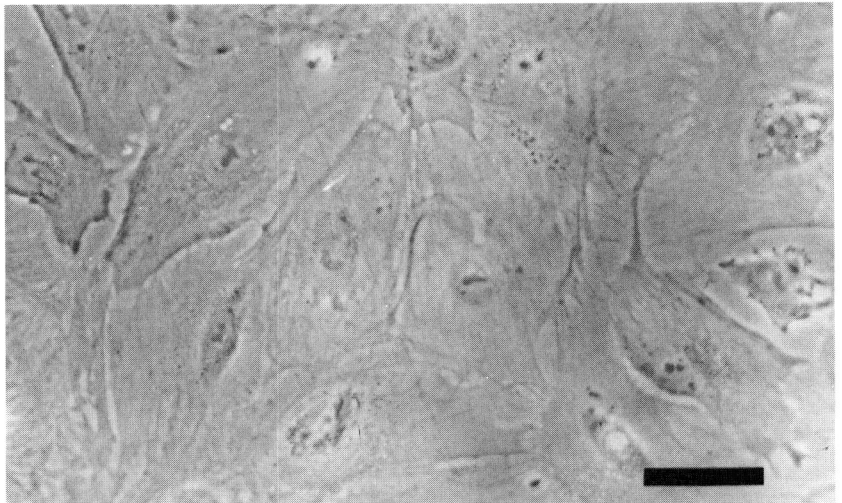

Figure 7.3 Dispersed cell cultures derived from 4−/4+ and 4−/4− aggregates. D3 ES cells were induced by either the 4−/4+ protocol or the 4−/4− protocol (in which RA was omitted). Induced aggregates were dissociated with trypsin, plated on laminin, and cultured for 5 days. Top, −4/4+; bottom, 4−/4−. Bar: 50 μm.

nomenclature, we also refer to these cells as NLCs. Many of the nonneuronal cells stain with glial fibrillary acidic protein and thus belong to the astrocytic lineage (Bain and Gottlieb, unpublished results). The ES-derived NLCs fire spikes that are blocked by tetrodotoxin (TTX). NLCs have functional glutamate, GABA, and glycine receptors (figure 7.4). During differentiation, a strong induction of the GAD_{65} and GAD_{67} genes occurs. When cultures of NLCs are examined in the electron microscope, structures with the appearance of synapses are seen with reasonable frequency (G. Bain, M. Yao, and D. Gottlieb, unpublished observations). Physiological recordings reveal that NLCs form functional synapses with each other (Finley et al., 1996; see figure 7.4). Thus, the NLCs in this system have many of the most basic features of neurons.

Advantages and Limitations of the P19 and ES Cell-Based Systems

In the final analysis, all cell lines are tools the purpose of which is to investigate biological systems present in the normal animal but unapproachable directly. Cell lines as well as primary culture systems are designed to provide improved access to cells for the study of biological questions. In nearly all cases, the manipulations required to gain control over the cells' environment will distort some aspects of their normal development. Therefore, each cell line or cell culture system must be evaluated for both advantages and limitations in making comparisons to other possible approaches. The P19 and ES systems have three great advantages relative to other cell lines. Several of these advantages are also the basis of important limitations.

The first fundamental advantage is that P19 and ES cells encompass a very broad range of embryonic development. At the beginning of the pathway are stem cells with the phenotype of inner cell mass and primitive ectoderm. At its end are NLCs with many—perhaps most—of the phenotypes of normal GABAergic and glutamatergic neurons. In principle, P19 and ES cells should allow studies of the major fate decisions (illustrated in figure 7.1) between these extremes. Very little is known about the mechanisms involved in these choices in mammals, in part because of lack of suitable models. P19 and ES systems have great potential to be such a model and shed light on basic events of early neurogenesis. In contrast, most of the commonly used neuronal cell lines are immortalized derivatives of progenitors from later stages of development having

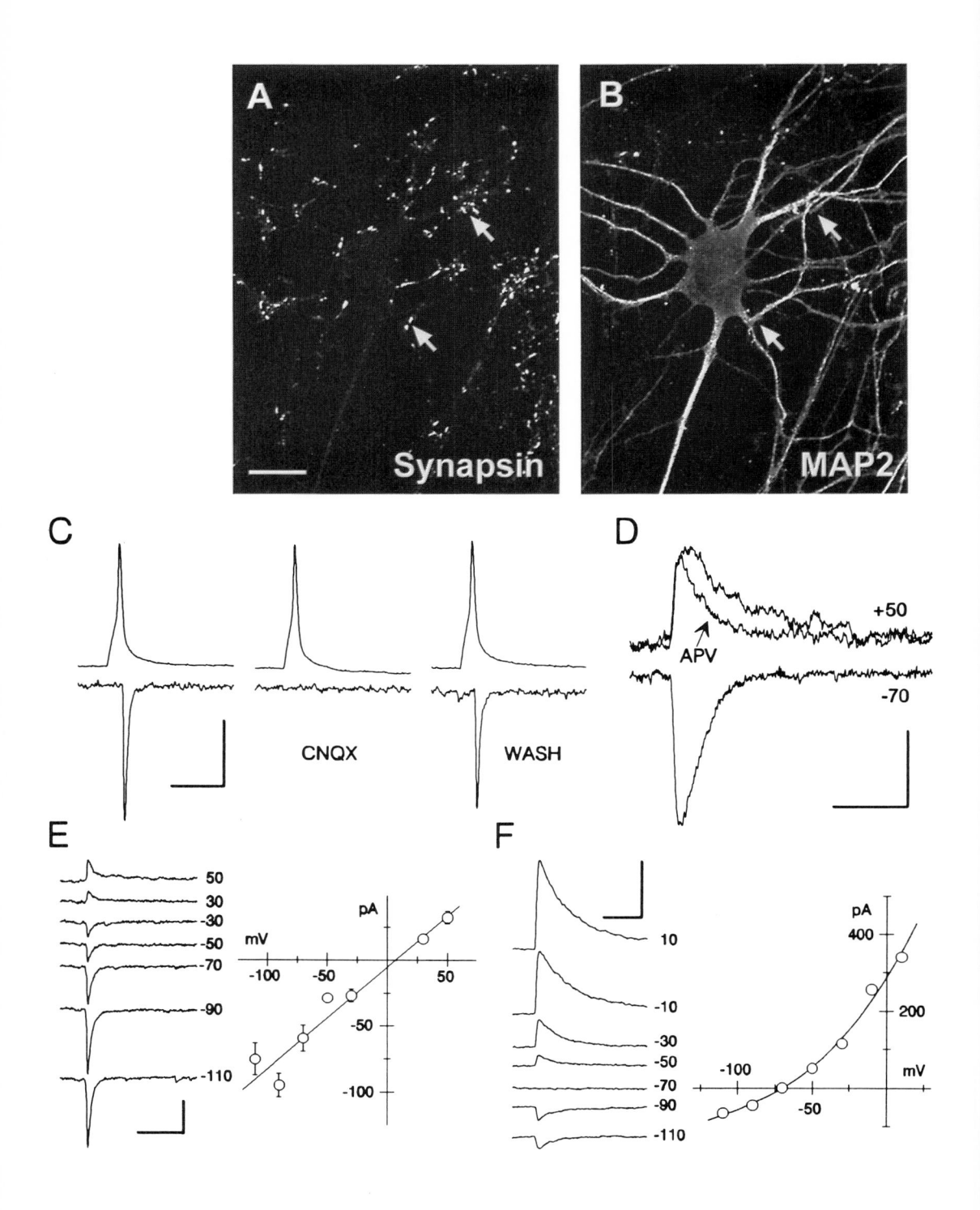

more restricted fates. For instance, PC12 cells and other neural crest–derived lines express crest-specific phenotypes but not those characteristic of the CNS. They are suited eminently for analyzing how decisions *within* the crest lineage are made but may not be appropriate models for studying the initial commitment to a crest fate. P19 and ES cells "traverse" this decision point and seem to go in a CNS-like direction, making them candidates for investigating how such decisions are made. The robust expression of GABAergic and glutamatergic phenotypes and the ability to form synapses are in dramatic contrast to most commonly used cell lines.

A second advantage of the P19 and ES systems is that the stem cells are amenable to genetic manipulation. This propensity is especially pertinent to the ES cell system. It is now possible to manipulate the genome of ES cells and then to analyze the impact of the change on NLCs. With the new in vitro induction method, many experiments can be done without the need to make chimeric mice. Most mammalian cell lines can be transfected with exogenous DNA and thus are potentially suited to genetic manipulation. However, the practical costs of realizing this potential may be very high. Protocols for transfection and selection of mutants, though simple in concept, are perfected only through laborious research, so that available methods are limited for many cell lines. ES cells have become the dominant cell model for mammalian genetics; in contrast to many cell lines, a rich collection of established genetic techniques is available. Also, a large and growing collection of altered ES cell lines is already available.

Figure 7.4 Anatomical and physiological evidence for synapse formation by P19 and ES cells. (*A, B*) Double immunofluorescence localization of synapsin and MAP2 in an ES cell culture 9 days after plating. Arrows point to synapsin-positive puncta adjacent to the cell body and dendrites of a MAP2-positive neuron. (*C–E*) Excitatory transmission similar to that observed in primary CNS neurons. (*C*) Action potentials elicited in a presynaptic P19 cell (top traces) evoke CNQX-sensitive postsynaptic currents in an adjacent cell (bottom traces) 12 days after plating. (*D*) In ES cell cultures, both NMDA and non-NMDA receptors contribute to the postsynaptic current. In medium containing Mg^{2+}, depolarization to $+50\,mV$ reveals a component of transmission that is blocked by $50\,\mu M$ APV (23 days after plating). (*E*) Peak synaptic current recorded in an ES cell 34 days after plating has a linear current-voltage relation typical of the excitatory postsynaptic currents recorded from CNS neurons. (*F*) The current-voltage relation for an inhibitory synaptic response shows rectification and a reversal potential consistent with chloride-selective channels (P19 cell, 14 days after plating). Scale bars: (*A, B*) $25\,\mu m$; (*C*) $40\,mV$ (top), $40\,pA$ (bottom), $15\,ms$; (*D*) $20\,pA$, $30\,ms$; (*E*) $40\,pA$, $40\,ms$; (*F*) $200\,pA$, $15\,ms$. (Parts *A, B, D, E* adapted from Finley et al., 1996; parts *C*, F Courtesy of M. F. A. Finley and J. E. Huettner, unpublished experiments.)

Currently, the most powerful approach to genetic modification of ES cells is the replacement of native genes with mutant alleles by homologous recombination. In early experiments, one of the two alleles was replaced in culture and knock-outs were generated by creating mice and crossing heterozygotes. Now it is possible to obtain diploid knock-outs directly in culture (Mortensen et al., 1991; Sawai et al., 1991; Field et al., 1992; Zhuang et al., 1992). Genes suspected of playing interesting roles in neuronal development or physiology can be knocked out, and the impact on NLCs can be determined.

Homologous recombination has other important uses. Its frequency is not influenced by the size of inserts between flanking regions of homology (Mansour et al., 1990). This finding means that relatively large inserts can be targeted to genes of interest. In this way, cDNAs can be inserted into a known locus; expression of the cDNA then comes under the control of the native "target" gene regulatory elements (Mansour et al., 1990). By use of this approach, it will be possible to direct ectopic expression of transgenes with precise control over levels, time, and cell type of expression. Such precise control is difficult with other systems of overexpression.

A third advantage of the ES system is that the cells are genetically normal and can be used to make mice. Many neuronal cell lines express oncogenes introduced in their creation, whereas others probably carry oncogenic mutations that have not been characterized. Results with these lines must be be interpreted against such known or suspected abnormal genetic backgrounds. These considerations make difficult the comparison of results between lines or between a cell line and the normal animal. ES cells avoid this complication. The relevance of mechanisms discovered in vitro to normal development and function is a persistent source of concern. The ES system makes it possible to bridge the gap between culture and the animal by making chimeras. An analysis may start with in vitro experiments; then, conclusions can be tested with appropriate lines in chimeric mice. In this way, the costly but crucial animal experiments can be used to maximal advantage.

The basic characteristics of the P19 and ES cell system impose a set of important *limitations* on their use. As stem cells do not express neuronal properties and have to be induced into neurons, certain productive strategies used with differentiated cell lines are not applicable. For instance, transient expression of promoter-reporter constructs is a powerful way of mapping *cis*-acting gene

control elements. This method cannot be used with P19 and ES cells because transfection must be performed in the stem cells and, by the time induction is finished, expression ceases (Bain and Gottlieb, unpublished observations). Lines such as PC12, wherein the dividing cells express neuronal properties, are suitable for direct selection of mutants in neuronal phenotypes. In pluripotent cell systems, only indirect and clumsy methods can be used to select mutants.

The fact that the in vitro differentiation of ES cells and P19s appear to mimic the natural pathways also may present problems of interpretation. Many cell lines give relatively homogeneous populations of cells, which greatly facilitates experiments with a biochemical end point, as the results can be interpreted in terms of a single type of cell. In the P19- and ES-based systems, multiple neuronal as well as glial cell types are produced, so biochemical results must be interpreted with great caution. At this point, it is not clear how many distinct types of neurons and glial cells can be derived from ES or P19 cells; however, the fact that multiple cell types are produced should not be considered abnormal. Lineage studies in vivo show that neurons and glial cells can be sister cells even at the final rounds of cell division during neurogenesis. Therefore, it is to be expected that pluripotent precursor cells will have the potential to yield a wide range of cell types. Indeed, we view this as one of the great strengths of the P19 and ES cell systems. Study of the action of candidate differentiation factors on properties of NLCs should yield insights into the various cues that determine the phenotype of neuronal subpopulations. Use of this approach eventually may make possible the guidance of the stem cells along subpathways of differentiation as we learn more about the genes and factors that cause neurons to select particular fates.

Protocols

There are three steps in obtaining NLCs: culturing stem cells, induction under conditions that favor formation of aggregates, and dissociation of the aggregates and replating onto adhesive substrate. The conditions for culturing stem cells, cells undergoing induction with RA, and the resulting NLCs are very different from one another. For each stage, however, protocols for P19 and ES cells are similar. Accordingly, this section is divided into subsections on culturing stem cells, carrying out inductions, and

culturing NLCs, with protocols for P19 and ES cells in each sub-section. All culture steps are carried out at 37°C in a humidified incubator with 5% CO_2.

Culture of Stem Cells

P19 stem cells are available from the American Type Culture Collection (ATCC). In the case of ES cells, these cells are best obtained from laboratories currently using the ES cells to generate knock-out mice, as this is the best assurance of genetic normality. P19 stem cells and ES cells have normal karyotypes. However, in the case of ES cells wherein the issue has been studied systematically (Suda et al., 1987), variant clones arise at a measurable rate. Presumably, this also can occur in P19 cells; therefore, it is essential that lines used for in vitro differentiation be as close to canonical stocks as possible. On obtaining lines, frozen stocks should be established. Propagation of new stocks should proceed for a limited and defined duration only. We propagate P19 cells for approximately 1 month, then start with a newly thawed sample.

The technique for propagating P19 stem cells is straightforward. The methods described here are similar to those reviewed by Rudnicki and McBurney (1987). Cells are grown in standard tissue-culture flasks; T25 flasks are most convenient. We use a medium formulation (Jones-Villeneuve et al., 1982) consisting of αMEM (GIBCO, Gaithersburg MD, no. 12571-014) with 7.5% newborn calf serum and 2.5% fetal calf serum, which we designate P19 growth medium (P19GM) (table 7.1). Good results are obtained with ordinary serum lots from GIBCO; it has not been necessary to prescreen serum.

P19 cultures are started from a frozen stock by seeding cells into a T25 flask with 5 ml of P19GM and allowing cells to reach near-confluency. At this point, the cultures have 5 to 8×10^6 cells total. Cells are passaged so that one-tenth of the cells in a near-confluent flask are seeded into a new T25 flask in 5 ml of P19GM. Cells then are passaged at 2-day intervals, again using one-tenth of the cells to seed each new flask. To passage, cells are removed from the culture flask surface with a trypsin solution (0.25% trypsin with EDTA in Hank's salts (GIBCO-BRL no. 15050). Growth medium is aspirated, and 1 ml of the trypsin solution is used to cover the cells. Incubation then is carried out for 10 min at 37°C. Four ml of P19GM is added to quench the trypsin, and the suspension is triturated

Table 7.1   Table of Media

P19 Growth Medium (P19GM)
αMEM (GIBCO no. 12571-014) 90%
Newborn calf serum 7.5%
Fetal calf serum 2.5%

P19 induction medium (P19IM)
αMEM (GIBCO no. 12571-014) 95%
Fetal calf serum 5%

ES growth medium (ESGM)
Dulbecco's MEM (high glucose plus L-glutamine minus pyruvate; GIBCO no. 11965-043) 79%
Fetal calf serum 10%
Newborn calf serum 10%
Nucleoside stock 1%
Leukemia inhibitory factor (LIF) final concentration $= 1000$ units/ml
β-Mercaptoethanol 10^{-4} M

Es induction medium (ESIM)
Same as ESGM but omits LIF and β-mercaptoethanol

MEM $+ 5\%$ rat serum
Eagle's MEM (GIBCO no. 11430-014)
plus:
Glucose 17 mM
Glutamine 250 μM
NaHCO$_3$ 26 mM
Rat serum 5%

Neurobasal medium
Neurobasal medium (GIBCO no. 21103-15)
B27 supplement (50× GIBCO no. 17504-010)
Glutamine 250 μM

Nucleoside stock
In 100 ml double-distilled water
Adenosine 80 mg
Guanosine 85 mg
Cytidine 73 mg
Uridine 73 mg
Thymidine 24 mg
Filter-sterilize; this is a 100× stock

---

through a 5-ml pipet to give a population of dispersed cells. Then 0.5 ml of this cell suspension is used to inoculate each new flask that contains 5 ml of P19GM. Cells are passaged routinely every 2 days.

Two aspects of this protocol bear special attention. At low densities, embryonal carcinoma lines, including P19 cells, differentiate spontaneously. To avoid this, flasks should be seeded at the minimal density cited earlier. Second, P19 cells do not regulate their replication in a density-dependent manner; at high densities, they continue to divide, and the overcrowded cultures become filled with lysed cells. It is imperative to passage cells before this condition occurs.

The broad outlines of ES cell culture are similar to P19, but important differences remain. For our work, we use a variant of the protocol widely used for routine maintenance of ES cell stocks. A detailed description of the standard method is available (Robertson, 1987). One of the advantages of the ES cell approach is the ability to work with cells with a normal genome (as determined by creating germ-line transmitting chimeras). For most of our work, we have used an isolate of the D3 ES line from a stock used to create knock-out mice and thus demonstrably normal (Veis et al., 1993). We also have used CC1.2 and RW1 derivatives, and they behave exactly as does the D3 line. As with P19 cells, ES cells are propagated for a limited time only (approximately 1 month) before starting with new, frozen stocks. This schedule avoids the problem of working with karyotypic variants. For making knock-outs, ES cells are grown on feeder cell layers. For in vitro differentiation, it is convenient to grow them on a gelatin-coated substrate without feeders. The substrate is formed by coating the bottom of tissue-culture flasks with 0.1% gelatin. We use a sterile 2% gelatin solution in water (Sigma no. 74H2346), which is diluted 20-fold in distilled water. Five milliliters is added to a T25 flask and is left overnight at room temperature. The gelatin solution then is aspirated, and the flask is ready for use. ES cells are cultured in the coated flask in a medium consisting of D-MEM [high glucose with L-glutamine, without pyruvate (GIBCO no. 11965-043)] with 10% fetal bovine serum and 10% newborn calf serum plus nucleoside stocks, leukemia inhibitory factor (LIF-ESGRO from BRL cat no. 13275-011; 1000 units/ml final concentration) and 10^{-4} M β-mercaptoethanol. This medium is designated ESGM (see table 7.1).

The nucleoside stock solution is made up by dissolving the following in distilled water at 37°C: adenosine, 0.8 mg/ml; guanosine, 0.85 mg/ml; cytidine, 0.73 mg/ml; uridine, 0.73 mg/ml; and thymidine, 0.24 mg/ml; stock is filter-sterilized. The nucleoside stock is 100 times the final desired concentration and is kept at refrigerator temperature; this causes nucleosides to precipitate, but they redissolve easily when the stock solution is warmed to 37°C. LIF and β-mercaptoethanol are essential to prevent spontaneous differentiation of ES cells. As with P19 cells, it is important to monitor the density of cultures and to keep them within established bounds. We passage flasks when they reach a density of approximately 2×10^7 cells per T25 flask. Cells are trypsinized by the same method used for P19 stem-cell cultures. New flasks are seeded with 5×10^6 cells. Routine passages are performed every 2 days.

Induction of Differentiation

For induction, P19 cells first are harvested from confluent flasks by the trypsinization protocol previously given. The induction is carried out in nonadhesive dishes to promote aggregate formation. P19 stem cells are very adhesive and even adhere to many non-tissue-culture dishes. We use 100×15 mm bacteriological Petri dishes (Fisher 8-757-13). Most lots work, but we have found occasional batches that are either toxic or too adhesive. The 1×10^6 freshly trypsinized cells are seeded in 10 ml of a medium consisting of αMEM plus 5% fetal bovine serum (P19 IM). The lower concentration of serum relative to P19GM seems to promote induction. Immediately after seeding, all-trans RA (Sigma, cat. no. R-2625) is added to final concentration of 5×10^{-7} M. A concentrated stock (1 mM) is prepared in 95% ethanol by dissolving 50 mg of RA in 156 ml of 100% ethanol and adding 8 ml distilled water. The stock is stored in a dark bottle in the refrigerator and is stable for several months. Aggregates form after 1 day in culture; a few aggregates adhere to the dish, but this does not cause problems. After 2 days, the medium is changed by transferring the suspension of aggregates to a 15-ml conical centrifuge tube, allowing the aggregates to settle for 10 min, aspirating the medium, and replacing it with new medium of the same composition (including fresh RA). The aggregates and fresh medium are returned to the culture dishes, and culture is continued for another 2 days. At this point, the cells are induced and ready for plating.

Induction of ES cells is carried out by a variant of this protocol. ES cells are harvested from standard growth flasks that have been cultured for 2 days since plating using the same trypsinization protocol described earlier. ES cells are harder to dissociate than are P19 cells. We find that if we trypsinize them extensively enough to yield a single cell suspension, they do not form aggregates as consistently as do cells trypsinized more mildly. Therefore, we quantitate the input of cells for induction by using a standard fraction (one-fourth) of the cells from a 2-day postplating flask that (as described earlier) is near confluency; this technique gives an estimated 5×10^6 cells per induction. These cells are seeded into 10 ml of medium identical to ESGM except that LIF and β-mercaptoethanol are omitted (ESIM) (table 7.1); this medium is used throughout the induction procedure. Omission of LIF is essential because it is a powerful suppressor of ES cell differentiation. Cells are cultured in 100-mm nonadhesive Petri dishes wherein they form aggregates after 1 day, although the aggregates are at first smaller and more "ragged" than are P19 aggregates. After 2 days of culture, the medium is replaced with a fresh aliquot of the same medium using the sedimentation method descried earlier for P19 cells. After 4 days of culture, the medium is replaced by the same method, and 5×10^{-7} M RA is introduced. After 2 more days, the medium is replaced with fresh medium containing the same concentration of RA, and culture is continued for another 2 days. At this stage, the induction is finished, and the cells are ready to plate. We find that *4 days of culture as aggregates before the addition of RA greatly improves the extent of induction*, compared to adding RA immediately. An alternative method in which neurons are induced by exposure of aggregates to RA for the first 2 days has been described (Fraichard et al., 1995; Strubing et al., 1995). In one case, this yields 10% neurons (Fraichard et al., 1995), substantially lower than what we observe. The percentage of neurons obtained by Strubbing et al., (1995) is not documented. Further studies on the timing and levels of RA may reveal better induction methods.

Plating for Neuronal Differentiation

The protocols for the neuronal differentiation stage follow roughly those that are used for primary neuronal dispersed cell cultures. RA is not added after the induction step. This distinction is essential, because RA is an extremely powerful effector and its inclusion

after induction could have major effects on the cells. The protocols for P19 and ES cells are very similar. In the case of P19 cells, aggregates are harvested and washed once in αMEM without serum and are resuspended in 2 ml of 0.25% trypsin-EDTA to which DNAase (50 μg/ml) has been added to prevent formation of DNA gels. Cells are incubated for 10 min at 37°C; the tube is flicked every few minutes to ensure even suspension of the aggregates. Then 4 ml of P19SM is added to halt trypsin action. Cells are collected by centrifugation and are resuspended in 5 ml of P19SM. Next, cells are triturated to yield a single-cell suspension and are counted in a hemocytometer. Optimal neuronal differentiation is obtained by plating dissociated cells at a density of 7.5×10^5 cells in 2 ml of P19SM in a 35 mm dish or in larger dishes at proportional densities.

P19 cultures set up in this manner yield a population consisting of flat background cells and NLCs. For approximately 8 days, these cultures are stable and healthy. Past this point, extensive cell death occurs. The exact cause of the wave of cell death is not understood well. One probable factor is glutamate toxicity, as we have demonstrated that NLCs express glutamate receptors and that glutamate is cytotoxic to these cells (Turetsky et al., 1994). Recently, we have shown that NLCs differentiate very well when induced P19 cells are plated in N2 medium (Yao et al., 1995). Here too, a period of healthy growth is followed by a wave of neuronal cell death. This death can be prevented by switching the P19 cells from N2 medium to Neurobasal medium plus the B27 supplement (table 7.1) (Brewer et al., 1993) In this medium, the NLCs are stable for at least 3 weeks (Yao et al., 1995). Long-term cultures of P19 NLCs can be obtained also by an alternative method in which the cultures are plated onto a monolayer of rat astrocytes in P19GM. Preparation of astrocytes is detailed in Huettner and Baughman (1986). At 2 days postplating, the cultures are switched into MEM + 5% rat serum containing 10 μM cytosine arabinoside. Cells are fed with fresh MEM + 5% rat serum on the fourth day and then every 3 to 5 days.

The procedure for ES cells is very similar. Dissociation conditions are the same as those for P19 cells. Here, as with stock ES cultures, dissociation is not as complete as that for P19 cells, so true single-cell suspensions are not obtained. The dissociated aggregates from one induction yield enough cells for twelve 35-mm dishes.

Induced ES cells can be cultured on a gelatin-coated dish in ESIM (ESGM minus LIF and β-mercaptoethanol). The NLCs in such

cultures remain healthy for 5 to 7 days. To obtain long-term cultures, induced ES cells first are plated in ESIM. Then, on the third or fourth postplating day, cytosine arabinoside is added to a final concentration of 10 μm. The following day, half of the medium is replaced with Neurobasal medium. The cultures are fed every 3 to 5 days with Neurobasal medium.

Fully induced P19 or ES aggregates cultured as described earlier also can be plated without dissociating. The aggregates spread out over the surface after 4 to 5 days, revealing many differentiated neurons. These are particularly suitable for some physiological studies. Aggregate cultures are somewhat more forgiving than are dispersed cultures and should be considered as a way of obtaining neurons on the first few tries.

Characterization and Troubleshooting

P19 Cells

P19 stem cells are easy to grow and maintain if certain pitfalls are avoided. These cells do not stop replicating in a density-dependent manner and, thus, readily overgrow if not split on schedule. Overgrown cultures contain many dead cells and are not suitable for differentiation. Cultures used for induction should be relatively free of debris and should not have acid medium. Induction is carried out in 100-mm bacteriological dishes as previously described. Although most lots of dishes are suitable, we have encountered some degree of variability. Some are too adhesive, resulting in monolayers rather than aggregates. Others are toxic, resulting in suspensions of single dead cells. These dead cells are phase-dark, whereas living cells are phase-bright; viability can be ascertained also by trypan blue exclusion. It is essential to secure a supply of nonadhesive, nontoxic dishes.

Scaling the induction down is difficult. Smaller dishes tend to give a small number of very large aggregates that develop necrotic centers and do not give equally good inductions. It would be desirable to have objective standards to determine whether an induction was going well. Unfortunately, most of the characterization of cells in aggregates has been done by assays for gene expression, which are rather laborious (see Bain et al., 1994, for a list of genes turned on by the RA induction). The best way to determine

whether an induction is going well is to continue the procedure to the point at which differentiated neurons are obtained.

Once induction is complete, aggregates are dissociated with trypsin. The conditions described earlier yield suspensions of viable, competent cells with little cell death during trypsinization. A certain amount of "fine-tuning" is necessary to obtain good results. It is essential to remove all of the serum-containing medium from the aggregates to avoid blocking trypsin activity with the serum protease inhibitors. Trituration of the trypsinized cells must be done to the right degree. Major variables include the diameter of the pipet tip, the force used to express the cell suspension, and the number of rounds of trituration. These items need to be determined by trial and error. Cell viability can be determined by trypan blue exclusion.

Once the induced cells are plated as dispersed cells, the system crosses the boundary from a cell line to terminally differentiated cells. As mentioned earlier, the NLCs have many of the basic features of CNS neurons grown in primary culture and must be treated as such to obtain successful cultures. The differentiated status of the cells can be judged by their overall morphological makeup, which is a reliable indicator. If desired, status can be checked by a number of antibodies including neuron-specific endase, neunofilament-200, GAP43, and MAP2, all of which give a staining pattern similar to primary neurons in culture. NLCs are sensitive to glutamate toxicity. To avoid this danger, cultures should be switched to specialized media approximately 5 days after plating. To avoid glutamate toxicity, long-term cultures should be maintained in medium with little or no exogenous glutamic acid, such as Eagle's MEM plus 3 to 5% serum (Turetsky et al., 1993) or Neurobasal medium +B27 (Yao et al., 1995; Finley et al., 1996)

ES Cells

ES cells can be maintained in the undifferentiated state either by culture on feeder cells or by culture on gelatin in medium supplemented with LIF. To obtain good inductions, it is important to minimize the number of feeder cells, because they secrete LIF, which blocks differentiation even of cells grown in aggregates (Shen and Leder, 1992). Feeder cells used to support ES cells are treated first with radiation or chemicals to prevent further division. We greatly reduce feeder cells simply by passaging cultures twice

on gelatin (in the presence of LIF, of course); the few remaining feeder cells do not interfere with differentiation. This procedure is especially important in bringing new ES cells into a laboratory. Ignoring the feeder cell issue could lead to the erroneous conclusion that a clone of ES cells (mutant or otherwise) does not differentiate properly.

Trypsinization of undifferentiated ES cultures is a troublesome step. Overdigesting leads to single-cell suspensions, which do not aggregate well. Underdigestion results in large clumps, which fail to differentiate well. A certain amount of trial and error is necessary to strike the happy medium. A day after plating, suspension cultures are a mixture of small, irregular aggregates, single live cells, and dead cells. The aggregates are phase-bright but with irregular outlines. They increase in size over the next 2 days. By day 5, the aggregates have the characteristic outer cell layer and underlying basement membrane of embryoid bodies that can be seen (although imperfectly) in phase optics.

Current Uses of the P19 and ES Cell Systems

The P19 system is well-established and is being used for many types of studies of neural development; because of space limitations, only a few can be reviewed here. One exciting use is to screen for genes that are regulated strongly and rapidly in response to RA. Bouillet et al. (1995) have used a subtractive hybridization cloning strategy to clone 50 genes that are regulated rapidly in response to RA; 40 of these genes are novel. Using a similar strategy, Wijnholds et al. (1995) have cloned a gene called *neuronatin*, which appears to be involved selectively in hindbrain formation. Other studies exploit the fact that P19 stem cells can be transfected so as to express cDNAs. Overexpression of the notch gene in P19 cells leads to a suppression of neuronal differentiation (Nye et al., 1994). The effect is specific in that differentiation of glial cells occurs normally. Ectopic expression of the secreted regulatory protein Wnt-1 perturbs the normal progression of the neuronal pathway (Smolich and Papkoff, 1994). The data suggest that Wnt-1 plays a role in the differentiation and stabilization of a precursor-type cell. In another study, the function of the retinoblastoma (Rb) family of proteins was perturbed by transfecting P19 cells with the adenovirus E1A protein that binds and inactivates Rb protein (Slack et al., 1995). Clones of P19 cells overexpressing E1A undergo

apoptosis when induced with RA. These results illuminate a new facet of Rb protein function.

Efficient neuronal differentiation of ES cells has been possible only for the last year. In one of our laboratories (that of D.G.), the system has been used to discover novel genes that are expressed early in embryonic development. Subtraction cloning was used to isolate genes expressed in RA-induced aggregates but not in undifferentiated ES cells. At least eight novel sequences have been discovered and are being characterized (W. J. Ray, G. Bain, and D. Gottlieb, unpublished data). We also are analyzing the expression of genes involved in regional specification of the nervous system. In one set of experiments, we are using a lacZ knock-in to the BF-1 locus. Preliminary results indicate that the BF-1 gene is regulated highly in the in vitro system (D. Gottlieb and E. Lai, unpublished observations).

8   Culturing the Large Neurons of Aplysia

Daniel J. Goldberg and Samuel Schacher

People study *Aplysia* neurons in culture for the same basic reasons they study them in situ: size and individuality. Enormous cell bodies exist in the *Aplysia* nervous system. R2, which may be as large as a millimeter in diameter, is the largest neuronal soma yet described in any animal, and all the major ganglia that constitute the central nervous system of this marine slug have some cell bodies measuring in the hundreds of microns. The demonstration by Arvanitaki's group nearly 50 years ago that some of these cells could be recognized reproducibly as unique individuals by position in the ganglion and firing pattern made apparent their potential usefulness to neurophysiologists. Kandel and colleagues have made *Aplysia* one of the best-known names in neurobiology through their studies of cellular and molecular changes underlying simple forms of learning (Kandel, 1976; Kandel et al., 1983). The relatively small number of neurons involved in particular behaviors, along with their size and identifiability, made it possible to describe many components of the circuitry responsible for those behaviors and, thus, to pinpoint some of the loci of plasticity during learned modifications of the behaviors.

Although behavior is not the immediate focus of experiments in which *Aplysia* neurons are studied in culture, the culturing of identified nerve cells can serve as a tool for analyzing the mechanisms of the identified cellular and molecular changes underlying behavioral plasticity. For example, it has been possible to reconstruct in the culture dish the critical circuit element mediating sensitization of the gill withdrawal reflex, the synapse of mechanosensory neuron onto gill motor neuron (Rayport and Schacher, 1986). This work has allowed experiments that have defined a brief period of time during the training regimen when protein synthesis must occur for long-term conditioning to result (Montarolo et al., 1986; Castellucci et al., 1989). Morphological changes in the axonal tree of the sensory neuron, thought to be important in the plasticity (Bailey and Chen, 1988), could be detected by repeated injections of a fluorescent dye that fills the cell body and neuritic processes

(Glanzman et al., 1990). Furthermore, the large cell bodies facilitate the injection of proteins or constructed genetic probes to examine the molecular bases for short- and long-term synaptic plasticity (Dash et al., 1990; Kaang et al., 1993; Alberini et al., 1994).

One can reconstruct this circuit element in culture because the neurons form appropriate chemical synapses. In fact, cultured *Aplysia* neurons can be used for examining the mechanisms underlying specificity of synapse formation. For example, L10 forms chemical synapses with left—but not right—upper-quadrant cells in culture, matching the specificity displayed in the abdominal ganglion (Camardo et al., 1983). The culture dish is a good place in which to study the distribution of surface molecules and to test their potential importance in generating this specificity, for example, by the use of antibodies as stains or pharmacological blocking agents (Keller and Schacher, 1990; Mayford et al., 1992; Zhu et al., 1994).

In addition to selective synapse formation, certain other phenomena important in the growth of axonal trees and the formation of patterns of connectivity have been reproduced in *Aplysia* cultures and analyzed in ways that would be difficult or impossible in situ. One example is "competition" among sensory neurons for postsynaptic space on the axonal tree of the L7 motor neuron (Glanzman et al., 1991; Bank and Schacher, 1992). Another is the remote effect on growth of one of the two main branches of the giant cerebral neuron (GCN) axon triggered by contact of the other axon with postsynaptic targets (Schacher, 1985). The large size of these axonal branches allowed the use of video-enhanced contrast–differential interference contrast (VEC-DIC) microscopy to measure the relative amounts of transport of membrane-bound organelles in the two branches before and after contact (Goldberg and Schacher, 1987).

VEC-DIC microscopy also has revealed certain *Aplysia* growth cones in culture to be particularly fine specimens for analyzing the intracellular events underlying axonal elongation and steering (Goldberg and Burmeister, 1986; Burmeister and Goldberg, 1988; Forscher and Smith, 1988; Goldberg, 1988; Burmeister et al., 1991). It is not difficult to find growth cones that are 10 to 30 µm across, though the size of *Aplysia* growth cones is not as exceptional as that of the cell bodies (and there is no close correlation between those sizes). Intracellular organelle movement is very well-defined

because these growth cones are particularly rich in vesicles and because the numerous peptidergic neurons (e.g., bag cells, right-upper-quadrant cells, B1 and B2) have vesicles that are larger than 100 nm in diameter. Also, the preparation is viewed at room temperature rather than at 37°C and, thus, events probably are slowed considerably.

In summary, *Aplysia* neurons in culture have afforded the opportunity to study simplified manifestations of neuronal plasticity and development in a format wherein analysis (e.g., video microscopy or electrophysiology) and manipulation (e.g., intracellular injection or restricted placement of targets) are relatively easy.

Protocol for Preparing Cultures of *Aplysia* Neurons

Single Cells or Dispersed Cells?

Two basic methods have been used for culturing *Aplysia* neurons: dispersion of entire ganglia or removal of neurons singly. The former, simply an extension of procedures used for culturing vertebrate neurons, was developed originally in Strumwasser's laboratory to allow electrophysiological measurements in the small neurosecretory bag cells in isolation (Kaczmarek et al., 1979). The advantage of this procedure is speed. Hundreds of neurons can be collected in the several minutes it takes to dissect a few neurons individually. We have used dispersion to prepare cultures for video microscopic observation of growth cones or for biochemical analysis, such as assays of cAMP.

Several features of the single-cell culture of *Aplysia* neurons (Camardo et al., 1983; Schacher and Proshansky 1983; Rayport and Schacher, 1986) make it the preferred technique for many experiments. First, one can pick out specific, identified neurons. For example, if one wished to study why cell X forms chemical synapses with cell Y but not cell Z, one could not use the dispersion method. Second, neurons can be removed from the ganglion with long lengths of their axons, whereas the axon usually is lost in the dispersion method. Features of the axonal tree can be retained in culture. For example, the GCN, also known as a *metacerebral cell*, is monopolar, as is the case with many invertebrate neurons, with fine dendritic processes coming off the most proximal 1 mm of the

axon. The axon is bifurcate, and the branches exit the ganglion in different nerves. We can remove this neuron routinely from juvenile animals with an axonal tree that has long lengths of both major branches, dendrites, and even sometimes a secondary branch of one of the major branches. Thus, GCN in culture is well-suited for studies of differential synapse formation and differential growth of the branches of the same axonal tree (Schacher, 1985; Goldberg and Schacher, 1987). Third, giant neurons can be obtained reliably only by the single-cell dissection method. It may be that these cells do not tolerate the loss of axon that occurs during dispersion. Last, dishes of cells prepared by individual dissection are much "cleaner" than those prepared by dispersion, in that they contain far fewer nonneuronal cells and very little acellular debris.

Ganglia from juvenile or adult animals (1.5–80 g) can be used for both types of cell culturing; larger animals (>100 g) can be used only for dispersion, as the cells are embedded too firmly in the ganglia to allow them to be pulled out individually. With both procedures, cells can be grown either in medium containing *Aplysia* hemolymph or in protein-free defined medium, provided the culture dish has been pretreated with *Aplysia* hemolymph. Hemolymph contains an unidentified high-molecular-weight activity that binds to the substratum and is required for good growth of these neurons (Burmeister et al., 1991). Cultured neurons survive in its absence, but growth is slow and looks abnormal. In this respect, *Aplysia* neurons are like many vertebrate neurons, which need proteins such as laminin and fibronectin on the substrate to exhibit vigorous neuritic growth. However, no such vertebrate protein that we have tested works with *Aplysia* neurons.

Acquisition of Animals

Aplysia californica, which is found in abundance off the coast of southern California, is the main species used for culturing. *Aplysia depilans*, which is available from the Mediterranean, is also suitable (Spira et al., 1993; Ziv and Spira, 1993). Specimens of *A. californica* can be purchased weekly from a few companies for $9 to $15 each (plus air freight charges).[1] They can be kept for up to a few weeks in aerated aquaria of cooled artificial seawater, needing no more than feedings of seaweed. Juveniles should be segregated in small cages within the aquarium and fed separately, with live seaweed much preferred to dried sheets. Adult animals are avail-

able year-round, though their quality and abundance often decline during the summer, when many are believed to be in the last stage of their life cycle in the wild. Juveniles are available from the wild only for part of the year. The mariculture facility at the University of Miami (formerly the Howard Hughes Medical Institute Mariculture Facility) rears *Aplysia* entirely in the laboratory and can supply juvenile *Aplysia* and adult animals throughout the year.

Sterile Technique

One advantage of working with cultures from *Aplysia*—and probably from other invertebrates—is that less tendency exists for them to become contaminated with microorganisms. This proclivity probably applies because the cultures are stored at 18°C and are used within a week and because the concentration of salt in the medium is relatively high. Sterile dishes and medium are used, and the culturing is done in a horizontal laminar flow hood. However, there are lapses in the sterile technique. For example, the micropipettes used for removing individual cells are not sterile, nor are either the steel pins used for fixing the ganglia to the dissecting dish or the forceps used for removing connective tissue. Often, we have viewed an open dish on the video microscope for a few hours and then returned it to the 18°C incubator without signs of contamination appearing over the next several days. On occasion, the entire culturing procedure has been done on an open bench, and the preparation has been found satisfactory the next day.

Preparation of Culture Medium and of Hemolymph

We use as our protein-free defined culture medium an L-15 medium supplemented with salts to bring the ionic concentrations up to those in seawater (SL-15). Each liter of SL-15 is made by dissolving sequentially 1 powder pack of L-15 (modified, with glutamine) and then salts, sugar, and antibiotics, as described in box 8.1. The medium is sterile-filtered and refrigerated in sterile, reusable glass bottles. We try to use the medium within 3 weeks, as glutamine is unstable in solution. Alternatively, salts, sugar, and antibiotics are added to L-15 (liquid) without glutamine, which is added as needed to aliquots of the SL-15. If cultures are to be maintained for more than 2 days, it is advisable to use 50% hemolymph:50% SL-15 as the culture medium. Cell survival seems

Box 8.1   Preparation of Supplemented L-15 (SL-15) Culture Medium

Ingredient	Amount	Final Concentration (mM)*
NaCl	17.93 g	444
KCl	0.344 g	10
$MgCl_2 \cdot 6H_2O$	5.7 g	28
$MgSO_4 \cdot 7H_2O$	6.24 g	27
$NaHCO_3$	0.194 g	2
D-glucose (dextrose)	6.24 g	35
HEPES·Na	3.74 g	15
$CaCl_2 \cdot 2H_2O$	1.488 g	11
Streptomycin	1 ml of 0.2 g/ml stock	
Penicillin	0.4 ml of 250,000 U/ml stock	

PROCEDURE

Dissolve one package of L-15 powder (GIBCO cat. no. 430-1300EB) in ~950 ml of water. Then dissolve sequentially the ingredients listed above. Adjust the pH to 7.4–7.5 by using NaOH and bring the final volume to 1 L.

*This concentration includes salts present in the packaged L-15 mix.

prolonged with this medium. In this case, the substrate need not be preexposed to hemolymph.

Hemolymph is a convenient source of growth-promoting activity because it can be obtained easily in large quantities. The 500 to 1500-g *Aplysia* can yield up to half their body weight in hemolymph. To collect hemolymph, the large animal is left in a beaker of artificial sea water at 4°C for an hour to anesthetize it. Then it is held gently and tilted so that hemolymph flows to the head. A small (1-cm-long) slice is made through the body wall on the dorsal midline between the eyes. The hemolymph spurts out and is collected in a beaker. (For a discussion of the anatomy and many other aspects of *Aplysia*, see Kandel, 1976.) It should take less than a minute to collect the hemolymph after the cut is made. Gentle squeezing of the posterior of the animal can increase the recovery, but it is important that the hemolymph not be contaminated with ink or mucus. The hemolymph, which should be colorless to pale purple, is centrifuged for 10 min in a refrigerated Sorvall centrifuge at approximately $10,000 \times g$ to pellet cells and large particles, and the supernatant is sterile-filtered and then stored for as long as necessary in 5- to 10-ml aliquots at −75°C.

Preparation of Culture Dishes

Neurons are placed in culture in plastic 50×9–mm Petri dishes with tight-fitting lids (Falcon, cat. no. 1006). Specimens can be viewed with DIC optics only on glass, so we modify the culture dishes for those experiments using DIC by placing inserts of glass coverslips in the dishes. Securing the plastic dish with a custom-made holder, we use a drill press or punch to cut a hole in the bottom of the dish. We make two different types of dishes. In one, the hole is a rectangle (18×33 mm) with arched rather than straight short sides. In the other, used in experiments in which we want to conserve reagents (e.g., fluorescent antibodies), the hole is a circle (13 mm in diameter) which, in some cultures, is connected by narrow channels (2.5×6 mm) on opposite sides to smaller circles (4 mm diameter) to permit perfusion. The edges of the hole are sanded manually inside and outside the dish, debris is blown out of the dish with jets of compressed air, and the dish is submerged in 70% ethanol overnight to remove organic residues from the cutting procedure.

No. 1 rectangular (24×40 mm) or circular (24-mm) glass coverslips (German glass, Carolina Biological) are cleaned specially prior to mounting. They are submerged in a beaker of 50% nitric acid that is heated to 90°C on a hotplate in a chemical fume hood and then are removed from the hotplate and left overnight. Coverslips then are briefly immersed successively in tap water, 10 changes of deionized, double-distilled water and, finally, 70% ethanol and then are wiped dry with Kimwipes. This cleaning procedure is derived from those originally developed for culturing vertebrate cells. We move the cover slips individually from solution to solution with a forceps, but it would clearly be much more efficient to use racks. It may not be necessary to go through this elaborate cleaning procedure at all. We have found neurites to grow well on coverslips used straight from the box, but those just starting with *Aplysia* culture might want to establish good cultures with the rigorous procedure before getting lax.

The coverslip is glued to the underside of the dish to seal the bottom of the hole, using silicone plastic (Sylgard, Dow Corning). Uncovered dishes are sterilized in the laminar flow hood by exposure for 30 to 45 min to ultraviolet light [Sylvania 8W germicidal lamp (G8T5)] 8–15 inches away). Approximately 30 dishes can be sterilized at once. After sterilization, they are capped with new sterile lids.

We perform high-resolution video microscopy on an inverted microscope, entailing the use of a short-working-distance, oil-immersion condenser. For such experiments, an acid-washed 24×40–mm no. 1 coverslip is positioned atop the hole in the plate so that the neurons lie at the bottom of a covered chamber that is 1 mm deep (the thickness of the bottom of the Petri dish). To allow perfusion of this chamber, the top coverslip is positioned so that the chamber is only partly covered, with open wells at either end. The top coverslip is added to the dish just before the video observations are to be made. It is placed on the surface of the culture medium and then lowered by withdrawing medium until it rests atop the hole and medium remains only in the chamber.

All culture dishes, with or without the glass inserts, are pretreated before adding the neurons by exposure first to a solution of polylysine in sodium borate. Sodium borate (0.1 M, pH 8.0–8.2) may be stored in the refrigerator for several weeks. A solution of 0.25–1 mg/ml poly-D-lysine hydrobromide (mol. wt. >300,000; Sigma cat. no. P-1024) is made on the day it is to be used, is sterile-filtered, and is added to each dish to cover the bottom. Lidded dishes are left at room temperature for anywhere from overnight to over a weekend, although occasionally we have left them for as little as a few hours without noticeable problems arising. The polylysine solution is aspirated through a sterile Pasteur pipette connected to a vacuum line, and the dishes are rinsed five times with sterile, deionized, double-distilled water. If necessary, hemolymph then is added to cover the bottoms of the dishes, and the dishes are left at room temperature for 3 to 24 h. The hemolymph is removed, the dishes are rinsed once with our defined culture medium, then 2.5 to 3.0 ml of culture medium is added.

Dissection

REMOVAL OF GANGLIA AND DESHEATHING
If ganglia from more than one animal will be needed for the planned experiments, all are removed and treated simultaneously with protease, then stored in SL-15 to be worked on individually (see the following). Animals up to 20 g are anesthetized by submersion for approximately 30 min in 0.35 M $MgCl_2$. Larger animals must receive an injection of perhaps a fourth to a half of their body weight of $MgCl_2$ solution into the body cavity. The injection should

be made through the side of the animal just rostral to the parapodia (the two large flaps on the dorsal surface of the animal), with the 20-gauge needle pointing rostrally.

The anesthetized animal is pinned foot down to a Petri dish containing a layer of Sylgard, is placed on a stereo dissecting microscope, and is viewed at 13× magnification with epiillumination. A fine Vannas scissors is used to make an incision rostrally on the dorsal midline from close to the parapodia to the tip of the animal. This exposes the digestive tract, connected via the esophagus to the buccal mass, a red ball that occupies much of the head and serves as the chewing apparatus (figure 8.1). Astride the juncture of esophagus and buccal mass is the orange cerebral ganglion, a few millimeters across and easily visible. (All the ganglia are

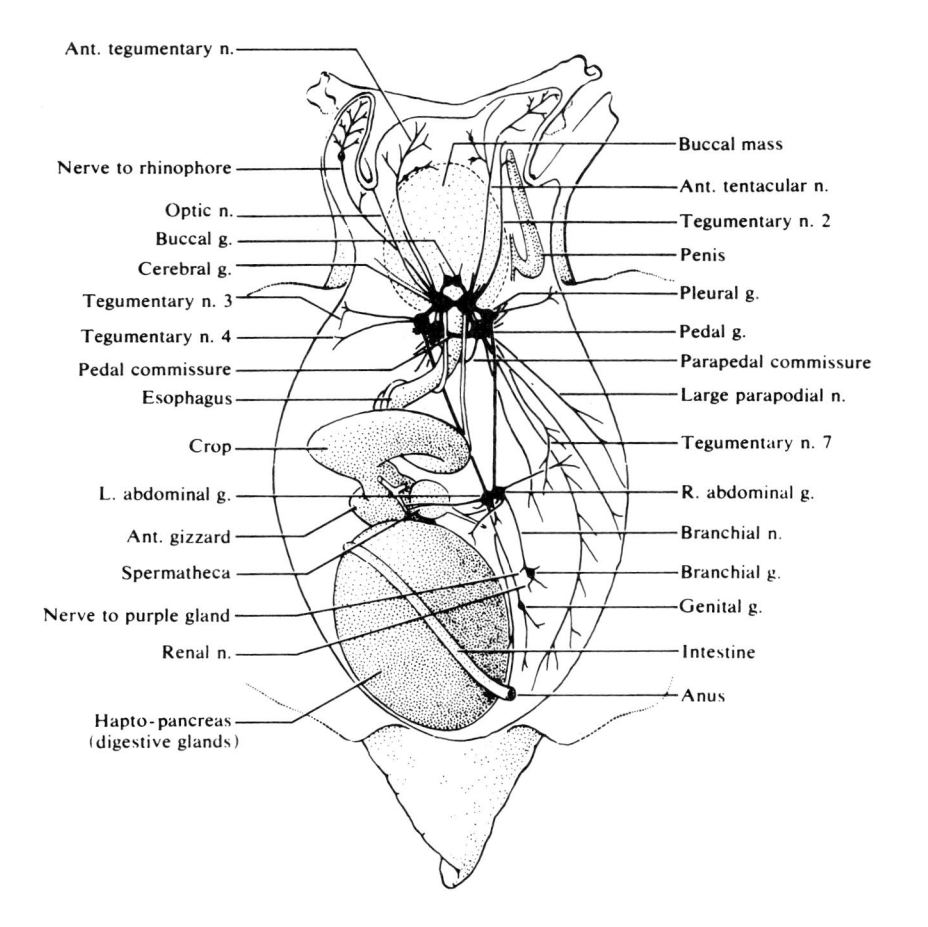

Figure 8.1 Nervous system in relation to internal organs of *Aplysia*. (Reprinted with permission from Kandel, 1976. Copyright 1976 W. H. Freeman and Co.)

orange.) Connectives from the cerebral ganglion encircle the esophagus and connect on each side to a pleuropedal ganglion; the smaller pleural is fused to the pedal ganglion but can be separated from it. The two pedal ganglia are joined by a commissure that lies beneath the esophagus, so nervous tissue completely rings the esophagus. The long pleuroabdominal connectives (right and left) exit from the pleuropedal ganglia and extend distally along the esophagus to the abdominal ganglion.

After removal of the abdominal ganglion (if desired), the esophagus and salivary glands are grasped with a blunt no. 5 Dumont jeweler's forceps, are pulled away from the head, and are severed with the scissors as close as possible to the cerebral ganglion. By cutting connectives and peripheral nerves, one can remove the desired ganglia. We use several different ganglia for different purposes and thus generally take the entire ring structure plus the fused pair of buccal ganglia that lies underneath (and is connected to) the cerebral ganglion.

The connective tissue capsules of the ganglia are softened by incubation with protease (type IX from *Bacillus polymyxa*, Sigma cat, no. P-6141). The ganglia from several animals are combined in one plastic Petri dish containing 8 ml of sterile-filtered protease solution (7 units/ml in SL-15) and are incubated at 34° to 35°C in a dry oven. The duration of incubation varies according to the size of the animals. For 1.5- to 4-g animals, we usually use 90 to 100 min, and for 4- to 10-g animals, perhaps 105 min. Larger animals (75–150 g) would require 120 to 150 min. In any case, it is important to remember that the thickness and composition of the connective tissue sheath may vary during the year and among animals obtained from different sources. Therefore, the digestion times suggested may not give consistent optimal softening of the sheath, so expect that they will require empirical adjustment. An overdigested sheath is one that has disintegrated to such a degree that scarcely any manipulation is needed to expose the neurons, which themselves will appear mushy rather than like firm grapes.

After digestion, the ganglia are transferred to SL-15 and kept at room temperature or, preferably, at 18°C until one is ready to dissect out the cells. It is probably best to start the cell removal as soon as possible, but we frequently allow digested ganglia to remain for 2 to 3 h before dissection without noticeable effect on the success of the culturing.

DISPERSION OF CELLS IN GANGLIA

Usually, we obtain ganglia from 2- to 5-g juveniles, but ganglia from larger juveniles or even adults can be used by increasing the duration of protease treatment and subdividing the ganglia more before trituration (see later). We favor the pedal ganglia, for they are the largest in the animal and have a high percentage of the small and medium-sized neurons that survive the dispersion procedure. The small pleural ganglion is attached closely to each of the two pedal ganglia and should be removed before desheathment. In addition, the mechanosensory cell cluster in the pleural portion of the pleuropedal ganglion can be dissected out after desheathing and can be dissociated into single cells via trituration. Approximately 150 to 200 sensory cells can be harvested from each cluster. Ganglia are transferred to a sterile 50-mm glass Petri dish the bottom of which is covered with Sylgard and which contains either 1% fetal bovine serum (Whittaker Bioproducts) or 10% to 50% hemolymph in SL-15. The primary purpose of the serum probably is to provide a proteinaceous coating of the surfaces of the neurons and the micropipettes used for dissection, making them less sticky. In fact, recently we have found that 1% bovine serum albumin works satisfactorily.

While a ganglion is being viewed at 32× magnification with a stereo dissecting microscope, it is pinned to the Sylgard by 0.1-mm-thick stainless steel minuten pins (Carolina Biological) the blunt halves of which have been cut off with a wire cutter to shorten the pins to a length of several millimeters. Two pins are placed through nerve stumps radiating from opposite edges of the ganglion so as to stretch the connective tissue capsule (figure 8.2). Then, under viewing with 8× magnification, the connective tissue capsule is ripped off, exposing the cell bodies. Techniques vary here. It is most efficient first to tear the capsule by pinching it with the sharp tips of two Dumont no. 5 "biologie" model forceps close to each other. Then the capsule is grasped by slipping one prong of each forceps under it and is peeled back. Done by a practiced hand, the desheathing can take less than a minute. Sheath and axon stumps are trimmed away with a fine Vannas scissors, leaving the naked clump of cells of the ganglion. This clump is cut into two or three pieces (or a specific cluster is removed), depending on the size of the ganglion.

The divided clumps from two ganglia are taken up with approximately 15 to 20 µl of medium into a length of capillary tubing (30 µl

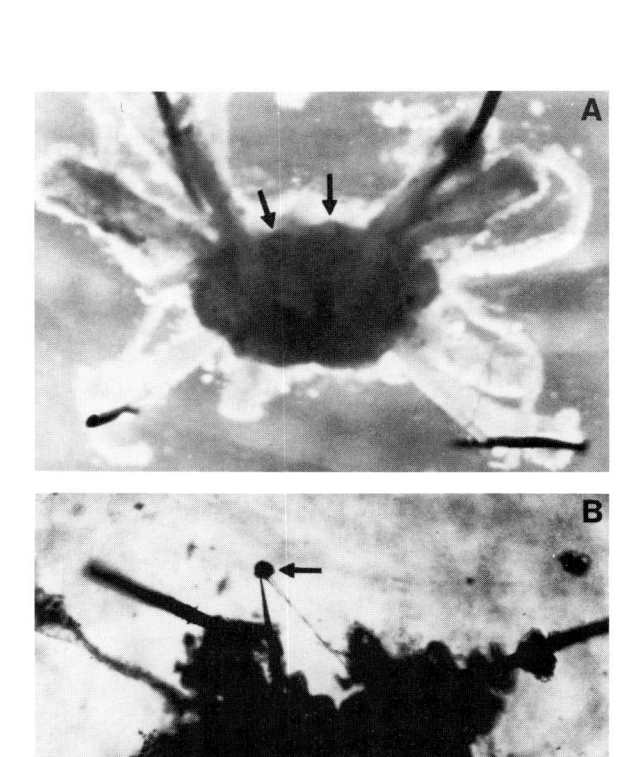

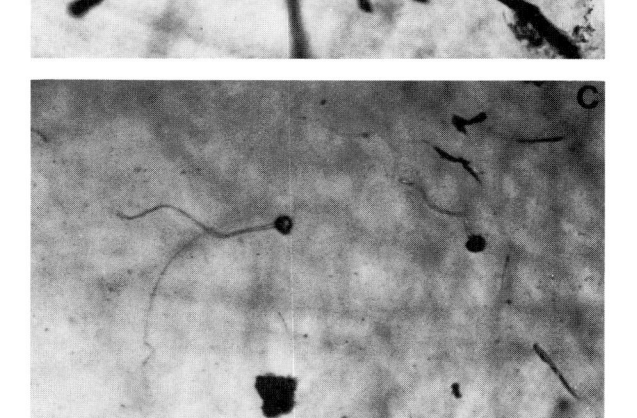

Figure 8.2 Removal of giant cerebral neuron (GCN) from cerebral ganglion of *Aplysia*. (*A*) A ganglion is shown pinned to the dish before desheathing, with the pair of GCNs visible near the top (arrows). (*B*) A GCN (arrows) is pulled out from another cerebral ganglion with a micropipette, the axon trailing the cell body. (*C*) After removal from the ganglion and release from the micropipette, the neurons rest at the bottom of the dish. The two main axonal branches of the GCN on the left are well-separated. Scale bar: 250 μm.

Drummond microcap, Fisher Scientific) for transfer to a plastic, capped, conical microcentrifuge tube (0.5 ml, no. 72.699, Sarstedt, Princeton, NJ) containing 0.2 ml of SL-15. These clumps are triturated rapidly by inspiring them into and expelling them from a plastic tip on an adjustable pipette (Gilson P-200 Pipetman) set for 0.1 ml. Thirty to forty cycles usually are sufficient to disaggregate the clumps thoroughly. An additional 0.25 ml of SL-15 then is added to the tube, and it is capped and centrifuged at room temperature for 10 min at low speed (no. 3 setting) in a table-top IEC (International Equipment Co.) clinical centrifuge to collect the dissociated cells near the bottom of the tube, without actually pelleting them.

From the bottom of the tube of cell suspension, 50 to 100 µl then is drawn off using the Pipetman with a fresh tip, and is placed as a large droplet in the center of a culture dish. The dish is covered and allowed to sit undisturbed for 5 to 10 min, allowing the cells to settle and stick to the substratum. When many of the cells have stuck, SL-15 is added gently to the final desired volume, which can be as little as 0.75 to 1.0 ml to fill only the central chamber or as much as 3 ml to cover the entire bottom of the culture dish. We add cells to the dish in this manner so as to confine them to the central region of the dish. If the cells are added to a dish that already contains a large volume of medium, they tend to disperse too widely.

REMOVAL OF INDIVIDUAL NEURONS
Though adult animals may be used as source material for cultures of dispersed cells, generally they are not used for removal of individual neurons. Typically, we use 2- to 5-g juvenile animals, though on occasion we have used juveniles as large as 30 g. For generating cocultures of mechanosensory and motor neurons (see the foregoing), abdominal or pleural ganglia are dissected from 70- to 90-g animals as a source of the individual presynaptic sensory cells (cell bodies of 50–70 µm in diameter), whereas postsynaptic motor cells are isolated from small juveniles as described further.

The sheath is removed from the ganglion as described earlier, with some additional considerations. First, to remove identified cells, one must pin the ganglion to the dish with the appropriate surface up; cell bodies are found on both dorsal and ventral surfaces, surrounding a core of neuropil. Second, the ganglion must remain pinned firmly to the dish while the individual cells are extricated. So, though two opposite pins are sufficient to stretch

and secure the buccal ganglion pair, the larger, more squarish cerebral ganglion needs a pin at each of its four corners (see figure 8.2),
as do the abdominal and pleuropedal ganglia. (The pleural and
pedal ganglia need not be separated in this procedure.) Third, the
sheath is pulled back merely to expose the cell bodies, rather than
being detached from the ganglion. Last, one does not detach the
nerve stumps from the ganglion. If the lengths of the axon stumps
of the neurons to be extricated are inconsequential for the experiment, the nerves should be cut only long enough to allow pins to be
inserted. The shorter the axon stump, the easier it is to remove a
neuron. However, some experiments may require neurons with
long axon stumps, thus requiring the nerves containing those axons
to be cut far from the ganglion during removal from the animal. We
have pulled out neurons with axon stumps as long as 2 mm.

Individual neurons are removed by using glass micropipettes
with very long, fine tips. We make them from microelectrode glass
with a 1.5-mm outer diameter and an internal glass filament (World
Precision Instruments, New Haven, CT), using a Narishige PE-2
vertical microelectrode puller. The tapering tip should be approximately 15 mm of the total 65-mm length of the micropipette, and its
orifice should be so small (probably <0.5 μm) as virtually to prevent
liquid from entering by capillarity when submerged. If liquid starts
rising substantially in the tip at any point during the microdissection procedure, it means that some of the tip has broken off,
and the micropipette should be discarded.

The neuron of interest is removed by touching it with the tip of
the micropipette, preferably near the edge opposite to the direction
in which the cell will be pulled out of the ganglion. The neuron
should adhere and can then be slowly extracted, its axon(s) trailing
(see figure 8.2B). It is preferable to pull the cell away from the
nerves that contain its axonal branches, but this approach is not
always possible, as some cells have branches that exit the ganglion
in opposite directions. When the neuron has been pulled free of
the ganglion, it is dislodged from the micropipette by flicking the
latter against a piece of micropipette tip that has previously been
embedded upright in the Sylgard at a convenient distance from the
ganglion. Discarded micropipettes often are used to make these
"posts."

The neuron gradually settles to the bottom when dislodged from
the micropipette (see figure 8.2C). If the neuron has multiple axonal
branches that might have to be kept apart in the culture dish, it

is imperative to separate them at this point. This is done with the tip of the micropipette, but it is essential that the tip be unbroken (one may have to change micropipettes a few times), because the branches tend to stick to broken tips. If the branches have intertwined, find a separation, insert the tip of a micropipette, and knock it forcefully against the branches repeatedly to separate them gradually. It is surprising how hard the branches can be hit without injuring them if they are floating freely in the medium.

Neurons are transferred to the culture dish in a 30-µl microcap. Unlike the procedure with dispersed cells, the bottom of the culture dish is covered completely with culture medium (2.5 ml) when cells are added. To take up cells for transfer to the culture dish, allow medium to come up the microcap more than halfway by capillarity and then expel it completely, using the bulb supplied with the microcaps. This process coats the inside of the microcap with protein, thereby reducing sticking of the neurons. Then, viewing the preparation with 80× magnification, bring the tip of the microcap close to the neurons, holding it at an angle of 40° to 70° to the bottom. The neurons should be drawn gently into the microcap by capillarity; a few can be transferred in one microcap. If they do not enter immediately, draw more medium into the microcap by reducing the angle at which it is held. The uptake of the neurons should be strictly by capillarity. If one tries to suck them up by using the bulb, it will be very difficult to transfer them subsequently to the culture dish. The bulb should be used only for expelling medium (and neurons) from the microcap.

Neurons are expelled into the culture dish by submerging the tip of the microcap in the medium and gently squeezing the bulb. This action is performed under viewing at low power so that the neurons can be seen moving down the microcap. Sometimes a neuron sticks to the wall of the microcap. Often it can be dislodged by moving the medium rapidly up and down a short distance within the microcap. Never allow the meniscus to overtake the stuck cell; exposure to air will destroy the cell immediately. Usually we try to culture 5 to 15 identified neurons per dish, concentrated in the center (without overlapping), but the number and arrangement of neurons in culture dishes will depend on personal needs. For example, it is possible to culture a single sensory cell with a single motor cell target. After the motor target is placed in the center of the well and is allowed to adhere to the surface, an individual sensory cell can be added by pipetting the cell carefully near the motor target.

Once in the dish, a cell and its axonal branches can be positioned rather precisely, if desired. Use an unbroken micropipette that has been dipped in 1% serum, bovine serum albumin, or hemolymph to keep the neuron from sticking. The most difficult aspect of this fine positioning, which is done at high magnification, is getting the axonal branches to stay put. Until the endings stick to the substrate, the branches tend to move in the currents in the medium generated by the vibrations of the laminar flow hood. If positioning is important, the dish must remain on the microscope stage overnight to allow axonal growth to begin, which will help tack the neurons down.

Care of Cultures

We store cultures in an incubator set at 17° to 18°C. (No special atmospheric conditions are needed in the incubator.) There is nothing sacred about this temperature. In the wild, *A. californica* experiences temperatures ranging from 12° to 25°C (Kupfermann and Carew, 1974). We store animals in our laboratory aquaria at 11° to 14°C. Often we leave cultured neurons at room temperature (20°–22°C) for a few days, apparently without inhibiting neuronal growth. However, most of the data in the literature on *Aplysia* neurons in culture are derived from cultures stored at 17° to 18°C. If cultures are to be stored for several days, it is advisable to change part of the medium every day by gently adding 1 ml of hemolymph:SL-15 to one edge of the dish, then immediately withdrawing 1 ml from the other edge. Substantial contamination of cultures with microorganisms rarely is observed. Culture dishes should be moved gingerly, as cell bodies and original axonal stumps sometimes will be attached only weakly to the substrate.

Progression of Cultures

Neuritic growth sometimes can be detected within a few hours of culturing the cells. By the next day, one should see several neurites that are a few hundred microns long (figure 8.3). Most of the growth is from the ends of the original axonal stumps of neurons that were pulled out individually. Typically, many thin neurites emerge from the end of the stump. Some processes may emerge from the region of the cell body, more so if the original axon is very short. Neurons cultured by dispersion usually do not retain their axonal stumps.

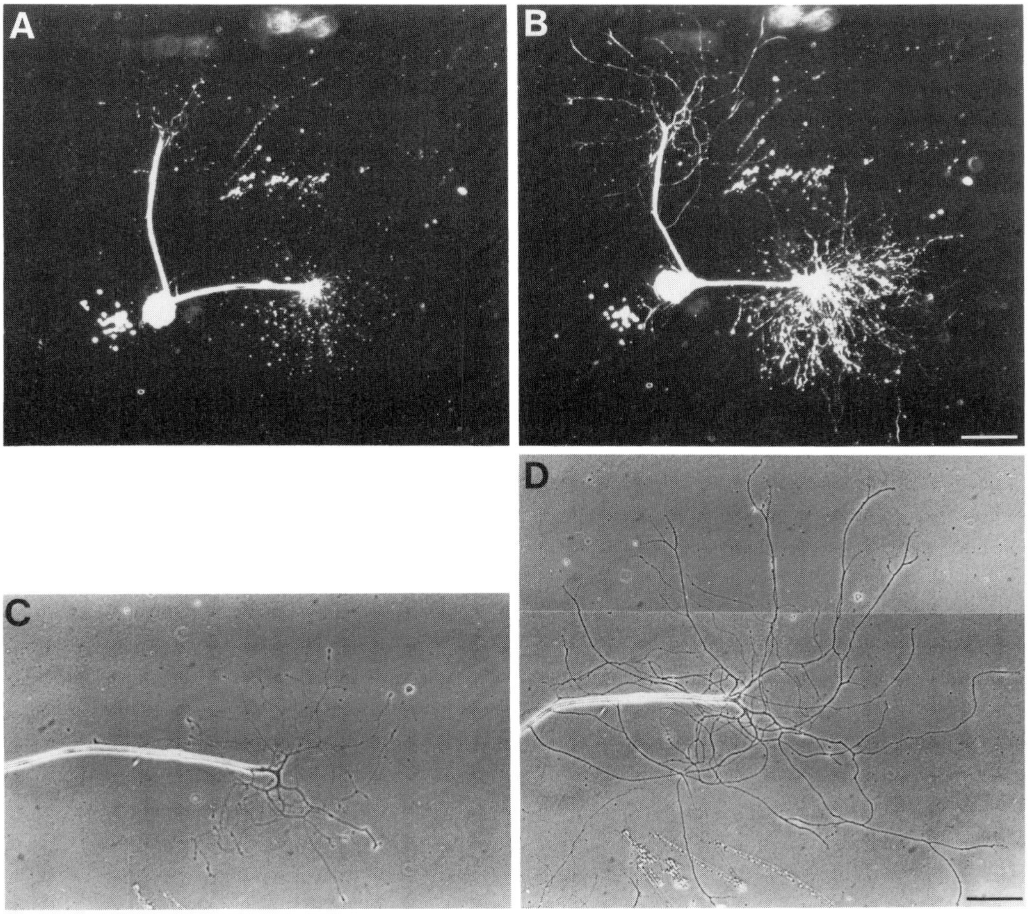

Figure 8.3 Neurite outgrowth from a giant cerebral neuron in culture. Outgrowth from the ends of the original axonal stumps is evident after 1 day (*A, C*) and is more extensive after 5 days (*B, D*). (*C, D*) Views of the lip nerve at higher magnification. Also, some neuritic outgrowth is evident from near the cell body. Scale bar: (*A, B*) 250 μm, (*C, D*) 100 μm.

Neurites grow out from the cell body, much as is seen with vertebrate neurons. Usually, a few thick processes grow, and these later branch to form thinner neurites. We do not have a lot of experience with dispersed cultures, but it is our impression that substantial growth is somewhat slower in starting in them than in cultures of neurons dissected individually, as might be expected, as new axons must be initiated. However, there should be some growth within a day of placing the cells in culture and, with both types of culture, growth should continue for 3 to 7 days (see figure 8.3). Chemical synapses between neurons are electrophysiologically detectable as

early as 12 h after coculture. Although neuritic growth stops within 1 week, electrophysiological properties of the neurons are maintained for up to 3 weeks. Neurons obviously are dying when beading of their neurites is visible.

Contamination with glial cells of individually dissected neurons has never been a problem. A few undefined nonneuronal cells adhering to the cell body often are transferred to the culture dish with the extricated neuron, but their aggregate volume is far less than that of the neuron and they do not seem to proliferate during the few days of culture. Many more nonneuronal cells are, of course, present in cultures obtained by ganglion dissociation but are not enough to be a significant problem during the few days of use of the cultures.

Problems

Unsatisfactory cultures occur because of poor cell survival or poor neuritic growth. Poor synapse formation parallels poor neuritic growth. Poor cell survival most often results from excessive treatment of the ganglion with protease. A properly treated connective tissue capsule should look a little ragged, but it should not tend to fall apart of its own accord; it should be necessary to rip it off with forceps or by stretching the ganglion with pins. The neuronal cell bodies should look firm and well-defined in the ganglion, like a cluster of grapes. The mushy cell bodies of an overdigested ganglion are more likely to be ripped open by the great stress of being pulled from the ganglion. (Even cell bodies of healthy neurons will deform considerably while the neuron is being pulled from the ganglion.) Also, a greater likelihood exists that the initial segment of the axon will be damaged, causing the cell to die during dissection or in culture.

Poor neuronal growth (or synapse formation) is a somewhat more common and vexing problem. The three most common causes are overtreatment of the ganglion with protease, bad hemolymph, and bad animals. Neurons from an overdigested ganglion often will survive in the culture dish. However, if the axons are very wrinkled or "feel" stiff when tapped with a micropipette, chances are good that growth will be poor. One would think that, once things are going properly, treatment of ganglia with protease for a consistent amount of time would never result in overdigestion. Sad to say, this is not true, probably because of variation in the thickness of con-

nective tissue capsules among batches of animals even of the same size. However, this should not be a frequent problem. Hemolymph with little growth-promoting activity rarely is a problem if it is collected from large animals. The activity of each batch of hemolymph should first be tested in a few cultures. If satisfactory, the hemolymph can be frozen in aliquots and used as needed. One large animal provides enough hemolymph to treat a few hundred culture dishes.

Bad animals is the default explanation for poor axonal growth—but with reason. Some periods of poor axonal growth in our laboratories have coincided with periods of poor growth in other laboratories. Occasionally, the ganglia from an entire batch of animals simply do not look right. Often, the cell bodies have excessive pigmentation (deeper orange-to-red color with reflective illumination). Probably the only recourse is to try obtaining animals from a different source or of a different size.

Other Invertebrate Neurons in Culture

Three other invertebrates whose neurons have been studied extensively in culture—addressing issues of axonal growth, synapse formation, and plasticity—are the medicinal leech *Hirudo medicinalis* and the pond snails *Helisoma trivolvis* and *Lymnaea stagnalis*. Though the neurons of these animals are not as large as the giant neurons of *Aplysia*, some are quite respectable in size: the Retzius neuron of the leech is approximately 100 μm in diameter, and the average *Helisoma* growth cone is at least as large as those of *Aplysia*. Leech neurons can form specific chemical synapses in culture and have been studied electrophysiologically (Ready and Nicholls, 1979; Chiquet and Nicholls, 1987). Cultured identified leech neurons have been used also to assess how specific cell-cell interactions and second-messenger cascades influence the formation of specific connections and the development of pre- and post-synaptic properties (Drapeau, 1990; Catarsi and Drapeau, 1993; Merz and Drapeau, 1994). *Helisoma* neurons have been used primarily to study the regulation of growth cone activity by neurotransmitters and second messengers (Haydon et al., 1984; Cohan et al., 1985, 1987; Rehder and Kater, 1992) and the role of intercellular and intracellular signals in synapse formation and plasticity of specific connections (Zoran et al., 1990; 1991; Funte and Haydon, 1993; Durgerian et al., 1993). The *Lymnaea* preparation

has been used to study both the individual cell and network properties of small ensembles of neurons in vitro (Syed et al., 1990; Bulloch and Syed, 1992).

Our Work with Cultured *Aplysia* Neurons

We have used *Aplysia* neurons in culture to study intracellular events underlying axonal growth and synapse formation and modulation, and how these events are modified by the environment. VEC-DIC microscopy was used to study initial events in the formation of growth cones by observation of *Aplysia* axons transected in culture (Goldberg and Burmeister, 1992). Events within the growth cone underlying axonal elongation were analyzed by using VEC-DIC observation of the growth cones of B1 and B2, a pair of giant peptidergic neurons of the buccal ganglia (Goldberg and Burmeister, 1986). We were able to obtain a more detailed record (in real time) of these events than previously had been possible with optical procedures providing much less magnification and resolution. An idea of the increase in detail obtained by connecting the microscope to the special video camera used for VEC-DIC microscopy is provided by figure 8.4. Axonal elongation was seen to consist of a series of three morphological transformations in the growth cone: protrusion of flat plasma membrane poor in cytoplasm and membranous organelles; engorgement of this membrane with membranous organelles and cytoplasm moving in from proximal regions of the growth cone; and consolidation of this spread swollen region into a cylindrical neurite. The large size of many *Aplysia* growth cones allowed microapplication of Ca^{2+} to small areas of the peripheral region of the growth cone to assess its role in the protrusion step (Goldberg, 1988).

Video microscopic observation of *Aplysia* growth cones is providing insight into the interaction of the growth cone with environmental cues. Hemolymph was found to accelerate axonal growth by facilitating specifically the engorgement step of the elongation sequence (Burmeister et al., 1991). Subsequent work on vertebrate growth cones showed that laminin works similarly (Rivas et al., 1992), suggesting this route as a common mode of action for substrate-binding growth promoters. Video-intensified fluorescence microscopy demonstrated that phosphotyrosine is concentrated heavily at the tips of *Aplysia* growth cone filopodia when the neurites are growing slowly on a polylysine substrate but not when

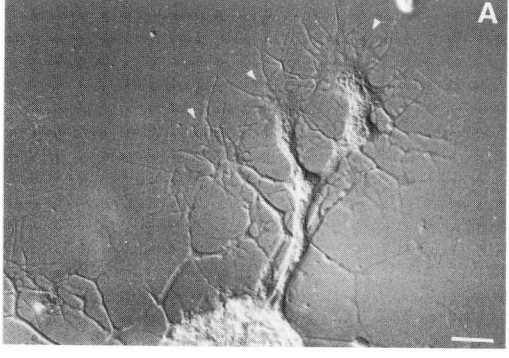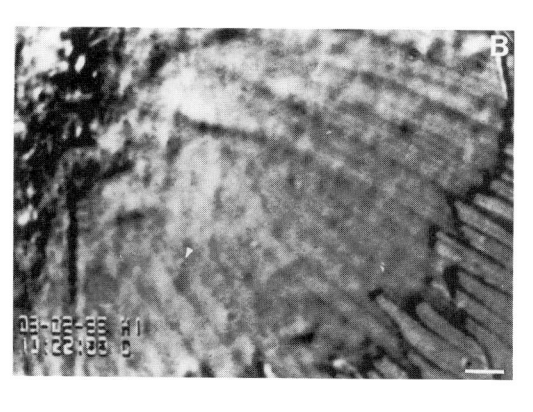

Figure 8.4 Growth cones of *Aplysia* neurons in culture. (*A*) Three large growth cones (arrowheads) viewed with differential interference contrast (Nomarski) microscopy. Neurites have emerged recently from the swollen end of the axonal stump, partially seen as the bright object at the bottom. Scale bar: 10 µm. (*B*) Distal portion of another large growth cone viewed with video-enhanced contrast-differential interference contrast microscopy. Bundles of actin filaments can be seen projecting back from filopodia through the large lamellipodium. Membranous organelles are clustered in the central region at top left. This technique allows the detection of individual vesicles. Scale bar: 1 µm.

neurites are growing rapidly on a substrate preexposed to hemolymph (Wu and Goldberg, 1993). Filopodia are perhaps the most important elements of the growth cone for interacting with environmental cues that direct neuritic growth, but how they are specialized to perform this function is understood poorly. Our findings suggest the importance of protein-tyrosine phosphorylation and, once again, are proving relevant to vertebrate growth cones. In addition, video microscopical observation of *Aplysia* growth cones responding to substrate cues in culture suggests that some neurite turning during growth occurs by a withering of inappropriately directed small processes, a small-scale version of the pruning that shapes developing axonal trees (Burmeister and Goldberg, 1988).

As mentioned earlier, we were able to use *Aplysia* neurons also in culture to gain some insight into the intracellular events that underlie differential growth of different branches of an axonal tree. Here, the ability to remove long lengths of the axonal tree and to reconstruct in culture some of the in situ circuitry was critical. GCN, whose axon splits into two major branches, can be placed in culture so that the ends of the branches are far apart. If appropriate target neurons are placed near only one branch, chemical synapses form, and the growth of neurites from that branch continues while growth from the other branch slows dramatically (Schacher, 1985).

We were able to detect, with VEC-DIC microscopy, a diversion of rapidly transported materials away from the slowly growing branch (Goldberg and Schacher, 1987). This change in the distribution of delivered materials may be an important factor contributing to the differential growth.

The ability of *Aplysia* neurons to reestablish chemical connections in vitro, including connections that form the basic circuit for a reflex behavior, has allowed us to begin to study the cellular and molecular mechanisms underlying both initial synapse formation and long-term modulation of mature connections. *Aplysia* mechanosensory neurons reestablish appropriate chemical connections that can be modified up (homosynaptic or heterosynaptic facilitation) or down (homosynaptic or heterosynaptic depression) for short or long durations (Montarolo et al., 1986, 1988; Rayport and Schacher, 1986; Schacher et al., 1990; Lin and Glanzman, 1994a,b). With repeated fluorescent dye injections, it has been possible to examine the morphological details of the initial interactions between the neurites of the presynaptic and postsynaptic cells and the changes in those interactions over time or after experimental manipulations that evoke long-term changes in synaptic efficacy. The results of these studies reveal that presynaptic neurons form more intimate contact with their target cells than with nontarget cells (Glanzman et al., 1989; Hawver and Schacher, 1993; Zhu et al., 1994a; figure 8.5). These initial interactions can be modulated by neurotransmitters, by the activation of specific second-messenger systems, or by adding specific monoclonal antibodies that recognize cell-surface adhesion molecules (Peter et al., 1994; Zhu et al., 1994a; Wu and Schacher, 1994). The results suggest that diffusible substances activating specific intracellular second-messenger cascades can influence cell-cell interactions by altering the distribution or expression of cell adhesion molecules on either the presynaptic or postsynaptic cell.

Similar mechanisms may be involved in the long-term modulation of the behaviorally relevant sensorimotor synaptic connection in vitro. Both long-term facilitation with serotonin and long-term inhibition with the neuropeptide FMRFamide are accompanied by structural changes in the arbor of the presynaptic sensory cell that are dependent on the presence of the appropriate target cell and on changes in protein and RNA synthesis (Montarolo et al., 1986, 1988; Glanzman et al., 1990; Schacher and Montarolo, 1991; Bailey et al., 1992). Recent studies have concentrated on the role of specific

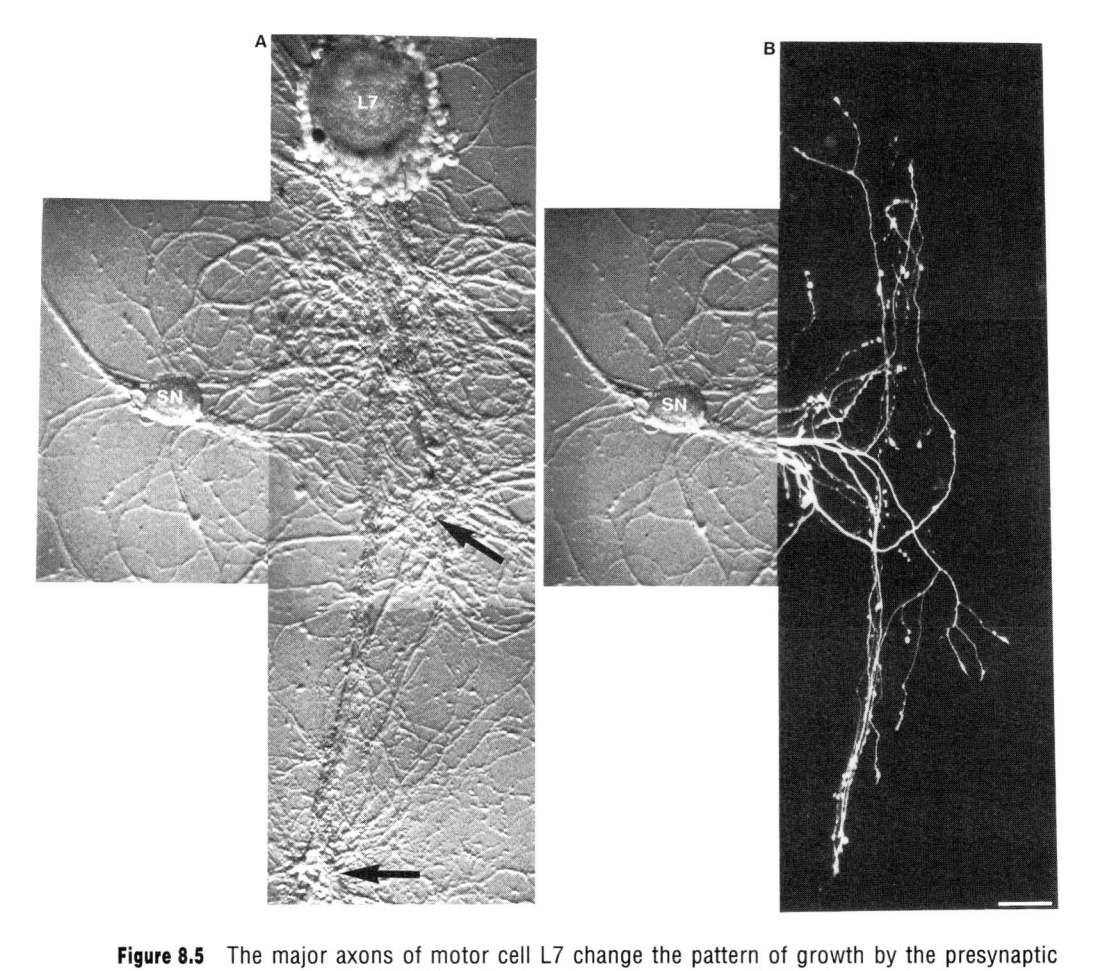

Figure 8.5 The major axons of motor cell L7 change the pattern of growth by the presynaptic sensory cell. (*A*) Differential interference–contrast (DIC) micrograph of a sensory neuron (SN) cocultured with motor cell L7 (L7) for 3 days. The axon stump of the sensory cell is approximately 200 μm from the middle region of the major motor axons that emerge from the cell body of L7 and extend toward the bottom of the photograph. The stumps of the L7 axons are indicated by the arrows (at the bottom of the photograph and in the middle of the photograph at the level of the sensory cell and its axon). (*B*) Collage of DIC view of the sensory neuron and epifluorescence view of the sensory neurites emerging from the stump of the sensory neuron and interacting with motor neurites and axons following intracellular injection of carboxy-fluorescein. Note that the sensory neurites extend primarily as thick bundles until reaching close to or following contact with the major axons of L7. Sensory neurites then form many branches studded with varicosities and extend primarily both up (toward cell body) and down (away from cell body) the major axons of L7. Scale bar: 50 μm. (Reprinted with permission from Zho et al., 1994a.)

second-messenger cascades and cell-surface adhesion molecules in effecting these changes in synaptic function and structure (Keller and Schacher, 1990; Mayford et al., 1992; Schacher et al., 1993; Peter et al., 1994; Wu and Schacher, 1994; Zhu et al., 1994a,b). The results are consistant with the hypothesis that some of the same mechanisms associated with the initial formation of specific connections are reused during the modulation of those connections in the mature nervous system with behavioral plasticity.

Note

1. The following companies supply *Aplysia* collected off the coast of southern California: Marinus, Long Beach, CA (310) 435-6522 ($10.50 per animal); Marine Specimens, Pacific Palisades, CA (310) 459-8083 ($10.00); Alacrity, Redondo Beach, CA (310) 372-4950 ($10.00). Marinus has the most extensive diving capability and thus would be the best source for juvenile animals obtained by collection. Juvenile and adult animals that have been reared entirely in the laboratory are available from the mariculture facility at the University of Miami, Miami, FL (305) 361-1037 (prices range from $5 for small juveniles to $20 for adults).

9 Culturing Spinal Neurons and Muscle Cells from Xenopus Embryos

Nacira Tabti, Janet Alder, and Mu-ming Poo

Dissociated cell cultures of embryonic nerve and muscle tissues provide useful systems for studying various aspects of neuron and muscle differentiation, neuromuscular synaptogenesis, and synaptic functions (Fishchbach, 1972; Spitzer and Lamborghini, 1976; Anderson and Cohen, 1977). Cultures derived from embryos of the clawed toad *Xenopus* offer several advantages: (1) The preparation of the culture is relatively simple, and the culture can be maintained at room temperature in simple medium, requiring minimal facilities; (2) the cells remain viable for many hours in open air at room temperature on the microscope stage, ideal for electrophysiological recordings; (3) the developmental stages of the *Xenopus* cells in vivo are well-characterized (Nieuwkoop and Faber, 1967), providing useful background information for identifying parallel development in culture; and (4) the early embryo is readily accessible to intracellular injection of chemicals.

To study the molecular events involved in a number of neuronal functions, including nerve growth and turning, synaptogenesis, and transmitter secretion, it is useful to manipulate the chemical composition of the nerve terminal. Unfortunately, this approach often is hindered by the inaccessibility of the small nerve terminal to experimental manipulation. Early *Xenopus* blastomeres, on the other hand, are large and are injected easily with molecules of interest. During the first few days of embryonic development, the *Xenopus* embryo undergoes successive cell divisions without substantial growth in its overall size. Thus, macromolecules that are injected into an early blastomere remain relatively undiluted throughout cell diversion, resulting in an effective loading of the molecules into all the progeny cells of the injected blastomere, including spinal neurons and myotomal myocytes. The method of overexpression or ectopic expression of messages by blastomere injection of *Xenopus* embryos has been used extensively to study the role of a number of proteins in embryonic development and morphogenesis, including basic fibroblast growth factor (Amaya et

al., 1991; Kimelman and Maas, 1992), homeobox proteins (Ruiz i Altaba and Melton, 1989; Niehrs et al., 1993), N-cadherin (Detrick et al., 1990; Fujimori et al., 1990), G protein α-subunits (Otte et al., 1992), and myogenic factors (Rashbass et al., 1992). Recently, we used this blastomere injection technique to study the roles of synapse-specific proteins by introducing exogenous protein, antibodies, or cRNA into the embryos (Lu et al., 1991; Alder et al., 1992; 1995; Schaeffer et al., 1994). Coinjection of the molecules of interest with a fluorescent marker, such as rhodamine-conjugated dextran, into identified embryonic cells, the lineage maps of which are well-known (Jacobson, 1982), is used to identify the progeny cells. Preparation of dissociated cell culture at a later stage of embryonic development allows one to obtain cells loaded with injected molecules for the study of cell-cell interactions in culture. Thus, by manipulating the levels or properties of specific neuronal components and by studying the consequences of that manipulation in culture, one can dissect molecular mechanisms underlying various neuronal functions.

During the first few days after cell plating, cultured *Xenopus* embryonic neurons and muscle cells undergo morphological and functional differentiation similar to that observed in vivo (Kullberg et al., 1977; Peng et al., 1979; Buchanan et al., 1989; Evers et al., 1989). A number of advanced techniques in video image processing and electrophysiology, which are difficult to apply to whole-tissue preparations, have been performed successfully on these cultures (Kuromi et al., 1985; Cohen et al., 1987; Harris et al., 1988). For example, young neurons can be presented with a stable gradient of a chemical, and their growth pattern can be imaged to determine whether the factor has chemotropic properties (Lohof et al., 1992; Zheng et al., 1994). In addition, the patch clamp recording technique has provided extensive information on the changes in neuronal and muscular ionic conductances during development (Brehm et al., 1984; Ribera and Spitzer, 1989). *Xenopus* muscle cells also can be brought into contact with other muscle cells or with neurons. This cell manipulation technique has facilitated studies of cell-cell interactions with accurate temporal resolution. It has been applied to study the appearance of gap junctions between muscle cells (Chow and Poo, 1984) and the properties of early synaptic potentials (Evers et al., 1989) as well as the ultrastructure of early synaptic specializations between nerve and muscle cells (Buchanan et al., 1989).

Under the culture conditions that we have established, muscle cells can be maintained in a healthy state for 2 to 3 weeks, but few neurons survive beyond 5 days in culture. This system is thus most useful for studying early events in neuronal and synaptic development. In our experience, a novice usually can obtain usable cultures after a few trials.

Protocol for Obtaining *Xenopus* Embryos

Obtaining Mature Oocytes

Male and female pairs of adult *Xenopus laevis* can be purchased from Nasco Fort Atkinson, WI, Xenopus I (Dexter, MI), or Carolina Biological, Inc. (Burlington, NC). The female is identified by her larger size and a distinct cloaca opening at the rear end. Embryos may be obtained either by conditioning the animals for breeding or by artificial fertilization. The former procedure requires two consecutive injections of human chorionic gonadotropin (HCG) hormone to both the male and female, spaced several hours apart. Embryos are available within 2 to 3 days, depending on the injection schedule and on the doses of HCG (Thompson and Franks, 1978). Artificial fertilization is less time-consuming and provides large batches of embryos at a similar stage of development. The oocytes are obtained from adult females following a single injection of HCG. The male is sacrificed, and the sperm required for fertilization are obtained from isolated testes. Here we describe the method of artificial fertilization that is used in our laboratory.

Many factors may contribute to successful spawning after the injection of *Xenopus* females. Big, healthy females are preferred and should be kept at approximately 20°C for 2 weeks before HCG injection. The light-dark cycle also must be controlled; 10 h of light seems to be an optimal choice. *Xenopus* females are housed in separate containers filled with 0.1% saline and labeled with dates of injections. Males can be kept in a common large tank. All animals are fed three times a week with fresh liver, and tank water is changed at 6 h following feeding.

During injection of hormone, the female is held firmly by placing her in a nylon net (with the head directly toward the closed end) and holding her body still with one hand. Subcutaneous injections of HCG are made along the back, into the dorsal lymph sacs that lie

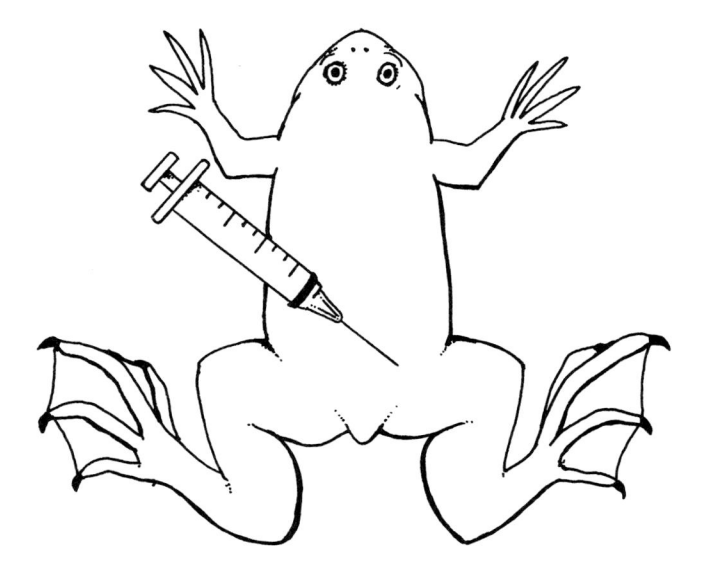

Figure 9.1 Injection of a *Xenopus* female with human gonadotropin hormone. The tip of the needle points to one of the bilateral sites at which the subcutaneous injection of HCG is made.

under the skin between the spine and the thigh joint (figure 9.1). A 25-guage 5/8-inch needle is inserted through the skin, and 1 ml of a solution containing 1000 IU of HCG (Sigma CG10) dissolved in sterile water is injected slowly. After the injection, the female is kept in a small tank of water and left in an undisturbed space until the first few eggs are noticed in the water. The time required for spawning is perhaps 12 h for 1000 IU hormone. The eggs are some 1 mm in diameter, brown at the animal pole and yellowish white at the vegetal pole. When natural spawning has begun, the testes are dissected from the male, and the eggs are fertilized (see further). The females are reused at a minimal interval of 3 months.

Artificial Fertilization

Fill two 5-ml test tubes with 10% Ringer's solution (100% Ringer's in mM: NaCl 115, KCL 2.6, $CaCl_2$ 2, HEPES 10, pH 7.6, 10% Ringer's: one part 100% Ringer's solution to nine parts H_2O) and store them in ice. Quickly decapitate and pith the male. Cut the ventral skin along the midline down to the pelvis and laterally on both sides. Push the skin aside to expose the abdominal muscles, then cut through them to expose the viscera. The paired testes are whitish ovoid structures (approximately 10 mm long and 3 mm wide) attached to the base of fat bodies (yellowish, with many

figurelike lobes). Carefully remove the testes and transfer each immediately to a 5-ml test tube. Rinse them a few times with 10% Ringer's solution to clean them of blood. The testes are stored on ice in a solution containing 80% of FCS and MMR (in mM: 100 NaCl, 2 KCl, 1 MgSO$_4$, 2 CaCl$_2$, 5 HEPES, 0.1, (EDTA), pH 7.8). It can be used for a few days, and a piece of tissue can be used for each fertilization.

When testes are ready for use, release the mature oocytes from the female by gently rubbing along her back down toward the cloaca. Collect oocytes in an empty 100-mm Petri dish. Depending on the number of eggs obtained at one time (which varies from tens to hundreds), a piece of testis tissue is crushed in a test tube homogenizer in 10% Ringer's solution to yield a cloudy solution. Cover the freshly obtained oocytes with this solution and spread the eggs into a monolayer by shaking the Petri dish. Fertilization should occur within 10 to 15 min at room temperature, as indicated by the rotation of the oocytes inside the vitelline membrane, bringing the darkly pigmented animal pole upward. Once fertilized, the eggs should be washed with 10% Ringer's solution and incubated in the same solution for further development. Soon after cleavage starts (perhaps 1.25 h after fertilization), embryos are sorted out under dissection microscope, and unfertilized or damaged embryos are removed from the incubation dish to prevent contamination of the healthy embryos. Staging of embryonic development follows Nieuwkoop and Faber (1967). Embryos from stage 19 (initial neural tube stage, with neural folds touching each other, 21 h after fertilization) to stage 22 (suture of neural tube completely closed, 24 h after fertilization) are used for nerve-muscle culture. These early stages are used because neural tube and associated myotomal tissues can be dissociated in calcium- and magnesium-free (CMF) solution without the use of enzymes. In addition, at later stages, most of the myoblasts already have acquired a spindle shape, and the proportion of round muscle cells, which are suitable for manipulation, becomes sparse.

Protocol for Early Blastomere Injection

Preparation

Prepare several good injection pipettes prior to fertilization of the eggs. Pull small glass pipettes (1-mm outer diameter, 0.5-mm inner

diameter; Drummond Microcaps, Novato, CA cat. no. 1-000-0060-65) on a one-step microelectrode puller (Sutter Instruments P-80 or equivalent) so that the length of the tapered shaft is no more than 5 mm. Under a dissecting microscope at high magnification and using a fine forcep (Dumont 5 or 55), break the tip of the pipette so that the opening is sharp and shaped like the tip of a needle, with an outer diameter of 6 to 10 µm.

Fertilize the eggs artificially as described earlier. After the embryos have undergone rotation in the vitelline membrane, manually remove the jelly coat of the embryos by using two fine forceps and place these embryos in a Petri dish (60 × 15 mm, Falcon 3002) containing 10% Ringer's solution. Use a Pasteur pipette with the tip cut to an opening slightly larger than the embryos to transfer them. The number of embryos injected per fertilization by one person usually is in the range of 20 to 50.

While waiting for the embryos to divide, you can prepare the solution for injection. Mix the solution containing the molecule of interest with one containing rhodamine-conjugated dextran (Sigma R-8881), so that the final concentration of dextran is perhaps 1 mg/ml. For cRNA injections, we start with 5 µl of 2 mg/ml cRNA and mix it 1:1 with rhodamine-dextran solution (15 mg/ml in dH_{20}). Centrifuge the dextran solution for 1 min before mixing to remove large aggregates of dextran that may block the injection pipette. Remember to use RNase-free techniques if you are injecting RNA.

Injection

When the first cleavage furrow is visible on the embryos (approximately 1.25 hours after fertilization), fill a pipette with the injection solution as follows. Put an injection pipette at the end of 1-mm tubing attached to a 10-ml syringe. Place a drop of solution (say, 5 µl) on a piece of parafilm and immerse the tip of the pipette in the drop of solution. Fill the pipette from the tip, using suction created by the syringe. If the tip becomes blocked, apply a small amount of positive pressure to unblock it, then continue to fill.

The pipette is attached to a pipette holder with a side opening for pressure input and is manipulated by a three-dimensional micromanipulator (Leitz or equivalent). To calibrate the pipette, pipette solution is injected into a shallow well filled with oil by applying pressure pulses through the pipette with a Picospritzer (General Valve Corp., Fairfield, NJ). The diameter of the injected droplet in

oil is measured by using an eyepiece micrometer. Increase the duration of the pulse until the volume of the droplet is some 2 nl (diameter of perhaps 0.06 mm). Clean the oil off the tip of the pipette by giving a few pulses in Ringer's solution.

For horizontal access of the injection pipette to the embryo, we use the top of a 96-well culture dish as an embryo container during injection. Because the vitelline membrane makes the embryos slippery, a suction pipette is used to keep them in place during injection. The suction pipette is made from a 100-µl pipette (VWR Micropipettes, Bridgeport, NJ, cat. no. 53432-921) that has been heat-polished so that the opening at one end is smaller than an embryo and then is attached to a micromanipulator (Leitz or equivalent). The suction pressure is provided by mouth through tubing attached to the pipette while individual embryos are injected. For an embryo that had not yet completed first division (i.e., one-cell stage), 16 nl (8 standard pulses) are injected. For a two-cell-stage embryo, 8 nl are injected; for a 4-cell-stage embryo, 4 nl are injected; and so on. In general, the volume of solution injected should not exceed 10% of the total cell volume. Injected embryos are kept separately in Petri dishes filled with 10% Ringer's solution and are marked properly (see also Gimlich, 1991, for a description of methods).

Protocol for Culturing Spinal Neurons and Muscle Cells

Preparation

Make culture medium and CMF Ringer's solution. One liter of culture Ringer's solution (made from 490 ml 100%), 500 ml Leibovitz L-15 medium (Gibco, Baltimore, MD), and 10 ml fetal bovine serum (Gibco). CMF solution consists of (in mM): NaCl 115, KCl 2.6, HEPES 10, EDTA 0.4 (pH 7.6).

Preparation of cultures is carried out in a hood via sterile technique. All solutions are sterilized by using 0.20-µm filter flasks (Nalgene 1850-090), and culture medium is filtered prior to the addition of fetal bovine serum (FBS). We do not use antibiotics routinely. However, if bacterial contamination becomes a frequent problem, one may add penicillin-streptomycin (5000 units and 5 mg/ml) to the 10% Ringer's solution and the CMF solution used during culture preparation. The number of embryos needed

depends on the number of cultures to be prepared; Usually, we use one embryo per culture dish.

Before starting the microdissection, fill one Petri dish (60 × 15 mm, Falcon 3002) with 70% ethanol, six Petri dishes (60 mm) with 10% filtered Ringer's solution, and one Petri dish (100 × 15 mm, Baxter D1906) with CMF solution. Cut the tips of autoclaved 5-inch Pasteur pipettes to an opening slightly larger than the embryos. To prepare dishes for cell plating, immerse coverglasses (no. 1, 22-mm square) in 95% ethanol, pick them up individually with forceps, and flame them in a glass burner. Rapidly transfer each coverglass to a culture dish (50 × 9 mm, Falcon 1006). When the coverglass has cooled down, add 2 to 3 ml of sterile culture medium and close the lid. Finally, prepare a 9-inch Pasteur pipette for dispersing the cells. Grasp the tip with one hand, hold it over a flame, draw it out to a long neck (8–10 cm), and break the neck at appropriate place to obtain a tip opening of some 0.2 mm. After you have become experienced, these preparations for cell plating can be performed during the period of cell dissociation (see further). The entire procedure for preparing one dozen cultures from 1 to 2 dozen embryos will take perhaps 1 h for an experienced person.

Microdissection and Cell Plating

Immerse the embryos (stages 20–22) in 70% alcohol for approximately 10 s to sterilize the jelly coat, then transfer them into one of the dishes containing 10% Ringer's solution. Under a dissecting microscope, release the embryos from the jelly coat and the vitelline membranes by pulling the membrane apart with two fine forceps (Dumont no. 5). The vitelline membrane is a thin, transparent membrane surrounding the embryo. Wash the bare embryos by transferring them successively through the five remaining dishes of sterile 10% Ringer's solution, using a new sterile pipette for each step. Transfer of solution from dish to dish should be minimized during this procedure. The cleaned embryos then are transferred to CMF solution, wherein the microdissection is carried out.

The neural tube and the associated myotomal tissue on the dorsal surface of the embryo are cut with microsurgical scissors (Moria MC19/B) (figure 9.2). The dissected tissue mass consists of approximately one-eighth of the total embryo. Keep the dissected tissue in the center of the dish, moving the remainder of the embryo to the

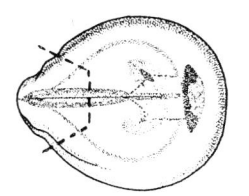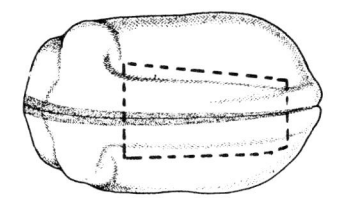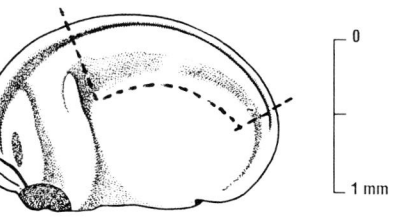

Figure 9.2 Microdissection of the embryonic tissue used for *Xenopus* nerve-muscle cultures. Schematic drawing of a stage 22 *Xenopus* embryo; the part to be dissected for culturing is delineated by dashed lines. From left to right: anterior, dorsal, and lateral views of the embryo. The dissected part consists of the neural tube and the associated myotomes. (Drawing adapted from Nieuwkoop and Faber, 1967.)

periphery. The cells become associated loosely after some 20 to 30 min exposure to CMF solution; the older the embryos, the longer the dissociation time required.

Near the end of the dissociation period, carefully peel the epithelial layer away with two tweezers and discard it. This tissue, which is easily identified because of its pigmentation, may detach spontaneously from the dissected neural tube-myotome during the period of cell dissociation. The tissue then is dispersed by aspiration into the narrowed Pasteur pipette. Fill the pipette by sucking up a small amount of culture medium from the culture dish, then quickly move it to the dish containing the embryos, pushing some culture medium out to prevent inflow of CMF solution into the pipette. As soon as the mouth of the pipette faces the dissected tissue, reverse the pipette pressure and suck the tissue up. After 20 to 30 min in CMF solution, aspiration of the tissue into the pipette should disperse most of the cells into a suspension. Move the pipette to the culture dish (containing culture medium) and gently expel the cell suspension, plating them onto the coverglass in parallel lines. The density of cell plating can be controlled by the amount of solution drawn into the pipette and by the speed of plating. Plating in lines helps to increase cell density for formation of nerve-muscle synapses and to locate the cells during the experiment. Avoid air bubble formation in the pipette when moving the pipette from the CMF to the culture dish, to prevent lysis of cells by air-water interfacial tension. After plating each dish, wash the pipette with culture medium to clean away yolk granules and cell debris from the pipette walls. Then repeat this procedure for each of the remaining pieces of neural tube and myotomes. When plating is complete, leave the culture dishes undisturbed for at least

15 min before moving them into a clean box. For the latter, we used plastic containers with tight lids. Keep the cells at room temperature and away from strong light sources and renew culture medium every 3 days. The cells also could be plated directly onto plastic culture dishes, or culture dishes coated with substrate molecules (e.g., laminin and collagen), which will influence the cell morphology greatly (see later).

Related Techniques and Alternative Methods

One of the early uses of nerve-muscle cultures from *Xenopus* embryos was to examine changes in the membrane ionic conductances during neuronal development (Spitzer and Lamborghini, 1976). Cohen and coworkers used similar cultures to study ACh receptor clustering during synaptic development (Anderson et al., 1977; Anderson and Cohen, 1977). The dissection procedures and compositions of the dissociation and culture media differ somewhat among these reports. Spitzer and coworkers dissociate the neural plate fragment in CMF Steinberg's solution containing 0.4 mM EDTA. The culture medium consists of Steinberg's solution and 0.1% bovine serum albumin; the pH of the medium is 7.8, and the calcium concentration may be as high as 10 mM (Spitzer and Lamborghini, 1976). Cohen and coworkers perform the microdissection in the presence of collagenase (1 mg/ml 60% L-15), and cell dissociation is performed in CMF medium containing EDTA (2 mg/ml) and trypsin (5 mg/ml). Cells are plated in a medium consisting of 60% L-15, 5% horse serum, and Holmes's à-1 protein (0.2 g/ml). They are maintained in the same medium devoid of serum, as the presence of 5% horse serum seems to cause muscle cell degeneration within 3 to 4 days (Anderson et al., 1977). These alternative methods yield cultures that show some difference in the appearance of nerve and muscle cells. For example, Cohen's method produces large, extended muscle cells that have been very useful in studying nerve-induced redistribution of muscle surface ACh receptors (see further). We have not, however, noticed any electrophysiological property of the neurons or muscle cells that is dependent on the culture method.

Muscle or nerve cells also can be grown separately. This activity is achieved by restricting the dissection to myotomal muscles or neural tubes and by optimizing the culture medium for each type of

cell. For instance, neurons grow better in serum-free medium and at higher calcium concentrations. Muscle cells, on the other hand, grow best in culture medium containing 2% FBS. For pure neuronal cultures, the dorsal pieces of the embryos are incubated in Steinberg's solution containing 1 mg/ml collagenase, which results in dissociation of myotomal muscle cells from the neural tube. The neural tube then is removed and further dissociated in CMF-Steinberg's solution before dispersion and plating (Peng et al., 1991). Neural tube explants can be cultured as well without further dissociation by cutting the neural tube into slice approximately 0.5 mm thick and plating them intact onto a substrate-coated coverglass or culture dish (Peng et al., 1991). These explants have the advantage of more extensive neuritic outgrowth and longer survival than do isolated spinal neurons. Cultures of myoblasts and multinucleated myotubes can be prepared by dissecting the limb buds of stages 50 to 55 tadpoles. These myotubes can be innervated in culture with neurons from the neural tubes of *Xenopus* embryos (Kay et al., 1988; Peng et al., 1991).

Culture Description

Within minutes after plating, cells begin to attach to the culture substratum. At this time, cells are roundish and heterogeneous in size, and cell types are difficult to distinguish. However, after the first few hours, muscle cells can be identified by a clear cytoplasmic protrusion, and spinal neurons can be determined by the emergence of thin processes from the cell (figure 9.3A). By 1 day in culture, at least four types of cells can be identified clearly: muscle cells, neurons, fibroblasts, and melanocytes. Depending on the substratum used for culture, the percentage of cells that eventually attach to the substratum may vary from 20% (uncoated coverglass) to 90% (polystyrene culture dish).

Muscle Cells

During the first day in culture, myoblasts contain a substantial number of yolk granules in their perinuclear cytoplasm. Most of the yolk granules are digested within the first few days as cells increase in size. In 1-day-old cultures plated on glass coverslips, myoblasts have two forms: spindle-shaped or round. Both spindle-shaped

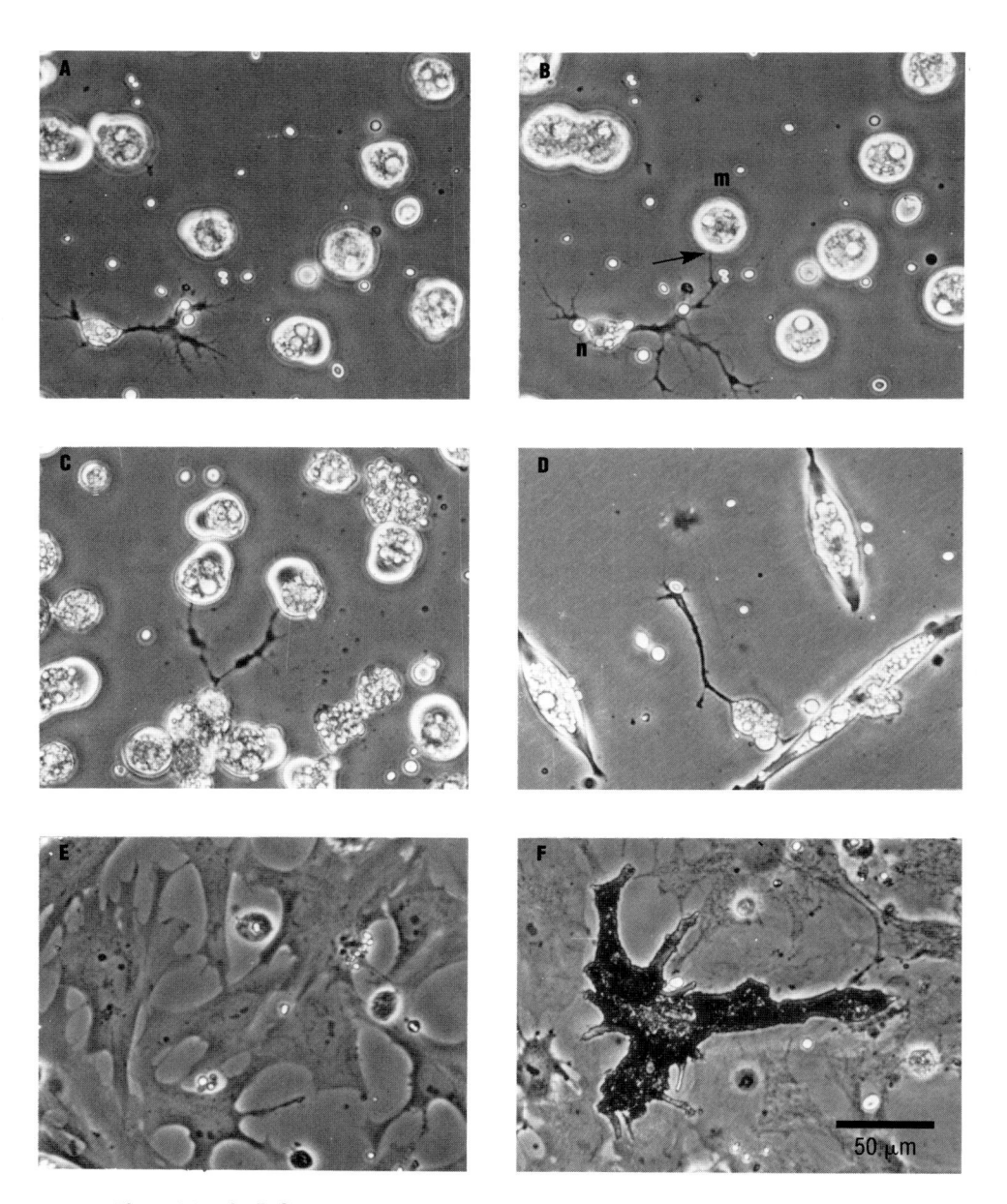

Figure 9.3   *A, B* Synaptogenesis in *Xenopus* cell culture. The same cells were visualized by phase-contrast microscopy and were photographed at 11 h (*A*) and 23 h (*B*) after plating, respectively. Notice the establishment of nerve-muscle contact (arrow) between the spinal neuron (n) and the myoball (m) and the change in the shape of the muscle cells from irregular (*A*) to spherical shapes (*B*). *C, D.* Effect of the substratum on the shape of the muscle cells. Cells were grown on a coverglass (*C*) and on the bottom of a polystyrene culture dish (*D*). Both photographs were taken 10 h after plating. *E, F.* Six-week-old cultures in which only fibroblasts (*E*) and melanocytes (*F*) have survived.

cells and rounded "myoballs" undergo a similar pattern of differentiation in culture and exhibit similar electrophysiological properties (Evers et al., 1989). The round shape of the myoball apparently is due to the lack of cell adherence to the glass substratum. Spindle-shaped muscle cells develop clear striations easily visible under the phase-contrast microscope by the second or third day after cell plating. The two types of muscle cells are useful for different types of experiments. The extended muscle cells have been used to investigate the influence of innervation on ACh receptor topography (Anderson and Cohen, 1977), and the round myoballs are suitable for voltage-clamp studies of synaptogenesis (Xie and Poo, 1986).

The predominance of spindle-shaped or round muscle cells is determined by at least four factors: (1) the presence and the concentration of FBS in the culture medium, (2) the age of the embryo used for culturing, (3) the type of culture substratum, and (4) the age of the culture. For example, when FBS is present in the culture medium at 1% to 2% and uncoated coverglasses are used as substratum, most of the myoblasts take the form of myoballs (see figure 9.3C), which can be detached easily from the substratum. However, under these conditions, the proportion of myoballs decreases if embryos are used at older developmental stages. When FBS is omitted, as in the procedure of Spitzer and Lamborghini (1976), spindle-shaped muscle cells predominate (see figure 9.3D). This variation also occurs when cells are plated directly onto polystyrene culture dishes coated with various substrate molecules (e.g., liminin, collagen, and polylysine) even in the presence of FBS. Finally, as muscle cells mature in culture, they tend to adhere more extensively to the substratum. Hence, by the fourth day in medium containing 1% FBS, myoballs have become sparse, and muscle cells display a wide variety of shapes, from round or ellipsoidal to spindle-shaped or stellate.

Proliferation of myoblasts has not been observed in these cultures. In contrast to muscle cells explanted from chick or rat embryos or from older *Xenopus* embryos, *Xenopus* myoblasts from stages 20 to 22 embryos do not fuse to form polynucleated myotubes in culture. They remain mononucleated as long as they survive. Under our standard conditions (1% FBS) and without renewing the culture medium, muscle cells survive for up to 2 weeks.

Spinal Neurons

Shortly after plating, spinal neurons appear as relatively small, spherical cells of perhaps 10 μm in diameter (figure 9.4A), the cytoplasm of which is filled with yolk granules. The neuronal population in this culture is heterogeneous, presumably consisting of sensory and motor neurons and interneurons. We have not yet been able to distinguish these cell types by their morphological characteristics. After 2 to 3 h in culture, the phase-bright cell bodies start extending phase-dark processes terminating in palm-shaped growth cones. Figure 9.4 shows an example of neuronal growth at different times after plating. The rate of neurite growth is maximal (up to 50 μm/h at 20°C) during the first 12 h in culture, and most of the neurite growth occurs during the first day. The relative proportion of muscle and nerve cells in each dish is variable. When uncoated coverglasses are used as substratum, a good culture may contain some 20 to 30 neurite-bearing neurons and 10 times as many muscle cells. This ratio also depends on the concentration of FBS added to the culture medium; the higher the concentration of serum, the fewer the neurons and the shorter their survival. In 1% serum, neurons may survive up to 4 days. In general, neurons that contact muscle cells survive longer, suggesting the existence of trophic interactions between these cells. For studying neurite outgrowth and synaptogenesis, we use the cultures during the first 2 days after plating. Nerve-muscle contacts are frequent in these cultures (see figure 9.3B, C) and can be observed soon after neurite outgrowth begins. When cells are plated in high density, the majority of muscle cells may be contacted by neuronal processes. In contrast to chick or rat muscle cells in culture, *Xenopus* muscle cells not contacted by neurons do not contract spontaneously. However, contact-induced spontaneous contractions are suppressed by curare, indicating that they are caused by spontaneous acetylcholine (ACh) release from the neurons. Interestingly, the development of cross-striations in the muscle cells is, in fact, accelerated by their contact with the cocultured neurons (Kidokoro and Saito, 1988).

Other Cell Types

In using the culture method described earlier, other cell types have seldom been observed during the first few days, although the identity of spherical cells that fail to attach to the culture substratum is

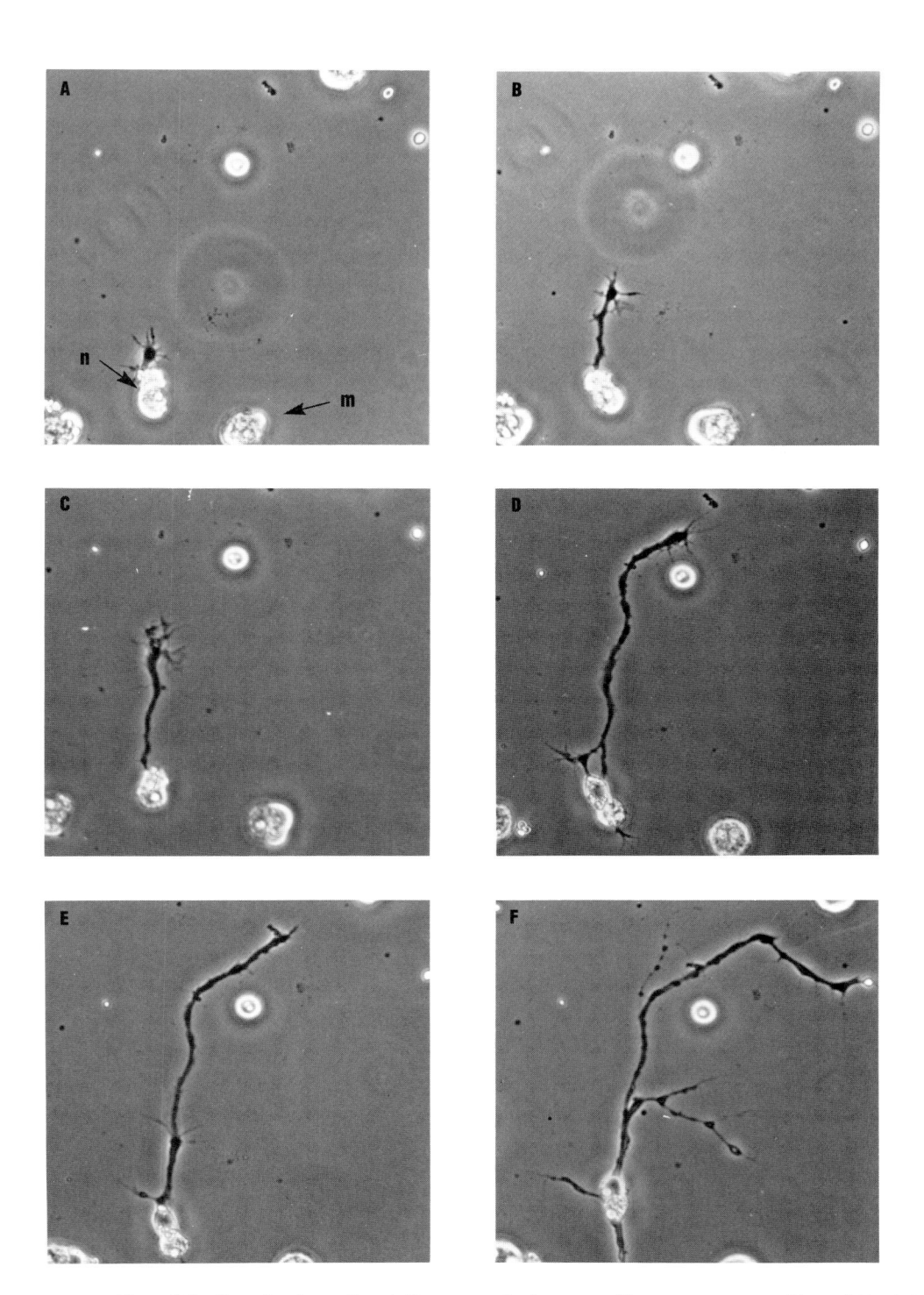

Figure 9.4   Growth of a cultured *Xenopus* spinal neuron. The same neuron with a phase-bright cell body and a phase-dark neurite was photographed at different times after plating. (*A*) 2 h; (*B*) 3 h; (*C*) 5 h; (*D*) 9 h; (*E*) 11 h; and (*F*) 23 h.

unknown. These cells can be washed away by renewing the culture medium. Also, many small yolk granules are visible in the culture and disappear over time. Fibroblasts and melanocytes, however, do attach and proliferate well in these cultures after a few days. Fibroblasts can be distinguished by their phase-dark cytoplasm and their extensive lamellipodia (see figure 9.3E); melanocytes are characterized by the presence of darkly pigmented melanophores in their cytoplasm (see figure 9.3F). Though initially present in low numbers, fibroblasts become predominant in these cultures after a few weeks. Eventually, they cover the entire surface of the culture substratum when most of the other cells have degenerated (see figure 9.3E).

Applications

Neuronal Differentiation and Growth

Xenopus spinal neurons in culture are useful for studying cellular mechanisms underlying neuronal differentiation and growth. This system has been employed successfully for studying the development of ion channels in neurons and their role in regulating molecular events of neuronal differentiation (see for reviews Ribera and Spitzer, 1992; Spitzer, 1994). Isolated neurons are useful also for examining intracellular signals associated with differentiation and neurite growth (Zheng et al., 1994; Gu and Spitzer, 1995). The following summary of our studies on the chemotropic turning of growth cones provides an illustration for the use of *Xenopus* cultures.

A gradient of extracellular molecules across the growth cone can be created in the culture dish by repetitive pulsatile ejection of picoliter amounts of test solution from a micropipette. This technique generates a relatively stable microscopic gradient of 5% to 10% concentration difference of the ejected chemical across a growth cone 10 µm in width within minutes after the onset of the gradient (Lohof et al., 1992). For this procedure, a micropipette (100 µl, VWR micropipettes 53432-921) is pulled on a two-stage pipette puller (Narishige, Sea Cliff, NY, cat. no. PP-83) and is heat-polished (Narishige MF-83) to reduce the inner diameter of the tip to between 1 and 2 µm. The pipette is filled with the solution containing high concentrations of the test chemical and is placed at a

distance of 100 µm from a neurite's growth cone and 45 degrees from the direction of neurite extension. The pipette is connected to an electrically gated pressure application system (Picospritzer II, General Valve Corp.). Positive pressure of 2 to 3 psi is applied to the pipette with defined frequency and duration (usually 2 Hz and 10 ms, respectively) by using a pulse generator (Grass SD9). The average volume of the ejected solution per pressure pulse is determined by measuring the volume of droplets ejected into oil for standard pipettes (0.3–0.7 pl). The images of the growth cone are recorded via a video camera and are stored in the videotape recorder at the onset and at various time points during the experiment. We found that the growth cone of *Xenopus* spinal neurons responds to gradients of membrane permeable cAMP analogues (Lohof et al., 1992), neurotransmitters (Zheng et al., 1994, 1996), and neurotrophins (Lohof, 1994) by turning toward the source of the chemical. For the turning in transmitter gradients, we observed an increase in cytosolic Ca^{2+} and in the number of filopodia on the side of the growth cone facing the source of transmitters prior to the turning, suggesting that these events may be linked causally to the turning response. The presence of extracellular Ca^{2+} and activation of Ca^{2+}-calmodulin-dependent protein kinase appeared to be required for transmitter-induced turning. Whether a cytoplasmic gradient of Ca^{2+} is sufficient for inducing the turning response and whether it is also necessary for turning induced by cAMP analogue or neurotrophins remain unknown. It is possible to combine the blastomere injection technique with the chemotropic turning assay to dissect the cellular events triggered by extracellular molecular cues. For example, the involvement of axon-specific protein GAP43 (Goslin et al., 1988; Skene, 1989) or other cytoskeletal proteins on neurite extension and chemotropic turning response at the growth cone may be revealed by manipulating the level of these proteins in the neuron.

Synaptogenesis

Xenopus nerve-muscle culture was used first by Cohen and co-workers in their classic work on the nerve-induced clustering of ACh receptors in postsynaptic muscle cells (Anderson et al., 1977). Taking advantage of the low density and the clear visibility of individual cells of this culture, Kidokoro and Yeh (1982) first examined synaptic activity during the initial period of nerve-muscle

contact. Nerve-evoked synaptic potentials were recorded from the myocyte with intracellular microelectrodes within minutes following visible neuromuscular contact. To define more precisely the timing for nerve-muscle contact, Poo and coworkers (Chow and Poo, 1985; Xie and Poo, 1986; Evers et al., 1989) took advantage of the fact that round myocytes (myoballs) can be detached from the culture substratum and moved toward a chosen target (figure 9.5A, B). Myoballs were impaled with a whole-cell patch recording electrode (simultaneously used for recording) and translocated into direct contact with the cocultured neuron. Miniature endplate currents were detected within seconds following neuromuscular contacts. Using an excised patch of muscle membrane in outside-out configuration as a probe for ACh release, Xie and Poo (1986) showed that the release of ACh from the growth cone was induced by the physical contact with the muscle cells in an apparently specific manner. Contact of the growth cone with the tip of a glass pipette or the cell body of a neuron was ineffective. When the neuron was stimulated to fire action potentials, evoked endplate potentials also could be detected within the first minute of contact. The rapid formation of functional synapses is possible in this system, presumably because the growing neuron has acquired the main cellular mechanisms for neurotransmitter secretion (Sun and Poo, 1987) before the synapse is differentiated morphologically (Buchanan et al., 1989). Early synaptic transmission has a high failure rate, but during the first 30 min of contact, the rate of failures of evoked responses drops substantially, whereas the amplitude of evoked responses becomes larger. Spontaneous synaptic potentials become more frequent, and their mean amplitude also increases within this period. This increase in synaptic efficacy apparently is related to the gradual stabilization of nerve-muscle adhesion, as indicated by the increasing difficulty in pulling the nerve and muscle cells apart over 30 min of contact. Clustering of nicotinic ACh receptors is a prominent postsynaptic specialization that follows initial nerve-muscle contact (Anderson et al., 1977). Other synaptic specializations include the appearance of postsynaptic densities, the basal lamina, and the clustering of synaptic vesicles all appear gradually during the first few days, in parallel with that observed in vivo (Kullberg, et al., 1977; Weldon and Cohen, 1979; Takahashi et al., 1987; Buchanan et al., 1989). Though many early events of synaptogenesis have been described, the molecular basis underlying these events are largely unknown. The blastomere injection tech-

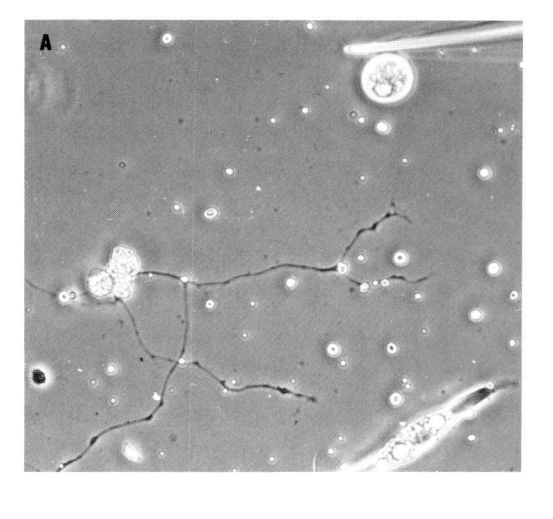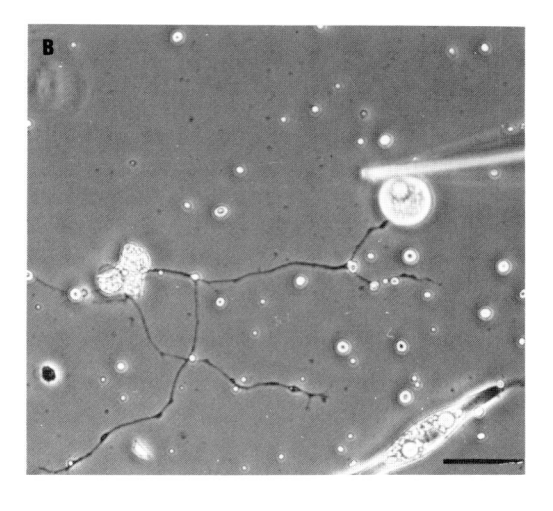

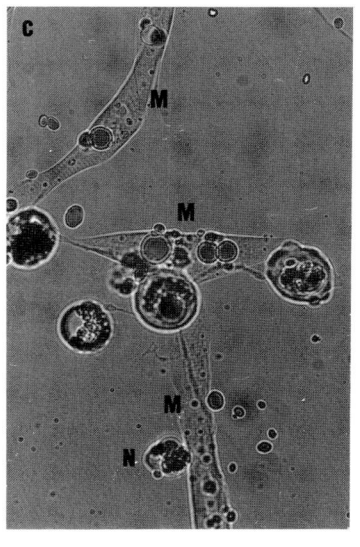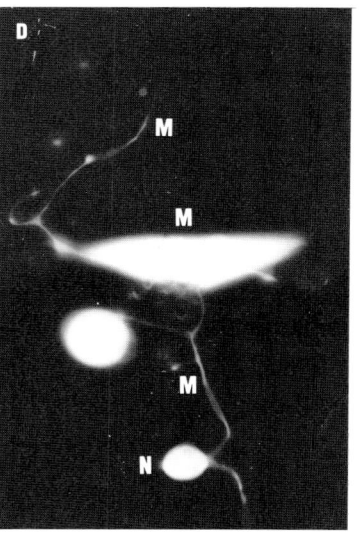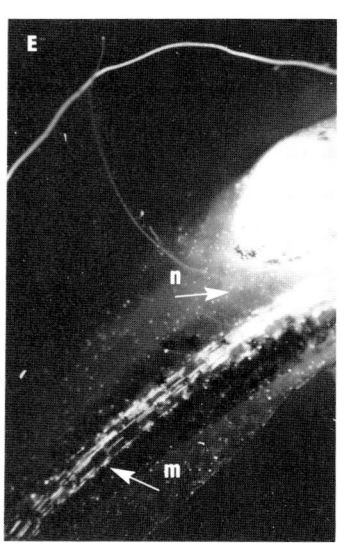

Figure 9.5 (*A, B*) Cell manipulation in 1-day-old *Xenopus* nerve-muscle culture. The myoball first is detached from the coverglass (*A*) and brought into contact with the neuronal growth cone (*B*). Functional synaptic transmission can be established within the first minute after contact (Evers et al., 1989). Scale bar: 50 μm. (*C–E*) Fluorescence labeling of the nerve and muscle cells by intracellular injection of rhodamine-dextran into one blastomere (of a 32-cell-stage embryo) known to give rise to muscle cells and motoneurons. (*C*) Phase-contrast micrograph of 1-day-old culture prepared from an embryo injected 1 day prior to cell culture. (*D*) Fluorescence micrograph of the cells shown in *C*. Notice that a labeled neuron (N) has innervated both fluorescent and nonfluorescent muscle cells (M). All fluorescent cells are derived from one injected blastomere. (*E*) Low-resolution fluorescence micrograph of a whole-mount 2-day-old *Xenopus* tadpole tail. The embryo has been injected with rhodamine-dextran in one of the blastomeres at the 32-cell stage, similar to the procedure followed for the culture shown in *C* and *D*. Cells in *C*, *D*, and *E* were, thus, of similar age. The labeled neurons (n) and myotomal muscle cells (m) are related clonally.

nique may be useful for further molecular studies. Because all the progeny cells of the injected blastomere, including both spinal neurons and myotomal myocytes, contain the exogenous molecules, it is possible to examine selectively the effect of either pre- or postsynaptic manipulation of the molecule on the structure and functional development of the synapse.

TRANSMITTER SECRETION

Recent progress in molecular cloning has led to the identification of a number of proteins in the synaptic vesicle (Bennett and Scheller, 1993; Kelly, 1993; Walch-Solimena et al., 1993). The blastomere injection method has been used to examine the role of three of these proteins—synaptophysin and synaptotagmin and synapsin—in the packaging, mobilization, and exocytosis of synaptic vesicles, using exogenous proteins, antibodies, or cRNA of these proteins into the early blastomeres of *Xenopus* embryos. The synaptic functions were assayed by physiological recordings in nerve-muscle cultures 1 day after plating (2 days after loading).

We found that loading of presynaptic neurons with antisynaptophysin antibodies reduced both the spontaneous and evoked ACh secretion at the synapses (Alder et al., 1992), whereas overexpression of synaptophysin by loading synthetic synaptophysin cRNA (figure 9.6 and color plate 5) produced enhanced ACh secretion (Alder et al., 1995). In the synapses overexpressing synaptophysin, the spontaneous synaptic currents showed a marked increase in frequency without significant change in the mean amplitude or rise time, as compared to control synapses, suggesting that synaptophysin enhances secretion but is not involved in determining the size of the ACh quanta. The impulse-evoked synaptic currents showed increase amplitude as well as reduced fluctuation and delay of onset.

Furthermore, the rate of tetanus-induced depression was faster in neurons overexpressing synaptophysin, suggesting that synaptophysin enhances the probability of vesicular exocytosis without a change in the rate of vesicle replenishment. In contrast, overexpressing synaptotagmins by injection of cRNA of rat synaptotagmin I or II reduced the frequency of spontaneous exocytosis without affecting the amplitude of either the quantal ACh packet or the evoked synaptic current (Morimoto et al., 1998). Interestingly, overexpression of synaptotagmin led to an increased amplitude of paired-pulse facilitation and augmentation of evoked synaptic

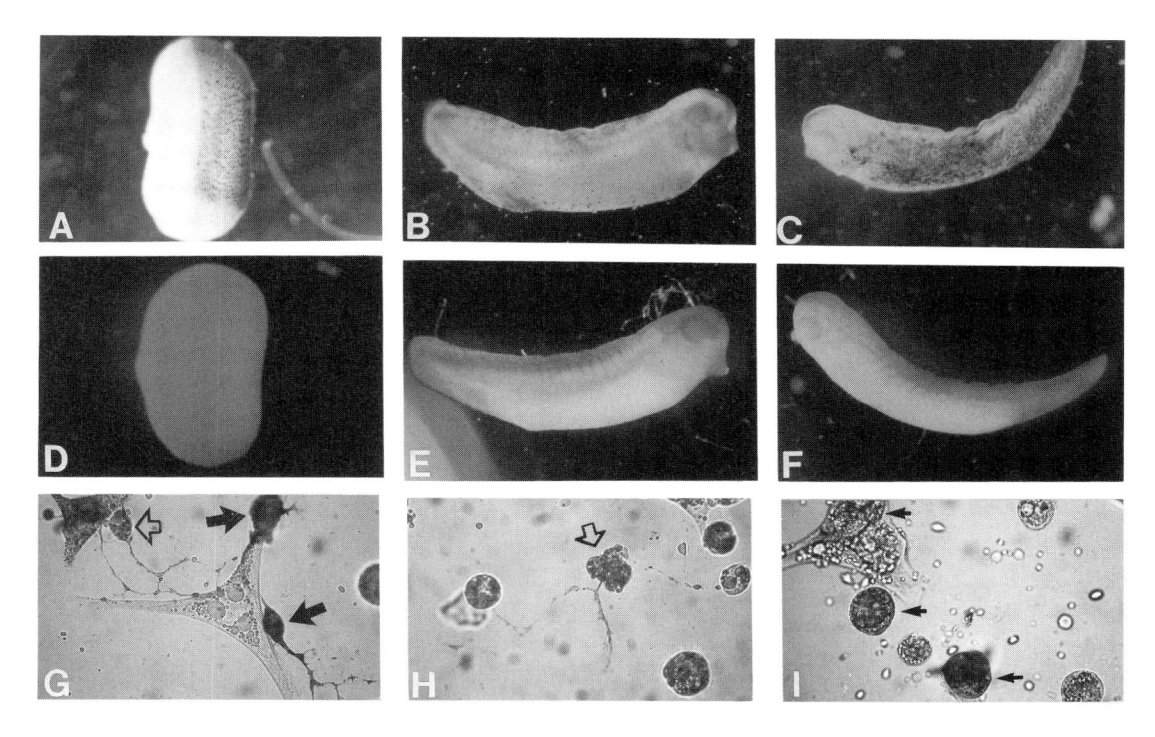

Figure 9.6 Overexpression of synaptophysin in *Xenopus* embryos injected with synaptophysin mRNA. Embryos were injected at the two-cell stage, and synaptophysin expression was examined by immunocytochemical staining via alkaline phosphatase-conjugated secondary antibodies. (*A*) Dorsal view of 1-day-old embryo showing positive staining for synaptophysin on one half only. (*B, C*) Lateral views of 2-day-old embryos, expressing exogenous synaptophysin only on one side. Left and right photographs are opposite lateral views of the same embryo. (*D–F*) Same as *A–C* except that the embryos were not injected with synaptophysin cRNA. In the 2-day-old embryo (*E, F*), weak staining was visible in the spinal cord and other neuronal structures, but no difference in staining intensity was found between the two sides of the embryo. (*G*) Nerve-muscle culture prepared from a 1-day-old embryo injected with synaptophysin cRNA. Some neurons and their processes (filled arrows) are more darkly stained than others (open arrows). Staining is also visible in some myocytes. (*H*) Culture prepared from a control, uninjected embryo. All neurons (open arrow) were stained with the same low intensity, and no myocytes showed significant staining. (*I*) Myocytes in nerve-muscle cultures prepared from embryos injected with synaptophysin mRNA. Some myocytes (arrowheads) express synaptophysin, whereas others (unmarked) are unstained. See plate 5 for color version.

currents under high-frequency stimulation, suggesting that synaptotagmin inhibits the spontaneous exocytosis while elevating
the supply of synaptic vesicles for high-frequency transmission.
Electron-microscopic studies showed that synaptophysin overexpression does not affect the density or distribution of synaptic
vesicles, whereas synaptotagmin expression increased the density
of synaptic vesicles at a region 100 to 300 nm from the presynaptic
membrane (Morimoto et al., 1998). The level of synapsin (I or IIa), a
peripheral synaptic vesicle protein, was elevated also in the presynaptic neuron by direct injection of the purified protein into the
early blastomere. Physiological assay of neuromuscular synapses in
culture showed an enhanced spontaneous and evoked ACh secretion. Unlike that observed after overexpressing either synaptophysin or synaptotagmin, the mean quantal size of the ACh packet was
increased in synapsin-loaded neuron, suggesting a potential role of
synapsins in the maturation of quanta in addition to their effects on
the rate of vesicle exocytosis (Lu et al., 1991; Schaeffer et al., 1994).
The differential functional effects resulting from manipulation of
various synaptic proteins illustrate the potential usefulness of the
blastomere injection method in molecular analysis of synaptic
processes.

Some Future Experiments

The blastomere injection method may be useful also studying the
role of certain proteins by inhibiting their expression through the
use of antisense technique. The injection of antisense oligonucleotides into *Xenopus* embryos results in the complete degradation of
the target mRNA, because RNase H becomes activated and specifically degrades the RNA that is bound to the oligonucleotides (Vize
et al., 1991). Because of the toxicity of antisense oligonucleotides
at high doses and their sensitivity to degradation even if they are
modified with phosphoamidate ($T_{1/2} = 15$ min) (Dagle et al., 1990),
it may be necessary to use full-length antisense RNA to inhibit
expression (Vize et al., 1991). It is also possible to inhibit protein
expression by adding antisense oligonucleotides directly to the
neuronal culture at the time of cell plating (Listerud et al., 1991;
Kosik et al., 1993), but this method has not been applied to
Xenopus cultures. The use of direct DNA injection into *Xenopus*
embryos is known to be limited by the low replication rate of
exogenous DNA and mosaic pattern of expression (Vize et al.,

1991). However, this mosaic pattern could prove useful for studies on the effect of exogenous proteins to particular regions of the embryo. Ultimately, the creation of a transgenic system for *Xenopus* embryos (perhaps using retroviruses for introducing DNA) may be necessary (Vize et al., 1991). Finally, the function of certain proteins may be revealed by the approach of dominant negative mutation (Amaya et al., 1991). Using blastomere injection of the protein or cRNA, one may overexpress a mutant version of a gene, the product of which effectively replaces the endogenous wild-type protein and perturbs a specific neuronal function.

10 Cultures from Chick Peripheral Ganglia

Carolyn L. Smith

People use cultures from chick peripheral ganglia to study the biology of peripheral ganglion neurons and for research on general neurobiological problems, such as the mechanisms of axonal outgrowth and the physiology of ion channels. One reason for the popularity of these cultures is that they are simple and relatively inexpensive to prepare. Fertilized eggs are readily available and can be stored in a refrigerator until needed. Embryonic development begins when the eggs are transferred to an egg incubator. Therefore, it is easy to maintain a continuous supply of embryos at appropriate stages for culture. Peripheral ganglia are simple to dissect, and each contains several thousands of neurons. The neurons grow well in several commercially available culture media and can be maintained in a chemically defined medium provided that they are supplied with an appropriate substrate and the neurotrophic factors they require for development.

The easiest type of culture to prepare—and the first to be used for neurobiological experiments—consists of whole ganglia grown as explants (Lewis and Lewis, 1912). The profuse outgrowth of neurites from explanted ganglia (see figure 2.6) makes them an ideal preparation in which to study the behavior of growing axons. Early work on such preparations helped establish the importance of growth cones in guiding growing axons, and more recent studies revealed some of the attractive and repulsive cues to which growth cones respond (Hughes, 1953; Nakai and Kawasaki, 1956; Levi-Montalcini and Angeletti, 1968; Kapfhammer and Raper, 1987; Luo et al., 1993). The observation by Levi-Montalcini and colleagues that a soluble factor produced by a mouse sarcoma promoted outgrowth of neurites from chick dorsal root and sympathetic ganglia led to the discovery of nerve growth factor (NGF), the neurotrophic factor that all sympathetic neurons and many sensory neurons require for survival and differentiation (reviewed by Levi-Montalcini, 1987).

Procedures for preparing dissociated cell cultures from chick peripheral ganglia were described by Nakai (1956) and by Levi-

Montalcini and Angeletti (1963), opening the way to new types of analyses and experimentation. The ability to visualize neurons in their entirety made it possible to trace all the processes of individual neurons. The effects of experimental manipulations on neuronal survival and differentiation could be assessed more easily than in explant cultures. Also, neurons were accessible for experimental manipulation, such as electrophysiological recording, microinjection, and immunolabeling. In addition to neurons, peripheral ganglia contain glial cells and fibroblasts. The presence of nonneuronal cells is not essential for survival of sensory neurons, and several methods have been devised for separating neurons from non-neuronal cells prior to plating (see later), thereby making it possible to study neurons isolated from other types of cells.

Peripheral ganglion neurons have several characteristics that make them attractive to cellular neurobiologists. They form axons within less than an hour after plating when they are grown on a substrate that promotes neurite outgrowth (such as laminin). Their axons have prominent growth cones at their distal ends and are competent to form synaptic connections with appropriate target cells (Role et al., 1987). The cell bodies of peripheral ganglion neurons have a diverse assortment of ion channels and neurotransmitter receptors (Nowycky, 1992; Hille, 1994; Zhang, Vijayaraghavan, and Berg, 1994) and are amenable to recording with micropipettes or patch clamp electrodes. The heterogeneity of the neurons with respect to biochemical phenotype (reviewed by Lawson, 1992) makes them a good model for research on neuronal differentiation.

The characteristic of peripheral ganglion neurons that has had the greatest impact on the neurosciences is their sensitivity to neurotrophic factors. Studies of chick peripheral ganglion neurons grown in vitro had an important role in the discovery not only of NGF (Levi-Montalcini, 1987) but also brain-derived neurotrophic factor (BDNF; Barde et al., 1982) and neurotrophin-3 (NT-3; Maisonpierre et al., 1990), essential for the development of certain types of neurons, and ciliary neurotrophic factor (CNTF; Barbin et al., 1984), which supports the survival of ciliary motoneurons and spinal motoneurons. NGF, BDNF, and NT-3 are members of a family of neurotrophic factors, the "neurotrophins," which are important for the development of subsets of neurons in the central nervous system and in peripheral ganglia (Korsching, 1993; Snider, 1994). Cultures from chick peripheral ganglia continue to be used for research on neurotrophic factors.

A limitation of dissociated neurons from chick peripheral ganglia as a model for neurobiological research is that they do not form dendrites. This is true even of sympathetic neurons, which *do* form dendrites in vivo. Lein et al. (1995) have shown that sympathetic neurons from rats can be induced to form dendrites by exposure to basement membrane material, serum, or purified osteogenic protein. These factors also may promote the formation of dendrites by chick sympathetic neurons but, to my knowledge, this has not been demonstrated.

Neurobiologists now have a large number of alternative culture preparations from which to choose, many of which are described in this volume. Each of these preparations is better suited for studying certain problems than are cultures from chick peripheral ganglia. However, with the exception of immortal cell lines, which have their own drawbacks, none of them is as simple and inexpensive to prepare as cultures from chick peripheral ganglia. For this reason, cultures from chick peripheral ganglia continue to be a popular model for neuroscience research. They also are an excellent culture preparation for use in laboratory courses and student projects.

Types of Peripheral Ganglion Neurons and Their Embryological Origins

Different types of peripheral ganglion neurons have distinctive biochemical characteristics and electrophysiological properties. The extent to which they express these distinctive traits in vitro depends on their stage of maturation at the time of removal from the embryo and the conditions under which they are grown. Each type of neuron requires specific neurotrophic factors for development and must be supplied with appropriate factors to survive in vitro. In addition, peripheral ganglion neurons are plastic with respect to some aspects of their phenotypes, so they may express different characteristics when grown under different conditions.

Dorsal Root Ganglia

In situ dorsal root ganglia contain several distinct types of sensory neurons that respond to different sensory stimuli and project to different neurons in the spinal cord. The sensory neurons that mediate different sensory modalities differ in size, biochemical phenotype, electrophysiological properties, and sensitivity to neurotrophic factors (Scott, 1992).

All sensory neurons in dorsal root ganglia are derived from the neural crest, a population of cells that migrates from the lateral margins of the neural primordium during formation of the neural tube. Neurons in brachial and thoracic dorsal root ganglia are generated during days 3 to 7 of incubation (E3 to E7; Carr and Simpson, 1978). Neurons in the more caudal, lumbar, and sacral ganglia probably are generated about 1 day later. Dorsal root ganglia can be dissected from embryos as young as E4.5. Sensory neurons from embryos at E4.5 do not require neurotrophic factors for survival, but they differentiate more rapidly in medium containing BDNF or NT-3 than in medium lacking neurotrophic factors (Wright et al., 1992).

After sensory neurons innervate peripheral targets (approximately E5–E8), they become dependent on neurotrophic factors produced by their targets: Nociceptive and thermoreceptive sensory neurons require NGF; proprioceptive neurons require NT-3; another subset of sensory neurons, probably including some low-threshold cutaneous mechanosensory neurons, require BDNF, which is present in peripheral tissues and in the central nervous system (reviewed by Snider, 1994). Sensory neurons undergo biochemical maturation after they innervate peripheral targets and may require contact with their targets to become fully mature (Marusich et al., 1986; Barakat and Droz, 1989).

Cranial Sensory Ganglia

Neurons in the sensory ganglia associated with the cranial nerves innervate diverse targets: The trigeminal ganglia and jugular ganglia contain cutaneous sensory neurons that innervate skin of the head; the petrosal and nodose ganglia are composed predominantly of interoreceptive neurons; and the geniculate, vestibular, and acoustic ganglia contain neurons that innervate specialized receptors in the gustatory, vestibular, and auditory organs. Most of the neurons in the jugular ganglia and the dorsomedial lobe of the trigeminal ganglia are derived from the neural crest and require NGF for development. Neurons in the ventrolateral lobe of the trigeminal ganglia and in the geniculate, vestibular, auditory, petrosal, and nodose ganglia are derived from ectodermal placodes and require BDNF (reviewed by Davies, 1987).

Sympathetic Ganglia

Sympathetic ganglia contain neurons that innervate autonomic targets, such as glands and smooth muscle, and receive synaptic input from cholinergic neurons in the spinal cord. Most sympathetic neurons are catecholaminergic, although some are cholinergic. Most (if not all) sympathetic neurons require NGF for development.

Sympathetic ganglia are formed by a population of neural crest cells that first migrate ventrally to a region near the dorsal aorta (E3) and then move dorsally to positions adjacent to the vertebral column (E6; Rothman et al., 1978). Sympathetic neuroblasts express traits characteristic of neurons, including traits specific to catecholaminergic neurons, before they cease proliferating (Rothman et al, 1978; Rohrer and Thoenen, 1987). The neuroblasts are insensitive to NGF but respond to NT-3 (Verdi and Anderson, 1994). Exposure to NT-3 causes them to cease proliferating and induces expression of the tyrosine kinase receptor for NGF. Generation of postmitotic sympathetic neurons begins at E3.5 and continues until hatching, although most neurons are generated before E12 (Rothman et al., 1978).

Sympathetic neurons grown in vitro are renowned for their plasticity with respect to neurotransmitter phenotype; they express catecholaminergic characteristics when they are grown under standard culture conditions in medium containing NGF but can be induced to express cholinergic characteristics by experimental manipulations, including treatment with leukemia-inhibitory factor or CNTF (Yamamori et al., 1989; Rao et al., 1992). Regulation of neurotransmitter phenotype in sympathetic neurons has been studied extensively in culture preparations, primarily with neurons from rats (reviewed by Patterson, 1990; Landis, 1994) but also with neurons from chick embryos (Ernsberger et al., 1989).

Parasympathetic Ganglia

The parasympathetic ganglia that are the easiest to dissect are the ciliary ganglia, which contain cholinergic motoneurons that innervate muscles of the iris, ciliary body, and choroid. Ciliary motoneurons are derived from the neural crest. They require neurotrophic factors present in the eye for survival and can be maintained in vitro in medium containing eye extract (Nishi and Berg,

1981) or purified neurotrophic factors. Several neurotrophic factors support the survival of ciliary motoneurons in vitro, including adult rat sciatic nerve CNTF (Manthorpe et al., 1986b), growth-promoting activity from chick sciatic nerve (Eckenstein et al., 1990), and basic or acidic fibroblast growth factor (Eckenstein et al., 1990).

Ciliary motoneurons resemble spinal motoneurons in several respects and, like spinal motoneurons, are competent for forming synaptic junctions with skeletal moscle. Ciliary motoneurons are easier to purify than are spinal motoneurons and, for this reason, they sometimes are used as an alternative to study formation of neuromuscular junctions in culture (Role et al., 1987).

Methods for Culturing Peripheral Ganglion Neurons

Explant Cultures

Explanted ganglia can be grown in a liquid medium on a solid substrate (the same types of media and substrates used for dissociated cells, described later) or in a semisolid medium, such as a collagen gel. Axons can be visualized more clearly in a liquid medium than in a collagen gel, but collagen gels are useful for studies concerned with the effects of diffusible factors on axonal growth, because they impede diffusion to an extent sufficient to allow the development of a concentration gradient (Ebendal and Jacobson, 1977; Lumsden and Davies, 1983). Procedures for setting up explant cultures in collagen gels have been described elsewhere (Ebendahl, 1989).

Dissociated Cell Cultures

CHOICES OF CULTURE MEDIA

The standard culture medium for culture of neurons from chick peripheral ganglia consists of a commercial stock medium supplemented with 10% horse serum or fetal bovine serum and with neurotrophic factors. Several familiar types of media have been used successfully as a base, including Ham's F12, Dulbecco's modified Eagle's medium, and Liebovitz's L-15. The consensus among many

researchers who routinely use a serum-supplemented medium is that the best base is F14 (Vogel et al., 1972), an enriched version of Ham's F12 available by special order from Gibco (Baltimore, MD). The length of time for which neurons survive depends on the growth substrate and other factors but, under optimal conditions, most neurons survive at least 48 h and many survive for a week or longer. Five percent chick embryo extract or 50% heart cell conditioned medium sometimes is added to the culture medium to promote neuronal differentiation and long-term survival (Mudge, 1977; Letourneau, 1979; Holz, et al., 1988).

Serum-free media for culture of neurons from chick peripheral ganglia have been devised by several investigators (Bottenstein et al., 1980; Wakade et al. 1982). The medium devised by Wakade et al. (1982), which uses F14 as a base, is just as good as a serum-supplemented medium for short-term culture of neurons and is better for long-term culture (Wakade et al., 1982a). We use a slightly modified version of this medium, recommended to us by Marusich et al., (1986 and personal communications). The medium consists of F14 with 10 μg/ml avian transferrin, 5 μg/ml insulin, 5 ng/ml selenium, and 1 mg/ml bovine serum albumin. With the exception of avian transferrin, all these components can be obtained from standard vendors of culture products. Avian transferrin can be obtained from InterCell Technology (Hopwell, NJ). Human transferrin is more widely available and less expensive than is avian transferrin and may be a suitable substitute (Wakade et al. 1982a).

CULTURE DISHES

Many of the applications for which people use cultures from peripheral ganglia require observing living neurons with a microscope. Preparing cultures suitable for observation with a low-power (dry) objective is simple: Neurons can be plated in standard plastic culture dishes and can be viewed on an inverted microscope. Neuronal cell bodies and axons are easily visible with a high-quality 20- to 40× objective and phase-contrast optics. However, neurons must be grown on glass coverslips for observation with a high-power objective or by optical techniques that require polarized light, such as differential interference contrast (DIC; Nomarski). Glass coverslips also are better for epifluorescence imaging and more convenient for immunocytochemistry.

Much of our work depends on observing neurons with a high-power objective, so we routinely grow our cultures on glass

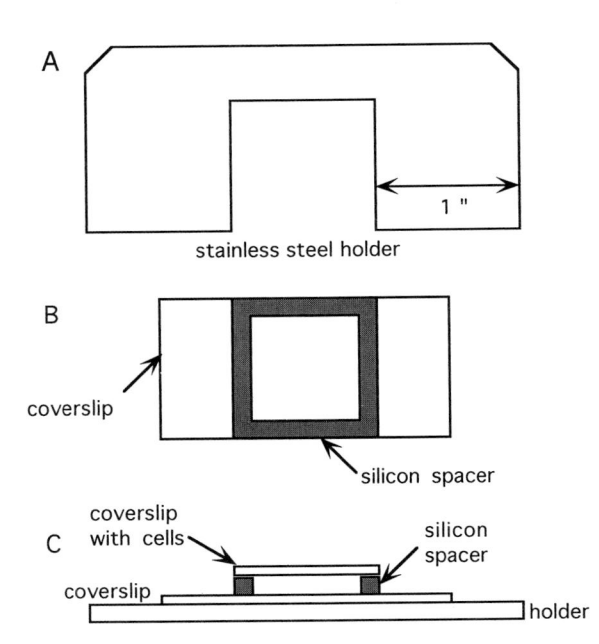

Figure 10.1 Design of chamber for maintaining cultures during observation by high-resolution microscopy. (*A*) Stainless steel holder. (*B*) A 22 × 40 mm coverslip with silicon rubber spacer. (*C*) Side view of the assembled chamber (not drawn to scale). The 22 × 40–mm coverslip is attached to the holder with tape. The silicon rubber spacer is sealed to the coverslips with silicon grease.

coverslips. We use 22-mm-square coverslips because they fit into standard 35-mm culture dishes and are a convenient size for microscopy. To prepare a living culture for observation on a microscope, the coverslip on which the cells are growing is mounted in a simple chamber (figure 10.1) consisting of the coverslip with attached cells, a second larger coverslip (22 × 40 mm), and a spacer made from a sheet of silicon rubber (0.02 inches thick, Reiss Corp., Blackstone, VA). The chamber is attached to a metal holder that fits on the stage of a microscope. It can be viewed with either an inverted or upright microscope and is sufficiently thin to accommodate a high-numerical-aperture (1.4 N.A.), oil-immersion condenser (required for high-resolution transmitted light imaging). More elaborate chambers, some having built-in heaters and ports for changing solutions, are available from commercial sources.

Another popular method for preparing cultures suitable for imaging with a high-power objective is to plate cells in glass-bottom culture dishes made by drilling a hole in the bottom of a

standard culture dish and gluing a glass coverslip under the hole. Cells growing in glass-bottom dishes can be viewed on an inverted microscope with a condenser that has sufficiently long working distance to accommodate the sides of the dish. These dishes are a good choice for applications that require an open dish, such as electrophysiological recording or microinjection.

POSSIBLE SUBSTRATES

Laminin is used widely as a substrate for culture of neurons from peripheral ganglia because it promotes survival of neurons and elicits rapid outgrowth of axons (Manthorpe et al., 1983; Edgar et al., 1984). Peripheral ganglion neurons grow well also on several other types of native substrate proteins, including fibronection, N-cadherin, or L1/NgCAM (Letourneau, 1979; Manthorpe et al., 1983; Gundersen, 1987; Zheng et al., 1994a). Axons grow at different rates on these substrates, and these differences in growth rate are associated with variations in the sizes and morphological make up of the growth cones (Gunderson, 1988; Payne et al., 1992, Zheng et al., 1994; C. Smith, unpublished observations). Protein substrates can be applied directly onto tissue-culture dishes or clean glass coverslips, but they adhere more strongly to dishes or coverslips that have been coated with a positively charged substance, such as polyornithine (Collins, 1978). Neurons grown in a serum-supplemented medium can form axons on uncoated culture dishes or coverslips or on a surface coated with polyornithine alone. However, neurons grown in a serum-free medium form axons slowly or fail to form axons on these substrates.

Our Approach

The protocol in this chapter describes procedures that we use to prepare dissociated cell cultures from chick dorsal root and sympathetic ganglia for studies concerned with the mechanisms of axonal outgrowth. We use neurons from dorsal root ganglia for experiments in which it is helpful to have neurons with large-diameter cell bodies but prefer neurons from sympathetic ganglia for most purposes, because they are more uniform in morphology and behavior. Also, sympathetic ganglia contain a higher percentage of neurons relative to nonneuronal cells. Generally, we prepare cultures from embryos at E8 to E12 because ganglia from embryos

at these stages are easier to dissect and contain fewer nonneuronal cells than do ganglia from older embryos. However, neurons from older embryos have larger cell bodies and growth cones.

Dorsal root and sympathetic ganglia are present in most spinal segments of a chick embryo (~38 segments), but some of the ganglia are small and difficult to dissect. The ganglia that are easiest to dissect are those from the lumbosacral spinal segments. The dorsal root ganglia in segments L1 through S3 (eight ganglia per side) are large because they innervate the hindlimbs. In a chick embryo at E9, each lumbosacral dorsal root ganglion contains ~40,000 cells, although only ~8000 of the cells are neurons. The lumbosacral sympathetic ganglia (two bilateral chains of interconnected ganglia) contain ~300,000 cells, of which ~90% are neurons. We plate neurons at fairly low densities (1000–40,000 neurons per 35-mm culture dish), so a single embryo provides enough neurons for many dishes.

An experienced person can dissect the dorsal root or sympathetic ganglia from a chick embryo at E8 to E12 in less than 15 min. Dissociation of the ganglia (by digestion in trypsin and trituration with a fire-polished pipette) takes just a little more than 30 min. Cultures can be set up in approximately 1 h, provided that the culture dishes and all the necessary solutions have been prepared in advance. Preparation of pure neuronal cultures, which requires separating the neurons from the nonneuronal cells, takes more time (1–12 h, depending on the method used). The method described in this chapter adds 3 to 4 h.

Our procedures for culturing dorsal root and sympathetic ganglion neurons are essentially identical, and the same procedures can be applied successfully to neurons from other types of ganglia. The neurons are grown in a chemically defined medium (Marusich et al., 1986) on glass coverslips coated with polyornithine followed by laminin. Neurons grown on laminin begin to form axons soon after plating and, by 24 h after plating, most neurons have axons several hundreds of micrometers long. Our work focuses on early stages in axonal outgrowth, so generally we examine cultures within less than 24 h after plating. For studies that require maintaining cultures for longer periods, it might be better to plate the neurons on a more adhesive substrate, such as plastic culture dishes coated with polyornithine, although neurons grown on this substrate form axons less rapidly than do neurons on laminin.

Protocol

Preparations

EGGS

We purchase fertilized chicken eggs (White Leghorn) from a local supplier. The eggs can be stored for up to 2 weeks in a refrigerator at 55°F, but storage for longer times reduces viability. The embryos begin to develop when the eggs are placed in an egg incubator. The eggs should be set with their blunt ends up so the embryos will float to the top and be easy to remove. They do not have to be turned. The temperature in the incubator should be 99.5°F, and the atmosphere should be kept humid. Our incubator (GQF Manufacturing Corp., Savannah, GA) comes with an "automatic humidifier," which consists of a tray of water connected by rubber tubing and a float-valve to a reservoir placed on top of the incubator.

COVERSLIPS

Sources

We use 22-mm-square Gold Seal coverslips (no. 1.5 thickness) for routine purposes but use special coverslips (Bellco; cat. no. 1916-92525, Gaithersburg, MD) that have a grid pattern photoetched on their surfaces for experiments that depend on observing the same cells on multiple occasions. The grid pattern is visible by phase-contrast or DIC optics and helps to relocate the cells.

Cleaning

Coverslips must be cleaned before they are used, otherwise cells adhere poorly to them. Our procedures for cleaning coverslips (box 10.1) are time-consuming but produce substrates that promote neuronal growth more consistently than do simpler procedures that we have tried. The racks and vessels into which the coverslips are placed for cleaning should be acid-resistant, because one step of the procedure involves soaking the coverslips for 2 days in concentrated nitric acid. We put the coverslips in polypropylene racks (Fluoroware, cat. no. A66-0603 Chaska, MN). Each rack has 25 slots but can hold ~50 coverslips in such a way that they do not stick together. Two racks of coverslips fit into a standard, rectangular glass staining dish (11 × 13 cm). To keep the coverslips from

Box 10.1 Cleaning Coverslips

1. Soak coverslips for 30 min in warm water with Alconox (approximately 1/2 tsp/L).
2. Rinse in running water and three changes of distilled water.
3. Soak for 2 days in concentrated HNO_3.
4. Rinse five times in distilled H_2O (over several hours).
5. Rinse two times in sterile, glass-distilled H_2O.
6. Dry in a laminar flow hood.
7. Sterilize by 5-min exposure to a short-wave ultraviolet(UV) lamp. (UV Products, no. R526, San Gabriel, CA) at a distance of 3 in.
8. Place each coverslip in a 35-mm tissue-culture dish and sterilize by 5-min exposure to UV.
9. Replace lids on the dishes and store them in a clean container. (e.g., a 245 × 245 × 20–mm plastic Petri dish; Nunc no. 240835).

floating away when the racks are submerged in the cleaning solutions, we place a polypropylene screen (Fluoroware no. A25-02-0603) and weight (a $\frac{5}{8}$-inch wafer carrier; no. AA16-01) on top of the racks.

Coating with Polyornithine

For sterility, subsequent steps should be carried out in a laminar flow hood. Prepare a solution of 0.5 mg/ml polyornithine (Sigma Chemical Corp., St. Louis, MO; cat. no. P-8638) in sterile borate buffer (61.5 mM; pH 8.3). The polyornithine solution can be stored at 4°C for up to 6 months. Keep the coverslips in the culture dishes in which they were placed after cleaning. Use an adjustable volume pipetter to put a drop of the polyornithine solution in the center of each coverslip. Generally, we use a 200-µl drop, which covers an area 1 to 1.5 cm in diameter (the area of the coverslips in which cells can be observed most easily). Cover the dishes and place them in a 37°C tissue-culture incubator for 2 to 24 h. Remove the polyornithine solution by aspiration with a pipette and rinse the dishes five times (over several hours) with sterile, glass-distilled water. Agitate the dishes several times during rinsing to ensure that water passes under the coverslip, otherwise the coverslips may stick to the plastic and be difficult to remove. Allow the coverslips to air-dry in a laminar flow hood, then sterilize under ultraviolet light (UV) for 5 min. Coated coverslips may be stored at room temperature for up to a year.

Box 10.2 Preparation of Calcium- and Magnesium-Free HBSS

Ingredients for 1 L 10× HBSS

4.0 g	KCl
0.6 g	KH_2PO_4
76.5 g	NaCl
3.5 g	$NaHCO_3$
0.48 g	$NaHPO_4$
23.8 g	HEPES

Dissolve ingredients in 900-ml glass-distilled H_2O. To make HBSS with glucose, also add 10 g glucose (dextrose). Adjust pH to 7.2 with NaOH. Add distilled H_2O (dH_2O) to bring volume to 1.0 L.

Filter-sterilize. Put 45-ml aliquots in 50-ml plastic centrifuge tubes. Store at −20°C. Dilute to 1× with dH_2O before use.

Coating with Laminin

Stock solutions of laminin (1 mg/ml; Gibco no. 23017-015) are delivered in glass vials on dry ice. The solution should be thawed slowly at 4°C because rapid thawing causes the laminin to precipitate. Thawed laminin can be divided into aliquots and refrozen. Dilute the laminin solution to 10 μg/ml with sterile calcium- and magnesium-free HEPES buffered balanced salt solution (HBSS; box 10.2) prior to use. Coverslips should be coated with laminin no more than 24 h before cells are plated on them. Put a 200-μl drop of diluted laminin in the center of each coverslip. Leave the laminin on the coverslips for 2 to 24 h in a 37°C culture incubator. Remove the laminin solution and rinse the coverslip three times in HBSS. After the last rinse, flood the coverslip with culture medium. Store the dishes in a CO_2 incubator while preparing the cells for plating.

CULTURE MEDIUM

Culture Media

F14 can be purchased by custom order (50-L minimum) from Gibco. The most economical way to purchase it is in dry packages (50 × 1 L). The standard formula (no. 78-5248) contains phenol red, a pH indicator, and L-glutamine but lacks sodium bicarbonate. Formula no. 89-5177, which lacks phenol red, is a better choice for applications that depend on observing cells with a high-intensity lamp (e.g., epifluorescence or high-magnification DIC imaging), because photooxidation of phenol red can be injurious to cells.

Box 10.3   Medium Supplements

1.   Nutrient mixture

A.   BSA/INSULIN/SELENIUM STOCK
Add to 50 ml F14:

4 g BSA (Sigma no. A-9647)
20 mg insulin (Collaborative Research no. 40205)
20 µl selenium solution (1 mg/ml; Collective Research no. 40201)

Add sufficient additional HEPES buffered F14 to bring volume to 80 ml.
Filter-sterilize. Divide into 20-ml aliquots. Store at −20°C.

B.   NUTRIENT MIXTURE WITH TRANSFERRIN
Add to 20 ml BSA/insulin/selenium stock 10 mg avian transferrin (Intercell
Technology, Hopewell, NJ). Divide into 1 ml aliquots. Store at −20°C.

2.   Antibiotic mixture
Reconstitute one vial lyophilized penicillin-streptomycin (Gibco no. 600-5075;
100,000 units penicillin; 100,000 µg streptomycin) in 18 ml sterile distilled
H_2O. Add 2 ml Fungizone 250 µg/ml; Gibco no. 600-529AE). Divide into 0.5 ml
aliquots. Store at −20°C.

3.   Neurotrophic factors

7s-NGF (Sigma no. N0513)
BDNF (R&D Systems no. 248-BD; Promega no. G-1491)
NT-3 (R&D Systems no. 267-N3; Promega no. G-1501)

Dissolve neurotrophic factors at 50 µg/ml in F14 with 0.1% BSA. Divide into
aliquots (20 µl for NGF; 5 or 10 µl for BDNF and NT-3). Store frozen, preferably
below −70°C.

To reconstitute F14, dissolve the contents of one package in 900 ml glass-distilled H_2O. Stir until the F14 is dissolved completely, then add 1.94 g $NaHCO_3$. The pH should be ∼7.3; adjustment usually is not necessary, but it is wise to check. Bring the volume to 1 L and filter-sterilize, preferably by a positive-pressure filtration system (Sterivex-G5 peristaltic pump; Millipore). Reconstituted F14 can be stored at 4°C for several months. To prepare complete culture medium, to 50 ml F14 add one aliquot of each of the medium supplements described in box 10.3: nutrient mixture with transferrin, antibiotic mixture (optional), and neurotrophic factors. NGF is reasonably inexpensive and is available from most standard vendors of cell culture products. It supports the survival

of essentially all sympathetic neurons but only ~40% of dorsal root ganglion neurons. Addition of 1 to 10 ng/ml BDNF and NT-3 (Promega, R&D Systems) results in the survival of a larger proportion of dorsal root ganglion neurons, but these neurotrophic factors are expensive, so generally we do not add them. Complete culture medium can be stored at 4°C for up to 5 days. Before cells are added to the medium, the temperature and pH should be brought to physiological levels by placing the medium in a 37°C incubator with an atmosphere containing 7% CO_2.

Medium for Microscopy
As it is inconvenient to keep cultures in an atmosphere with 7% CO_2 during observation on a microscope, we transfer them to a culture medium that maintains a physiological pH in air. The medium we use for microscopy contains the same supplements as does our standard culture medium but is made from F14 lacking phenol red (formula no. 89-5177) and is buffered with 10 mM HEPES (pH 7.4) rather than sodium bicarbonate. The supplements are prepared with HEPES buffered F14.

SYLGARD COATED DISSECTION DISH
Sylgard (Dow Corning Corp., Midland, MI) is prepared by mixing Sylgard Elastomer with Sylgard Curing Agent at a ratio of 10 parts to 1, by weight. The volume needed to coat the bottom of a 100-mm Petri dish is ~30 ml. Stir the mixture thoroughly, but try to avoid mixing in air, which forms bubbles. Then pour the mixture into the Petri dish. Some bubbles probably will be present, but they can be removed by placing the dish under a vacuum for 2 to 3 h (at room temperature) or by storing the dish at −20°C until bubbles rise to the surface, then bursting the bubbles with the tip of a pin. Cure the Sylgard for 2 to 3 days at room temperature or for 24 h at 60°C. Sylgard-coated dishes can be reused many times. Before using a dish for dissection, sterilize it by soaking for 10 min with 70% ethanol or by autoclaving.

Dissection and Plating

SETTING UP
Dissection and plating are performed in a laminar flow hood. The equipment and solutions you will need are listed in box 10.4.

Box 10.4 Equipment and Solutions for Dissection and Plating

1. Research-grade binocular dissecting microscope.
2. High-intensity lamp (preferably a halogen lamp with fiber light guides).
3. Adjustable pipetter (10–200 μl) and sterile pipette tips.
4. Sterile cotton-plugged Pasteur pipettes.
5. Alcohol burner or Bunsen burner.
6. Sylgard-coated dissection dish.
7. $\frac{7}{16}$-inch steel minuten pins (Carolina Biological).
8. 15-ml clear conical centrifuge tubes and rack.
9. 100-mm plastic Petri dishes.
10. Coarse forceps.
11. Two pairs of watchmaker's forceps (Dumont no. 5).
12. One small (4$\frac{1}{2}$-inch) pointed dissecting scissors.
13. Medium-fine iridectomy scissors (Tiemann, Hauppauge, NY: no. 160-158).
14. HBSS with glucose (~500 ml).
15. 2.5% trypsin (Gibco no. 15090-038).
16. HEPES buffered F14 supplemented with 10% horse serum (~5 ml).
17. Complete culture medium (~2 ml/dish).

Transfer with a pipette 5 ml F14 with 10% horse serum into a 15-ml centrifuge tubes and place the tube in a 37°C water bath. Pipette sufficient culture medium for the number of cultures to be made into a 100-mm Petri dish and store (covered) in a 37°C CO_2 incubator. Fire-polish the tip of a cotton-plugged Pasteur pipette so as to smooth the tip and reduce the opening by approximately one-third. Coat the inside with F14 with 10% horse serum and store it near the dissecting microscope; a convenient place to store it is in a 15-ml centrifuge tube. The pipette will be used to transfer ganglia and for trituration. Pour into a 100-mm plastic Petri dish and into the Sylgard-coated dissection dish ~50 ml HBSS with glucose (enough to submerge an embryo). Pour ~2 ml HBSS with glucose into a 15-ml centrifuge tube. Keep this tube near your dissecting microscope; it will be used to store the ganglia.

DISSECTION

Sterilize the blunt end of an egg by squirting it twice with 70% ethanol. Allow the egg to dry for a few minutes after each squirt. Make a small hole in the blunt end by piercing it with the tips of a coarse forceps. Then enlarge the hole and remove the white membrane over the air sac to expose the embryo. Using a coarse forceps, gently pick up the embryo by its neck and transfer the embryo to the 100-mm plastic Petri dish containing HBSS with glucose. De-

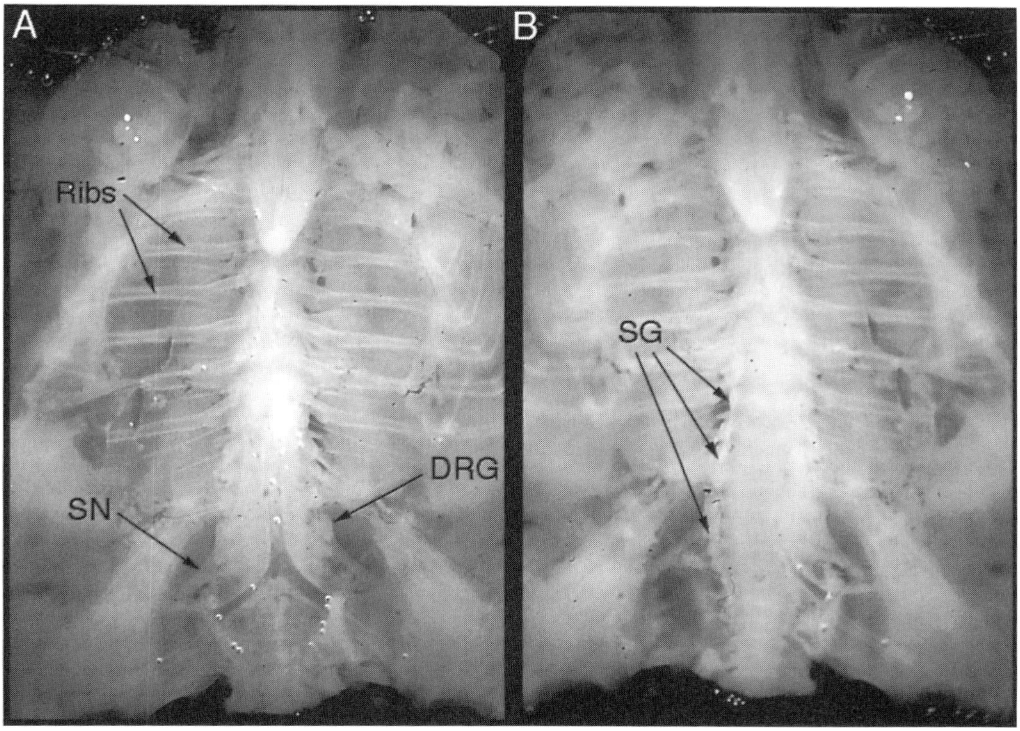

Figure 10.2 Dissection of lumbosacral dorsal root and sympathetic ganglia from a chick embryo at E11. (*A*) Ventral view of the vertebral column, ribs, dorsal root ganglia (DRG), and spinal nerves (SN) after removal of heart, lungs, and abdominal viscera. (*B*) Exposure of sympathetic ganglia by removal of the peritoneum. An incision was made in the peritoneum along the midline of the vertebral column, and the peritoneum on the left side was reflected laterally to reveal the chain of sympathetic ganglia (SG). See plate 6 for color version.

capitate the embryo with dissecting scissors and remove as much of the abdominal viscera as possible without damaging the area around the vertebral column. Then transfer the body to the dissection dish and pin it, ventral side up, to the Sylgard with minuten pins through the wings and legs.

Subsequent steps of the dissection are performed under a dissecting microscope. Put a piece of black paper or black rubber mat on the stage of the microscope and place the dissection dish on it. Adjust the lamp to illuminate the embryo at an oblique angle. Remove the breast muscle and bone and the underlying heart and lungs. Underneath will be seen the ribs and vertebral column (figure 10.2 and color plate 6). Cut off the tail and stretch the legs to make the embryo as flat as possible. Rinse the embryo by squirting it with a pipette containing HBSS. Remove the viscera from over

the lumbosacral region of the vertebral column (caudal to the rib cage). Along the lateral aspects of the lumbosacral vertebral column will be seen the distal portions of the dorsal root ganglia and the spinal nerves that project into the hind limbs (see figure 10.2). The lumbosacral chains of sympathetic ganglia may not be visible at this point. They are pale cordlike structures that lie behind the peritoneum (the membrane overlying the vertebral column). They are ventromedial to the dorsal root ganglia.

To dissect the sympathetic chains, first make an incision along the midline through the peritoneum. Pull the membrane flaps laterally to reveal the sympathetic chains medial to the dorsal root ganglia. Watch closely while pulling the membrane flaps, because the sympathetic chains sometimes stick to them. Pick up the caudal end of one chain with a fine forceps and use the iridectomy scissors to tease the intact chain gently from the embryo. The chain will be easy to remove up to the level of the second most caudal rib. Cut the chain at this level and transfer it with a fire-polished pipette to a centrifuge tube containing HBSS with glucose. Remove the second chain by the same procedures.

Dorsal root ganglia can be removed by plucking them out from the vertebral column with fine forceps. The author finds it easier first to remove the cartilage from the ventral side of the vertebral column, then to take out the spinal cord. This procedure makes the dorsal root ganglia easier to see and provides a cavity in which they can be stored until transfer to a centrifuge tube. To remove the ventral side of the vertebral column, make two longitudinal incisions in the cartilage ventromedial to the dorsal root ganglia. Begin the incisions at the caudal end and continue to the thoracic level. Cut the flap of cartilage at its rostral end and discard it. Underneath will be seen the spinal cord and, along the lateral edges of the vertebral column, the dorsal root ganglia. The large dorsal root ganglia in the eight spinal segments caudal to the ribs contain sensory neurons that innervate the hind limbs. Remove the spinal cord, taking care that no dorsal root ganglia are pulled out with it. Cut the lumbosacral dorsal root ganglia away from the vertebral column, then cut the spinal nerves emerging from the distal sides of the ganglia. Make the cuts close to the ganglia to minimize contamination of the cultures by nonneuronal cells from the nerve sheaths. Pluck the ganglia with a forceps and store them in the cavity in the vertebral column. After collecting several ganglia, transfer them with a fire-polished pipette to a centrifuge tube containing HBSS with glucose.

DISSOCIATION AND PLATING

When the dissection is completed transfer the ganglia to a centrifuge tube containing 0.25% trypsin in HBSS with glucose. Incubate the ganglia for 30 min in a water bath at 37°C, then transfer them to a tube containing F14 with 10% horse serum to inactivate the trypsin. Let the ganglia sink to the bottom of the tube and transfer them to a centrifuge tube containing 2 ml warm culture medium (from the Petri dish of culture medium already in the incubator). Dissociate the ganglia by drawing them into a fire-polished pipette, then expelling them along the side of the centrifuge tube. Avoid introducing air bubbles into the suspension, as air interfaces can damage the cells. Trituration should be energetic enough to dissociate the ganglia in 15 to 22 passages through the pipette.

Count the numbers of cells present in the cell suspension with a hemacytometer on a microscope with a 20× objective and phase-contrast optics. Neurons appear rounded and phase-bright and sometimes have processes. Nonneuronal cells are darker and irregularly shaped. Adjust the volume as required to give the desired plating density (<1000 neurons per coverslip for low-density cultures, up to 50,000 neurons for dense cultures). A volume of ∼1 ml will be needed to fill the bottom of a 35-mm culture dish, but cells can be conserved by plating a smaller volume (100–200 µl) in the center of the coverslip. If the smaller volume is chosen, it will require drying the edges of the coverslips and the bottom of the dishes before putting the cell suspension on the coverslips, otherwise the cells will flow off the coverslips. Avoid drying the laminin-coated regions of the coverslips. Cover the dishes and place them in a 37°C incubator with 7% CO_2. After 1 to 2 h, when the cells have attached to the substrate, add additional culture medium to each dish to bring the volume to 1 to 2 ml. One milliliter of culture medium is sufficient to maintain cultures for up to 12 h, but 2 ml should be used to maintain cells for longer times. The medium should be changed every 2 days if the experiment requires long-term culture of neurons.

Separating Neurons from Nonneuronal Cells

The presence of small numbers of nonneuronal cells in our cultures is not a problem for the types of experiments we perform. However, large numbers of nonneuronal cells are a nuisance, because they align with axons and obscure growth cones. Sympathetic ganglia contain sufficiently few nonneuronal cells relative

to the numbers of neurons so that we do not find it necessary to purify the neurons, but we do purify neurons from dorsal root ganglia. The procedure we use takes advantage of the differing adhesive qualities of neurons and nonneuronal cells to tissue-culture plastic (Barde et al., 1980).

This procedure results in loss of some neurons, so it is a good idea to start with perhaps twice as many neurons as are needed. Digest ganglia in 0.25% trypsin and rinse in F14 with 10% horse serum, following the procedures described earlier. Then transfer the ganglia to a tube containing 3 ml fresh F14 with 10% horse serum and dissociate by trituration. Transfer the cell suspension to a 60-mm tissue-culture dish and incubate for 2 to 4 h at 37°C under 7% CO_2. During this time, the nonneuronal cells adhere to the culture dish, but the neurons attach only weakly. To dislodge the neurons from the dish, incline the dish to an angle of approximately 45 degrees, draw medium from the dish into a fire-polished Pasteur pipette, then gently flush the bottom of the dish with medium from the pipette. Transfer the cell suspension to a 15-ml centrifuge tube and spin at 800 rpm for 5 min in a table-top centrifuge. Remove the medium from the pelleted cells and add approximately 100 µl of culture medium. Briskly thump the bottom of the tube with a finger to resuspend the cells, then add 2 ml culture medium and triturate the cells. Plate the neurons by the procedures described previously.

This procedure, although adequate for our purposes, does not produce pure neuronal cultures; some nonneuronal cells invariable are collected along with the neurons. A procedure for separation of neurons from nonneuronal cells, reported to be more effective (Davies, 1989), is effected by sedimentation in a glass dropping funnel containing F14 with 10% horse serum. Neurons and nonneuronal cells pass through the column at different rates, so they are retrieved from the funnel in different fractions.

The presence of even small numbers of nonneuronal cells may pose problems for experiments that require maintaining cultures for long periods. Nonneuronal cells continue to proliferate until they become confluent and may displace the neurons. Proliferation of nonneuronal cells can be inhibited by treating the cultures with antimitotic drugs (e.g., 1–5 µM cytosine arabinofuranoside), but these drugs may injure neurons. A better way to inhibit proliferation is to expose the cultures to gamma irradiation (5000 rads; Holz et al., 1988), which kills nonneuronal cells but has no apparent effect on the neurons. Another strategy that has been reported to be

effective is to grow the cultures for 2 days in F14 medium containing 10% horse serum (and the required neurotrophic factors), then to replace the medium with serum-free F14 medium. Although nonneuronal cells grow in either type of medium, transferring them from medium with serum to a serum-free medium apparently causes them to die, whereas neurons survive (Wakade, et al., 1982b).

Characteristics of the Cultures

Freshly dissociated sympathetic neurons or dorsal root ganglion neurons have rounded cell bodies and multiple, thin filopodia (<0.2 µm). Most neurons lose their axonal and dendritic branches during dissociation, although some retain remnants of these branches. Neurons adhere to the substrate within a few minutes after plating. Their cell bodies flatten slightly as they attach (figure 10.3A–D) and typically are ovoid, with the nucleus displaced to one side of the main mass of cytoplasm (though nuclei are not in the plane of focus in figure 10.3). Sympathetic neurons from embryos at E9 have cell bodies 7 to 14 µm in diameter. The diameters of dorsal root ganglion neurons are from 7 µm to some 18 µm.

Sympathetic neurons often begin to form neurites within less than 10 min after attachment to the substrate (see figure 10.3A–D). By 1 hour after plating, many neurons have several neurites longer than 50 µm (see figure 10.3E). Dorsal root ganglion neurons take a little longer to form neurites, but most begin within 1 to 3 h. The neurites grow intermittently, with periods of elongation interrupted by periods of retraction, and some neurites disappear. Twenty-four hours after plating, most neurons have two or more neurites several hundred micrometers in length. We assume that the neurites are axons rather than dendrites, because of their lengths and fairly constant diameters. Also, immunocytochemical studies have shown that processes with this appearance have compositions characteristic of axons (Lein and Higgins, 1989; also see chapter 13). The neurites fasiculate when they come into contact and eventually form a complex network unless neurons are plated at very low densities. The best time to observe growth cones (see figure 10.3F) is between 6 and 24 h after plating, before neurites become extensively intermingled.

Cultures from sympathetic ganglia of embryos at E7 to E9 contain, in addition to differentiated neurons, neuroblasts that retain

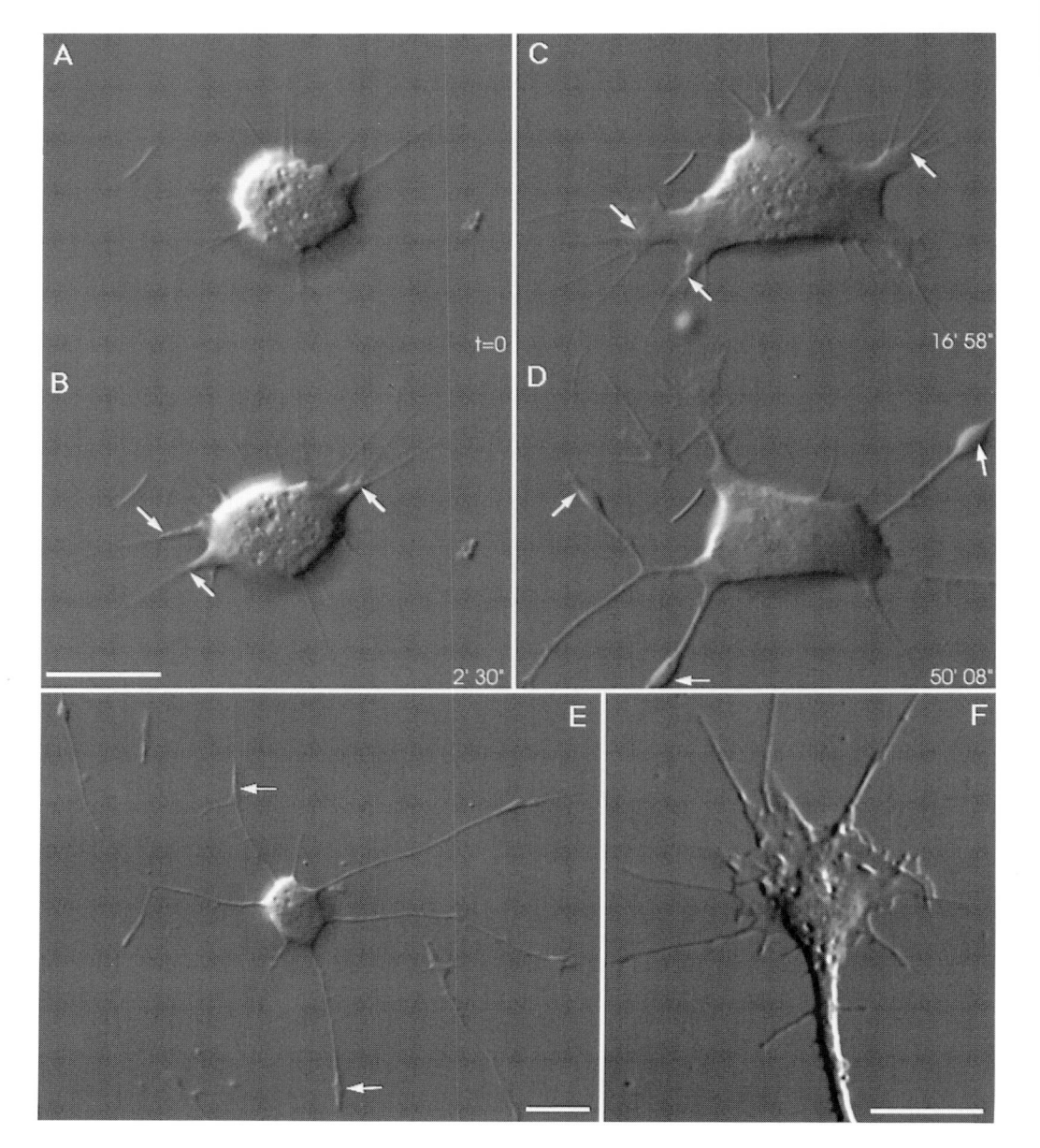

Figure 10.3 Stages in neurite formation by dissociated peripheral ganglion neurons grown on coverslips coated with polyornithine followed by laminin. Neurons were visualized by video microscopy with differential interference–contrast (Nomarski) optics. (*A–D*) The initiation of neurite outgrowth by a sympathetic neuron. Five minutes after plating (*A*; $t = 0$), the neuron was attached to the substrate and had multiple filopodia. Two and a half minutes later (*B*), proximal portions of three filopodia thickened, owing to invasion by cytoplasm (arrows). The cytoplasmic protrusions widened as they advanced and engulfed several adjacent filopodia (*C*; arrows). After 50 minutes, the neuron had definitive neurites with growth cones at their distal ends (*D*; arrows). (*E*) Sympathetic neuron one hour after plating. The neurites have bulbous growth cones (arrows), as is characteristic of fast-growing neurites. (*F*) Growth cone of a dorsal root ganglion neuron 12 h after plating. Scale bars: 10 μm.

the ability to divide in vitro. The neuroblasts resemble neurons in that they form long processes, with growth cones at their distal ends. Before neuroblasts divide, their processes shorten and shrink in diameter to widths comparable to those of filopodia. After cytokinesis, the processes thicken and resume growing. We have not attempted to determine the fraction of cells that are neuroblasts as opposed to neurons, but our studies of cultures by time-lapse video microscopy suggest that it is in the order of 1 cell in 10. Neuroblasts are present in cultures from dorsal root ganglia of embryos at E4 to E7 but, unlike sympathetic neuroblasts, sensory neuroblasts do not form processes or express other traits characteristic of neurons (Rohrer and Thoenen, 1987).

The most prevalent type of nonneuronal cells in cultures from embryos at E11 or later are spindle-shaped cells that align with axons; we presume that these are Schwann cells. Schwann cells differentiate later than do neurons, so fewer Schwann cells are present in cultures from embryos at E7 or E8 than from older embryos. In addition, the cultures contain fibroblasts, distinguishable by their characteristic flattened shapes.

Applications

Studies of chick peripheral ganglion neurons grown in vitro have made many important contributions to our understanding of axonal outgrowth. The pioneering work of Bray, Wessells, Letourneau, and others helped to reveal the roles of microtubules and actin filaments in axonal elongation and growth cone motility (reviewed by Bray, 1992), and more recent work by Heidemann and colleagues has provided information about the cytomechanics of axonal growth (reviewed by Heidemann, 1996). In addition, much has been learned about the types of cues that can guide growing axons (Letourneau, 1979; Kapfhammer and Raper, 1986; Gunderson, 1987; Kuhn et al., 1991; Letourneau, 1992; Luo et al., 1993). Our work has focused on a less extensively studied aspect of axonal development: the initial outgrowth from the cell body (Smith, 1994a,b).

Cultures of freshly dissociated sympathetic neurons provide a particularly favorable system in which to study this process, because sympathetic neurons form axons in a highly stereotyped manner. Freshly plated sympathetic neurons have multiple filopodia, thin processes that contain actin filaments. Axons form by invasion of filopodia with microtubules, organelles, and other

components of axoplasm. In cultures plated on laminin, filopodia often are invaded by cytoplasm as soon as they attach to the substrate (see figure 10.3A–D). However, in cultures plated on polyornithine, filopodia are invaded only when their tips attach to a three-dimensional object, such as another cell or a large, polystyrene bead coated with an adhesive substance (figure 10.4). Beads coated either with polyornithine and laminin or with polyornithine alone can trigger invasion of a filopodium by cytoplasm.

A filopodium can be invaded by cytoplasm only as long as the object to which it has become attached remains anchored to the substrate. Generally, cells remain anchored, but beads do not. If a bead detaches from the substrate while a filopodium is being invaded by cytoplasm, the cytoplasm immediately stops advancing and retracts back into the cell body (see figure 10.4A). Also, if a bead is placed on a filopodium (with laser tweezers) and released, the bead does not initiate invasion of the filopodium by cytoplasm but, instead, is transported over the surface of the filopodium to the cell body.

A clue as to why neurons on laminin form neurites spontaneously—whereas neurons on polyornithine do not—was obtained from experiments in which neurons were examined by time-lapse microscopy with an optical technique (laser-scanning interference reflection microscopy) that shows the spatial separation of cells from the substrate (figure 10.5). Filopodia of neurons on laminin are not apposed closely to the substrate along most of their lengths, although their distal tips often are in close contact (see figure 10.5C,D). By contrast, filopodia on polyornithine are in close apposition along their entire lengths (see figure 10.5A,B). However, when the tip of a filopodium attaches to a cell or large bead, the filopodium straightens and lifts off the substrate (see figure 10.5A,B), suggesting that it is under tension. The filopodium typically begins to be invaded by cytoplasm within 5 to 15 min after it lifts off the substrate.

Our interpretation of these observations is that filopodia must be under tension to be invaded by cytoplasm. Tension can develop when the tip of the fiopodium is attached to an immobile object but not when the entire filopodium is attached to a substrate (as occurs on polyornithine). Additional support for the idea that tension plays a role in neurite formation comes from studies that showed that dorsal root ganglion neurons can be induced to form an axon

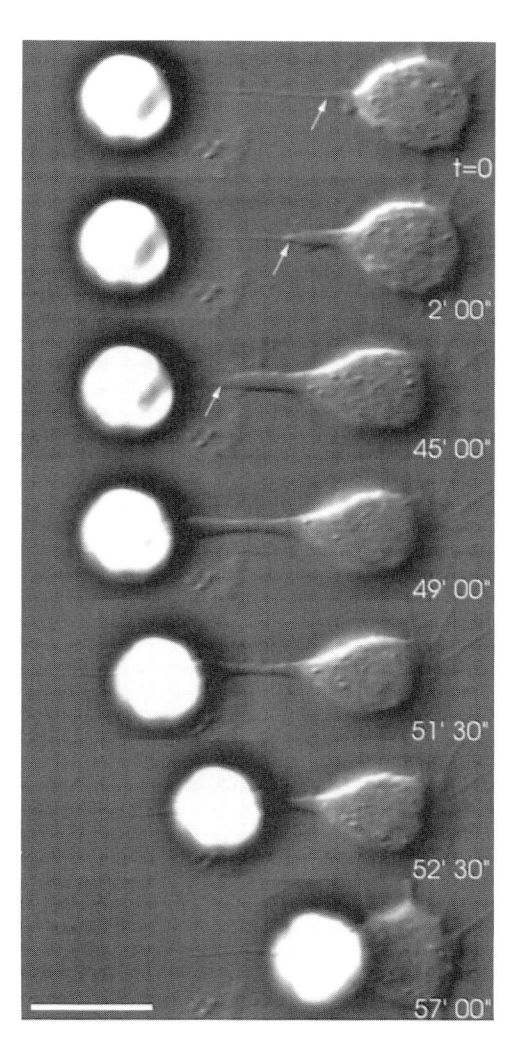

Figure 10.4 Video images of a sympathetic neuron following attachment of a filopodium to a large polystyrene bead. Between t = 0 and t = 49 minutes, the filopodium was invaded by a column of cytoplasm, the first stage in neurite formation. Simultaneously, the cell body moved toward the bead. Between t = 49 minutes and t = 51 minutes 30 seconds, the bead detached from the substrate. Then, the column of cytoplasm retracted into the cell carrying the bead with it, and the cell body returned to its original position. Scale bar: 10 μm.

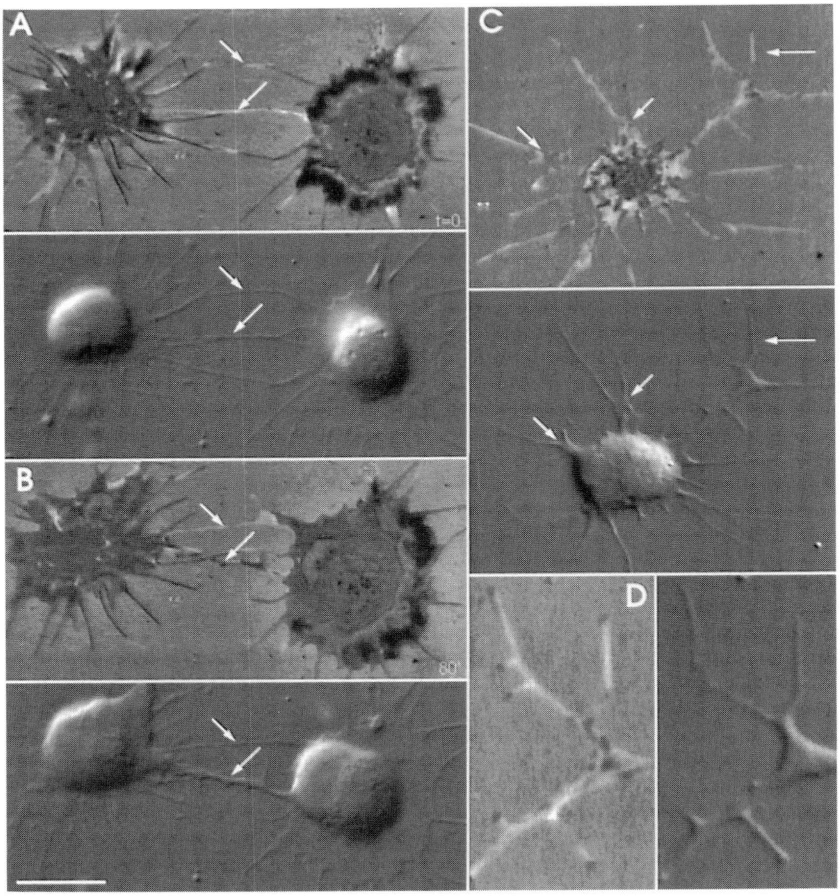

Figure 10.5 Interactions of neurons with the growth substrate during the initiation of neurite outgrowth, as visualized by interference reflection microscopy (IRM) and differential interference–contrast (DIC) laser-scanning microscopy. In IRM images, areas of the cells that are apposed closely to the substrate appear *dark*, whereas less closely attached areas appear *light*. The left column shows IRM and DIC images of a pair of neurons on polyornithine before (*A*) and after (*B*) filopodia were invaded by cytoplasm. Most filopodia were apposed closely to the substrate and were not invaded by cytoplasm. However, two filopodia that emerged from the neuron on the right were apposed only loosely, as evident from the brightness of the IRM images (upper panels) and from their movement relative to the substrate. These filopodia were invaded by cytoplasm (*B*). (*C*) IRM and DIC images of a neuron on laminin after some of its filopodia were invaded by cytoplasm (arrows). The filopodia indicated by the *long arrows* are shown at higher magnification (*D*). Note that these filopodia are apposed loosely to the substrate along most of their lengths (*C, D*) but that their tips are apposed closely (*D*). Scale bar: 10 μm.

by attaching a pipette to their margin and pulling it outward (Bray, 1984; Zheng et al., 1991).

The processes that occur in neuronal cell bodies during the initiation of axon outgrowth closely parallel processes observed in growth cones when one of their filopodia contacts another cell (O'Connor et al., 1990; Lin and Forscher, 1993). In both situations, attachment of the tip of a filopodium to an object triggers invasion of the filopodium by cytoplasm and establishes the future path of the neurite. The process where by adhesion of a filopodium initiates movements of cytoplasm and the identity of the molecular motors that produce these movements are subjects of current interest.

These experiments illustrate some of the advantages of cultures from chick peripheral ganglia for studies on axonal outgrowth and on other aspects of neuronal development. The neurons behave in a stereotyped and predictable manner because essentially they are uniform in phenotype. They are sufficiently hardy to withstand a variety of experimental manipulations, including manipulations that require keeping the neurons outside a culture incubator for extended times, and they grow well at low densities, thereby making it possible to study the behavior of isolated neurons. The culture conditions can be controlled precisely by growing the neurons in a chemically defined medium. Moreover, the ease and low cost of preparing them make it practical to set up new cultures daily, thereby providing a steady supply at the desired stage of development.

11 Culturing Mammalian Sympathoadrenal Derivatives

Nagesh K. Mahanthappa and Paul H. Patterson

The neural crest gives rise to a variety of cell types during vertebrate development, including the sympathoadrenal lineage, one of the most thoroughly characterized neuronal lineages in vertebrates (Anderson, 1993). Sympathoadrenal derivatives include the neurons constituting the sympathetic branch of the peripheral nervous system and the chromaffin cells of the adrenal medulla. Both these cell types can be maintained readily as homogenous populations in vitro (figure 11.1). By virtue of the ease of their dissection and homogeneity, cultured sympathetic neurons have provided a particularly robust system for the study of neuronal development and physiology. As examples, sympathetic neurons have been used to study growth factors (Mains and Patterson, 1973), ion channels, and receptors (Furshpan et al., 1976), neurite outgrowth (Pittman and Buettner, 1989; Mahanthappa and Patterson, 1992a,b), determination of neurotransmitter phenotype (Yamamori et al., 1989), and apoptosis (Martin et al., 1988). Cultured chromaffin cells have proved very useful for studying exocytosis and adrenal physiology and as a unique system in which to study transdifferentiation. Under appropriate conditions, primary adrenal chromaffin cells can be converted into cells indistinguishable from sympathetic neurons (Doupe et al., 1985a). The ability to induce such a phenotypic switch under well-defined conditions has provided developmental insights and also makes available cellular material of value for neural transplantation (Mahanthappa et al., 1990).

Although there are many variations on the culture methods used successfully to maintain these cell types, we focus on methods that have been developed over the last 35 years for the study of sympathetic neurons and adrenal chromaffin cells from neonatal rats. Simple modifications and technical alternatives also are discussed briefly. It should be noted also that the progenitors of the sympathoadrenal lineage have been isolated and cultured successfully (Carnahan and Patterson, 1991), as have rat neural crest cells (Stemple and Anderson, 1992).

A

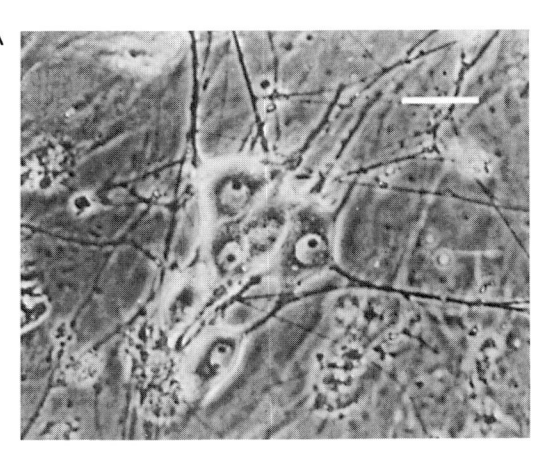

B

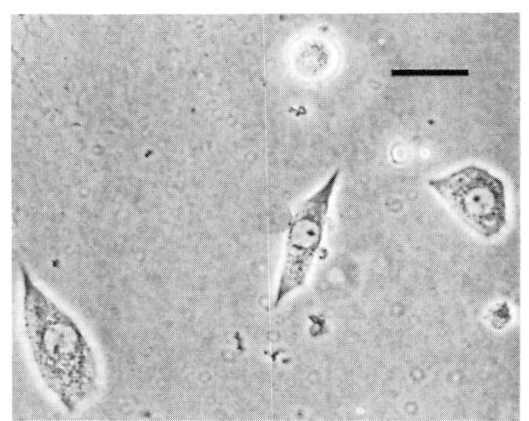

Figure 11.1 Representative photomicrographs of sympathetic neurons (*A*) and adrenal chromaffin cells (*B*) cultured from the neonatal rat. Scale bar: 50 μm for neurons, 25 μm for chromaffin cells. (Reproduced with permission from (*A*) P. H. Patterson, L. F. Reichardt, L. L. Y. Chun, Biochemical studies on the development of primary sympathetic neurons in cell culture. Cold Spring Harb. Symp. Quant. Biol. 1975; 40: 389–397; and (*B*) A. J. Doupe, S. C. Landis, P. H. Patterson, Environmental influences in the development of neural crest derivatives: glucocorticoids, growth factors, and chromaffin cell plasticity. J. Neurosci. 1985; 5: 2119–2142.)

Culture Media and Substrates

L-15 Basal Medium (L-15-Air)

With certain modifications, Leibovitz's L-15 medium was found to be among the best media for the culture of rat sympathetic neurons (Mains and Patterson, 1973). As most laboratories are not prepared to make their own medium from scratch, it probably is easiest to start with liquid L-15 medium (GibcoBRL, Gaithersburg, MD, and others). Note that this medium's commercial formulation is for use with atmospheric CO_2 concentrations (not the 5–10% CO_2 normally used in tissue-culture incubators), thus we refer to the modified form as *L-15-air*. We use this medium primarily for holding cells after dissection or for maintaining neurons in the absence of dividing nonneuronal cells (in incubators with atmostpheric levels of CO_2; Mains and Patterson, 1973). This medium also is modified further to produce the growth medium described later. The primary changes made in the commercial L-15 medium involve adjusting the osmolarity and adding additional nutrients. To a single 500-ml bottle of standard L-15, two additions are made: 2.5 ml of stable vitamin mix (box 11.1) and 37.5 ml of tissue-culture-grade water containing 60 mg of imidazole. It is highly recommended to use either double-distilled water (water that has been glass-distilled after passage though ion-exchange resins) or water that has been passed freshly through a purification system, such as the MilliQ (Millipore Corp., Bedford, MA). Alternatively, tissue-culture-grade water can be purchased (Sigma Chemical Co., St. Louis, MO, being one source). The additives are stirred into the medium until dissolved, and the pH is adjusted to 7.35 to 7.40 by using 1 M HCl. The medium can be sterile-filtered (0.22 µm pore size) through any of a number of disposable bottle filter systems (e.g., Corning, Costar, etc.) but, in the case of media containing bicarbonate (see further), the application of a vacuum to the medium environment can result in marked shifts of pH. Thus, if possible, it is recommended that positive pressure systems driven by pressurized nitrogen be used. In this case, the medium is filter-sterilized via a large 0.2 µm filter (Gelman or Nalgene disposible units, or reusable Millipore unit) through which boiling water has been passed to remove the detergent. Glass bottles (detergent-free) are used to collect medium from the positive pressure appartus; these bottles must be rinsed exhaustively and autoclaved with pure water in them.

Box 11.1 Preparation of Stable Vitamin mix

Stable vitamin mix (SVM) is prepared as a 200-fold concentrate.
Weigh out:

L-Aspartic acid, free acid	0.6 g
L-Glutamic acid, free acid	0.6 g
L-proline, hydroxyproline-free	0.6 g
L-cystine	0.6 g
p-Aminobenzoic acid, free acid	0.2 g
β-Alanine	0.2 g
Vitamin B_{12}	0.08 g
Myo-inositol	0.4 g
Choline, chloride salt	0.4 g
Fumaric acid, free acid	1.0 g
Coenzyme A, free acid	0.016 g
d-Biotin	0.08 mg
DL-6,8-Thioctic acid, oxidized form	0.02 g

Dissolve into a final volume of 200 ml by using tissue-culture-grade water, aliquot, and store at −20°C. All the components of SVM are available from Sigma Chemical Co.

Complete Growth Medium

Growth of cells for long-term culture uses the L-15-air medium buffered for a 5% CO_2 atmosphere (L-15-CO_2). To make L-15-CO_2, 170 ml of sterile 150 mM $NaHCO_3$ is added to 850 ml of L-15-air. Immediately before use, the following additives are blended with 100 ml of L-15-CO_2: 2.0 ml glucose (30% wt/vol solution), 1.0 ml glutamine (200 mM solution), 1.0 ml penicillin-streptomycin (10,000 units/ml and 10 mg/ml, respectively, in a single solution), 1.0 ml fresh vitamin mix (box 11.2), and 5.0 ml adult rat serum (see later). This complete growth medium can be stored at 4°C for up to 2 weeks. For purposes of convenience, we premix the glucose, glutamine, and antibiotics and store at −20°C as single, 4-ml aliquots.

Rat serum is preferable for these cultures, as other sera, notably fetal bovine serum, can be significantly more mitogenic for non-neuronal cells (contaminating the cultures) and also can be toxic for the neurons (Mains and Patterson, 1973). If fetal bovine serum must be used, it is recommended that the serum lots be prescreened and selected for minimal mitogenic activity on contaminating cell types. We produce our own rat serum from the females that are

Box 11.2 Preparation of Fresh Vitamin Mix

> Fresh Vitamin mix (FVM) is prepared as a 100-fold concentrate.
> Weigh out:
>
> | | |
> |---|---|
> | 6,7-Dimethyl-5,6,7,8-tetrahydropterine | 1.0 mg |
> | Glutathione, reduced form | 5.0 mg |
> | Ascorbic acid | 200.0 mg |
>
> Dissolve by using tissue-culture-grade water, adjust pH to 5–6 by using
> 0.5 M KOH, and bring to a final volume of 20 ml. Filter-sterilize, aliquot, and
> store at −20°C. The dimethyltetrahydropterine is available from Calbiochem,
> Inc.

delivered with the pups used for dissection (Hawrot and Patterson, 1979).

Serum-Free Growth Medium

The robust survival of sympathetic neurons and chromaffin cells in culture is maintained readily in serum-containing medium, but experimental design may dictate that the cells be maintained in the absence of serum. Such long-term growth and survival of sympathoadrenal derivatives can be maintained in defined, serum-free conditions (Wolinsky et al., 1985). Glucose, glutamine, antibiotics, and fresh vitamin mix are added to L-15-CO_2 as described earlier, but rather than adding serum, additional components are added as described in box 11.3. For short-term, serum-free growth (1–2 days), only transferrin and insulin are necessary.

Substrates

The traditional substrate for sympathoadrenal derivatives is type I collagen. This substrate may be either bovine, and thus readily purchased from a variety of suppliers, or prepared fresh from rat tail tendons. An abbreviated protocol for the extraction of the latter follows. Tail is removed from freshly killed adult rat and is cleaned by brief washing in 70% ethanol (ETOH). After removal of skin, the tendons are stripped with sterile needle-nose pliers and placed in a sterile Petri dish, where they are rinsed briefly with sterile water. Tendons are transferred to a sterile flask containing an autoclaved,

Box 11.3 Additives for Serum-Free Medium

	Final Concentration	Stock Solution Concentration
Transferrin, "holo" form	100 μg/ml	10 mg/ml (in PBS)
Insulin, Zn salt	5 μg/ml	2.5 mg/ml (in 5 mM HCl, keep at 4°C)
Putrescine, free base	16 μg/ml	1.6 mg/ml (in PBS, store at 4°C)
Progesterone	20 nM	20 μM (in ethanol, store at 4°C)
Selenious acid	30 nM	30 μM (in water, neutralized with NaOH

magnetic stir-bar and approximately 250 ml of 0.1% acetic acid for each 0.5 g of tendon. The flask is stirred overnight at 4°C, then centrifuged at 10,000 rpm for 30 min. The top half of the solution is pipetted off carefully, and this final product may be stored at 4°C for several weeks or aliquoted and stored at −80°C for several months. The collagen solution is diluted 1:3 with water before use and is air-dried on culture-dish surfaces. A more detailed discussion of collagen preparation may be found in this volume in Chapter 19.

Composite substrates that incorporate rat tail collagen also have been used. In one variation, rat tail collagen is diluted it 1:1 with water, then mixed 1:1 with 1 mg/ml poly-D-lysine. Thus, the final concentrations are 0.5 mg/ml polylysine and 1:4 dilution of collagen. One drop of this solution per 35-mm dish is spread with a bent Pasteur pipette and allowed to dry overnight at 37°C. The following day, each plate is incubated with 1 ml of 20 μg/ml laminin in L-15-air for 1 to 2 h at room temperature. The laminin solution then is removed and replaced with L-15-CO_2 medium; the plates are maintained in a tissue-culture incubator for a few hours to condition them prior to use. The actual amounts of the solutions used can be scaled in proportion to the surface area to be coated.

Alternative substrates include pure laminin, plasma fibronectin, and Matrigel (an Engelbreth-Holm-Swarm sarcoma basement-membrane extract; Becton Dickinson Labware Collaborative Biomedical Products, Bedford, MA). It should be noted, however, that most of what is known about the cell biology and biochemistry of these cells in culture has been determined on a simple collagen substrate; this is to say that alternative substrates well may support

or induce altered cellular phenotypes. Note too that polylysine alone can be toxic for these cells if used in serum-free conditions.

Numerous culture vessels can be coated with the foregoing substrates. In addition to traditional tissue-culture dishes, a configuration that is optimal for microscopy involves using a lathe-like device to bore a hole of variable diameter (4–10 mm) through the center of a 35-mm tissue-culture dish. A coverslip (plastic or glass) then is applied to the underside of the dish by using melted paraffin, petroleum jelly, or a mixture of the two: The coverslip thus seals the hole. This procedure creates a "mini-well" with optical properties superior to conventional tissue-culture plastic. Furthermore, choosing an appropriate-bore diameter allows a minimal number of cells and a minimal amount of experimental reagents to be used for individual cultures. Additional cell plating configurations are discussed later.

Culturing Neurons from the Superior Cervical Ganglion

Dissection

The superior cervical ganglion (SCG) is the largest ganglion of the sympathetic chain and is the most easily dissected. Neonatal rats are killed either by a blow to the head or by lethal injection with pentobarbital sodium (0.2–0.3 ml per pup at 6 grains/ml). Decapitation of the sacrificed pup provides most direct access to the SCG. With the head fixed ventral side up, the trachea, the ventral tissue surrounding the trachea, and the entire lower mandible are removed. This procedure reveals the upper palate and, immediately caudal to it, two bilaterally symmetrical, longitudinal muscles. Lateral to the muscles on each side, one readily can identify the carotid arteries (figure 11.2). The SCG lies somewhat underneath and medial to the carotid artery and appears as an off-white, slightly translucent, oblong structure with connectives (nerves) coursing rostrally and caudally from it. A potential difficulty with this dissection is confusion between the SCG and the nodose sensory ganglion. The latter is thinner and longer than is the SCG and projects more dorsally and deeper into the head as the dissector views it. It should be noted that the proximity of these two ganglia also provides an opportunity for culture of different types of peripheral neurons from a single dissection. Moreover, nodose neurons can be

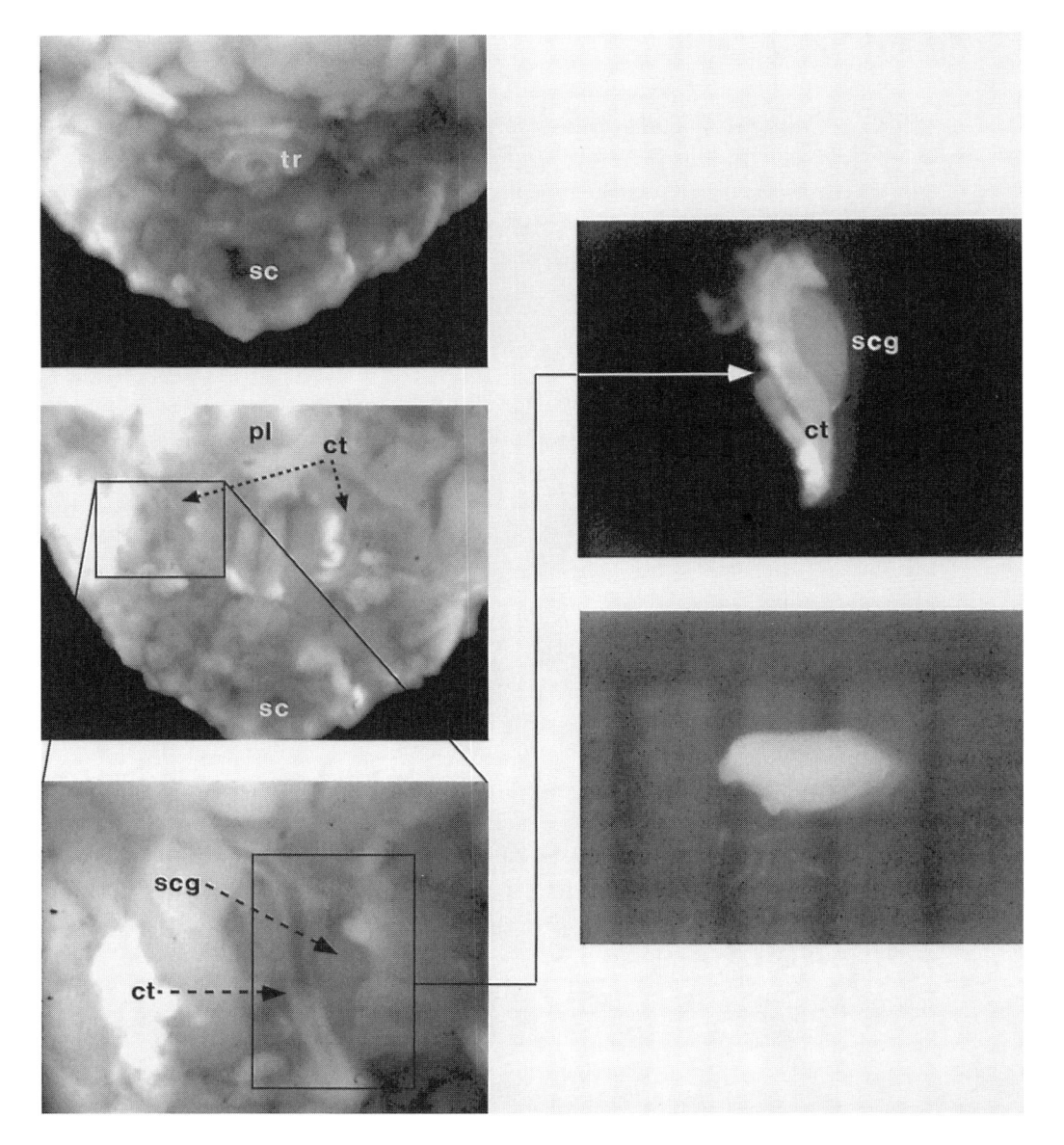

Figure 11.2 Video images from the dissection of a superior cervical ganglion. (*A*) View of the neck region of a decapitated rat pup. After removal of the trachea along with the entire lower mandible (*B*), the carotid arteries are exposed. Immediately medial and somewhat deeper than the carotids lie the superior cervical ganglia (*C*). Dissected away with surrounding tissue, the relationship of the ganglion to the artery is more evident (*D*). When the surrounding tissue has been removed and the ganglion has been cleaned of connective nerves, the ganglion appears as an oblong structure 1–2 mm long, indicated by the millimeter markings below the plane of focus (*E*). ct, carotid artery; pl, palate; scg, superior cervical ganglion; tr, trachea; sc, spinal column.

grown under the same conditions as those required for the sympathetic neurons.

With practice, it is possible to remove the ganglion alone, but the novice may first wish to dissect the SCG with surrounding tissue attached, then cut away the nonganglionic tissue in a dish containing L-15-air and under higher magnification. During the dissection, ganglia are held in a sterile Petri dish containing L-15-air on ice. When all ganglia have been collected, they are cleaned of nonganglionic tissue. Care should be taken to remove as much of the connecting nerves as possible; failure to do so will result in a large increase in contaminating nonneuronal cells (Schwann cells and fibroblasts). Clean ganglia are placed in a second dish containing L-15-air.

Dissociation and Plating

MECHANICAL METHOD
Ganglia may be dissociated either mechanically or enzymatically. The former approach produces extremely pure preparations of neurons, but the yields are rather poor (1%–10% of the 25,000 neurons present in the ganglion). Enzymatic dissociation provides yields of >80%, but additional steps are necessary to reduce contamination by nonneuronal cells.

The first step in mechanical dissociation is the peeling away of the ganglion sheath with a very fine forceps (e.g., Dumont no. 5). The extent to which this is successful is a function of the investigator's experience and patience. Once the sheaths have been removed, they are taken out of the dish, and the remaining tissue is teased apart on the bottom of the dish. Pieces of ganglia are shredded with a fine forceps, following which the entire solution is triturated gently by passing it several times through a hypodermic needle (23-gauge) or a Pasteur pipette, the bore of which has been flame-polished and narrowed to a small opening. Care should be taken to avoid introducing air bubbles during this process. The solution then is transferred to a 15-ml centrifuge tube, and the undissociated material is allowed to settle for approximately 5 min. The supernatant then is transferred to a new centrifuge tube and is spun at 800 to 1000 $\times$ g for 10 min. The pellet is resuspended in the desired volume of complete or serum-free growth medium and is plated. Cultures are maintained at 37°C in a 5% CO_2 incubator and,

for standard cultures, the medium is replaced every 3 to 4 days. Nerve growth factor (NGF) is added to the medium to a final concentration of 10 ng/ml to maintain normal sympathetic neuron survival. Recombinant NGF (available from a number of suppliers) is best stored at −80°C in aliquots containing 1 mg/ml bovine serum albumin; consult the supplier's specification sheet for further details. Should any residual nonneuronal cells appear in these cultures, they can be eliminated by use of the antimitotic drugs described after.

ENZYMATIC METHOD

The most commonly used dissociation method is the enzymatic. Before transfer of cleaned ganglia to a 15-ml centrifuge tube, they are each cut into two to three pieces with small iridectomy scissors to improve enzyme access to the tissue. These fragments then are transferred to a tube and are allowed to settle to the bottom; the L-15-air is replaced with dissociation solution prepared freshly as the fragments are settling. All methods in this section reflect volumes of materials and reagents appropriate for the dissociation of up to approximately 40 SCGs (the result of dissecting 20 pups). The dissociation solution is prepared as follows. In a 15-ml centrifuge tube, 1 ml of 10× concentrate calcium-magnesium-free Hank's balanced salt solution (CMF-HBSS; available from most suppliers of tissue-culture medium) is mixed with 8 ml of tissue-culture-grade water. Then 10 mg of collagenase (collagenase A, from Boehringer Mannheim) is added and mixed gently until dissolved. Next, 0.1 M NaOH is added dropwise until the color of the phenol red indicator dye in the CMF-HBSS turns a color approximating that of L-15-air. The final volume of the solution is brought to 10 ml with tissue-culture-grade water, yielding a final collagenase concentration of 1 mg/ml. The solution is sterilized by passing it through a 0.22-μm syringe filter and is added to the SCG fragments. The capped tube is incubated at 37°C in a water bath, and the contents periodically and gently are mixed over the course of approximately 40 min. Dissociation is facilitated by a brief, gentle trituration, five times with a 5-ml tissue-culture pipette, after 20 min. After 40 min, the tube is spun at 800 to 1000 × g for 10 min. The supernatant is removed gently and carefully, and the pellet is resuspended in 1 ml of complete or serum-free growth medium via a flame-polished Pasteur pipette, the bore of which has been some-

what reduced. The solutions then are made up to 10 ml with the same medium, mixed gently, and centrifuged again to remove remaining enzyme. After removal of the supernatant, cells are resuspended in a final volume of 10 ml.

The cell suspension at this point contains neurons, Schwann cells, macrophages, fibroblasts, and traces of other cell types. Preplating in an important step in purifying the neurons and makes use of the fact that they do not adhere to tissue-culture plastic. The cell suspension is plated into two 60-mm Petri plates for 1 h at 37°C in a 5% CO_2. After this incubation, the plates are swirled gently, and the medium is transferred to two more 60-mm tissue-culture plates and returned to the incubator for 30 additional min. The first preplating removes primarily macrophages and some fibroblasts, and the second preplating removes primarily fibroblasts and Schwann cells. A single 1.5 to 2-h preplate on tissue-culture plastic also will work, but serial preplating is more effective. Larger volumes of medium and more plates are needed if larger numbers of ganglia are being processed, because higher cell densities result in neuron loss through secondary adhesion to Schwann cells and the like. At the end of 30 min, the plates are swirled, and the medium is transferred to a 15-ml tube and is centrifuged as before.

Cells are resuspended with NGF-containing medium in a volume appropriate for plating into the desired number of dishes. The few remaining nonneuronal cells will be a concern only if the experimental design requires that the neurons be maintained for 2 to 3 days. For longer-term, neuron-alone cultures, nonneuronal cells are eliminated by a cycle of treatments with antimitotic agents. Historically, cytosine arabinoside and fluorodeoxyuridine have been the agents of choice, but recent work has shown aphidicoline (4 µg/ml) is less toxic for the neurons (Wallace and Johnson, 1989). With the use of serum-free medium, nonneuronal cells divide little and may not require antimitotic treatment. If serum is used, the standard course of action is to allow the cells to adhere for 24 h and then to cycle them in and out of 10 µM cytosine arabinoside or 10 µM fluorodeoxyuridine at 24-h intervals for 3 days: day of plating, out; day 1, in; day 2, out; day 3, in; and day 4 onward, out. Under optimal conditions, neuron-alone cultures can be maintained many weeks. Cocultures with nonneuronal cells also can be maintained for long periods, but there can be problems with the carpet of cells peeling from the dish surface. Nonneuronal cell proliferation also can

be stabilized by irradiation with a source of Co^{60} (Hawrot and Patterson, 1979). This treatment does not appear to harm the neurons.

Special Culture Formats

Though a variety of culture paradigms have been used with sympathetic neurons, two are of particular note. The first uses multiple compartments to separate physically parts of a single culture from each other. The Campenot chamber (Campenot, 1977) separates neuronal cell bodies from their distal neurites through the use of a Teflon insert machined to a particular form (figure 11.3A). The insert is attached to a collagen-coated, grooved substrate with vacuum grease. In its usual use, neurons are plated in the central compartment, and neurites are guided by the grooves under the grease into the side compartments. When assembled correctly, little exchange of fluids or solutes takes place between compartments. Thus, such cultures lend themselves to experiments in which various agents are presented preferentially to neuronal cell bodies or distal neurites and growth cones. For example, retrograde transport of the cytokine leukemia-inhibitory factor from neurites to cell bodies was demonstrated (Ure et al., 1992; Ure and Campenot, 1994). Compartment cultures also allow sampling of media for molecules secreted or shed preferentially by the cell bodies or neurites. In an alternative compartment system, Pittman (1985) made use of concentric glass rings adhered to a substrate with vacuum grease to create separate compartments containing cell bodies, axon, and growth cones (see figure 3B). In this manner, it was shown that proteases are secreted preferentially by advancing growth cones rather than by the axons. A comprehensive review of the compartment technique has been written by Campenot (Campenot, 1992), and specialized equipment for the production and assembly of these cultures now can be purchased (Tyler Instruments, Inc., Edmonton, Canada).

The second culture format of special interest is noted for its use of very small numbers of neurons, either for conservation of materials and animals or for the study of individual neurons. For single-cell electrophysiology and microscopy, sympathetic neurons can be grown on islands of cardiac myocytes (figure 11.4) (Furshpan et al., 1976). This type of preparation is tedious but can provide data not otherwise available. For instance, such cultures were used to

A

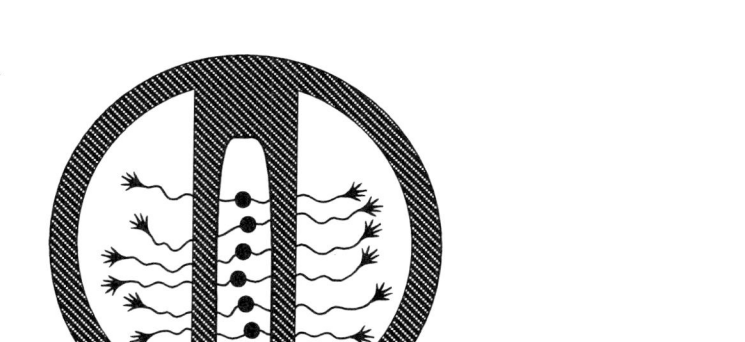

B

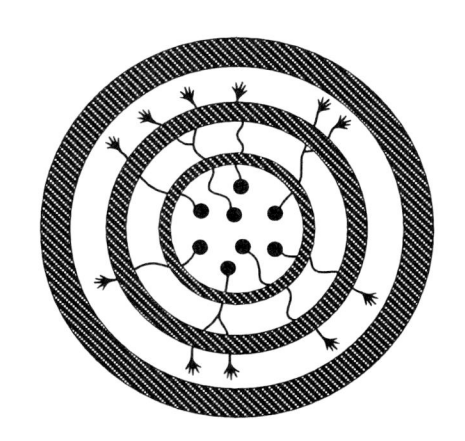

Figure 11.3 Barrier configurations for establishing compartmented cultures. The design of Campenot (Campenot, 1977) allows separation of cell bodies and distal neurites (*A*). This barrier device can be used also to create distinct compartments containing cell bodies, axons, and growth cones. Alternatively, the barrier configuration designed by Pittman (1985) (*B*) can be used also to establish a three-chambered culture environment. Axons grow under the barriers (hatched areas). See text for details. (Reproduced with permission from (*A*) Campenot, 1977, and (*B*) Pittman, 1985.)

prove that individual sympathetic neurons can change their synaptic phenotype over time in vitro (Furshpan et al., 1976). For some experiments, it is useful to identify individual cells in a mass culture so as to be able to return to them repeatedly. One successful approach is to plate cells on substrates on which a small, labeled grid has been imprinted so that they can be identified in the microscope (e.g., see Stemple et al., 1988). For biochemical purposes in which good optics are not a factor, 96-well plates (Falcon, Oxnard, CA) can be used. Cultures of a single to a few thousand neurons can be grown in these small wells and can be assayed for

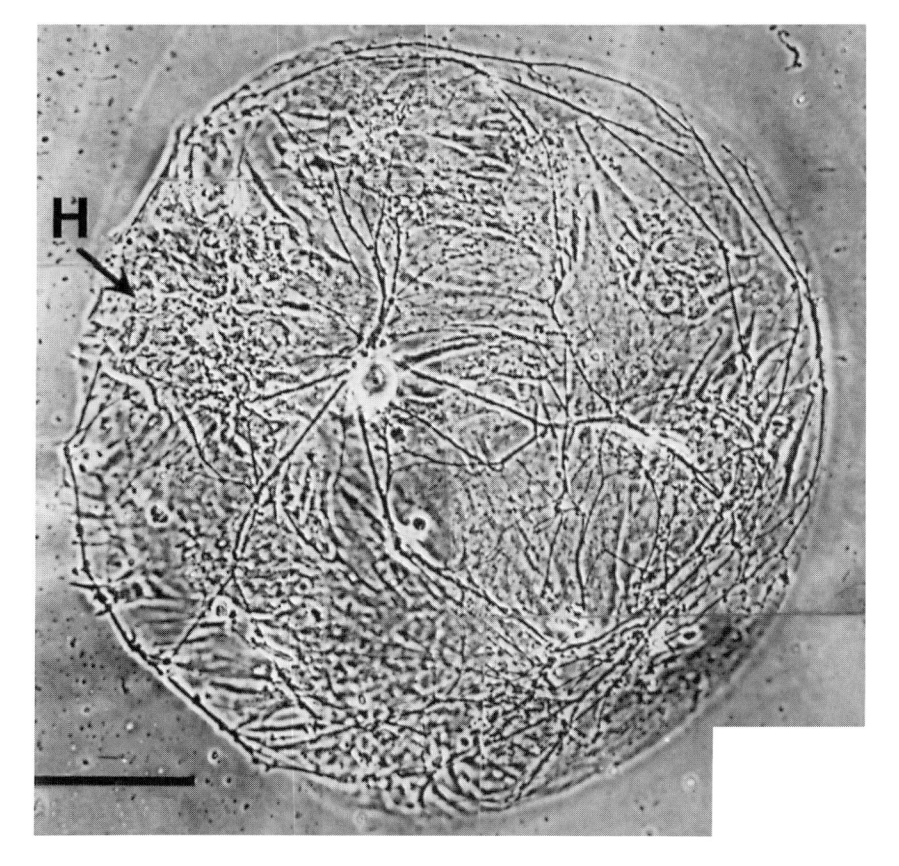

Figure 11.4 A microculture containing a solitary sympathetic neuron growing on a cluster of cardiac myocytes (H). This partiuclar culture was photographed after 19 days in culture. Scale bar: 100 μm. (Reproduced with permission from Furshpan et al., 1976.)

neurotransmitter synthesis (Reichardt and Patterson, 1977) or mRNA expression by reverse transcriptase–polymerase chain reaction (Fann and Patterson, 1993).

Culturing Chromaffin Cells from the Adrenal Medulla

Dissection

Though cells of the adrenal medulla may be grown successfully and cultured from rats of any age, we recommend using 1- to 7-day-old rats, as this practice decreases contamination of the cultures by nonchromaffin cells. The animals are killed and placed ventral side down on the dissection surface. The entire adrenal gland is dissected easily by making cuts with small scissors parallel and im-

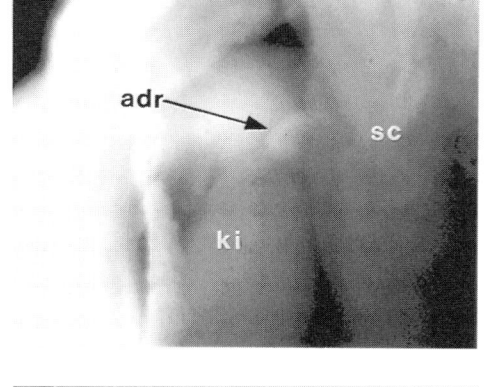

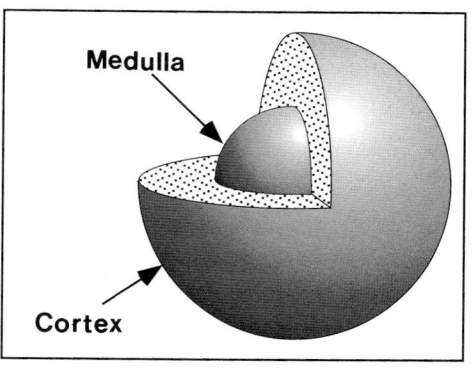

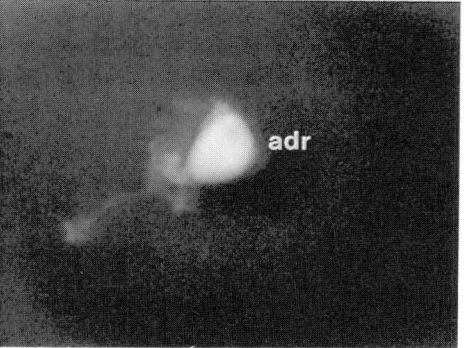

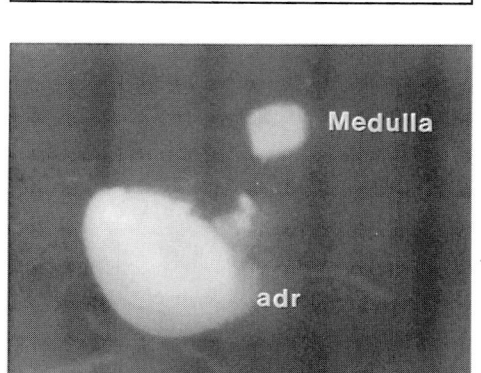

Figure 11.5 Video images from the dissection of the adrenal medulla. After an incision is made along the sides of the spinal column and the body wall is retracted, the adrenal gland can be observed sitting on the rostral end of the kidney (*A*). When cut free, the adrenal appears as a small, spherelike structure (*B*), the interior of which contains the medullary tissue as schematized in *C*. Though the entire neonatal adrenal may be 1.5–2 mm in diameter, the medulla freed of cortical tissue is ≤ 0.5 mm in diameter, indicated by the millimeter markings below the plane of focus (*D*). adr, adrenal; ki, kidney; sc, spinal column.

mediately adjacent to the spinal column, at the level of the kidney. With practice, the kidneys can be exposed readily to the dissection microscope; the adrenal gland is situated on the rostral end of the kidney (figure 11.5). The glands are small globular structures pinkish-white in color. Fatty tissue also may be present but is amorphous and yellow. A grasp with fine forceps of the connective tissue that surrounds the adrenal gland allows the gland to be removed intact by gentle pulling. During the dissection, glands are maintained on ice in L-15-air, as described earlier. Unlike SCG neurons, which show robust viability in vitro even after several hours of being stored on ice, chromaffin cells are more delicate, and the dissection should proceed as rapidly as possible.

Dissecting the medulla away from the surrounding cortex requires practice and patience. The medulla has a diameter one-third to one-half of the diameter of the entire gland. The dimensions can be appreciated best by cutting a gland in half: The inner medulla is much pinker than the outer cortex. With this knowledge as a guide, under a dissecting microscope, the cortex can be cut away from the intact gland by grasping some of the connective tissue with fine forceps and using sharp and fine scissors. It is best to err to the side of cutting away some medullary tissue to remove cortical cells rigorously. The collected medullae are placed in a second dish containing L-15-air for later transfer to a 15-ml centrifuge tube by pipette.

Dissociation and Plating

The dissociation of adrenal medullae is essentially the same as the enzymatic method used for the dissociation of sympathetic ganglia. The only modifications are as follows: (1) It is not necessary to cut the medullae into smaller pieces prior to enzymatic dissociation; (2) the total time in collagenase solution is 30 min, and a trituration step during the enzymatic incubation is not necessary; and (3) preplating proceeds for 1 h only, on tissue-culture plastic. To maintain the normal chromaffin cell phenotype and promote survival, these cells require glucocorticoids. Therefore, the medium for final plating is supplemented with dexamethasone to a final concentration of 10 µM. Dexamethsone is dissolved in ethanol and stored at $-20°C$ as a stock solution at a concentration of 10 mM.

Transdifferentiation of Adrenal Chromaffin Cells

A culture variation of interest to developmental neurobiologists is the conversion of chromaffin cells into sympathetic neurons. Both cell types are derived from the sympathoadrenal progenitor (Anderson, 1993), and application of the appropriate growth factors can drive this phenotypic decision (Doupe et al., 1985b). The decision to become a chromaffin cell is reversible, however, and removal of glucocorticoid and addition of NGF can transdifferentiate these cells into neurons (Unsicker et al., 1978; Doupe et al., 1985a; Lillien and Claude, 1985) (figure 11.6). Interestingly, it was found

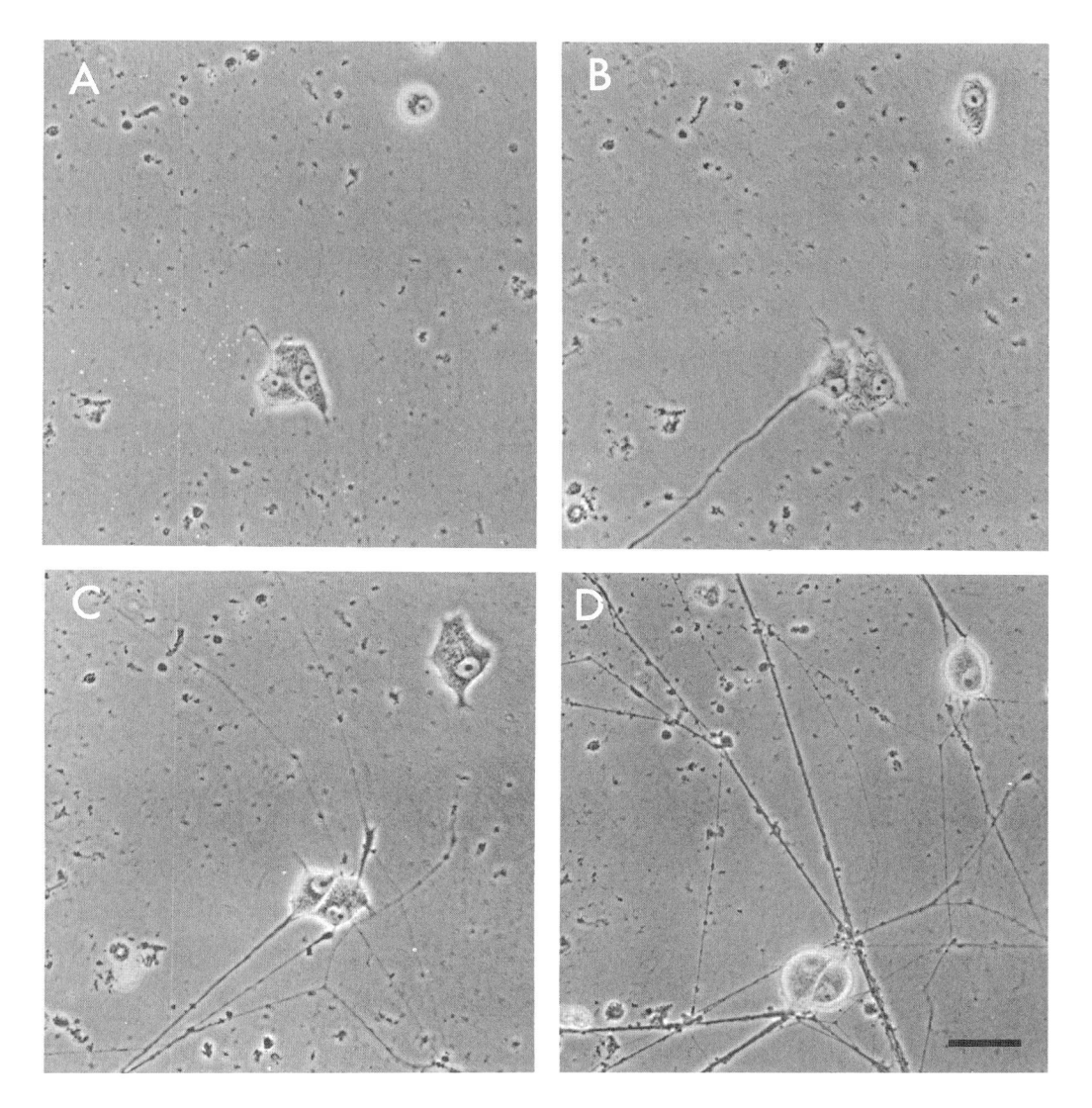

Figure 11.6 Adrenal chromaffin cells transdifferentiating in response to nerve growth factor (NGF). (*A*) Chromaffin cells on the day of dexamethasone withdrawal and addition of NGF. (*B*) The same cells after 1 day in NGF. (*C*) After 3 days. (*D*) After 13 days. Scale bar: 50 μm. (Reproduced with permission from A. J. Doupe, P. H. Patterson, S. C. Landis, Small intensely fluorescent (SIF) cells in culture: role of glucocorticoids and growth factors in their development and phenotypic interconversions with other neural crest derivatives. J. Neurosci. 1985; 5: 2143–2160.)

also that fibroblast growth factors (FGFs) also can drive neuronal differentiation of chromaffin cells (Claude et al., 1988; Stemple et al., 1988), but that this FGF-induced differentiation includes the onset of NGF dependency (Stemple et al., 1988). In the presence of glucocorticoids, however, basic FGF acts as a chromaffin cell mitogen rather than as a differentiation agent; thus, chromaffin cell numbers can be amplified in vitro by this coadministration of factors. The manipulation of adrenal chromaffin cells in this manner is of particular interest for the generation of graftable material for use in animal models of neurodegenerative disease (Mahanthappa et al., 1990; Chalmers et al., 1995; Niijima et al., 1995). It is worth noting also that a third cell type, the small intensely fluorescent cell, is related closely to both sympathetic neurons and chromaffin cells and also can be converted into either derivative in culture through manipulation of the same environmental cues (Doupe et al., 1985b).

Comments

The relative ease with which these neurons can be grown in vitro, in addition to their phenotypic homogeneity, is a great benefit to those who wish to make use of primary cultures rather than of neural cell lines. Thus, sympathetic neurons have served as paradigm neurons for a variety of molecular, biochemical, and cell biological studies of neuronal behavior. The culture systems described here have been used successfully also for nodose, dorsal root, and trigeminal ganglion neurons (Pittman, 1985). The ready availability of numerous trophic factors today, however, no longer constrains one to study NGF-dependent neurons. The culture systems described here can be adapted readily to fit the needs of a variety of mammalian neurons by modifying the trophic factors and the culture substrates. Similarly, the use of primary adrenal chromaffin cells can continue to serve as a diagnostic tool for assessing the roles of various factors in neural development and as tissue for the study of graft-mediated repair.

Acknowledgments

The authors thank Doreen McDowell for her unflagging technical support during more than 20 years of making the components used

by numerous students and researchers to culture sympathoadrenal derivatives. Thanks to David Anderson for providing the composite substrate recipe. Thanks to Mario Pita and Lee Margolin for providing valuable graphics assistance. Finally, thanks to all the people who have passed through the laboratories of Edwin Furshpan, David Potter, Story Landis, and Paul Patterson over the years, making contributions to the methods described here.

12 Mass Cultures and Microislands of Neurons from Postnatal Rat Brain

Michael M. Segal, Robert W. Baughman, Kenneth A. Jones, and James E. Huettner

We use dissociated cultures of postnatal neurons to study receptor pharmacology, synaptic transmission, and neuronal properties in simple circuits. Our effort is concentrated mainly on the visual cortex and hippocampus of the rat, although the protocols described in this chapter are widely applicable to postnatal neurons from many different brain areas.

The use of cell cultures for investigating synaptic function provides several advantages. One of them is the ability to record simultaneously from both the presynaptic and postsynaptic cells of a synaptic pair. Another advantage is the easy access to the cell membrane in culture, with the resulting ability to vary the composition of the perfusion medium precisely and rapidly, allowing localization and pharmacological characterization of synaptic receptors on the cell surface. Such approaches are difficult or impossible in vivo, and even tissue slices are not satisfactory in many cases.

On the other hand, with in vitro cell cultures, several concerns arise. For example, it is necessary to test whether all the relevant cell types from the tissue of origin have survived and differentiated appropriately in vitro. For a heterogeneous tissue, such as cerebral cortex, it also is important that methods be available allowing for reliable identification of specific cell types. In this regard, cultures prepared from postnatal animals appear to offer several clear advantages over those prepared from younger, embryonic animals. By the time of birth, cortical and hippocampal neurons already are differentiated substantially, and they appear to continue to express properties as they would in vivo. Furthermore, in postnatal animals, it is straightforward to label projection neurons with vital markers by retrograde axonal transport. This approach makes it possible to study systematically one class of cell in a diverse culture by permitting the unambiguous identification of labeled neurons over a period of many weeks.

In "mass cultures," which contain many neurons, the frequency of synaptic coupling between cortical or hippocampal neurons is

not high, perhaps 20% to 40%. A much higher frequency of connections can be achieved in microisland cultures, which contain one or several neurons growing in a small area, isolated from other neurons. Such a simplified system offers important advantages in studying synaptic connections and the physiology of small networks of neurons.

Microisland cultures were developed first to study the synaptic functions of sympathetic neurons (Furshpan et al., 1976, 1986). This simplified system displayed several important advantages:

- Synaptic interactions in the microisland cultures invariably are intense, presumably because the growing, branching axons are confined to a limited area and make many synapses on each target cell.
- Monosynaptic (including autaptic) interactions can be identified unambiguously because one can record from all neurons in the network.
- In solitary neuron microisland cultures, all the synaptic terminals stem from the same neuron, providing a uniform population of terminals to study.

The microisland culture techniques used with sympathetic neurons were difficult to apply to culturing central neurons because of the properties of central glial cells, which accompany the neurons in dissociated cell suspensions. The central nervous system glia migrate onto virtually any substrate and spread out to form bridges between microislands, resulting in one large mass culture.

One approach to this glial bridging problem is to use very-low-density cultures to separate solitary neurons from other cells (see chapter 13). However, microisland cultures have several advantages over sparse cultures as a way of simplifying the numbers of neurons in a circuit. Sparse cultures contain few neurons and have difficulty with neuronal survival owing to a paucity of trophic or contact effects of nearby neurons and glial cells. Though the trophic effects can be overcome by strategies to condition the medium (e.g., see chapter 13), an additional protection may accrue from physical wrapping of neuronal processes by glial cells (Harris and Rosenberg, 1993) as is achieved in microisland cultures (A. Yee and M. Segal, unpublished), resulting in protection from glutamate toxicity (Rosenberg et al., 1992). In addition, in sparse cultures that contain glial cells, it is difficult to know if a neuron truly is isolated from others, because neuronal processes are not visible under phase-contrast microscopy when they are wrapped by glial cells.

Therefore, constructing microisland cultures offers important advantages for many experiments.

The first success in restricting growth of central neurons and glial cells to small areas came by using Sylgard (Dow Corning, Midland, MI) as a nonadhesive substrate to define the borders of "mini-island cultures" containing 50 to 100 neurons (Huettner and Baughman, 1988). However, Sylgard is a viscous liquid that is difficult to apply in a fine pattern, making it impractical to use this technique to create microislands with fewer than 10 neurons. In addition, though glial cells have a lower adhesivity for Sylgard than they do for biological substrates, glial cells can grow on Sylgard reasonably well (Segal and Furshpan, 1990).

These technical problems were overcome by using agarose as a substrate. Agarose is virtually nonadhesive for glial cells (Costăchel et al., 1969; Grinnell et al., 1972; Westermark et al., 1978; Pontén and Stolt, 1980). Why cells avoid agarose is not clear. It might be owing to the negative charge of agarose (Costăchel et al., 1969), to specific chemical groups on the agarose, or to the high water content of the rehydrated agarose. Using a layer of agarose led to success in creating cultures in which cortical neurons and glial cells are restricted to microislands (Segal and Furshpan, 1990). Techniques derived from this approach are described in this chapter.

Microisland cultures have proved useful for studies of synaptic action. The corelease of two classic transmitters by a neuron was first demonstrated using peripheral nervous system microisland cultures (Furshpan et al., 1976, 1986). The central nervous system (CNS) microisland culture technique led to the first monosynaptic recording of GABA$_B$ synaptic action from one neuron onto another (Segal and Furshpan, 1990) and has enabled the demonstration that excitatory neurons and not inhibitory neurons are the cells that receive GABA$_B$ connections in hippocampal cultures (Segal, 1991). Microislands with a solitary neuron have been useful for recording miniature synaptic events. All events arise from the same presynaptic neuron and impinge on the same postsynaptic neuron (Bekkers and Stevens, 1991; Segal, 1991).

Microislands have been useful also for studying the electrophysiology of small circuits. It has even been possible to model one of the classic network phenomena in biology—seizures—in microislands that have only one or two neurons yet display the classic epileptiform activity found in brain slices and intact cortex (Segal, 1991, 1994).

General Culture Protocols

Our presentation here focuses on what we consider to be core techniques for preparing cultures of postnatal neurons. We also discuss alternative approaches that may be useful in specific circumstances, and we highlight particular situations in which each of us uses a slightly different methodology. Preparation of mass cultures is described first, then the modifications needed to create microisland cultures are outlined.

In general, the preparation of successful cultures requires three main elements: (1) an appropriate substrate for cell adhesion and growth, (2) an appropriate growth medium, and (3) a procedure for gentle dissociation and plating of viable neurons. In many cases, the goals of the experiments in which cultured cells are to be used will dictate one or more of these elements. However, when first setting up a new culture system, we begin by searching for conditions that optimize cell survival.

Culture Substrate

In our experience, both neurons and glial cells survive poorly, if at all, without an acceptable substrate for cell attachment—even when culture medium and dissociation conditions are optimal. In selecting a substrate, it is important to consider both the physical support, which is usually either glass or plastic, and the surface coating to improve cell adhesion.

For studies that do not require visualization of cells and neurites at high magnification, it may be acceptable to grow cells directly on the plastic bottom of 35-mm tissue culture dishes. We routinely obtain excellent survival on Corning dishes (no. 25000) to which we have added one of the surface coatings described later. We have not compared these dishes systematically to other brands.

For most of our electrical recording experiments, it is desirable for cells to be grown on a physical support of glass coverslips. Glass provides superior optical properties for visualization of cells by a variety of microscopic techniques. For example, the short working distance of many objective lenses used in fluorescence microscopy can preclude the use of thick plastic coverslips or the use of cells grown directly on the bottom of ordinary culture dishes. In addition, plastic coverslips or dishes can degrade seriously the quality of differential interference contrast images and can result in scatter

Box 12.1 Cleaning Glass Coverslips

1. Place coverslips in ceramic staining racks (Thomas Scientific) and immerse in concentrated HNO_3 for 24–48 h.
2. Rinse thoroughly with double-distilled water (DDW), then immerse in DDW and bring to a boil.
3. Place racks in an empty Pyrex beaker, cover with foil, and autoclave.
4. Warm the beaker on a hot plate for several hours to dry the coverslips.
5. In a sterile hood, transfer the coverslips to sterile 35-mm dishes.

and autofluorescence using epifluorescence microscopy. Plastic that degrades the differential interference contrast image can be recognized by its optical behavior when placed between two "crossed" polarizing filters (i.e., filters oriented at the angle at which the minimal amount of light passes). When rotated between crossed polarizing filters, a plastic that is incompatible with interference contrast microscopy will produce colored patterns and change substantially the amount of transmitted light when rotated to different angles.

Over the years, we have used a number of different sources for glass coverslips and a number of different surface coatings. Banker and colleagues (chapter 13) have highlighted the enormous variability in the properties of commercially available coverslips, in particular the empirical ability to support viable low-density cultures. It is our general impression that mass cultures, which include a mixture of glial cells and neurons, are more forgiving with respect to glass quality than are very-low-density cultures of isolated neurons. If cultures are surviving poorly on glass, however, often it is useful to test cells on tissue-culture plastic to determine whether the glass is to blame. We use either Fisher (no 12-548) or Gold Seal (no. 2406) glass coverslips, typically no. 1 thickness. Coverslips may be used as received, or they may be cleaned in concentrated nitric acid (box 12.1). For microisland cultures, in which the coverslips are coated with a layer of agarose, the properties of the coverslip appear to be less important.

For cultures that will be used for physiological recordings, generally we attach the coverslip to the outside of a 35-mm dish that has had a hole (1 cm in diameter) cut in its bottom. In this configuration, the plastic bottom of the culture dish forms a shallow well that helps protect the cultured cells during routine feedings. We

use a small lathe (Jensen Tools no. 334B840) to cut the hole and Sylgard (Sylgard 184, Dow-Corning) to attach the coverslips. Sylgard must be cured before culture medium is added to the dish. Usually, we cure dishes for 72 h at room temperature or for 48 hours at 40° to 50°C; above 50°C the plastic dishes will begin to melt. Sterilization is carried out by exposing the open dishes to ultraviolet (UV) light (GE 630T8; 30 min, 15 cm) prior to coating the glass surface for cell attachment. Fixing the coverslip to the dish improves the stability of long-term physiological recordings. With practice, a razor blade can be used to remove coverslips that have been attached with Sylgard. However, in situations where a free coverslip is the desired end point, we simply place the sterile coverslips into unmodified 35-mm dishes, apply a sterile surface coating, then plate dissociated cells. This approach is particularly useful when the culture will be processed for immunocytochemistry, because the coverslip is removed easily for mounting to a microscope slide. In addition, loose coverslips can be placed in chambers designed for physiological recording.

A number of companies offer specialized 35-mm culture dishes that incorporate a glass or modified plastic substrate. Although these dishes tend to be relatively expensive, their use may be justified for specific experiments. For example, Milian Instruments (Geneva, Switzerland, and Columbus, OH) manufactures a 35-mm plastic dish that features a 1.2-cm-diameter central well containing a labeled grid (no. PEG-351). We find the grid to be especially useful for quantitative measurement of neuronal survival and for identifying the locations of specific neurons (Lukas and Jones, 1994). In addition, the thickness (~ 0.2 mm) of the plastic in the central well permits the use of short working-distance objectives.

Surface Coating

Although freshly dissociated cells eventually will attach and spread on bare glass or tissue-culture plastic, they tend to stick to one another, resulting in large aggregates of cells unless the substrate is conducive to attachment. Therefore, the survival and uniformity of the cultures necessitate that the glass or plastic receive some type of coating that promotes cell adhesion. For mass cultures, we typically employ one of the following coatings on either glass or plastic:

- Poly-DL-ornithine (Sigma no. P0546) is dissolved at 10 mg/ml, filtered[1] at 0.22 µm, and stored in 1-ml aliquots at −20°C. For coating glass or plastic surfaces, the polyornithine is thawed, diluted 1:50 in sterile water, and applied immediately to the culture surface. The dishes are maintained overnight in a humid atmosphere (the incubator), then rinsed once with sterile water and once with balanced saline. In general, the coating does not work as well if applied for shorter times or if the polyornithine is diluted in balanced salt solutions.

- Poly-D-lysine and laminin (both from Collaborative Biomedical Products, no. 40210 and 40232) are dissolved in water at 0.1 mg/ml and 33 µg/ml, respectively. The solution is filtered, and 5-ml aliquots are stored at −70°C. The thawed solution is applied to the culture surface, and the dishes are placed in the incubator overnight. Before cell plating, the dishes are rinsed three times with 3 ml of sterile water, filled with growth medium, and equilibrated for 1 to 2 h at 37°C, 5% CO_2.

- Matrigel (Collaborative Biomedical Products no. 40234), a commercial extracellular matrix preparation, arrives frozen. It is thawed on ice, divided into 200-µl aliquots, and stored at −20°C. A frozen aliquot is thawed on ice, diluted with 5 ml of ice-cold saline, and dispensed immediately onto the culture surfaces. The dishes are incubated for 30 min at 37°C, free liquid is aspirated from the surface, and dissociated cells then are plated.

- Rat tail collagen (Collaborative Biomedical Products no. 40236) diluted to 0.5 mg/ml in DDW, approximately 30 µl, is added to the well to provide a uniform coating after evaporation at room temperature in a sterile hood. Before plating, the dishes are resterilized with UV light.

Each of these coatings offers advantages and disadvantages. The polymers of ornithine and lysine provide very strong attachment. On the other hand, preparation of such polycation surface coatings is relatively time-consuming. The polymers should be applied for at least 12 to 24 h to ensure adequate bonding to the culture surface. In addition, survival will be poor unless the dish surface is rinsed extensively before the cells are plated. The addition of laminin helps to promote neurite outgrowth on the polycation substrates, although one of us (JEH) has observed weaker attachment to surfaces coated with polylysine plus laminin in long-term cultures (i.e., >2–3 weeks).

Matrigel coatings can be prepared in less than 1 h and do not need to be rinsed, but both the concentrated stock and the final dilute solution must be maintained at 4°C or the matrix will form a gel. Neurons plated onto Matrigel or collagen sometimes migrate together to form small clusters of cells; this rarely occurs on polyornithine or polylysine. According to the manufacturer, Matrigel contains a number of different growth factors and, therefore, might be inappropriate for studies of neurotrophic agents or for other specific experiments.

Purified collagen is a simpler matrix preparation that provides an adequate substrate for glial cells and early postnatal CNS neurons. In general, it is much less adhesive than is polyornithine or polylysine and is relatively less adhesive than is Matrigel. These properties make collagen particularly useful for the generation of microisland cultures. As described later, droplets of collagen applied to a nonadhesive surface provide a consistent and uniform substrate for glial attachment; islands prepared with more adhesive substrates typically exhibit much greater variability.

Glial Feeder Layers

Long-term survival of CNS neurons is enhanced by the presence of glial cells. For early postnatal neurons (P0–P5), usually it is sufficient to plate freshly dissociated cells directly onto an appropriate substrate; glial cells within the cell suspension quickly multiply to confluence. Neurons from older animals (P5–P15), however, survive better when seeded onto a preexisting layer of glial cells.

Glial feeder layers are established from 3- to 6-day-old Long Evans rat pups; pups are swabbed with 70% ethanol and are sacrificed by decapitation. The skull is unroofed, the meninges are removed, and rectangular blocks of tissue approximately 5 × 6 mm from both cortical hemispheres are dissected with a scalpel. Cuts are made into the dorsal surface of the cortex to a depth of 3 mm, and the block of cortex is lifted out with a thin spatula. The tissue is transferred to a sterile 35-mm culture dish containing 1.5 ml of growth medium (see later), is chopped into small pieces with a scalpel, and is dissociated mechanically in a 15-ml conical tube by repeated trituration with a 2-ml glass serological pipette (e.g., Fisher no. 13-678-27D) held near the bottom of the tube. Undissociated clumps of cells are allowed to settle, and the turbid supernatant is transferred to a clean tube. Trituration of the remaining

Box 12.2 Passaging Glial Cells

1. Remove growth medium by aspiration.
2. Rinse the cells with 5 ml divalent cation-free solution.
3. Incubate for 5–15 min in divalent cation-free solution containing protease XXIII (Sigma no. P4032).
4. Transfer the cell suspension to a 15-ml conical tube and triturate to break up sheets of cells.
5. Centrifuge for 10 min at 300 $\times$ g and remove the supernatant.
6. Resuspend the cells in 10 ml of growth medium and plate onto coverslips. Cells from one confluent 25-cm^2 flask are used to seed 40 coverslips, 22 mm square.

Divalent cation-free solution (200 ml stock)

Component	Volume (ml)
Sterile DDW	170.4
10$\times$ Earle's balanced salt solution without Ca and Mg (Life Technologies no. 14160-022)	20
30% glucose	2.4
50 mM EDTA, pH 7.4	2
1 M NaHCO$_3$	5.2

clumps is repeated two or three times with 1 to 2 ml of fresh growth medium each time. Feeder layers may be established by plating the dissociated cells directly onto coverslips at a density of approximately 8×10^4 cells per cm^2. Alternately, the resulting cell suspension may be plated in a tissue-culture flask or 10-cm culture dish. In this case, we find it convenient to coat the culture surface for cell attachment with 0.1% gelatin prepared in sterile DDW from a 2% commercial stock solution (Sigma no. G1393). It is difficult to estimate the yield of glial cells, but tissue from a single rat pup will seed 40 to 60 dishes (0.8 cm^2 per dish) or one or two 25-cm^2 culture flasks. After several days of growth, the glial cells are removed from the flasks by brief enzymatic treatment in divalent cation-free solution (box 12.2). Although it is possible to passage the glial cells into new flasks and continue to expand the population, typically we prepare feeder layers after a single passage.

Whether freshly dissociated or passaged from a flask, glial cells begin to divide within a few hours after plating. When the glial layer has become perhaps 70% to 80% confluent (4–8 days, depending on the initial density), further cell division is halted by the

Box 12.3 Growth Medium

Component	Volume (ml)
Sterile water	39.85
10 × MEM (Life Technologies no. 11430-014)	5
Penicillin-streptomycin (Life Technologies no. 15075-013)	0.25
30% glucose	0.6
1 M NaHCO$_3$	1.3
50 mM glutamine (Sigma no. G3126)	0.5
Serum	2.5

Procedure

Add the listed stock solutions, in order, to the sterile water. Bubble with 95% O$_2$/5% CO$_2$ at 37°C, then add the serum and filter (0.22 μm). Rat serum typically is the serum used for neuronal cultures. The glucose and NaHCO$_3$ solutions are prepared with sterile water, filtered through 0.22-μm filters, and stored at room temperature in sterile polystyrene flasks. The glutamine solution is prepared in sterile water, filtered, divided into 0.25-ml aliquots, and stored in 1-ml polypropylene vials at −70°C to prevent nonenzymatic breakdown to glutamate; a fresh tube is thawed each time medium is prepared.

addition of cytosine-arabinoside (Ara-C, Sigma no. C6645; 10^{-5} M, final concentration). Ara-C appears to reduce the number of microglia in the cultures and to promote the flattening of GFAP-positive type I astrocytes.

After the feeder layer of glial cells has become nearly confluent, it is ready to receive freshly dissociated neurons. Typically, we rinse the dish with balanced salt solution and feed with growth medium (box 12.3) several hours before neurons are plated. It is important to note that vanishingly few neurons survive the procedures just described. This is particularly true for glial cells that have been passaged with divalent-free solutions. To eliminate any neurons that have managed to survive, the glial layers can be treated for several hours with 1 mM glutamate, rinsed three times with MEM (Life Technologies no. 11430-014, used at 1×), and refed with fresh growth medium.

Neuronal Growth Medium and Rat Serum

The growth medium for neurons, prepared according to the protocol in box 12.3, consists of Eagle's MEM with 0.5 mM glutamine, 20 mM glucose, 100 units/ml penicillin, and 0.1 mg/ml strepto-

mycin. For long-term survival of neurons, this medium must be supplemented with serum. Typically, we use 5% adult rat serum, prepared in-house, although commercial lots of calf or horse serum also may be used for this purpose. Three of us (RWB, KAJ, and JEH) routinely use growth medium supplemented with 5% commercial bovine fetal serum (Gibco, Gaithersburg, MD) for the preparation and maintenance of glial feeder layers, but we use rat serum for neuronal cultures. One of us (MMS) finds heat-inactivated iron-supplemented calf serum (Hyclone, Logan, UT, A-2151-L) to be best for all cultures.

Rat serum is prepared from retired male breeder C/D rats (Charles River, Wilmington, MA, or Harlan, Indianapolis, IN) by cardiac puncture with 10-ml Corvac integrated serum separator Vacutainer tubes [Sherwood Medical no. 8881-302015 tubes and 881-610037 needle holders] on a 21-gauge, 1-inch Monoject needle unit (Becton Dickinson no. 7212). The rats are anesthetized with 100% CO_2 for 2 min. The needle is introduced immediately below the sternum. In rats larger than 300 g, the 1-inch tip allows reliable intracardiac penetration when fully inserted rostrally into the thoracic cavity. Typically, two tubes containing some 8 ml each are collected from each rat. Small rotations or slight withdrawal—or, in some cases, reinsertion of the needle—may be required to achieve maximum collection. After 30 min at room temperature, the tubes are centrifuged at 2500 rpm at 4°C for 15 min. The serum is pooled and recentrifuged at 20,000 × g for 30 min to remove fibrin, which pellets. Aliquots of 2.5 ml are frozen in sterile 5-ml screw-cap polypropylene tubes and are stored at −70°C.

When prepared fresh, the growth medium contains approximately 15 µM glutamate, which comes from the added serum and from spontaneous decomposition of glutamine. This amount is enough to be neurotoxic. We observed that confluent glial cells are able to reduce the concentration of glutamate and aspartate below 0.5 to 1 µM over a period of several hours; therefore, usually we condition medium to be used for neurons by incubating it overnight with a confluent glial culture. To a 10-cm culture dish of confluent glial cells, 25 ml of freshly prepared medium is added, complete with rat serum. Following overnight incubation at 37°C (5% CO_2) the medium is removed and filtered (0.22 µm). Normally, the conditioned medium is used immediately but, after 2 days at 4°C, the glutamate level remains below 1 µM.

Dissociation and Plating of Neurons

Four solutions are prepared ahead of time: dissection medium, enzyme solution, heavy inhibitor, and light inhibitor (box 12.4). The ionic composition of the dissection medium is designed to prevent rundown of ionic gradients during handling of the tissue (Furshpan and Potter, 1989). Rat pups 6 to 10 days old are injected intraperitoneally with 100 mg/kg ketamine to block NMDA receptors and thereby to minimize excitotoxicity during dissection and to provide anesthesia. The head is swabbed with 70% ethanol and 3 min after the ketamine injection, the animal is sacrificed by cervical dislocation, the skull is unroofed, and the meninges are removed. For visual cortex cultures, one or two pieces of cortex (2 × 3 mm; ~6 mg) are removed from the posterior dorsal surface. For cultures from other brain areas, the following recipes assume use of an equivalent amount of those tissues and must be adjusted for different amounts.

The block of cortex is placed in dissection medium in a 35-mm dish, and a series of partial cuts is made to aid penetration of nutrients and enzyme. The block is transferred to a sterile, glass 20-ml liquid scintillation vial in a 30° to 32°C water bath, and 3.3 ml of papain enzyme solution is added. Gentle motion of the tissue blocks is provided by a stirring bar that is placed in the water bath and taps the 20-ml vial periodically. After 30 min, the enzyme solution is replaced with a fresh 3.3 ml and, after 30 additional min, is replaced with a final 3.3 ml of enzyme solution. After a total of 90 min exposure to enzyme, the tissue is transferred to a 15-ml conical tube wherein it is washed twice with occasional gentle swirling with 2.5 ml of heavy inhibitor for 30 s, three times with light inhibitor, and two times with growth medium. This extensive rinsing with inhibitor is required to remove the enzyme completely.

The tissue then is triturated gently in 1.5 ml of growth medium with a 2-ml glass serological pipette (e.g., Fisher no. 13-678-27D) for 40 passes or until the tissue mass has been reduced by perhaps one-third in size. After 1 min of settling, the supernatant is transferred to a new 15-ml tube. This sequence is repeated with two more 1.5-ml portions of growth medium, after which the tissue should be dissociated fully. After 2 to 3 min to allow for settling of large debris, the supernatants are combined and appearance and density of cells is evaluated in a hemacytometer (figure 12.1A). Typically, the yield is 10^5 cells per milligram of tissue. The cells are plated at a density of 10,000 to 40,000 cells per 1-cm-diameter

Box 12.4 Dissection and Dissociation Solutions

Dissection solution (100 ml stock):

Component	Volume (ml)	Final Concentration (mM)
Double-distilled water	91.175	
1 M MgCl$_2$	0.58	5.8 mM
1 M CaCl$_2$	0.025	0.25 mM
0.5 M HEPES	0.32	1.6 mM
0.5% Phenol red	0.2	(0.001%)
0.1 N NaOH	0.2	0.2 mM
2 M Na$_2$SO$_4$	4.5	90 mM
1 M K$_2$SO$_4$	3.0	30 mM
0.1 M Kynurenic acid	1.0	1 mM
5 mM APV	1.0	0.05 mM

Procedure
Combine the components in the order given, filter at 0.22 μm, store at 4°C.
Water is purified by reverse osmosis, glass-distilled, and autoclaved. Three of
us (MMS, KAJ, and RWB) prepare enzyme and inhibitor solutions using the
dissection stock solution described earlier. One of us (JEH) uses Earle's salt
solution (divalent cation-free solution as described in box 12.2, with
1.5 mM CaCl$_2$ and 1 mM MgCl$_2$) and equilibrates all solutions with 95% O$_2$/5%
CO$_2$ immediately before use.

Enzyme Solution (10 ml)
Warm 10 ml of dissection solution to 30°C–32°C.
Add 200 units of papain (no. LS03124, Worthington Biochemical Co., Free-
hold, NJ) and 1.6 mg of L-cysteine (Sigma no. C-7880).
Adjust pH to 7.4, with approximately 14 μl of 0.1 N NaOH.
Incubate for ∼30 min until the solution clears to activate the papain.
Filter at 0.22 μm and keep at 30°C–32°C.

Heavy Inhibitor (4 ml)
Add 40 mg of BSA (Sigma no. A7030) and 40 mg of trypsin inhibitor (Sigma
no. T-9253) to 4 ml of dissection solution.
Adjust pH to 7.4, with approximately 20 μl of 0.1 N NaOH.
Filter at 0.22 μm and keep at room temperature.

Light Inhibitor (10 ml)
Combine 1 ml of heavy inhibitor with 9 ml of dissection solution.

APV, 2-amino-5-phosphonovaleric acid.

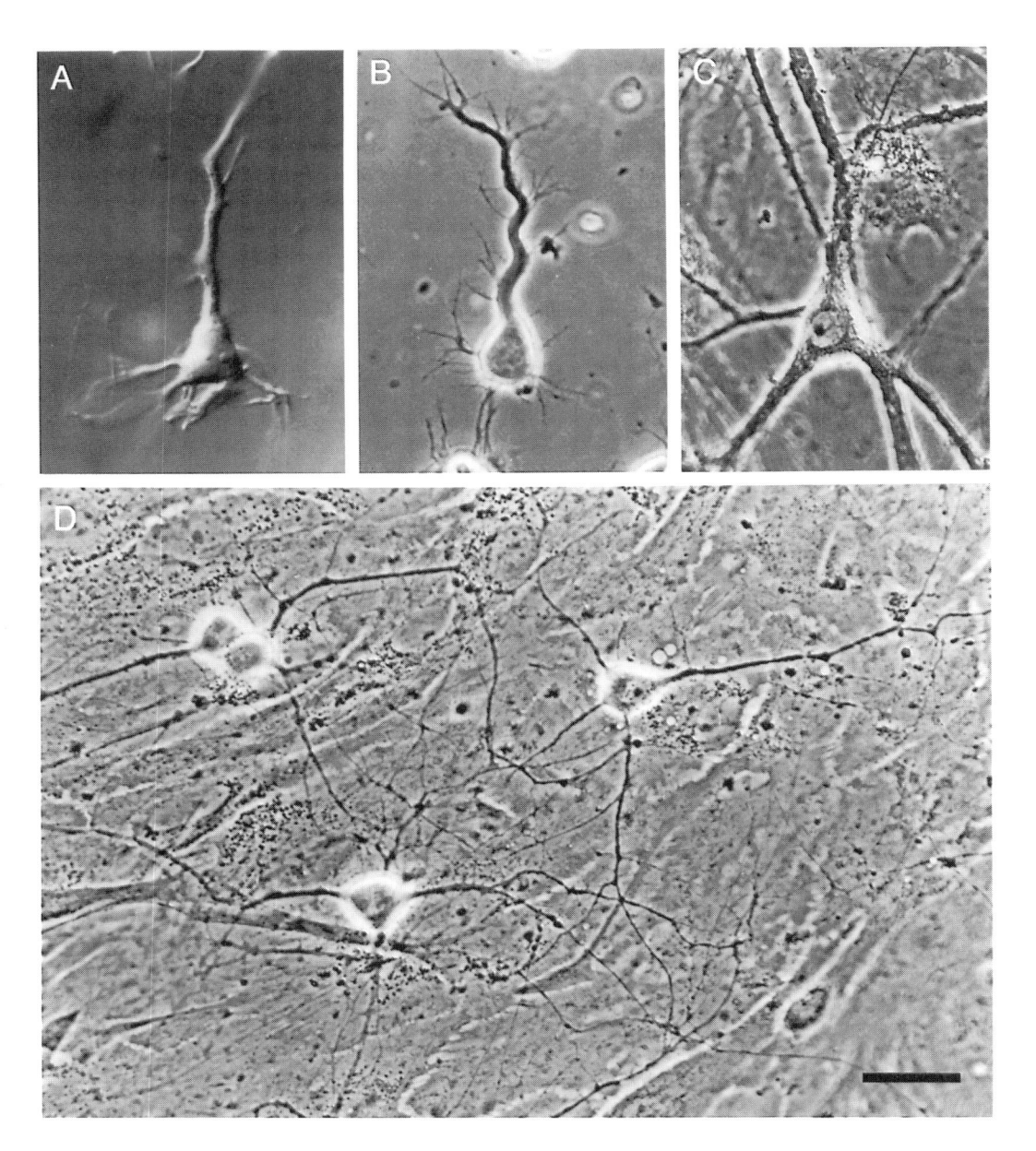

Figure 12.1 Dissociated neurons from animals aged 3 days (*D*), 7 days (*B*), 8 days (*A*), and 15 days (*C*). *A*. A freshly dissociated neuron immediately after trituration. *B–D*. Neurons in culture for 3 h (*B*), 16 days (*D*), and 19 days (*C*). Scale bar: 30 μm. (Reproduced with permission from J. E. Huettner, R. W. Baughman, Primary culture of identified neurons from the visual cortex of postnatal rats. J. Neurosci. 1986; 6: 3044–3060.)

well in 60 µl of growth medium. Medium in the dish, including that in the 1-cm well, is aspirated immediately (1 s) before the cells are added. In plating onto plain dishes or free coverslips, a sterile glass ring (Thomas no. 6705-R12) is used to confine the freshly dissociated cells to the center of the dish. After 2 h, each dish receives 1.25 ml of conditioned growth medium, and the cultures are fed with 1.25 ml of fresh conditioned growth medium every 5 to 7 days thereafter.

One obvious but very important warning is to avoid tilting the dishes once they contain a full layer of growth medium. Tilting can wet the top edge of the Petri dish with growth medium and allow fungi to enter the dish. This appears to be the most common cause of microbial contamination.

As mentioned, usually we plate cells from animals P5 or older onto an established monolayer of glial cells. In this case, Ara-C is added to the dishes 24 to 48 h after cells have been plated (10^{-5} M final concentration). With younger animals, freshly dissociated cells can be plated directly onto a coated substrate. Glial cells within the mixed cell suspension will divide and form a monolayer over a period of 4 to 6 days, at which point cell division can be halted.

If a gamma ray source is available, it may be preferable to arrest glial division by irradiation rather than with Ara-C. Although approximately one-third of the neurons die several hours after irradiation, the remaining nerve cells appear to survive longer and remain healthier than do cells in cultures treated with Ara-C. We have used dosages of 1000 rads, delivered either as a 10-min exposure to a cesium 137 gamma source or as a 1-min exposure to a cobalt 60 source. Glial feeder layers are irradiated after 4 days, allowing for sufficient proliferation of astrocytes. Neurons plated onto glial cells are irradiated after 1 day.

Special Procedures for Microisland Cultures

The basic principle of making microisland cultures is to prepare islands of a substrate adhesive for neurons on a background of a nonadhesive substrate. The protocol described here uses islands defined by what we believe to be the best adhesive substrate—glial cells—on a background of what we believe to be the most nonadhesive substrate—agarose. The methods presented here are based on those of Segal and Furshpan (1990).

Preparing Dishes

The goal in preparing dishes is to have a surface with islands of substrate on a background of agarose. In the method described here, glass coverslips are attached to plastic dishes that have a central well cut out of the plastic. It is not possible to use this approach on unattached glass coverslips, as the agarose will detach following the slightest disturbance, such as changing a solution.

The basic plan is to prepare glass coverslips coated with agarose, attach the coverslips to Petri dishes, add islands of the collagen, and sterilize the dishes. Attaching the agarose-coated coverslip to the plastic dish serves to fasten down the film of agarose. When glial cells are added later, they form islands on the collagen.

The most critical feature is creating a thin layer of dried agarose and attaching it firmly to a dish so that it will not tear or move once it is hydrated. It is essential to avoid touching the agarose layer with any tools or dirt. Small imperfections in the agarose will expand once the agarose is rehydrated, resulting in the agarose flapping around or even floating away.

As an alternative procedure, if the experimental aim does not require the superior optical qualities provided by a glass substrate, agarose can be spread directly on the bottom of a plastic culture dish (Mennerick et al., 1995). Agarose bonds more strongly to plastic than to glass, and detachment after rehydration is much less common. We expect that agarose could be used also to coat unattached plastic coverslips, but we have not tested this.

Preparing Glass Coverslips Coated with Agarose

The procedure described next should be started at least 3 days before the dishes are needed, to allow time for the agarose to dry overnight and for the Sylgard to cure completely. The coverslips are placed in the bottom of 150-mm plastic Petri dishes, 12 to a dish, in a culture hood. Care must be taken to reject any coverslips with dust on the surface, as they will result in a defective agarose layer. A 0.2% (wt/vol) solution of agarose (Sigma agarose IIA, no. A-9918) is prepared by mixing the agarose powder with water and autoclaving the bottle for at least 10 min (with the top loose to prevent explosion or implosion). When the dissolved agarose is removed from the autoclave, the solution is swirled to ensure that it is mixed completely. The bottle then is placed in a 60°C water bath or on the top of an inverted 100-mm plastic Petri dish to reduce the

rate of heat loss, because the agarose solution will gel once it cools to near room temperature.

With a 1-ml pipette, agarose solution is placed on each of several coverslips, typically four at a time. The drop of agarose should be big enough to cover the central part of the coverslip, such that when the coverslip is placed over the well in the culture dish, the dried drop will cover the entire well generously, allowing for alignment errors. On the other hand, the drop should not be so large that it reaches the edge of the coverslip. Because the agarose becomes hydrated when cultures are grown in the dish, it could provide a pathway for fluid to leak from the dish. The object is to create a very thin film of dried agarose. This effect is achieved by removing most of the agarose several seconds after it is applied, while it is still liquid, leaving only a thin film of agarose that will dry on the coverslip. The removal of the agarose is performed with the same pipette as is used to apply it. Remove perhaps a third of the agarose at a time, as trying to remove it all in one step usually causes the solution to bead up, failing to cover enough of the coverslip. The removed agarose is discarded. Unused agarose solution can be reused another day, after autoclaving.

The coverslips are allowed to dry overnight in a location protected from dust, such as a hood. Faster drying in an oven can cause the agarose to crack. The choice of type of agarose used usually is not crucial: Similar results were obtained with several types of agarose that differ in their electroendosmosis and sulfate groups, (including Sigma agarose types IV, IVA, VIII, and SeaKem ME agarose, FMC Bioproducts, Rockland ME). Agarose solutions more dilute than 0.2% bead up too often instead of forming a continuous layer. More concentrated agarose solutions produce thicker layers that are more likely to buckle and detach from the underlying glass coverslip. Attempts to use GelBond plastic (to which agarose has been chemically bonded; FMC Bioproducts, Rockland ME) were associated with widespread death of cells within days.

Preparing Holes in Dishes

Culture dishes are cut as described earlier in the section on mass culture methods, but smaller holes are used. Wells of 8 mm may be the optimal size: Smaller wells result in too few microislands, but large wells can result in the agarose detaching due to exposure of free edges of the agarose or random imperfections in the agarose.

A vacuum cleaner is used to suction off stray bits of plastic formed during cutting. Then the holes are deburred with a rotating large spherical drill bit, both on the inside and outside of the dish, and the surfaces are vacuumed again to get off all debris. It is important to avoid plastic fragments in the dishes, because the fragments can damage the agarose surface.

Attaching Coverslips with Sylgard

Coverslips with the agarose coating are attached to the plastic Petri dishes by Sylgard, as described for attaching coverslips in the mass culture technique. However, several extra precautions are advisable in using the agarose-coated coverslips. Coverslips with agarose are attached only after the agarose has dried to a thin film. Fine forceps are used to hold the coverslip, and it is important not to contact the agarose layer. It is most important to center the coverslips accurately on the holes in the plastic dishes so as not to have free edges of the agarose film exposed to the solution in the culture dish well. It is also important to place enough Sylgard on the coverslip so that a tight seal is formed to hold down the agarose well. However, there should not be so much excess Sylgard that a large amount leaks into the well after the coverslip is attached.

Applying Substrate to Culture Dishes

The core method that will be described is spraying collagen onto the agarose to form tiny islands of adhesive substrate. Spraying should be done in a sterile environment, such as a culturing hood. Aluminum foil is placed in the hood to provide a disposable surface under the 35-mm plastic dishes when the collagen is sprayed. Collagen (Vitrogen 100, approximately 3 mg/ml, cat. no. 0701, Collagen Corporation, Palo Alto, CA) is used undiluted. Approximately 2.5 ml of the collagen solution is pipetted into an atomizer sprayer (Thomas Scientific no. 2753-L10), taking care not to break the small glass tube inside the sprayer.

Six 35-mm culture dishes are placed together on the foil, with their tops removed. The sprayer is held horizontally, some 15 cm above and 25 cm lateral to the open dishes. Collagen then is sprayed with blasts of air produced by squeezing the rubber bulb of the atomizer. The size and number of collagen dots will depend on the force of spraying, the distance to the dishes, the humidity, and

the number of sprayings. The size and number of dots can be checked between sprayings by placing a dish under a dissecting microscope in the hood. Often, it is necessary to tilt the dish or adjust a light source to see the collagen dots on the agarose. Typically, the dots should be perhaps 100 to 200 µm in diameter and should be numerous, but not so numerous as to have most dots having neighbors within a few hundred micrometers, as this accumulation will lead to bridging of neurons between islands to form a mass culture. More collagen can be sprayed until the right density of dots is achieved. Figure 12.2A shows a typical density of microislands in a portion of an 8-mm well in a completed culture.

After all the dishes have been sprayed, the remaining collagen is discarded, and the small amount of collagen that remains in the glass tube of the sprayer is ejected with several air blasts. The sprayer then is washed several times with 1 ml of dilute (0.3 M) HCl. With each wash, the added HCl is discarded and residual HCl is sprayed out into a sink or trash can with blasts of air. The inside of the sprayer then is washed twice with 70% ethanol in a similar manner.

The dishes sprayed with collagen can be used the same day or stored for at least several days at room temperature before use. On the day of culturing, dishes are UV-sterilized as described for mass cultures.

Alternative Substrates for Microislands

Substrates other than collagen have been used for microislands. Such substrates as polylysine and laminin also can be sprayed in a fashion similar to that for the collagen (Segal and Furshpan, 1990; Bekkers and Stevens, 1991). The main advantage of using polylysine and laminin is that neurons stick to these substrates better than to collagen, making it possible to plate neurons and glial cells in a single step. The one-step approach has been particularly valuable in culturing brain cells from mutant mice, the genotype of which is not known at the time of culturing (e.g., Geppert et al., 1994), as a two-step procedure would result in mixing cells of different genotype. Disadvantages also accrue to the one-step approach. One problem is that it is more difficult to control the amount and adhesiveness of these substrates in contrast to collagen, which forms a dried layer with uniform properties. This variability with polylysine and laminin results in many islands having

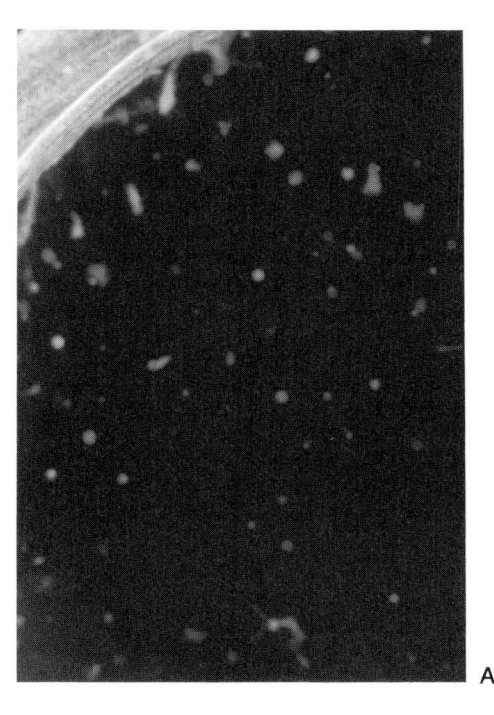

A

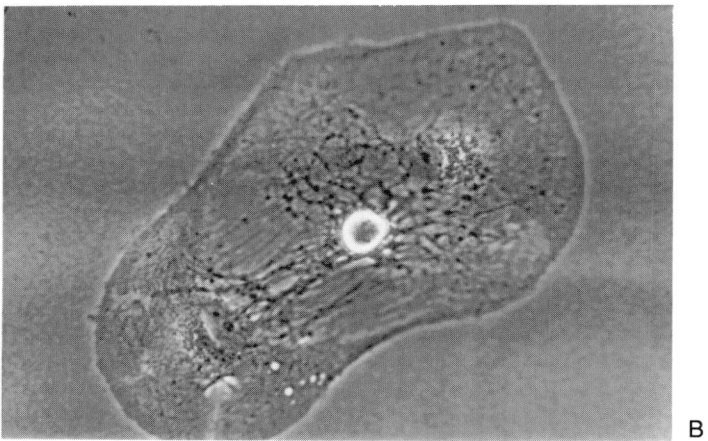

B

Figure 12.2 (*A*) A portion of an 8-mm well containing numerous microislands. (*B*) A single-neuron microisland visualized via phase-contrast microscopy. The neuron was growing for 24 days on an island formed from two overlapping collagen dots. The narrowest part of the island is 100 μm. Lucifer yellow injection of the same neuron (not shown) demonstrates filling of the processes that are visible in the phase-contrast view. (Reproduced with permission from M. M. Segal, Epileptiform activity in microcultures containing one excitatory hippocampal neuron. J. Neurophysiol. 1991; 65: 761–770.)

too many or too few neurons. Another problem with the one-step approach is that the resulting microisland cultures have fewer astrocytes, which could result in decreased neuronal survival (Rosenberg et al., 1992).

Plating Cells to Make Microisland Cultures

The methods of culturing to make microisland cultures are very similar to those described for mass cultures. The preparation of dissociated neurons is identical, with glass rings used to restrict the spread of the cell suspension in both the initial and second plating. In addition, after the cells are plated, the cultures are washed with growth medium to clear debris from the area between islands, so as to reduce bridging between microisland cultures.

INITIAL (GLIAL) PLATING

For the initial plating of glial cells, passaged glial cells can be used as described for mass cultures. Alternatively, the same suspension of cells from the dissociation can be used for the initial plating and the second plating, as few neurons will attach to collagen, and those few that do attach typically do not survive the addition of neuronal suspension in the second (neuronal) plating 1 or 2 weeks later. Before cells are plated, sterile forceps are used to place glass rings encircling the well that is formed by the hole in the plastic dish. The ring provides a much higher well into which the cell suspension can be deposited, resulting in a more uniform density of cells and a higher percentage of microislands containing the desired number of neurons. The glass rings should have an internal diameter equal to or larger than the outer dimension of the well and be several millimeters high (e.g., Thomas no. 6705-R12). The suspension of triturated cells is pipetted inside the rings, typically 0.15 ml per well. The fluid is added after first touching the inside of the glass ring to prevent the liquid from beading up into a central drop that will result in uneven cell dispersal. After the addition of cell suspension inside the glass rings, the culture dishes are placed in the incubator.

WASHING AWAY UNATTACHED CELLULAR MATERIAL

The washing step is done 2 h after the cells are plated. The glass rings are removed with sterile forceps. For the culture dishes receiving their initial plating of glial cells, the wells now contain a small volume of solution that carried the cells. One milliliter of new

growth medium is added, dripped directly onto the central well of each dish, at approximately two drops per sec. This step is one of the most important parts of the microisland culture protocol, as it determines how many cells are left on the microislands and between the islands. When the dish is positioned to catch the light correctly, one can see the debris being removed by the falling drops. One continues to drop fluid, if necessary from higher up, until most of this macroscopic debris is gone. It is important to wash the central well enough to remove almost all the debris that might produce bridging between microislands. It is equally important not to wash too much, because this will reduce the number of neurons on the islands. Once the proper amount of cellular material has been removed, the remaining part of the 1 ml of medium is expelled into the 35-mm dish away from the well. The next step is to remove the medium outside the well, typically using a pipette connected to a collection bottle with vacuum applied. A new pipette is used for each 150-mm dish containing six 35-mm dishes, so as to reduce the possibility of cross-contamination. New medium (1.5 ml) is added to each dish, typically outside the well, though it is sometimes necessary to drip some of this medium onto the central well if debris remains. The cultures are irradiated at day 4 or 5 after the first plating, a time at which the glial cells on the microislands are confluent.

SECOND (NEURONAL) PLATING
Second (neuronal) plating can be performed any time after astrocytes have covered the microislands, which typically happens in perhaps 4 days. For practical purposes, this step often is accomplished 1 or 2 weeks later, at the time when the initial plating is being performed on a new set of dishes. The dishes to receive the neuronal plating already contain 1.5 ml of medium. Before adding the new cell suspension, clean glass rings again are placed around the central wells in a sterile fashion to contain the applied cells to the area of the central well. The new cell suspension is added (typically 0.15 ml). After 2 h in the incubator, the glass rings are removed and the central wells are washed as was done for the first plating. As discussed earlier, it is very important to monitor the washing visually.

SURVIVAL AND FEEDING
Survival depends very much on the types of cells and the protocol for feeding. Survival is improved by the use of glial-conditioned

medium (described earlier) or the inclusion of glutamate antagonists in the cultures (Furshpan and Potter, 1989). Survival of a large number of microcultures for 4 to 6 weeks is typical in using the glutamate antagonist method (Segal and Furshpan, 1990). Cultures can be fed by replacing part of the medium each week, by adding new medium, or simply by beginning with a large excess of medium when the cultures are plated. Replacing part of the medium each week is particularly benign if glial-conditioned medium is used, as little glutamate exists to produce excitotoxicity. Alternatively, if medium is not replaced, it is particularly important that the incubator have a water pan located near the air input and that any antimicrobial solution, such as potassium dichromate, put into the water pan be dilute enough (<20 mOsm) so as not to draw moisture from the cultures.

Dialysis membrane can be used to isolate cells from direct contact with the medium in the rest of the culture dish. This may improve cell survival if the cultures are to be fed with serum- or glutamine-containing medium that has not been conditioned previously by using glial cells. The technique (Furshpan and Potter, 1989) will not be described in detail here, but involves securing wetted dialysis membranes (Spectra/Por no. 132498, 33 mm diameter, MW cutoff 12–14,000) fastened to specially made glass rings (O.D. 22 mm, I.D. 19 mm, height 8 mm) using rubber gaskets (2.5 mm Sykes-Moore gaskets, no. 1943-33325, Bellco Glass, Vineland, NJ). These membrane assemblies, filled with growth medium, are placed on the cultures within a day of plating the neurons, and excess growth medium is vacuumed away.

Troubleshooting

Probably the most important requirement for success in culturing postnatal neurons is to obtain viable cells from the dissociation procedure. We recommend careful examination of dissociated cells *immediately* after trituration. Healthy, viable cells will be phase-bright and typically will retain a significant dendritic tree if dissociated with papain (see figure 12.1A). Cells that remain intact but have a uniformly gray or granular appearance are likely to be dead. It may seem obvious, but there is little point in attempting to improve a culture medium or substrate until healthy dissociated cells can be produced. In our hands, papain consistently yields results superior to any other enzyme or combination of enzymes, including trypsin, dispase, collagenase, or protease XXIII. In instructing

new laboratory staff members to perform dissociations, often we find it helpful for them to practice once or twice without attempting to maintain sterility. Sterile technique can slow down the procedure and reduce cell viability. In addition, significant activity may be lost if the enzyme solution is filtered before the papain has dissolved completely. Therefore, a streamlined (i.e., nonsterile) dissociation may help to diagnose problems with the dissociation methods.

Failure of healthy dissociated cells to survive in vitro indicates a problem with the substrate or the growth medium. When things are working well, we obtain excellent results with polyornithine or polylysine on glass coverslips. Neurons plated on these surfaces are well-dispersed, and they develop elaborate dendritic trees. Occasionally, however, a complete plating of healthy cells will die in less than 24 h. We have been unable to determine whether these occurrences result from incomplete rinsing, inadequate bonding to the glass, or some other factor. Survival on Matrigel has been more consistent, and plating onto an established layer of glial cells also is highly reliable. In using Matrigel and glial cells, it is particularly important to inhibit completely the papain with the trypsin inhibitor ovomucoid (Sigma no. T9253), as uninhibited papain will digest matrix proteins and detach the glial monolayer.

Problems with growth medium often result in toxicity subsequent to feeding. It can be very informative to examine cultures an hour or two after feeding and compare them to sister cultures that were not fed. As mentioned, the use of conditioned medium, feeding by partial replacement, or reducing the frequency of feedings can help to minimize this toxicity. In some cases, we find it helpful to triturate and plate cells by using a simple balanced salt solution (e.g., Life Technologies no. 24010-027 plus 20 mM glucose) rather than complete growth medium. Cortical and hippocampal neurons from P0 to P5 rats will survive and begin to grow for 24 to 36 h in the absence of serum and the other additives found in complete medium. This approach can help to distinguish between a problem with medium and marginal viability of the freshly dissociated cells.

In addition to the preceding general comments, several problems are specific to the microculture technique.

- *Agarose detaching:* Try being more careful to avoid dust and gelled agarose in placing the agarose layer on coverslips. Be careful not to

let forceps or plastic debris touch the agarose. Ensure that no exposed free edges remain in the agarose layer in the well (a result of using agarose drops that were too small). Try using a thicker layer of agarose or using a more concentrated agarose solution.

- *Too few microislands:* Ensure a supply of enough microislands immediately after spraying. The microislands must be large enough ($\sim$100–200 μm) to support cell growth. The force, the distance, or the number of sprayings of substrate may have to be changed.
- *Too many cells on microislands:* Dilute the cell suspension or increase the force of the washing step. Do the opposite if too few cells remain.
- *Too much bridging between microislands:* Wash more vigorously after plating. If water-soluble substrates are being used, consider changing to collagen.

Properties of Cultured Neurons

Development of Neurons in Mass Cultures

Neurons begin to extend processes within a few hours after settling and, with time, form a complex network of interconnections (see figure 12.1). Synaptic transmission can be detected first after 1 or 2 days in culture. The complexity of synaptic connections increases progressively over the next few weeks. Well-established neurons in culture should be phase-bright, without granularity in the soma. In many cells, the nucleus and nucleolus are easily visible. Typically, neurites course across the glial feeder layer although, in dense cultures, fibers may dive beneath the nonneuronal cells for variable distances.

Long-term survival of plated cells depends on several factors. In general, cells prepared from younger animals appear to survive better than do those from animals 10 to 15 days old (which is the practical age limit in using our methods). Neurons survive best when the plating density is at least 20,000 to 40,000 cells per square centimeter; survival does not improve at higher densities but often is noticeably worse in sparsely plated cultures. Successful recordings have been obtained from neurons in cultures 90 days old. Such older cultures are more sensitive to glutamate toxicity, and the use of glutamate-free conditioned medium is accordingly more important to promote survival over long periods. With careful

treatment, at least 50% of the initially plated neurons will survive for more than a month.

Extensive characterization of these cultures suggests that they provide faithful expression of many neuronal properties. These include the presence of an apparently complete selection of neuronal and nonneuronal cells; a full repertoire of electrophysiological, pharmacological, and synaptic responses; and expression of typical morphological and ultrastructural elements.

Development of Neurons in Microisland Cultures

Figure 12.2B shows a microisland made with collagen on agarose. The grainy, cell-free background is the surface of the agarose. The round cell-containing area was defined by a drop of collagen sprayed onto the agarose. To this microisland of collagen, glial cells attached during the first plating, then neurons attached during the second plating. The selectivity of the cells for the islands is very strong. Occasional fibers that bridge over the clear agarose surface can be detected easily via phase-contrast microscopy, owing to the different optical properties of axons and bulk solution (not shown).

In the first 3 weeks after plating of neurons in microisland cultures, neuronal processes are clearly visible but, afterward, only the cell bodies of the neurons remain visible, though the extensive processes can be demonstrated by injection of fluorescent dyes (Segal and Furshpan, 1990; Segal, 1991). After an initial period of neuronal loss during the first 3 weeks, relatively stable survival of neurons in microisland cultures is observed for more than 10 weeks, including many microislands that contained three or fewer neurons. Survival of neurons in microislands is not as robust as in mass cultures, even when microisland cultures and mass cultures are present in the same dish. This finding presumably relates to some deficiency in cellular contacts or electrical signals in the microisland cultures.

Identification of Cultured Neurons

A number of different strategies can be used to identify specific cell types within a heterogeneous culture. For definitive identification of neurons with long-distance projections, we have used in vivo retrograde transport of fluorescent markers to label the neurons prior to dissociation. To label cells in layer 5 of the cortex that

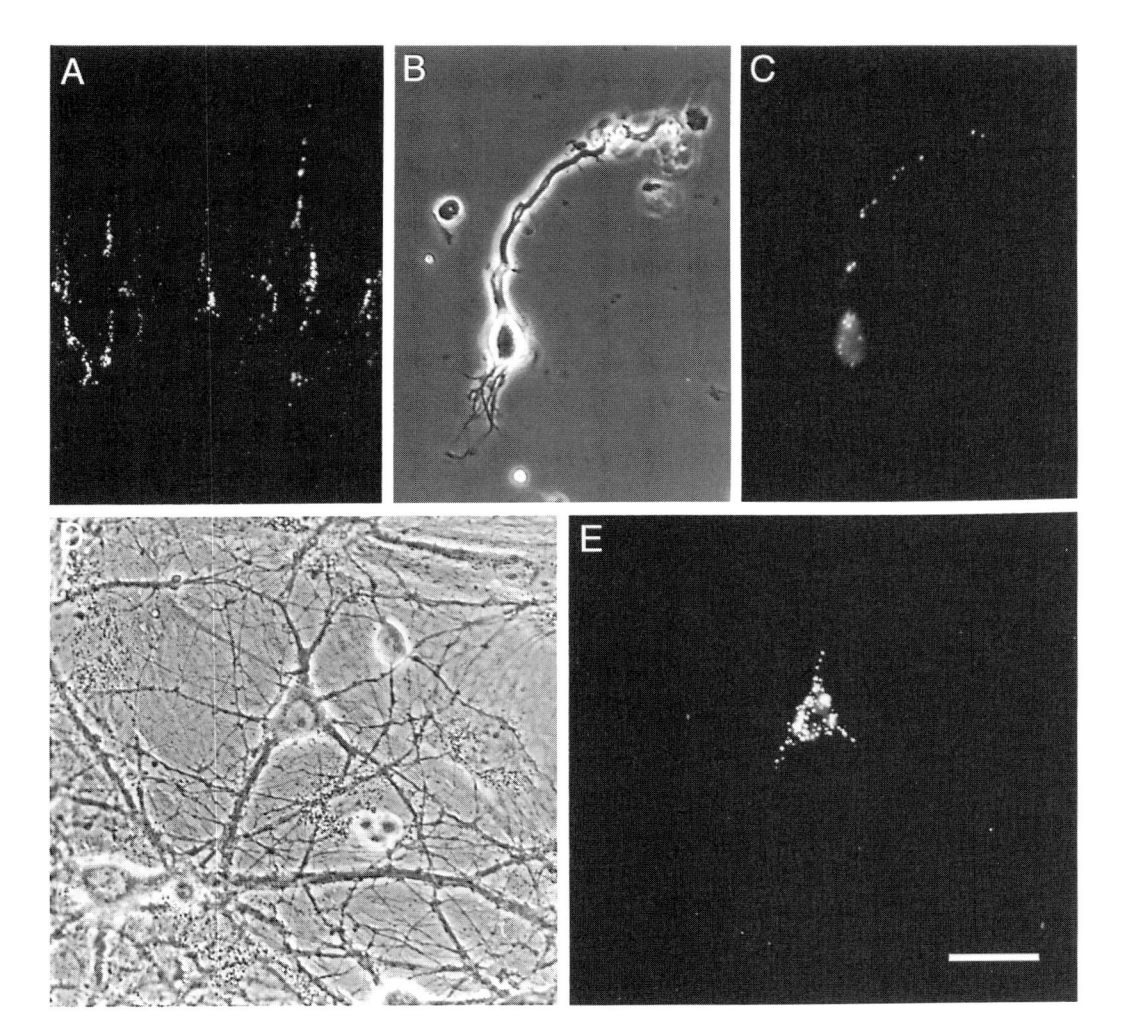

Figure 12.3 Neurons labeled with fluorescent microspheres in vivo (A) and in vitro (B–E). A. Pyramidal cells in layer 5 of visual cortex are labeled brightly in this coronal section prepared 2 days after an injection of microspheres in the superior colliculus. Phase-contrast (B) and fluorescence (C) micrographs of a freshly dissociated, labeled neuron. Phase-contrast (D) and fluorescence (E) micrographs of a labeled neuron after 34 days in culture. Scale bar: 65 µm (A); 38 µm (B, C); 40 µm (D, E). (D and E reproduced with permission from J. E. Huettner, R. W. Baughman, The pharmacology of synapses formed by identified corticocollicular neurons in primary cultures of rat visual cortex. J. Neurosci. 1988; 8: 160–175.)

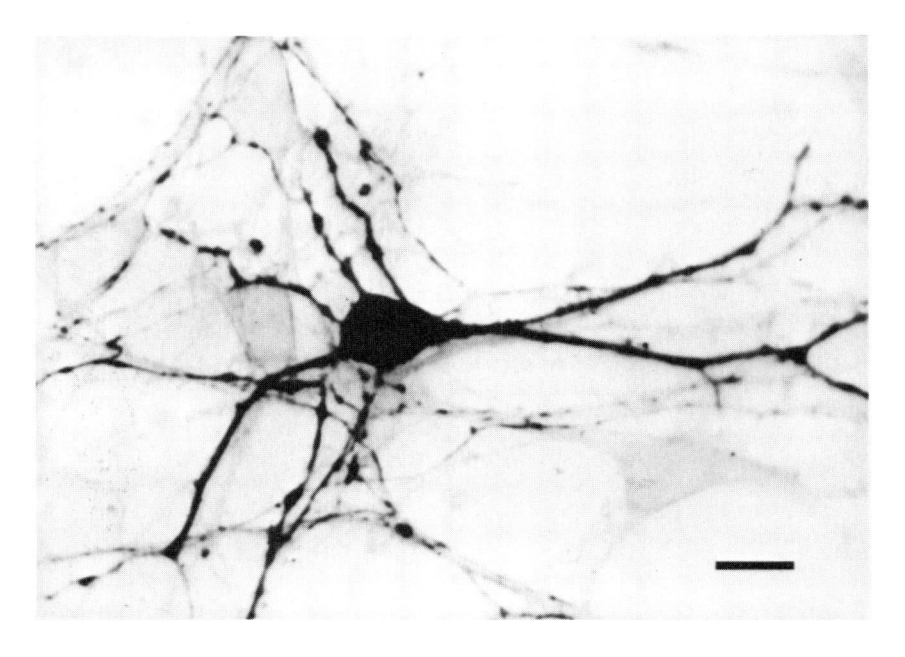

Figure 12.4 GABA-like immunoreactivity visualized after 29 days in a cortical mass culture. This field contains one positive cell and four unstained neurons. Scale bar: 25 μm.

project to the superior colliculus, fluorescent latex microspheres (Katz et al., 1984) are injected into the colliculus on postnatal day 5 or 6. Rat pups are anesthetized with halothane, and a suspension of microspheres (Lumifluor, Inc., New York, NY), used as received, is pressure-injected (5–20 psi) from a 2-μl microcap (BoLab, Lake Havasu City, AZ, no. BB101-2) pulled and broken to a 10- to 20-μm tip diameter. A small piece of skull bone is removed, and injections are made through the dura at a depth of 0.4 to 0.8 mm by using a micromanipulator to position the pipette. The scalp incision is closed with cyanoacrylate glue. After 24 to 48 h to permit retrograde transport to occur, visual cortex is dissociated and plated as described. Labeled neurons can be visualized immediately after dissociation and for many weeks in culture (figure 12.3). Illumination to visualize the fluorescent label appears to be innocuous to the cells.

Careful characterization of neurons in culture can reveal additional methods for cell type identification. For example, in hippocampal microislands, it is possible to distinguish neurons to some extent by size and, more definitively, by the physiological properties of the synaptic connections that they make on themselves or onto other neurons. In solitary neuron microislands, excitatory rat

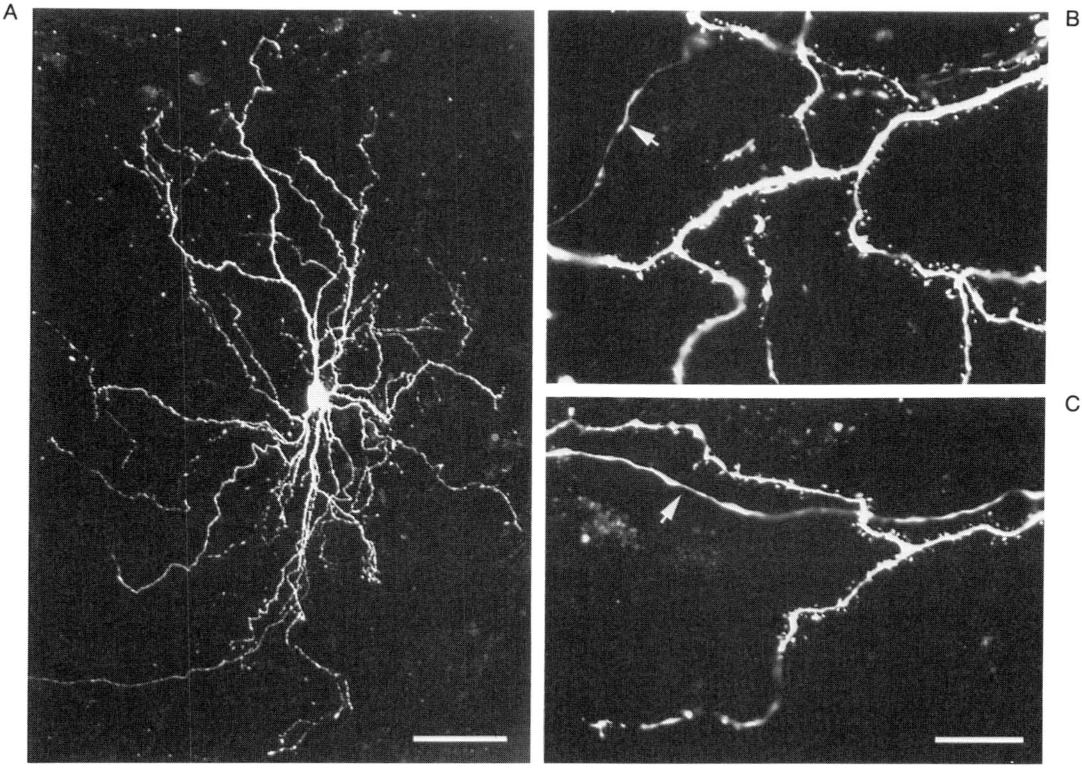

Figure 12.5 A corticocollicular neuron injected with Lucifer yellow (*A*) after 42 days in vitro. (*B*, *C*) High-magnification images of neurites from two different cells. Spine-bearing dendrites can be distinguished from the thinner, aspinous axons (arrows). Scale bar: 75 µm (*A*); 15 µm (*C*). (A with permission from J. E. Huettner, R. W. Baughman, Primary culture of identified neurons from the visual cortex of postnatal rats. J. Neurosci. 1986; 6: 3044–3060.)

hippocampal neurons were 20.8 µm in diameter (±3.0 µm SD), whereas inhibitory neurons were 16.2 µm (±2.2 µm) (Segal, 1991). Based on autaptic physiology and pharmacology, the transmitter type of 95% of hippocampal neurons alone in microislands could be established (Segal, 1991). The ability to guess transmitter type from neuronal size raises the yield of choosing microisland cultures with particular cell type mixtures—such as one excitatory neuron and one inhibitory neuron—that helps with the success rate for certain experiments.

In rat cortical cultures, excitatory and inhibitory neurons can be identified with reasonable certainty on the basis of their action-potential width (Huettner and Baughman, 1988). As first described in cortical tissue slices by McCormick and colleagues (1985), in-

hibitory neurons have much narrower action potentials than do excitatory neurons. Cells with action potentials of less than 0.9 ms at half-height are almost exclusively inhibitory, whereas cells with action potentials greater than 1.2 ms at half-height are almost exclusively excitatory.

Immunocytochemistry and Visualization of Neurite Patterns in Living Neurons

In addition to physiological analysis, a variety of immunocytochemical or morphological techniques can be used to characterize cell types present in cultures or to localize particular antigens on cells (e.g., Huettner and Baughman, 1986; Jones and Baughman, 1988). Staining for GABA is illustrated in figure 12.4.

For some studies, such as localization of neurotransmitter receptors, it is helpful to visualize the dendrites or axons of individual cells. Intracellular injection of Lucifer yellow (Sigma no. L0259) allows detailed visualization of neurites (figure 12.5), but this dye causes phototoxic damage and is poorly soluble in many internal solutions. We found the red dye sulforhodamine (Sigma no. S9012) to be more satisfactory, especially when ascorbic acid (200 μM; Sigma no. A7631) was added to the medium to reduce photooxidation (Jones and Baughman, 1988). The dye was added at 15 μM to the filling solution of whole-cell tight-seal electrodes. The use of an image intensifier allowed full visualization of neurites with no sign of phototoxicity or other effects on membrane properties.

Acknowledgments

Research in our laboratories has been supported by National Institutes of Health grants NS30888 to JEH, EY03502 to RWB, and K08 NS-01407 to MMS, and fellowships from the Dana Foundation and the Klingenstein Fund to MMS.

Note

1. Regarding filtration, most 0.2-μm filters contain a surfactant that appears to be toxic to cells. The effect of the surfactant can be seen by the frothing that occurs on shaking in a test tube of DDW that has passed through the filter. We minimize this problem by using nylon filters that contain very little surfactant (Corning no. 21062-25) and by washing each filter with sterile DDW before use, typically 10 ml for a 25-mm syringe filter.

13 Rat Hippocampal Neurons in Low-Density Culture

Kimberly Goslin, Hannelore Asmussen, and Gary Banker

The hippocampus is a structure that has fascinated neuroscientists for generations. Its anatomical organization is strikingly precise and beautiful (Amaral, 1987; Swanson et al., 1987; Brown and Zador, 1990), and it exhibits a remarkable capacity for activity-dependent changes in synaptic function, such as long-term potentiation (Hawkins et al., 1993; McNaughton, 1993; Malenka, 1994). Further, the hippocampus frequently is a source of seizure activity that can spread throughout the cortex, and its cells are highly susceptible to ischemia. Many of these characteristics are believed to reflect the specific endogenous properties of hippocampal neurons. For example, both the capacity for plasticity and the susceptibility to anoxia have been linked to the unique properties of NMDA receptors, which are expressed at particularly high levels by hippocampal neurons (Rothman and Olney, 1987; Malenka and Nicoll, 1993; Westbrook, 1993). What better approach to study these properties than in the accessible and controlled environment of cell culture?

To be honest, our own interests in the hippocampus are more prosaic. For us, the hippocampus is a source of a relatively homogeneous population of neurons with well-characterized properties typical of central nervous system (CNS) neurons in general. Pyramidal neurons, the principal cell type in the hippocampus, have been estimated to account for 85% to 90% of the total neuronal population. The CA1 and CA3 regions of the hippocampus contain pyramidal cells that differ from one another in some of their physiological properties and in some aspects of their connectivity and can be cultured separately. However, they are similar in many fundamental respects and, for our purposes, we make no attempt to distinguish between them. A variety of interneurons also have been described in the hippocampus (Swanson et al., 1987; Brown and Zador, 1990; Buzsaki and Chrobak, 1995), but they are few in number compared with pyramidal cells. Cells from the dentate gyrus, which lies adjacent to the hippocampus, are excluded rou-

tinely from most culture preparations (see later). Until recently, comparatively few studies have examined dentate neurons in culture (Boss et al., 1987a; Brewer and Cotman, 1989); the last few years have seen renewed interest in such cultures (e.g., Patel and McNamara, 1995; Lopez-Garcia et al., 1996; Tong et al., 1996).

Hippocampal pyramidal cells exhibit other features of interest for cell biological studies. For example, they have a characteristic, well-defined shape. Like most CNS neurons, they have a single axon and several dendrites, and their dendritic arbor is distinctive, consisting of a single long apical dendrite and several shorter basilar dendrites, all highly branched and studded with dendritic spines. In addition, hippocampal pyramidal neurons make direct connections with one another (via recurrent and Schaeffer collaterals and commissural projections) and with the population of endogenous interneurons. Thus, in culture, where sources of extrinsic afferent fibers are absent, hippocampal neurons still can make extensive, presumably appropriate, synaptic connections with one another.

Hippocampal cultures typically are prepared from 18- to 19-day fetal rats or from fetal mice at a comparable stage of development. At this age, the generation of pyramidal neurons, which begins in the rat at about E15, is essentially complete, but the generation of dentate granule cells, which largely occurs postnatally, scarcely has begun (Schlessinger et al., 1978; Bayer, 1980). The tissue still is easy to dissociate, the meninges are removed readily, and the number of glial cells still is relatively modest.

Detailed studies of the early development of pyramidal neurons in the rodent hippocampus have not been performed, but reasonable conjectures can be made about their development on the basis of data from other species or from other regions of the cortex (Shoukimas and Hinds, 1978; Nowakowski and Rakic, 1979; Anton et al., 1996). At the stage when cultures usually are prepared, most of the developing neurons lie within the intermediate zone and are in the process of migration from the ventricular surface, where they arise, to the pyramidal cell layer, their final destination (Banker and Cowan, 1977). Some of these cells already may have begun to extend axons, even though they have not completed their migration. Migrating cells sometimes have additional processes, somewhat suggestive of dendrites in shape, but the relationship of these processes to definitive dendrites or axons is uncertain. Older cells that have reached the pyramidal layer probably already have de-

veloped axons and have begun to extend apical dendrites, whereas cells still at the ventricular zone have not yet begun process outgrowth. Despite such variations in the stage of development of individual neurons, when the earliest generated or the most recently generated hippocampal neurons are labeled selectively with ^{3}H-thymidine before being placed into culture, both groups of cells develop axons and dendrites according to the same general sequence of morphological events (Fletcher and Banker, 1989).

The Rationale for Our Approach to Culturing Hippocampal Neurons

Many of our investigations require following the development of individual cells by time-lapse microscopy or by examining the differential distribution of antigens within single cells. For these purposes, culture conditions must permit the growth of cells at low density, so that individual neurons can be observed easily. Such conditions are routinely possible for peripheral neurons cultured in the presence of the appropriate growth factors, which promote the growth and survival of neurons from spinal and sympathetic ganglia. Despite much recent progress in identifying factors that enhance the growth of CNS neurons (Ghosh, 1996), thus far it is not routinely possible to obtain long-term survival of low-density CNS cultures by the addition of purified growth factors.

Glial cells are thought to be a source of neurotrophic substances and, in practice, most protocols for culturing CNS neurons depend on high cell densities and the rapid proliferation of endogenous glia to support neuronal survival and development. However, the complexity of such cultures precludes the possibility of following the development of processes emerging from single cells. Our approach is designed to circumvent the requirement for high cell densities (figure 13.1). We first prepare monolayer cultures of cortical astrocytes and allow them to grow until they reach confluence. Cultures of hippocampal neurons then are prepared separately on glass coverslips. Once the neurons have attached, the neurons and glia are combined to make a tissue-culture "sandwich," arranged so that the neurons on the coverslip face the glial cells on the Petri dish but are separated from them by a narrow gap. Although the two cell types do not contact each other, soluble substances can diffuse between them. This approach eliminates the requirement for endogenous glia and permits long-term survival of hippocampal neurons at very low cell densities. It has proved useful also for

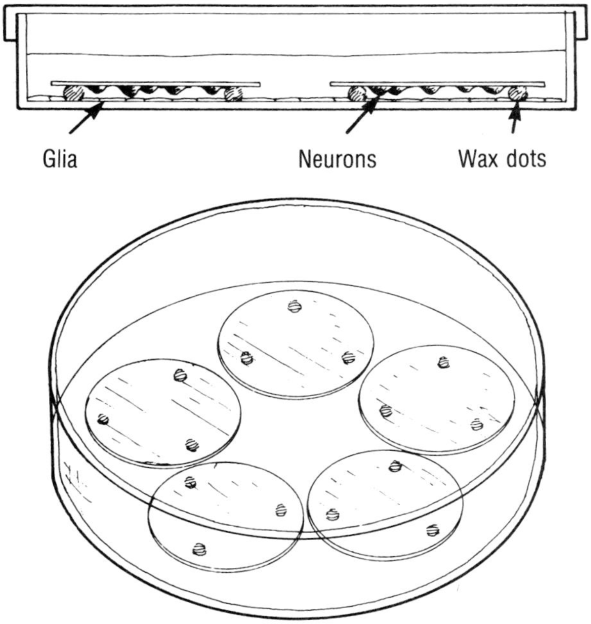

Figure 13.1 Dishes used for hippocampal-glial cocultures. Hippocampal neurons are cultured on glass coverslips, which are inverted so that they face the monolayer of glial cells. Paraffin dots attached to the coverslips support them above the glia.

culturing neurons from the cerebral cortex (Rosenberg and Dichter, 1989).

For experiments that do not require observation of living cells, we simply remove the neuron-bearing coverslips at the desired stage of development and manipulate them as experiments dictate. For viewing living neurons and for experiments involving micro-manipulation or microinjection of single cells, these coverslips can be transferred to special chambers designed for live-cell micro-scopy. Suitable chambers are available commercially, although the chambers we use were custom-made in local university machine shops.

Using our approach, it is relatively easy to obtain good short-term cultures, but long-term survival and dendritic maturation at the low cell densities we use require attention to detail, dedication, and some tolerance for frustration. Perhaps as a reflection of these qualities, the methods we have come to adopt are rather "fussy" and require some effort in preparation of materials and in planning ahead. Optimal results are attained when cultures are prepared on a regular basis, week in and week out, so that all steps become

routine. Presumably these difficulties arise because the conditions that are ideal for our experiments—low cell density, few glial cells—are so contrary to the cells' natural inclination for gregarious association.

Other Approaches for Culturing Hippocampal Neurons

If the special conditions of our cultures are unnecessary for your experiments, alternative approaches for preparing hippocampal cultures are available. Protocols developed in the late 1970s and early 1980s by John Peacock, Steve Rothman, Menahem Segal, and their collaborators (Peacock et al., 1979; Rothman and Cowan, 1979; Segal, 1983; Rothman, 1984) have served as models for many of the procedures for culturing hippocampal neurons subsequently adopted in other laboratories. In these protocols, hippocampi from fetal rats or mice are dissociated mechanically or by trypsin treatment, plated at relatively high densities onto collagen- or polylysine-treated substrates, and maintained in serum-containing media. Under these conditions, which favor glial proliferation, the neurons develop atop the forming glial monolayer. This approach has been a mainstay for physiological studies of hippocampal neurons. Alternatively, cultures can be prepared by plating hippocampal neurons directly onto a feeder layer of glia (Forsyth and Westbrook, 1988; Yamada et al., 1989). When combined with appropriate dissociation methods (Huettner and Baughman, 1986), this approach permits cultures to be prepared from postnatal animals (Jahr and Stevens, 1987; Bekkers and Stevens, 1989; Yamada et al., 1989). This approach is particularly valuable for physiologists because, after birth, the demarcation between CA1 and CA3 regions of the hippocampus can be discerned readily, and the two areas can be dissected and cultured separately. Such cultures have proved remarkably fruitful for physiological studies; when combined with appropriate imaging methods, they even allow measurements at the level of resolution of individual synaptic boutons (Bekkers and Stevens, 1989; Liu and Tsien, 1995).

Recently, Brewer and his colleagues (Brewer and Cotman, 1989; Brewer et al., 1993) have explored new, serum-free culture media that permit the development and survival of CNS neurons in the near-absence of glial cells. Originally developed for the culture of dentate neurons, these media have also been used successfully for

the culture of neurons from many regions of the the brain, including the hippocampus (Brewer 1995; Apperson et al., 1996; Xiang et al., 1996).

Protocol for Preparing Low-Density Hippocampal Cultures

Preparations

COVERSLIPS

Because much of our work uses microscopic techniques, which are difficult to apply to cells grown directly in plastic culture dishes, we plate hippocampal cells onto glass coverslips that have been treated with poly-L-lysine to enhance cell adhesion. The glass and its preparation seem to be quite important for the proper attachment, survival, and maturation of the neurons. For most purposes, we use 18-mm round coverslips (Fisher Scientific, Pittsburgh, PA: 18-mm circles, cat no.12-545-100-1D); for microscopy, we sometimes use coverslips 25 mm in diameter. We specify that coverslips be manufactured from a glass designated "1D," which has been tested and found to support neuronal growth. We also adhere religiously to the following protocol for cleaning and sterilizing coverslips, even though it is quite elaborate. This practice is consistent with our belief in the "black magic" of nerve cell culture: "Don't ask why, it just works." An abridged version of the protocol, together with our typical weekly preparation schedule, appears in box 13.1.

Coverslips are cleaned and sterilized in porcelain racks (Thomas Scientific, Swedesboro, NJ, cat. no. 8542-E40) that hold up to 23 coverslips in such a way that they do not stick together. Coverslips are handled most conveniently with Dumont-style forceps. Place the coverslips in staining racks and rinse them in distilled water to remove dust and residual detergent from the manufacturing process (2 rinses, 10 min each). Transfer the racks to concentrated nitric acid and leave for 18 to 36 h. Next, rinse them in tissue-culture-grade water (five changes over 2 h) and remove excess water, either by tapping the racks against a flat surface or by vacuum aspiration. Then transfer the racks to beakers, cover with aluminum foil, and sterilize with dry heat (225°C for 6 h) in a clean oven. Cool to room temperature.

Box 13.1   Preparation of Materials for Hippocampal Cultures

Preparative Step	Typical Schedule
1. Place coverslips in racks and rinse in water. Clean in concentrated nitric acid for 18–36 h.	Monday
2. Rinse two times for 1 h, then two times for $\frac{1}{2}$ h in milliQ or comparable-grade H_2O. Tap off excess H_2O.	Wednesday
3. Place racks in beakers, cover with foil, and sterilize with dry heat (225°C for 6 h).	Wednesday
4. Place coverslips in 60 mm plastic Petri dishes, five per dish, and apply three small drops of sterile, melted paraffin. They keep the coverslips from resting directly on the glial cells during coculturing. Sterilize by UV irradiation for 30 min.	Thursday
5. Dissolve polylysine (1 mg/ml) in borate buffer and filter-sterilize. Cover each coverslip with polylysine solution (about 6 drops will do) and leave overnight.	Thursday
6. Rinse coverslips with sterile H_2O, two changes, 2 h each.	Friday
7. Remove final rinse and add 4 ml of plating medium. The hippocampal neurons will be plated into these dishes.	Friday
8. The day before you plan to prepare hippocampal cultures, select the glial dishes to be used for coculturing. Remove the medium from these dishes, add 6 ml of maintenance medium, and return to incubator.	Monday
9. Set out cultures (see text and box 13.2)	Tuesday

All succeeding steps must be performed in a laminar flow hood. Transfer the coverslips to 60-mm plastic Petri dishes, five of the 18-mm per dish, or three of the 25-mm, arranged so that the overlap is minimal. Use microbiological dishes (e.g., Falcon no. 1007) rather than tissue culture dishes for this will ensure that the poly-L-lysine solution beads up over the coverslips rather than spreading over the entire dish. (This saves money—substrates are expensive.) To support the coverslips above the glial cells, during cocult
uring, three dots of paraffin (about 0.5 mm high) are placed near the outer edge of each coverslip at an equal distance from each other. Ster-ilize the paraffin (Paraplast embedding medium, Fisher no. 12-646-106) by autoclaving in a suitable bottle, then place the bottle on a hotplate to maintain the temperature between 90° and 110°C. Dip a Pasteur pipette into the hot paraffin until it fills, then touch the pip-ette tip to the coverslip. A small drop will form and harden almost

instantly. The size of the drop can be controlled by holding a finger over the bulb end of the Pasteur pipette. By working rapidly, it is possible to dot two or three coverslips before the paraffin in the pipette hardens. Then place the pipette back in the hot paraffin and continue. The temperature of the paraffin is important—if it is above 110°C, it spreads too thinly, if it is below 90°C, the dots do not adhere well and are likely to float off when they become wet. For safety's sake, sometimes we resterilize the coverslips at this stage by ultraviolet irradiation (30 min, within 6 inches of a 15-W germicidal lamp). Avoid exposing coverslips to ultraviolet light after treatment with poly-L-lysine.

Dissolve poly-L-lysine hydrobromide (MW: 30,000–70,000, Sigma P-2636), 1 mg/ml, in 0.1 M borate buffer (1.24 g boric acid and 1.90 g sodium tetraborate in 400 ml H$_2$O, pH 8.5) and filter-sterilize. The poly-L-lysine solution is freshly prepared for each use; 1 to 2 ml per dish will be needed. Cover each coverslip with poly-L-lysine solution and let stand for 12 to 24 h. When properly cleaned, the coverslips should be hydrophilic so that the poly-L-lysine solution spreads over their surface rather than beading up. Remove poly-L-lysine and rinse coverslips with sterile water (two washes, 2 h each). After the final rinse, add 4 ml of neuronal plating medium (box 13.2) and place the dishes in an incubator (where they can be stored for several days before use). At one time, we routinely allowed the coverslips to dry after the final rinse, so that they could be prepared ahead and stored. We have since concluded that better dendritic development is obtained when medium is applied immediately after rinsing the coverslips with water.

MEDIA

Tissue is dissected and dissociated in Hepes-buffered, calcium- and magnesium-free Hank's balanced salt solution (HBSS). Neurons are plated into serum-containing medium, then transferred to serum-free medium (N2.1) after they have attached to the substrate. Astroglia are cultured in serum-containing medium. Instructions for preparing these media are given in box 13.2.

When cultures are intended for low-light-level fluorescence microscopy, it is important to use mininum essential medium that does not contain phenol red (e.g., Gibco BRL no. 51200-038). Phenol red is endocytosed by the cells and can contribute significantly to fluorescence background and to phototoxicity.

Box 13.2   Media

NEURONAL PLATING MEDIUM

Component and Source	Volume (ml)
Minimum Essential Medium with Earle's salts [Gibco BRL no. 11095-080] (4°C)	430
Pyruvic acid, 100 mM [Sigma no. P-2256] (4°C)	5
Glucose, 20% (4°C)	15
Horse serum [Gibco BRL no. 26050-070 or JRH Biosciences no. 12449-78P] (−20°C)	50

N2.1 NEURONAL MAINTENANCE MEDIUM

Component and Source	Volume (ml)
Minimum Essential Medium with Earle's salts [Gibco BRL no. 11095-080] (4°C)	430
Pyruvic acid, 100 mM [Sigma no. P-2256] (4°C)	5
Glucose, 20% (4°C)	15
Ovalbumin, 1% in MEM [Sigma no. A-5503] (−20°C)	50
N2 supplement (−20°C)	50

N2 SUPPLEMENT

Component and Source	Amount
Insulin, 5 mg/ml in 0.01 N HCl [Sigma no. I-5500] (−20°C)	1 ml
Progesterone [Sigma no. P-0190]. Dissolve at 630 µg/ml in ethanol, then dilute 1:100 in H_2O (−20°C)	1 ml
Putrescine, 16.1 mg/ml [Sigma no. P-7505] (−20°C)	1 ml
Selenium dioxide [Sigma no. S-9379]. Dissolve at 330 µg/ml in H_2O, then dilute 1:100 in H_2O (−20°C)	1 ml
Transferrin, human [Sigma no. T-2252]	100 mg
Minimum Essential Medium with Earle's salts [Gibco BRL no. 11095-080] (4°C)	96 ml

GLIAL MEDIUM

Component and Source	Volume (ml)
Minimum Essential Medium with Earle's salts [Gibco BRL no. 11095-080] (4°C)	430
Glucose, 20% (4°C)	15
Penicillin-streptomycin [Gibco BRL no. 15145-014] (−20°C)	5
Horse serum [Gibco BRL no. 26050-070 or JRH Biosciences no. 12449-78P] (−20°C)	50

Box 13.2 **(continued)**

CMF-HBSS (CALCIUM- AND MAGNESIUM-FREE HANK'S BSS)

Component and Source	Volume (ml)
Hank's balanced salt solution, Ca-Mg-free, 10 × [Gibco BRL no. 14186-012] (4°C)	50
HEPES buffer, 1.0 M, pH 7.3 [Gibco BRL no. 15630-080] (4°C)	5
Penicillin-streptomycin [Gibco BRL no. 15145-014] (−20°C)	5
H_2O	To 500

General Instructions:
Media are prepared from sterile components and stored at 4°C. Except as noted, all stock solutions are prepared in milliQ-grade H_2O and filter-sterilized. They are either refrigerated (4°C) or aliquoted and frozen (−20°C), as indicated.

Astroglial Cell Cultures

OVERVIEW

Primary cultures of type 1 astroglia, prepared from the brains of postnatal rats, are used to support the survival of hippocampal neurons in low-density cultures. Cell suspensions can be plated directly into the dishes that will be used to hold the neuronal coverslips or they can be expanded in T-flasks, harvested, then replated or stored frozen until needed. By allocating 10% to 20% of the cells to dishes (for immediate use) and the rest to flasks (for freezing), a single litter of pups can provide sufficient astroglia to support hundreds of neuronal cultures.

Most laboratories that work with astroglial cells grow their cultures in medium supplemented with fetal bovine serum. In our hands, glial cells proliferate almost as rapidly in horse serum, and the resulting cultures work well in our protocols. Given the huge difference in price, we prefer horse serum.

PREPARING PRIMARY GLIAL CULTURES

Sacrifice 1- to 2-day-old postnatal rat pups by using an approved method of euthanasia. Generally, we use an entire litter of postnatal pups (10–12) for a single glial cell preparation. Decapitate the rat pups, remove the brains, and transfer them to a dish containing HBSS. All subsequent steps should be performed in a laminar flow hood. Under a dissecting microscope, isolate the cerebral hemi-

spheres (figure 13.2) and carefully strip away the meninges with fine forceps. Mince the tissue into small pieces with scissors, then transfer it to a 50-ml centrifuge tube in a final volume of 12 ml of HBSS. Add 1.5 ml each of 2.5% trypsin (Gibco BRL no. 25095-019) and 1% DNAse (Sigma no. DN-25) and incubate at 37°C for 15 min, swirling the mixture periodically. Remove the supernatant containing the dissociated cells and add it to a 50-ml centrifuge tube containing 3 ml of serum (to stop the trypsin activity). To the undissociated tissue remaining in the flask, add additional HBSS and enzyme solutions and incubate for 15 min more. Remove the supernatant, add it to the first supernatant, and filter the combined supernatants through a 72-μm nylon mesh (NITEX 100% polyamide Nylon Fiber, TETKO Inc.) to remove any undissociated tissue. Centrifuge at 1000 rpm for 5 min to pellet the cells, resuspend them in several milliliters of glial medium, and determine the cell density using a hemacytometer.

The cell yield should be on the order of 10 million cells per brain. The yield from one brain is enough to plate 20 to 40 dishes (Falcon no. 3002) or one T75 flask (Falcon no. 3084). Our standard density, which results in confluent monolayers in 10 to 14 days, is 80,000 cells per milliliter. Dilute the cells into a sufficient volume of glial medium to give 4 ml per dish and 25 ml per flask.

PASSAGING AND FREEZING ASTROGLIAL CULTURES
When cells in T-flasks have reached confluence, they must be harvested for replating or freezing. Pour off the medium from the flask and wash the cell sheet with HBSS. Add 10 ml trypsin/EDTA (Gibco no. 25300-047) and incubate at 37°C for 5 min. Tap the flask gently, add 1 ml of serum, and stand the flask upright to allow the cells to slide to the bottom. Then pipette the suspension into a 15-ml centrifuge tube and centrifuge at 1000 rpm for 5 min. Pour off the supernatant and resuspend the cell pellet in glial medium. For plating directly into dishes, dilute the cells from one T-flask into sufficient glial medium to plate 30 to 40 dishes (4 ml per 60-mm tissue-culture dish). We do not passage the glial cultures further because of concern about the potential for alteration of cell phenotypes.

Alternatively, trypsinized glial cells can be frozen and stored for future use. For freezing, resuspend the cell pellet from each T75 flask in 1.5 ml of glial medium. Gently pipette the cell suspension into a cryogenic vial (Corning cat. no. 25702). Add dimethylsulfoxide to 10%, pipetting it gently on top of the cell suspension so

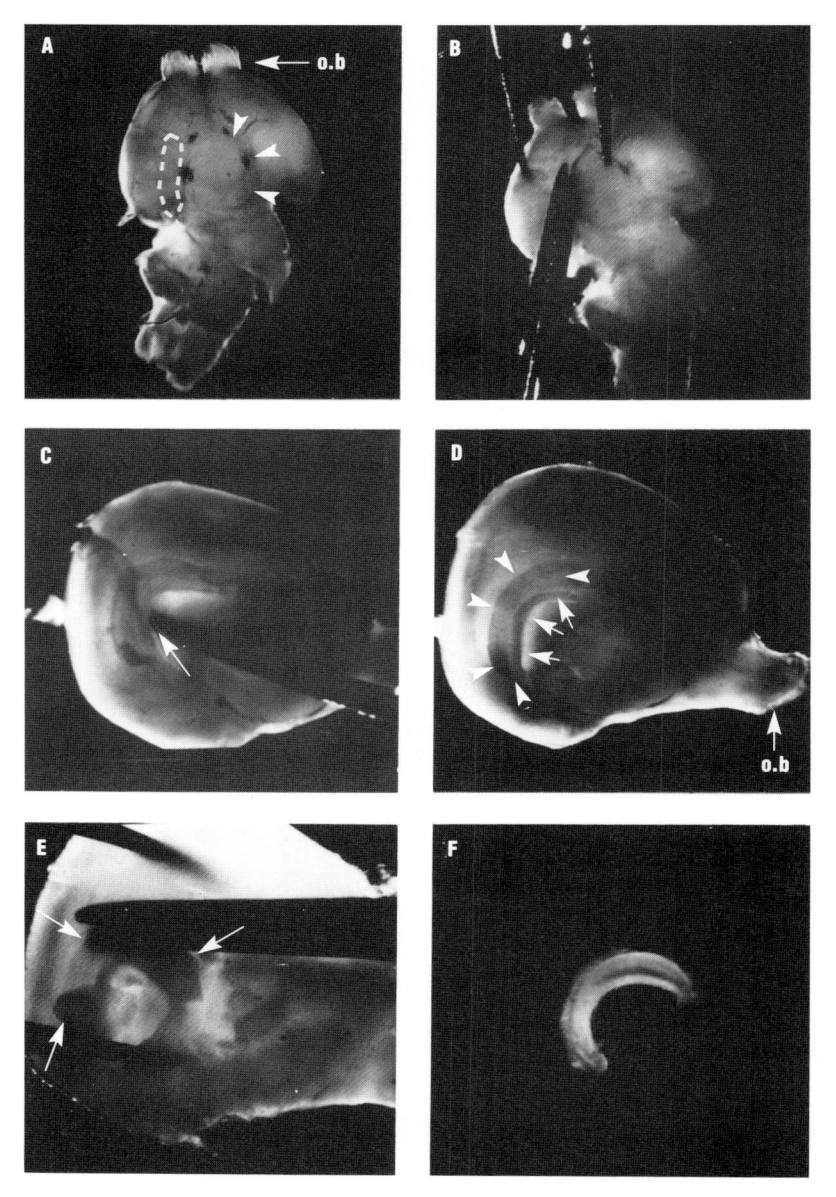

Figure 13.2 Dissection of the embryonic hippocampus. (*A*) Ventral aspect of the brain of an E18 fetus, with olfactory bulbs (o.b.) at the top. Arrowheads demarcate the junction between the diencephalon and the left cerebral hemisphere. The dotted line indicates the approximate position of the right hippocampus projected onto the ventral surface of the hemisphere. (*B*) Removal of the right cerebral hemisphere. Forceps are used to stabilize the brain; beginning posteriorly, fine scissors separate the hemisphere from the diencephalon. (*C*) Removal of the meninges from the left hippocampus. The left hemisphere is viewed from the midline, with anterior to the right. A pair of forceps (just out of view to the left) holds the meninges (black arrow), which have been removed from the rostral half of the hippocampus. The tip of another pair of forceps

that it mixes by diffusion. Place the vials in a styrofoam container (to ensure that the cells freeze slowly) and leave it in a −80°C freezer until frozen. Then transfer the vials to liquid nitrogen for long-term storage.

To thaw frozen cells, place the vial in a 37°C water bath just long enough to thaw the contents. Transfer the cell suspension to a 15-ml centrifuge tube that contains 1 ml of serum. Centrifuge for 6 min at 800 to 1000 rpm and resuspend the cells as described earlier.

MAINTAINING GLIAL CULTURES

When you first examine primary glial cultures the day after plating you are likely to think that the procedure did not work. You will see a huge amount of debris from the cells that did not survive and a woefully small number of flattened cells attached to the substrate. Don't despair! Those few glial cells will generate the culture you're hoping for.

Feed the cultures the day after plating (to remove most of this debris), then every 3 to 4 days (replacing the medium completely). The cultures generally reach confluence within 10 to 14 days after plating. We start using them for coculture when they reach at least 50% confluence, and we try to use them within a few days of the time they become confluent. One day before you plan to prepare hippocampal cultures, select glial dishes to be used for coculturing. Remove the medium from these dishes, add 6 ml of neuronal maintenance medium (N2.1), and return them to the incubator.

Some preparations of glial cells contain contaminating macrophages (or microglia). These may be recognized as round, phase-bright, loosely attached cells resting atop the glial monolayer. This problem is serious, because these cells release compounds that are highly neurotoxic. Once more than a few macrophages appear, they will continue to proliferate until the cultures become unsuitable for coculturing. If macrophages appear in flask cultures, usually they

(white arrow) passes beneath the fimbria into the lateral ventricle. (*D*) The left hemisphere after removal of the meninges. Arrowheads indicate the boundary between the hippocampus and the adjoining cortex. Small arrows mark the free edge of the hippocampus. (*E*) Removal of the left hippocampus. Forceps stabilize the hemisphere (arrows), while fine scissors cut around the convex margin of the hippocampus (arrows). (*F*) The left hippocampus after it has been removed. The fimbria appears as a light band along the concave aspect of the hippocampus.

can be dislodged by shaking the flask and can be removed by washing. If macrophages appear in cultures growing in dishes, not much can be done. Just throw them away and start over.

Setting out the Neuronal Cultures

TIMED PREGNANT RATS AND STAGING OF EMBRYOS
We obtain fetuses at embryonic day 18 (E18) from timed pregnant Sprague-Dawley rats (Taconic Farms, Germantown, NY). According to the convention we use, the day of sperm positivity is considered embryonic day 0 (E0), but be aware that some investigators, and some suppliers, consider this day 1; by their reckoning, we use animals at E19. To confirm the staging, we routinely record the length of the fetuses, measured from crown to rump. At E18, fetuses are approximately 25 mm long. Although this is the preferred age—and we believe it is important to be as consistent as possible in this regard—we have prepared cultures from animals ranging in length from 20 to 35 mm (roughly from E17 to E20) when fetuses of the desired age were unavailable. Expect an average of 10 to 12 fetuses per animal.

DISSECTION OF THE HIPPOCAMPUS
To minimize the time between sacrificing the animal and placing the cells in culture, it is important to be certain that all needed materials are ready before starting (box 13.3). With practice, it should be possible to complete the entire procedure in 1.5 to 2 h.

Once the brain has been removed from the skull, it must be immersed in HBSS at all times to prevent the tissue from drying. During the dissection, the brain is visualized best if placed in a clear dish containing a layer of Sylgard resin so that it can be illuminated from below. If possible, we suggest this approach, at least until you become familiar with the dissection. However, for convenience, we often dissect in small dishes partially filled with paraffin, using illumination from above. Such dishes have a soft surface, a slight depression in the center that helps to keep the brain in one position, and can be discarded after use. They are prepared from 35-mm plastic Petri dishes, which are filled about half-way with sterile melted paraffin and allowed to cool in a laminar flow hood. You can also use a plastic Petri dish containing sev-

Box 13.3   Dissection and Culture of Hippocampal Neurons

1. Euthanize the pregnant rat with halothane or other approved anesthetic, remove uterus, and place in a sterile Petri dish.
   The remaining steps are performed in a laminar flow hood.
2. Measure fetal length to confirm the embryonic age. The ideal stage is 18 days of gestation, when the fetus is about 25 mm from crown to rump.
3. Decapitate fetuses, dissect out the brains, and place them in calcium- and magnesium-free BSS.
4. Remove the hippocampi under a dissecting microscope. Strip away the meninges, then collect the dissected hippocampi in a small Petri dish in BSS.
5. Place all the hippocampi from one litter in a 15-ml centrifuge tube. Bring the total volume to 4.5 ml with BSS, then add 0.5 ml of 2.5% trypsin. Incubate at 37°C for 15 min.
6. Remove trypsin, add 5 ml of BSS, and let stand for 5 min. Repeat this step twice more, finally bringing the volume to 3–5 ml.
7. Dissociate the cells by pipetting up and down, first in a normal Pasteur pipette, then in a pipette with a tip fire-polished to nearly half the normal diameter. Continue pipetting until no chunks of tissue remain.
8. Determine the density of cells in a hemacytometer. The yield should be ~500,000 cells per hippocampus. Also determine the fraction of viable, trypan blue–excluding cells.
9. Add the desired number of viable cells to each of the dishes containing the polylysine-treated coverslips in MEM with 10% horse serum. Our standard plating density is 150,000 cells per 60-mm plastic Petri dish.
10. After 3–4 h, transfer the coverslips, with neurons attached, to dishes containing glial cells in maintenance medium. Turn the coverslips over so the neurons are facing down, toward the glial cells.
11. To reduce glial proliferation, add Ara-C (5×10^{-6} M) after 2–3 days.
12. Once a week, remove ~2 ml of medium and replace it with fresh maintenance medium.

eral drops of HBSS, as the most confident of the authors does, but any miscue will damage the tips of the forceps.

Euthanize the pregnant rat with halothane, carbon dioxide, or other approved means. Wipe the abdomen with 70% ethanol before making any incisions. To minimize possible contamination from the fur or skin, first cut through the skin alone and lay it back, then rinse the instruments with 70% ethanol and cut through the abdominal wall. Remove the two horns of the uterus and place them in a sterile Petri dish. The remaining steps should be carried out in a laminar flow hood.

Remove the fetuses from the uterus, decapitate them, and transfer the heads to a Petri dish containing HBSS prewarmed to 37°C.

Remove the brains as follows. Grasp the head firmly with a pair of Dumont-style forceps by inserting the tips of the forceps deeply into the orbits. With fine scissors, make a midline incision through the skin and skull, beginning at the level of the decapitation and continuing forward to the orbits. Then, with a second pair of forceps, reflect these tissues away to each side so that the entire cortex is revealed. Remove the brain by inserting the flat face of the forceps beneath the olfactory bulbs and working them caudally, separating the nerve connections that link the brain to the skull. Pick the brain up by the brainstem and transfer it to the dissecting dish.

The hippocampi are C-shaped structures on the medial aspect of the cerebral hemispheres and are removed under a dissecting microscope at 10 to 15× magnification (see figure 13.2). For this procedure, we use very fine, spring scissors (Castro-Viejo style with angled blades) and two Dumont-style forceps (no. 5). Begin by separating the cerebral hemispheres from the diencephalon and brainstem (see figure 13.2A,B). With the basal aspect of the brain facing up, cut along the boundary between the diencephalon and the cerebral hemisphere (roughly marked by the position of the blood vessels forming the circle of Willis). Place one blade of the scissors into the space between the hemisphere and diencephalon at the posterior pole, then cut forward and medially around the diencephalon (see figure 13.2B). Use a pair of forceps to spread the hemisphere away from the diencephalon, so that you can see the position of the hippocampus on the medial aspect of the hemisphere as you cut. Being careful not to damage the hippocampus, separate the hemisphere completely from the diencephalon. Repeat this procedure to remove the other hemisphere, then discard the brainstem and diencephalon.

Lay each hemisphere on its side, with the medial aspect facing up and the ventral surface toward you (see figure 13.2C). For orientation, the anterior pole of the hemisphere can be identified by the olfactory bulb. When viewed from the midline, the hippocampus forms a C in the left hemisphere and a reversed C in the right hemisphere. The outer, convex border of the hippocampus, which is continuous with adjoining regions of the cortex, often is delineated by blood vessels that run along the hippocampal fissure. The inner border, which is formed by the fiber tract called the *fimbria*, is free. The lateral ventricle lies immediately behind the hippocampus. Sometimes, when the hemispheres are separated, a chunk of thalamus remains attached, covering and obscuring the

hippocampus. Gently remove it with forceps to reveal the under-lying hippocampus.

The meninges and choroid plexus should be removed next (see figure 13.2C,D). The meninges form a thin layer covering the sur-face of the brain and can be recognized by the blood vessels that they contain. The choroid plexus, which also is highly vascular-ized, lies within the ventricle, attaching to the meninges at the fimbrial edge of the hippocampus. Stabilize the hemisphere with one pair of forceps, grasp a bit of the meninges with the other, and tug gently (see figure 13.2C). By beginning at one end of the hippo-campus, usually it is possible to pull away the meninges overlying the hippocampus as a single sheet. This must be done gently, or traction on the meninges will tear the underlying hippocampus, making its removal more difficult.

Once the meninges have been removed, the hippocampus can be cut out (see figure 13.2E). Because the inner edge of the hippo-campus is free and the lateral ventricle lies on its lateral aspect, only the outer edge and the anterior and posterior ends of the hip-pocampus have to be cut away from adjoining tissue. We find it easier to make these cuts if the scissors are held in one location, while the hemisphere is "steered" with the forceps to bring the hippocampus into the appropriate position for each cut. When the hippocampus has been cut free (see figure 13.2F), lift it with the tip of the closed scissors or forceps and transfer it to a dish containing HBSS.

DISSOCIATION AND PLATING

When all the needed hippocampi have been removed, use a Pasteur pipette to transfer them to a 15-ml conical centrifuge tube. Add more HBSS to bring the volume to 4.5 ml, then add 0.5 ml of 2.5% trypsin (Gibco BRL no. 25095-019) and tap the tube to mix. In-cubate the hippocampi with trypsin for 15 min in a water bath at 37°C. The hippocampi will settle to the bottom of the tube. After the incubation, gently pipette off the trypsin solution, add 5 ml of HBSS, shake the tube to mix, and let stand for 5 min. Repeat this twice more, to allow residual trypsin to diffuse from the tissue. Bring the final volume to 5 ml with HBSS (proportionately less if fewer than 10 fetuses have been used). Dissociate the tissue by pipetting vigorously up and down, first with a regular Pasteur pip-ette, then with a pipette with a tip that has been fire-polished to approximately half the normal diameter (i.e., to a little less than

1 mm). A pipette with a tip too small will damage the cells. To prevent foaming, push the HBSS out against the side of the centrifuge tube rather than into the liquid at the bottom. Pipette only as long as is necessary to obtain a homogeneous solution with no obvious particles of tissue remaining (usually about 15–20 times).

Determine the density of cells by using a hemacytometer. The yield should be some 500,000 cells per hippocampus, although this may vary depending on the strain of rat used (Boss et al., 1987b). Determine the fraction of viable, trypan blue–excluding cells. We prepare a stock solution of 0.8% trypan blue in 0.9% NaCl. This mix then is diluted 1:9 with HBSS, mixed 1:1 with a few drops of the cell suspension, and allowed to stand for 4 min before counting the fraction of dye-excluding cells. If everything has gone well, 85% to 95% of the cells should exclude trypan blue. Add the desired number of viable cells to each of the dishes containing the polylysine-treated coverslips in plating medium. Our standard plating density if 50,000 to 150,000 cells per 60-mm plastic Petri dish ($\sim$1500–5000 cells/cm^2), but cultures can be prepared at much lower and higher plating densities (Fletcher et al., 1994). Plating must be done rapidly to prevent the pH of the medium from becoming basic, which is highly deleterious to the cells. Remove a few dishes from the incubator at a time, add the appropriate volume of cells to each with a micropipette, and swirl the dishes to disperse the cells evenly. If the coverslips have become overlapped, separate them with forceps before returning the dishes to the incubator.

After 2 to 4 h, examine the cultures with an inverted microscope to ensure that most of the neurons have attached to the coverslips, then transfer the coverslips to the dishes containing glial cells in N2.1 medium. As the coverslips are transferred, turn them over so that the neuronal side, with the paraffin dots, is facing the glial cells.

FEEDING AND MAINTENANCE OF NEURONAL CULTURES
Cultures are maintained at 37°C in an atmosphere containing 5% CO_2. We routinely feed cultures once a week. When feeding, never change the culture medium completely; the neurons depend on a "conditioning" of the medium by glial cells for their long-term survival. We replace one-third of the medium at each feeding. To reduce glial proliferation, we usually add cytosine arabinoside

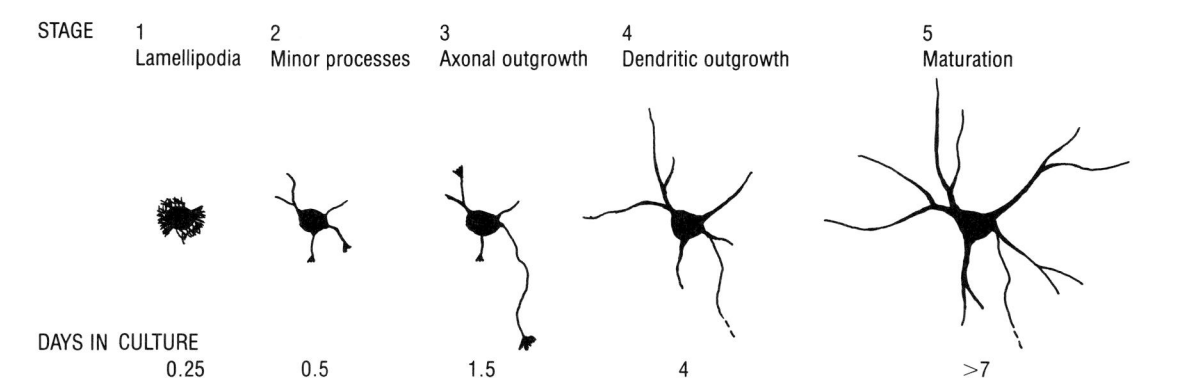

STAGE

1	2	3	4	5
Lamellipodia	Minor processes	Axonal outgrowth	Dendritic outgrowth	Maturation

DAYS IN CULTURE

| 0.25 | 0.5 | 1.5 | 4 | >7 |

Figure 13.3 Stages in the development of hippocampal neurons in culture. Approximate times for each stage of development are shown at the bottom. (Reproduced with permission from Dotti et al., 1988.)

(1-beta-D-arabinofuranosylcytosine) to the cultures 3 days after plating (5×10^{-6} M final concentration; Calbiochem cat. no. 251010).

Characterization of Cultures Prepared by this Method

We have emphasized that one of the unique features of our culture system is that it enables neurons to be grown at very low cell densities, even in the absence of intercellular contacts. By following individual cells plated at low density with time-lapse video microcopy and sequential photography, we have identified characteristic morphological changes that occur in the development of hippocampal neurons in culture (Dotti et al., 1988; Goslin and Banker, 1990). For convenience, we have divided the events of development into five stages, as summarized in figure 13.3. Not every cell follows this pattern of development, but this pattern is typical of those cells that come most closely to resemble hippocampal neurons in situ.

In stage 1, shortly after the cells have attached to the substratum, they become surrounded by flattened, motile lamellipodia. In stage 2, with time, the lamellipodia condense at several discrete sites along the cell's circumference; from these sites short, "minor" processes emerge. Minor processes, typically four to six in number, are roughly equal in length (20–30 µm), giving the cells a symmetrical appearance. They are highly dynamic, extending and retracting for short distances over a period of 12 to 24 h. Cells at this stage appear to be unpolarized; we have been unable to identify morphological,

electron-microscopic, or immunocytochemical characteristics that predict which of a cell's processes will become the axon. At stage 3, polarity first becomes evident when one of the minor processes begins to elongate continuously without retraction until it becomes much longer than the other processes. At this stage, the axon can be distinguished from the other processes on ultrastructural and immunocytochemical grounds (Goslin and Banker, 1990; Goslin et al., 1990; Deitch and Banker, 1993; Mandell and Banker, 1996). A representative stage 3 neuron with a single axon and several minor processes is shown in figure 13.4A. In a typical field from a culture at this age, one can identify cells at both stage 2 and stage 3 of development (see figure 13.4B). Occasional cells with multiple axons also are observed. A small number of nonneuronal cells also are present. Usually they have a flattened appearance but many form processes (see figure 13.4B). Throughout stage 3, the axon continues to grow at a rapid rate, but the remaining minor processes undergo little net elongation. In stage 4, after 2 to 4 days in culture, the remaining minor processes begin to elongate and to acquire the taper and branching pattern characteristic of dendrites. It is at this stage that presynaptic specializations first form on the cell body and dendrites (Fletcher et al., 1994) and the microtubule organization typical of mature dendrites first arises (Baas et al., 1989).

With subsequent development, the density of the axonal network increases, dendritic arbors become more elaborate and highly branched, synaptic contacts develop in large numbers, dendritic spines appear, and spontaneous electrical activity propagates throughout the neuronal network. These aspects of development reflect the continuation of processes begun at earlier stages of development. However, in contrast to the events of stages 1 to 4, which appear to be largely endogenously determined, many of these later aspects of neuronal maturation are highly dependent on cell interactions. To emphasize this important difference, we refer to this later period of development as stage 5.

An example of a cell at stage 5 of development is shown in figure 13.4C. The increase in the size of the cell body and in the diameter of the dendritic processes that occur in culture is apparent (compared with the 1-day-old cell in figure 13.4A photographed at the same magnification). The density of the axonal network that develops in culture is illustrated best at lower magnification (see figure 13.4D; compare with 1-day-old culture at the same plating density and magnification illustrated in figure 13.4B). In such cultures,

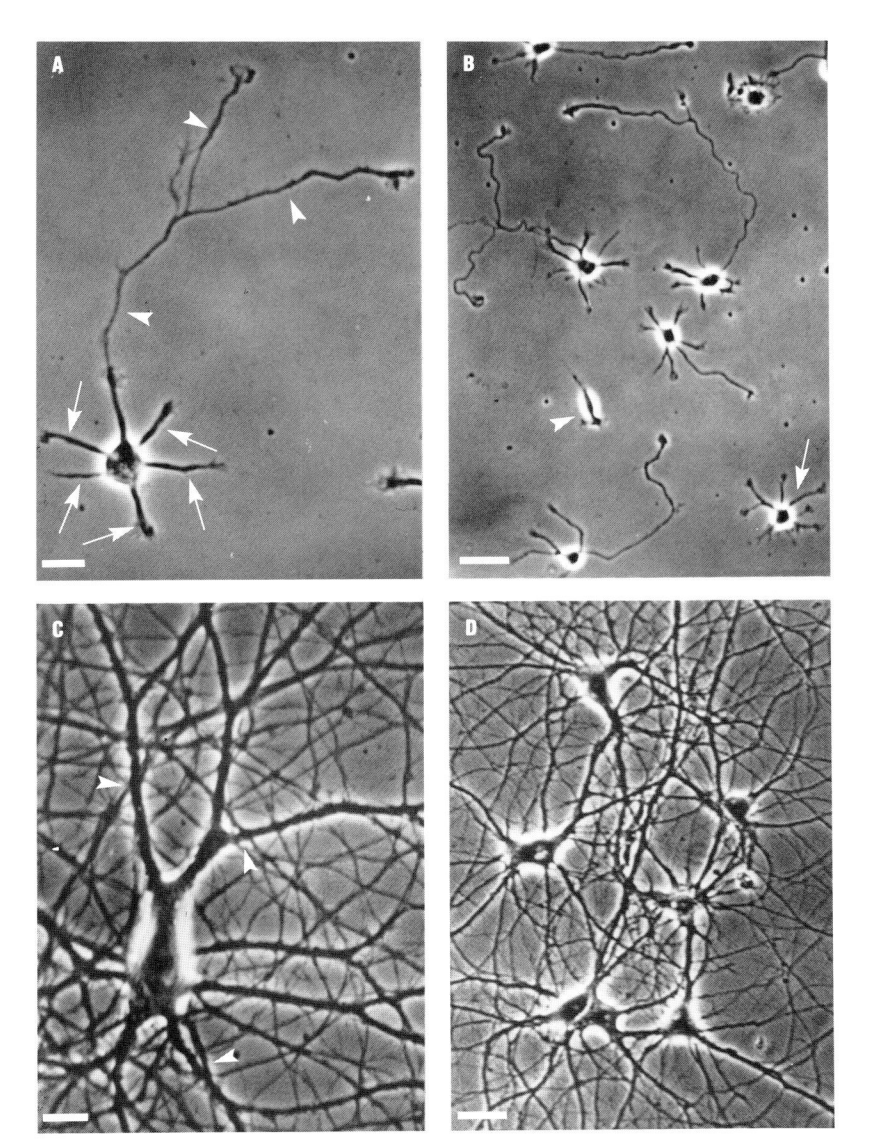

Figure 13.4 Representative examples of hippocampal neurons at various stages of development. (*A, B*) After 27 h in culture, most cells are at stage 3 of development; they have a single axon (arrowhead in *A*) and several minor processes (arrows in *A*) which later will become dendrites. Some stage-2 cells still are present (arrow in *B*), and occasional nonneuronal cells can be recognized (arrowheads in *B*). (*C, D*) After 4 weeks in culture, the increase in cell size and the complexity of the neuronal network are apparent. Arrows (*C*) indicate some of the prominent dendrites that emerge from this cell. Note that *A* and *C*, and *B* and *D*, are at identical magnifications. Scale bars: *A, C*, 10 μm; *B, D*, 50 μm.

dendrites can be identified readily as they emerge from the cell body because of their large diameter, but the thinner, distal portions of the dendrites become lost within the neuronal network, as does the cell's axon. In addition, axons frequently course along the dendrites and, by light microscopy, such axons cannot be distinguished from the underlying dendrites. These features can be resolved by intracellular injection of a fluorescent dye, such as Lucifer yellow, or by inducing the expression of a protein tagged with green fluorescent protein in a small fraction of the cells.

As an alternative, the development of immunocytochemical markers that selectively stain axons or dendrites has been a particularly important advance for identifying processes in cell culture and for studying their development. A list of the antibodies that we have found particularly useful for this purpose is presented in table 13.1. It is important to emphasize that these immunocytochemical markers do not necessarily exhibit their characteristic localization early in development. MAP2, for instance, is initially present throughout the cell (Caceres et al., 1986), becoming restricted to the dendrites only during stage 4 (figure 13.5); GAP-43 becomes preferentially distributed to the axonal domain at stage 3, but significant amounts remain in the processes that will become dendrites at stage 4 (Goslin et al., 1990). Experimental studies based on viral expression of test proteins indicate that the efficiency of sorting integral membrane proteins reaches mature levels only toward the end of the first week in culture (Jareb and Banker, 1995 and unpublished observations).

The presence of the machinery for protein synthesis in dendrites—but not in axons—offers an alternative and complementary method for distinguishing dendrites from axons and assessing their differentiation. Dendrites can be labeled by incubating cells with ^{3}H-uridine and allowing time for the labeled RNA to be transported throughout the dendritic tree, then localizing the label autoradiographically (Banker and Cowan, 1979; Davis et al., 1987, 1990). In situ hybridization can be used to detect dendritic rRNA or specific dendritic mRNAs (Kleiman et al., 1993a,b), and antibodies can be used to detect specific proteins that function in protein synthesis (Tiedge and Brosius, 1996). Other approaches that have been used to characterize axons and dendrites in hippocampal cultures have been reviewed elsewhere (Banker and Waxman, 1988; Craig and Banker, 1994).

Table 13.1   Useful Antibodies for Characterizing Hippocampal Cultures

ANTIGEN	LOCALIZATION	PROTEIN TYPE	ANTIBODY AND SOURCE
Neuron-specific tubulin isoform	All neuronal processes	Cytoskeletal	mAb TuJ1 (recognizes class III β-tubulin; Berkeley Antibody Co., Richmond, CA)
Tau	Axons	Cytoskeletal	mAb tau-1 (recognizes a dephospho-epitope; Boehringer Mannheim Indianapolis, IN)
GAP-43	Axons	Membrane-associated	mAb 9-1E12 (Boehringer Mannheim)
MAP2	Dendrites	Cytoskeletal	mAb AP20 (Sigma Chemical Co., St. Louis, MO)
Synaptic vesicles	Presynaptic specializations	Integral membrane	mAb SY-38 (antisynaptophysin; Boehringer-Mannheim)
GABA-A receptors	Postsynaptic specializations	Integral membrane	mAb bd17 (recognizes β2/3 subunit; Boehringer Mannheim)
Glutamate receptors	Postsynaptic specializations	Integral membrane	Rabbit anti-gluR1 (Chemicon, Temecula, CA) mAb 54.1 (anti-NMDAR1; Pharmingen, San Diego, CA)

Troubleshooting

Some All-Too-Familiar Problems

Even though we have used this protocol for several years and try to follow it religiously, we still suffer through periods in which cell growth is inconsistent. The problems we have encountered most frequently fall into three categories: poor cell survival, excessive fasciculation of processes, and abnormal development.

Poor cell survival is a self-evident problem. When things are going well, hippocampal neurons survive and remain healthy for 4 to 6 weeks under the culture conditions described. Over the first 2 to 3 weeks, cell death and process degeneration are slight. If most

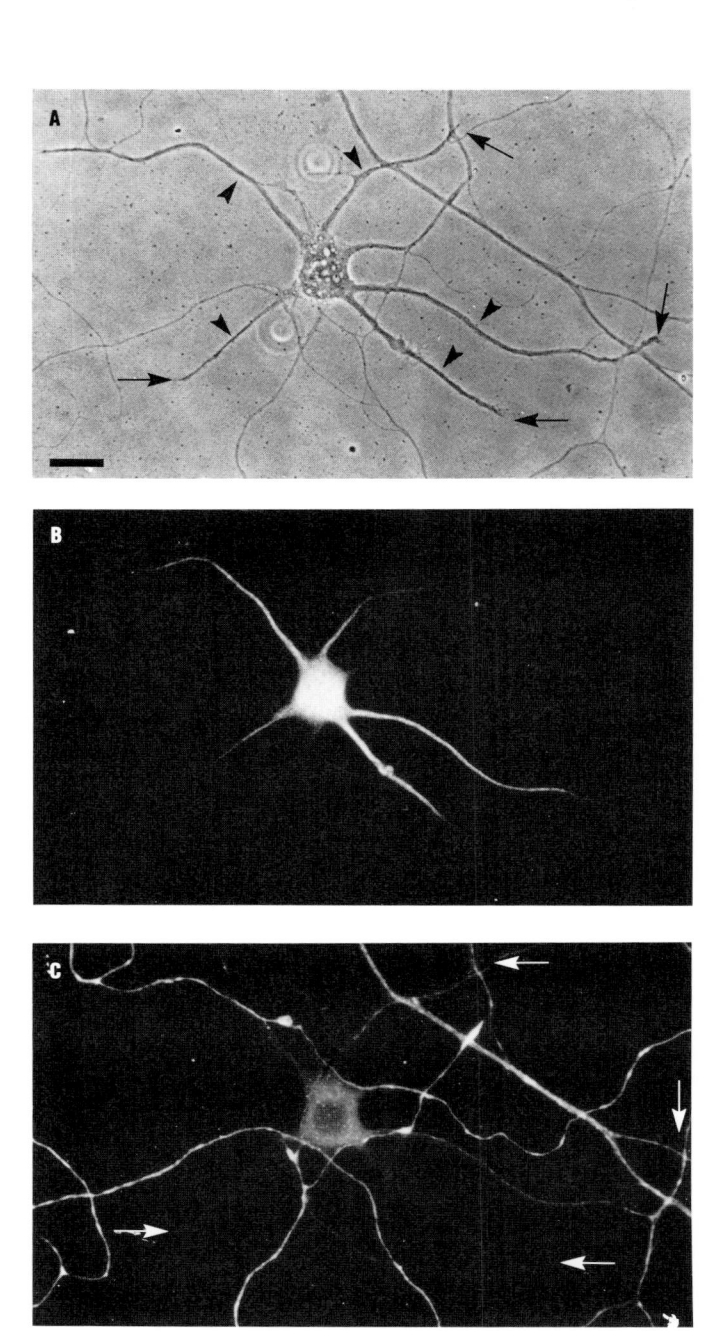

Figure 13.5 Simultaneous localization of MAP2 and GAP-43 in an 8-day-old hippocampal neuron. (A) Phase-contrast micrograph showing the five dendrites arising from this cell (arrowheads), four of which terminate in obvious growth cones (arrows). (B) MAP2 immunostaining is present throughout the dendrites, ending just proximal to the growth cones. (C) GAP-43 immunostaining is present throughout the axons that traverse the field but is absent from the dendrites and their growth cones. Scale bar: 15 μm. (Reprinted with permission from Goslin et al. 1988. Development of Neuronal Polarity. Nature 336: 672–674. Copyright © 1988 Macmillan Magazines Ltd.)

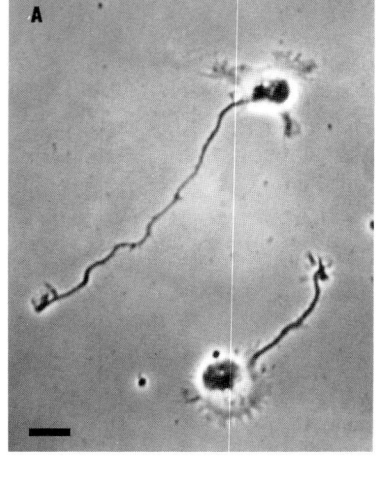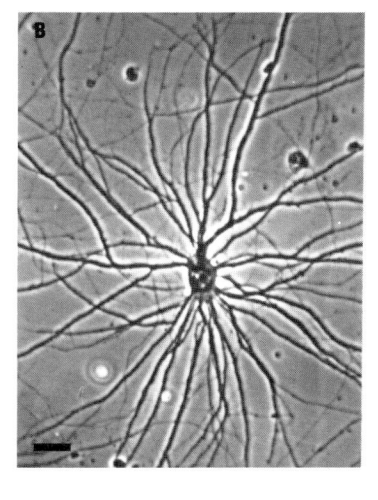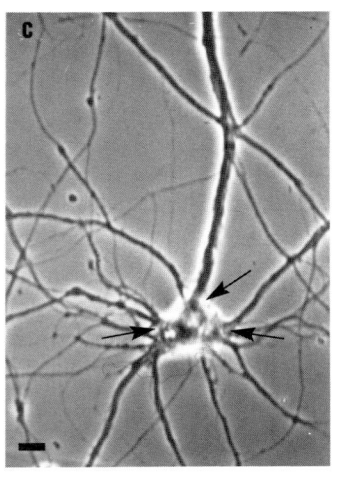

Figure 13.6 Examples of problems in culturing hippocampal neurons. (*A*) After 1 day in culture, some cells fail to extend minor processes and continue to be surrounded by flattened lamellipodia. The axon emerges directly from the cell body rather than elongating from a minor process. (*B*) Such cells later develop a large number of unbranched, poorly differentiated dendrites. The cell shown was cultured on an Aclar substrate for 3 weeks. (*C*) An example of a cell at 22 days in culture, showing the fasciculation that can occur. The dendritic taper normally observed is not apparent because dendrites are ensheathed by bundles of axons (arrows). The network of axons appears sparse because of the extensive fasciculation (compare with figure 13.4D). Scale bars: *A, C,* 10 μm; *B,* 25 μm.

cells do not survive for at least this long, something is wrong and must be corrected.

Another problem concerns fasciculation of processes. As cultures mature and the network of processes between cells becomes more extensive, some fasciculation inevitably occurs; an increasing proportion of axons tend to run along the surfaces of dendrites or of other axons rather than as individual processes attached directly to the substrate. In some culture preparations, this fasciculation occurs early in development and is exaggerated (figure 13.6C). In extreme cases, the cell bodies become clumped together, and thick, straight ropes of processes run between them. Presumably, fasciculation to this degree reflects a reduction in the adhesion of processes to the culture substrate. As one might expect, cells in such cultures frequently become detached or damaged during routine manipulations, such as fixation for microscopy.

Other problems, such as retarded or inconsistent development, are more subtle and potentially more troublesome for the beginner, who is less likely to detect them. Sometimes early development

seems retarded; 3-day-old cultures have cells that, judging from the lengths of their axons, one normally would find in a 1-day-old culture. We have been plagued also at times with cells whose pattern of dendritic development is distinctly abnormal: cells that develop an excessive number (more than a dozen) of radially oriented dendrites that are thin, of relatively uniform diameter, and usually unbranched (see figure 13.6). Often, the somata of such cells are extended and flattened, and their processes stain only weakly with antibodies against MAP2 and transport RNA poorly. We do not necessarily discard all abnormal cultures, but we are very cautious about interpreting experiments if we have concerns for the overall health of the cultures.

Possible Causes

In the face of a series of unhealthy cultures, any uncontrolled variation in the protocol must be suspect. To make matters worse, several problems can occur simultaneously. Nevertheless, some factors are more likely to be sources of poor cultures than are others: among these are the culture substrate, the glial cells used for coculturing, and the medium.

SUBSTRATE

In our experience, variability in the culture substrate is the most common cause of several of the problems that we have described, particularly fasciculation. The actual components that form the substrate for growth in our cultures are not known. Adsorption of substances from the serum onto the poly-L-lysine-treated substrate undoubtedly occurs and is an important determinant of subsequent neuronal development; the substrate may be modified further by adsorption of materials secreted by neurons or glial cells. Until the relevant substances have been identified and can be used in a controlled fashion, some variation in the characteristics of the substrate is inevitable. Thus, consistency in the preparation of coverslips is essential. We have found that seemingly minor changes in our standard protocol for cleaning and sterilization of glass coverslips can have dramatic effects on the cultures—rarely of a beneficial nature. We have observed also that coverslips obtained from different sources can differ considerably in their ability to support neuronal development and maturation. Some 5 years ago, the manufacturer of most of the coverslips sold under various brand names in

the United States began to purchase glass from an American rather than a German source. Several laboratories suddenly discovered that their apparently healthy neurons unexpectedly began to fasciculate and lift off the substrate after only a few days in culture. Coverslips prepared from the original, German glass are available again, but manufacturers have been reported to change their formulations periodically, so that sampling coverslips from several sources may be beneficial if problems are suspected. Falcon tissue-culture plastic dishes provide a consistently good substrate for the growth of hippocampal cells, when treated with poly-L-lysine according to the same protocol used for coverslips. They may provide a useful test substrate when problems with the preparation of glass coverslips are suspected.

Finally, it may be worth noting that substrates that minimize the problem of process fasciculation are not necessarily favorable for dendritic maturation. For example, polylysine-treated plastic coverslips cut from a fluorocarbon film (ACLAR 33C, Allied Chemical) are highly adhesive and foster vigorous axonal outgrowth, but dendritic development is consistently abnormal (as described in the preceding section).

ASTROGLIAL CULTURES

At the low cell densities we use, cultured hippocampal neurons survive and develop normally for only a few days in the absence of glial cells. Unfortunately, the factors produced by glia that are critical for the survival of hippocampal cultures are not known, nor is it understood how the culture environment affects their production. Because the glial cultures are comparatively rugged and easy to grow, one tends to overlook them as a source of variation that can contribute to culture problems. Contamination of glial cultures by macrophages or microglia is an obvious concern because they produce factors that are neurotoxic (see above, Astroglial Cell Cultures). Because batches of astrocytes may differ also in their ability to support neuronal cultures, we attempt to use astrocyte cultures at a consistent stage in their development, and we have come to prefer younger cultures before they have reached confluence.

Implicit in this discussion is the assumption that astrocytes release trophic substances into the culture medium. However, we have not found it possible to obtain good long-term survival of hippocampal neurons by using astrocyte-conditioned medium rather than the coculture approach. Because serum-containing

medium conditioned by astrocytes can support the growth of hippocampal neurons for at least 2 weeks in culture (Banker, 1980), it is possible that the production or stability of neurotrophins is reduced in the serum-free medium we now use. On the other hand, several other factors may contribute to the success of the sandwich technique. These might include neuronal stimulation of the glial production of neurotrophins, concentration of neuronally produced trophic substances in the small volume beneath the coverslip, uptake and metabolism of toxic substances by glial cells, production by glial cells of intermediary metabolites required by neurons, or reduction in oxygen tension (e.g., Selak et al., 1985b; Walicke et al., 1986b; Brewer and Cotman, 1989).

MEDIA

Although horse serum is present only during the period of cell attachment, we have had poor cultures that could be attributed to inadequate lots of serum or to serum that had deteriorated after prolonged storage. To avoid this problem, we routinely screen new lots of serum, scoring the percentage of cell attachment within an hour or so of plating. Because the culture medium itself lacks serum, variations in its composition should be minimal. Aside from frank errors in preparation, we have not experienced culture problems that could be attributed to culture medium. But don't ignore this possibility—mistakes do happen. We can confirm personally that glutamine is important for cell growth and can guarantee that medium mistakenly prepared with serum albumin instead of ovalbumin, especially serum albumin that has been stored so long it may contain traces of oxidized lipids, can make you old before your time.

Applications

Low-density cultures from the hippocampus offer a useful model system for cell biological studies of CNS neurons. Many of the questions that have motivated our work concern the development and maintenance of neuronal polarity. How do the structural and functional differences between axons and dendrites arise (Dotti et al., 1988; Goslin and Banker, 1989)? What cellular mechanisms underlie the selective sorting of proteins to axonal or dendritic domains (Dotti and Simons, 1990)? Much of this work, which has occupied us for more than a decade, has been reviewed recently

(Craig and Banker, 1994; Futerman and Banker, 1996; see also Cid-Arregui et al., 1995; Sharp et al., 1995).

More recently, it has become apparent that hippocampal cultures offer a promising model for studying the development and regulation of CNS synapses. Fletcher et al. (1991) demonstrated that antibodies directed against synaptic vesicle proteins offer a convenient means to visualize the distribution of presynaptic specializations on cultured hippocampal neurons and to monitor their development. They found that synapses could be detected first after 3 to 4 days in culture, near the time at which dendrites begin to mature but well after the first cell-cell contacts. By analyzing heterochronic cocultures, prepared by adding freshly dissociated neurons to cultures that had been allowed to mature for several days, Fletcher et al. (1994) found that newly formed axons that contact mature dendrites are capable of forming presynaptic specializations almost immediately. In contrast, the cell bodies and dendrites of hippocampal neurons are not capable of inducing the formation of presynaptic specializations until they reach a critical stage of maturation, which requires several days in culture.

Depolarization of hippocampal cultures evokes vesicle release at presynaptic terminals, which has permitted an analysis of exo- and endocytosis using imaging techniques. Active terminals can be labeled with lipophilic dyes such as FM1-43 (Ryan et al., 1993; 1996; Ryan and Smith, 1995) or with labeled antibody fragments directed against domains of synaptic vesicle proteins that become exposed to the external surface only after vesicle fusion (Kraszewski et al., 1995; Malgaroli et al., 1995). This approach has allowed detailed analysis of the dynamics of vesicle use and recycling (Ryan and Smith, 1995; Ryan et al., 1996) and visualization of individual boutons exhibiting long-term potentiation and has provided clues to the molecular machinery that mediates presynaptic endocytosis (Takei et al., 1996).

Hippocampal cultures are proving valuable also for analysis of postsynaptic receptor clustering and the molecular nature of the postsynaptic specialization. Staining with subunit-specific receptor antibodies can provide a comprehensive view of the postsynaptic receptor mosaic on the surface of an individual neuron (figure 13.7), a picture that would be very difficult to obtain from analysis of tissue sections (Craig et al., 1993, 1994; Eshhar et al., 1993). This analysis has shown that hippocampal neurons exhibit clusters of both glutamate and GABA receptors, which appear to be associated

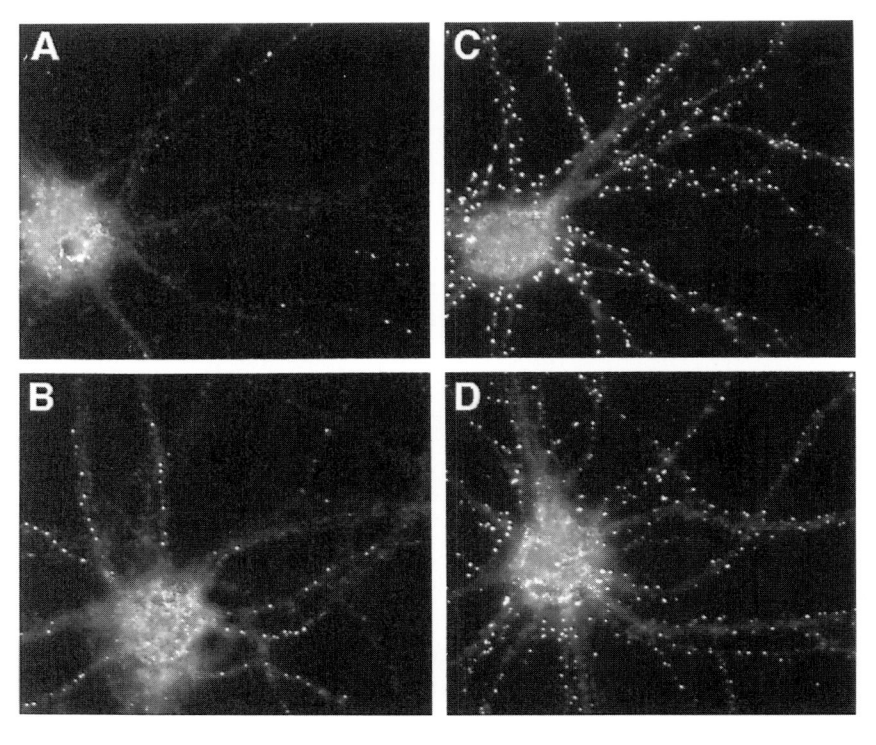

Figure 13.7   Treatment of hippocampal neurons with the NMDA receptor antagonist APV (2-amino-5-phosphono-valerate) changes the distribution of NMDA receptors. Hippocampal neurons were cultured at low density for 3 weeks in the absence (*A, B*) or presence (*C, D*) of APV, then were immunostained for NMDAR1. In the untreated, spontaneously active cultues, NMDAR1 is clustered at a few synaptic sites and at nonsynaptic sites (based on double-labeling for synaptophysin, not shown). Chronic receptor blockade induced a four-fold increase in the number of receptor clusters, with a greater proportion localized at synaptic sites (see Rao and Craig, 1997).

selectively with presynaptic terminals that release the corresponding neurotransmitter. Some aspects of the selective spatial distribution of synapses and receptors characteristic of hippocampal neurons in situ also are maintained in culture. GABAergic terminals are concentrated on cell bodies, whereas presumptive glutamatergic terminals are concentrated on dendrites (Benson and Cohen, 1996). Within the dendritic arbor, glutamate receptors are found both at shaft and spine synapses, whereas GABA receptors are restricted to synapses on shafts (Craig et al., 1994).

The last year has seen remarkable progress in identifying the molecular constituents that comprise the postsynaptic specialization and that may underlie receptor clustering (Gomperts, 1996;

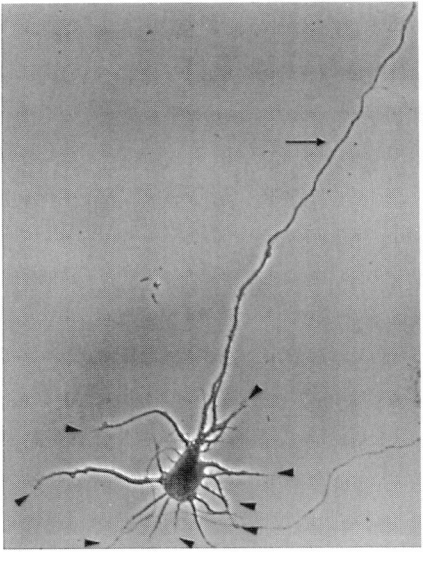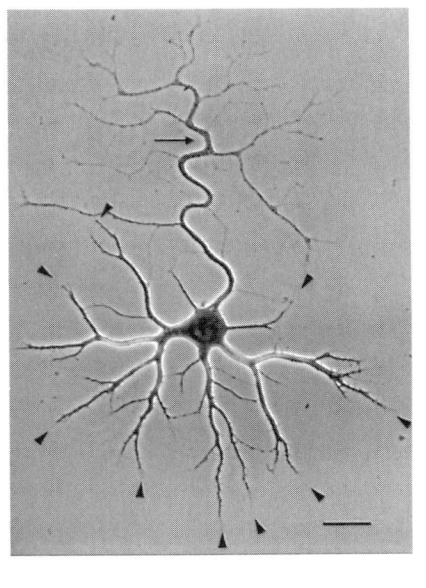

Figure 13.8 Accelerated development of dendritic arbor after osteogenic protein-1 (OP-1) treatment. Phase-contrast images of cultured hippocampal neurons that were maintained for 3 days in vitro, then were immunostained for MAP2. Cells were grown using our standard glial coculture paradigm (left) or in the presence of OP-1 without glial cells present (right). By comparison, the dendrites of the OP-1-treated cell are larger in diameter, more highly branched, and exhibit the taper characteristic of maturing dendrites. Arrowheads indicate the extent of the dendritic arbor; the arrow points to the axon. Scale bar: 20 μm.

Sheng, 1996). Double-staining hippocampal cultures has shown that members of the PSD-95/SAP-90 family of proteins are associated with the postsynaptic membrane at glutamatergic synapses (Kornau et al., 1995; Rao et al., 1996), as are CAM Kinase II, densin, and alpha-actinin (Apperson et al., 1996; Wyszynski et al., 1997). Gephyrin, a protein previously identified by its association with glycine receptors, is associated with GABAergic—but not with glutamatergic—synapses (Craig et al., 1996).

Hippocampal cultures can also be used to investigate the effects of global increases or decreases in electrical activity. This approach has been used to demonstrate that chronic blockade of electrical activity with tetrodotoxin does not prevent the formation of presynaptic specializations or the postsynaptic clustering of receptors (Fletcher et al., 1991; Craig et al, 1994; Benson and Cohen, 1996). In fact, treatment of cultures with the NMDA-receptor blocker APV selectively *enhances* the clustering of NMDA receptors (Rao

and Craig, 1997; see figure 13.7). Manipulations of activity also modulate MAP2 phosphorylation, as assessed by immunostaining with a phosphorylation-dependent monoclonal antibody, AP-18 (Halpain and Withers, 1995). In the presence of tetrodotoxin, this epitope is localized primarily at synapses but, within minutes of stimulation (e.g., 10 min after addition of the calcium channel agonist BayK), intense immunoreactivity is present throughout the dendritic tree. Similar manipulations increase the expression and dendritic transport of mRNA-encoding ARC, an immediate early gene product (G. Withers and C. Wallace, personal communication). Glutamate treatment also induces the expression of several other immediate early genes, which are mediated by calcium entry through NMDA receptors (Bading et al., 1995).

Finally, hippocampal cultures are proving useful for studies of dendritic development and spine formation. Immunostaining for MAP2 provides a convenient means to visualize and quantify the dendritic arbors of cultured hippocampal neurons, whereas diI labeling of a small number of cells allows visualization of living dendrites. We have used the former approach to demonstrate that osteogenic protein-1, a member of the transforming growth factor–beta superfamily, markedly accelerates the maturation of hippocampal dendrites (Withers et al., 1995, 1996), as originally described by Higgins and colleagues in their studies of sympathetic neurons (Lein et al., 1995). The tapering and branching that are the hallmarks of dendritic maturation, and which normally arise toward the end of the first week in culture, were observed as early as the first day in vitro in osteogenic protein-1-treated cultures (figure 13.8). DiI labeling has been used to visualize the dynamics of dendritic filopodia and dendritic spines in hippocampal cultures (Ziv and Smith, 1996) and to quantify changes in spine number and shape following manipulations of synaptic activity (Papa and Segal, 1996).

Despite the remarkable insights that have come from studies of the peripheral nervous system and neuromuscular junction, it is obvious that many important questions in neurobiology can be answered only by specifically studying neurons from the CNS. The goal of all our work with low-density cultures of hippocampal neurons has been to obtain a system for studying CNS neurons that is amenable to the same kinds of rigorous analyses that have been applied so successfully in cell culture studies of peripheral neurons and of nerve-muscle innervation.

Roseann Ventimiglia and Ronald M. Lindsay

The striatum (caudate nucleus and putamen) is the principal component of the basal ganglia, the major brain system through which cortical inputs involved with the voluntary control of movement are processed. The majority of striatal neurons ($\sim 90\%$) are characterized as medium spiny projection neurons and use the neurotransmitter γ-aminobutyric acid (GABA). These GABAergic neurons can be classified further on the basis of their neuropeptide content and their projection targets: striatal medium spiny neurons that project to the lateral globus pallidus contain enkephalin, whereas those that project to the medial globus pallidus or to the substantia nigra pars reticulata contain substance P. In turn, the striatum receives input from the dopamine neurons of the substantia nigra pars compacta via the nigrostriatal dopamine pathway. Some 10% of striatal neurons are classified as interneurons or intrinsic neurons whose axons do not project outside of the striatum. This group is comprised of large aspiny neurons that contain the neurotransmitter acetylcholine and small-medium aspiny neurons that contain the neuropeptides somatostatin and neuropeptide Y (Gerfen, 1992).

The function of the striatum is compromised in several neurodegenerative movement disorders, including Parkinson's disease and Huntington's chorea. Parkinson's disease is characterized by degeneration of the nigrostriatal dopamine system, resulting in bradykinesia (extreme slowness of movement and reflexes), rigidity, and uncontrollable tremor. Among neurodegenerative disorders, Parkinson's disease represents one example of a pathological state that has been well-characterized. Although the etiology of Parkinson's disease is not well understood and it is not yet possible to slow or reverse the degenerative process that underlies the disease, the symptoms of the disease may be alleviated partially by pharmacological intervention involving dopamine precursor or receptor agonist therapy. Furthermore, ongoing studies employing transplantation of fetal dopamine neurons (Lindvall et al., 1992) show promise as a therapeutic approach to Parkinson's disease. In

contrast to Parkinson's disease, significantly less progress has been made in developing therapeutic approaches to Huntington's disease. Huntington's disease is a progressive neurodegenerative disorder resulting in the loss of striatal medium spiny GABAergic projection neurons and is characterized by involuntary movements (choreas), cognitive deterioration, and emotional deficits. Although the gene defect that leads to Huntington's disease has been identified (Huntington's Disease Collaborative Research Group, 1993), no effective therapy currently exists for alleviating the symptoms or slowing the degenerative process in this disease.

One of our interests centers on assessing the neuroprotective potential of neurotrophic factors in degenerative processes that involve the loss of striatal neurons. In particular, we are interested in defining the responses of striatal neurons to treatment with various classes of neurotrophic factors, including the neurotrophins brain-derived neurotrophic factor (BDNF), neurotrophin-3 (NT-3), and neurotrophin-4/5 (NT-4/5), members of a family of neurotrophic factors related functionally and structurally to nerve growth factor (NGE) (Lindsay et al., 1994). Our specific aims are to examine the potential of neurotrophic factors to promote survival or differentiation of striatal neurons, to identify specific populations of striatal neurons that respond to neurotrophic factors, and to understand the nature of the biological responses induced by neurotrophic factor treatment.

Rationale

Considering the complexity of studying in vivo the responses of distinct populations of neurons to factors that may influence their survival or differentiation, we have developed a simplified in vitro system to examine at the cellular level the biological responses of embryonic striatal neurons to soluble growth factors. Such a simplified culture system permits evaluation of the specific effects of neurotrophic factors in a controlled environment. The disadvantages of using a dissociated culture system should be noted also: The cellular inputs to the striatum and its architectural organization no longer are present. For experiments whose aim is to examine cell-cell interactions or to develop a neurotoxicity model that approximates more closely the in vivo situation, one might choose to use an organotypic slice culture system. The organotypic slice culture of striatum has been used to characterize the neuro-

chemical differentiation of striatal neurons (Østergaard, 1993), whereas coculture of striatum with cortex (Whetsell and Schwarz, 1989) has been used to establish models of excitatory amino acid neurotoxicity.

To facilitate our studies, we developed a dissociated culture system derived from embryonic-day-17 (E17) rat striatum, a timepoint at which the majority of neurons in the striatum have been generated (Bayer, 1984; Marchand and Lajoie, 1986). Development of this culture system incorporated the following criteria:

- Dissociated neurons must be maintained at low density so as to minimize cell-cell contact and allow observation of single neurons.
- To avoid exposure of neurons to growth factors that may be present in serum, exposure to serum is kept to a minimum.
- The majority of cells present must be neurons.
- Neurons in culture must be identified by transmitter, enzyme, or other phenotypic marker to determine the specificity of neurotrophic factors toward different neuronal populations.
- Neurons must be attainable in sufficient numbers to permit analysis by biochemical or molecular approaches.

The culture system with the features previously described facilitates several lines of experimentation. The ability to culture striatal neurons at very low cell density permits the assessment of any general effects of neurotrophin treatment on neuronal survival by cell count analysis and allows the identification of the phenotypes of responsive neuronal populations by immunohistochemical means. Maintenance of striatal cultures in serum-free conditions reduces the proliferation of nonneuronal cells, thus making it possible to produce relatively pure neuronal cultures. Furthermore, the absence of serum from our culture medium ensures that observed biological responses are the result of exposure to the exogenously added neurotrophic factor and not due to any of the growth factors known to be present in serum.

We have found that these cultures are well suited to morphometric analysis (Ventimiglia, Jones, et al., 1995) and to analysis of physiological responses to neurotrophic factors, such as by patch-clamp recording (Maue et al., 1995). Considering the relatively homogeneous nature of striatal neurons (approximately 90% of neurons in the striatum are classified as medium spiny GABAergic projection neurons) and the fact that it is routinely possible to obtain large numbers of cells from dissection of a single litter of rat

embryos ($1.0–2.0 \times 10^6$ cells per embryo), use of this culture system permits analysis by biochemical means, such as neurotransmitter uptake assays, and molecular approaches, such as Northern blot analysis. Culture preparation for these various types of experiments simply requires modification of cell plating density and size of the tissue-culture plates used.

When undertaking the preparation of striatal cultures, the experimenter should consider not only the nature of the planned experiments but the duration of the required culture period. The nature of the assays of interest to us has been short-term (i.e., our assays generally are conducted after 7 or 8 days in vitro). For experiments that require long-term survival of neurons, the culture conditions that we describe may not be optimal. One then might wish to include an initial short exposure (up to the first 24 h of the culture period) of a fairly low concentration of serum or to modify the cell plating density to ensure adequate numbers of surviving neurons at the end of the culture period.

Protocol

Tissue Culture Plates

Because a great deal of our work involves the use of cell count assays to assess neurotrophin effects on cell number and morphometric analysis, we use 35-mm tissue-culture plates (Nunc, Naperville, IL, no. 174926) that are etched with 2-mm square grids. After experimentation with a variety of substrates, including laminin and fibronectin, we found that optimal cell adhesion, neurite outgrowth, and general culture "healthiness" was achieved when plates were coated with polylysine and merosin. Merosin is a basement membrane protein found in placenta, striated muscle, and Schwann cells (Leivo and Engvall, 1988). We adopted merosin after its successful use as a substrate for the establishment of embryonic rat ventral mesencephalic cultures (Hyman et al., 1994). One day prior to culture preparation, tissue culture plates are coated with poly-L-lysine (Sigma, no. P-6282, MW 70,000–150,000; 10 µg/ml, dissolved in sterile distilled water, approximately 1.5 ml per plate), and incubated at 4°C for 2 h. (Polylysine is made up as a 10× stock and is stored as aliquots at −20°C.) Plates then are washed three times with sterile water (10 min each) and allowed to

air-dry in the tissue-culture hood. Merosin (Chemicon, Temecula, CA, no. AA085, 1 μg/ml, dissolved in water and filter-sterilized through a 0.22-μm filter) then is added, and plates are incubated overnight in a 37°C, 5% CO_2 incubator. On the culture preparation day, the merosin solution is aspirated, and plates are incubated in medium composed of Dulbecco's modified Eagle's medium [D-MEM, high glucose, with sodium pyruvate, without glutamine (Irvine Scientific, Irvine, CA, no. 9033)], to which is added L-glutamine (2 mM; Cellgro/Mediatech, no. 25-005-LI), penicillin-streptomycin (25 IU–25 μg/ml; Mediatech, no. 30-002-LI), and 10% fetal calf serum (FCS; Hyclone, Salt Lake City, UT, no. A-1111-L) (box 14.1) for approximately 2 h before cell plating. Immediately before plating cells, D-MEM/FCS is aspirated, and plates are rinsed quickly with serum-free N2 medium. We find that this brief pre-incubation with D-MEM/FCS followed by rinsing improves cell adhesion, while keeping exposure to serum at a minimum.

Media

Cells are plated in serum-free medium (SFM) composed of D-MEM with glutamine (2 mM), penicillin-streptomycin (25 IU–25 μg/ml), and bovine serum albumin, 1 mg/ml (Sigma, St. Louis, MO, no. A-3059) and containing N2 supplements (Bottenstein et al., 1979): apotransferrin, final concentration 100 μg/ml (Sigma, no. T-1147); putrescine, 100 μM (Sigma, no. P-5780); progesterone, 20 nM (Sigma, no. P-8783); selenium, 30 nM (Sigma, no. S-5261); sodium pyruvate, 1 mM (Cellgro, no. 25-00-L1); and insulin, 5 μg/ml (Sigma, no. I-6634). We make up the N2 supplements in SFM as a 10× stock solution and store aliquots at −20°C. The 10× N2 stock is diluted in SFM (see box 14.1) prior to use. Insulin is made fresh at least weekly (see box 14.1) and added along with the 10× N2 stock to SFM. SFM and DMEM-FCS are used within 1 week of preparation.

Source of Animals

We obtain fetuses at embryonic day 17 from timed pregnant Sprague-Dawley rats supplied by Zivic-Miller (Zelienople, PA), with the day of sperm positivity considered E0. The pregnant rat is euthanized by carbon dioxide inhalation, and the area of the incision is soaked with 70% ethanol. The uterus is removed and

Box 14.1 Media Recipes

Calcium Magnesium-Free Hank's Balanced Salt Solution (CMF-BSS) for 400 ml

NaHCO$_3$ (3.5%)	1 ml
Hank's BSS (Gibco, no. 14180-012, 10×)	40 ml
Sterile water	to 400 ml

Serum-Free Medium (SFM) for 400 ml

Glutamine [Mediatech, no. 25-005-LI, 200 mM (100×)]	4 ml
Penicillin-streptomycin (Mediatech, no. 30-002-LI, 10,000 IU–10,000 µg/ml)	1 ml
Bovine serum albumin (BSA, Sigma, no. A-3059)	400 mg
Dulbecco's modified Eagle's medium (DMEM, Irvine Scientific, no. 9033) (with high glucose, with sodium pyruvate, without glutamine)	to 400 ml
Filter-sterilize.	

N2 Supplements (10 × Stock) for 100 ml

Apo-transferrin (Sigma, no. T-1147)	100 mg
Putrescine (Sigma, no. P-5780)	16 mg
Progesterone (Sigma, no. P-8783)	63 µg
Selenium (Sigma, no. S-5261)	104 µl of 50 µg/ml stock
Sodium pyruvate (Cellgro, no. 25-00-LI)	10 ml of 100 mM stock
Dilute in SFM; store aliquots at −20°C.	

Insulin for 1 ml

Insulin (Sigma, no. I-6634)	5 mg
SFM	900 µl
1 N HCl	100 µl
Filter-sterilize; use within 1 week.	
Keep at 4°C; do not freeze.	

N2 Medium for 100 ml

N2 10× stock	10 ml
Insulin stock	100 µl
SFM	to 100 ml
Filter-sterilize; use within 1 day.	

Box 14.1 (continued)

DMEM/FCS for 200 ml

Glutamine [Mediatech, no. 25-005-LI, 200 mM (100×)]	2 ml
Penicillin-streptomycin (Mediatech, no. 30-002-LI, 10,000 IU–10,000 µg/ml)	0.5 ml
Fetal calf serum (FCS; Hyclone, no. A-1111-L)	20 ml
Dulbecco's modified Eagle's medium (DMEM, Irvine Scientific, no. 9033) (with high glucose, with sodium pyruvate, without glutamine)	to 200 ml

---

placed in a sterile Petri dish, with care taken to avoid contamination by fur. The typical yield is between 10 and 14 fetuses per rat. Rat embryos at day 17 of gestation are approximately 20 mm in length, measured from crown to rump.

Dissection of the Striatum

Fetuses are removed from the uterus and decapitated. The heads then are transferred to a 100-mm Petri dish containing calcium-magnesium-free Hank's balanced salt solution (CMF-HBSS, prepared from 10× CMF-BSS, Gibco, no. 14180-012; see box 14.1). A pair of Dumont 45-degree angled forceps is used to anchor the brain while another pair of microsurgery straight-tip forceps (Dumont no. 5) is used to peel away the skin and skull, exposing the brain, which then is teased gently out of the skull and transferred to a new dish containing CMF-BSS. With the ventral aspect of the brain facing up, a thick coronal section is cut as described by Messer (1981) using 3-inch Vannas supreme microscissors (Roboz, Rockville, MD, no. RS-5620). A cut is made anteriorly through the level of the optic chiasm and posteriorly through the midpoint of the hypothalamus (figure 14.1A, step 1). For a more detailed illustration of the level of the dissection, the reader is referred to Altman and Bayer (1995). With the coronal section lying flat, the striatum (consisting of the caudate nucleus and putamen, including striatal neuroepithelium and subventricular zone) then is carved out using microdissecting knives (Fine Science Tools, Foster City, CA, no. 10055-12) (see figure 14.1A, step 2). Though every effort is made to dissect only striatal tissue, we cannot rule out completely

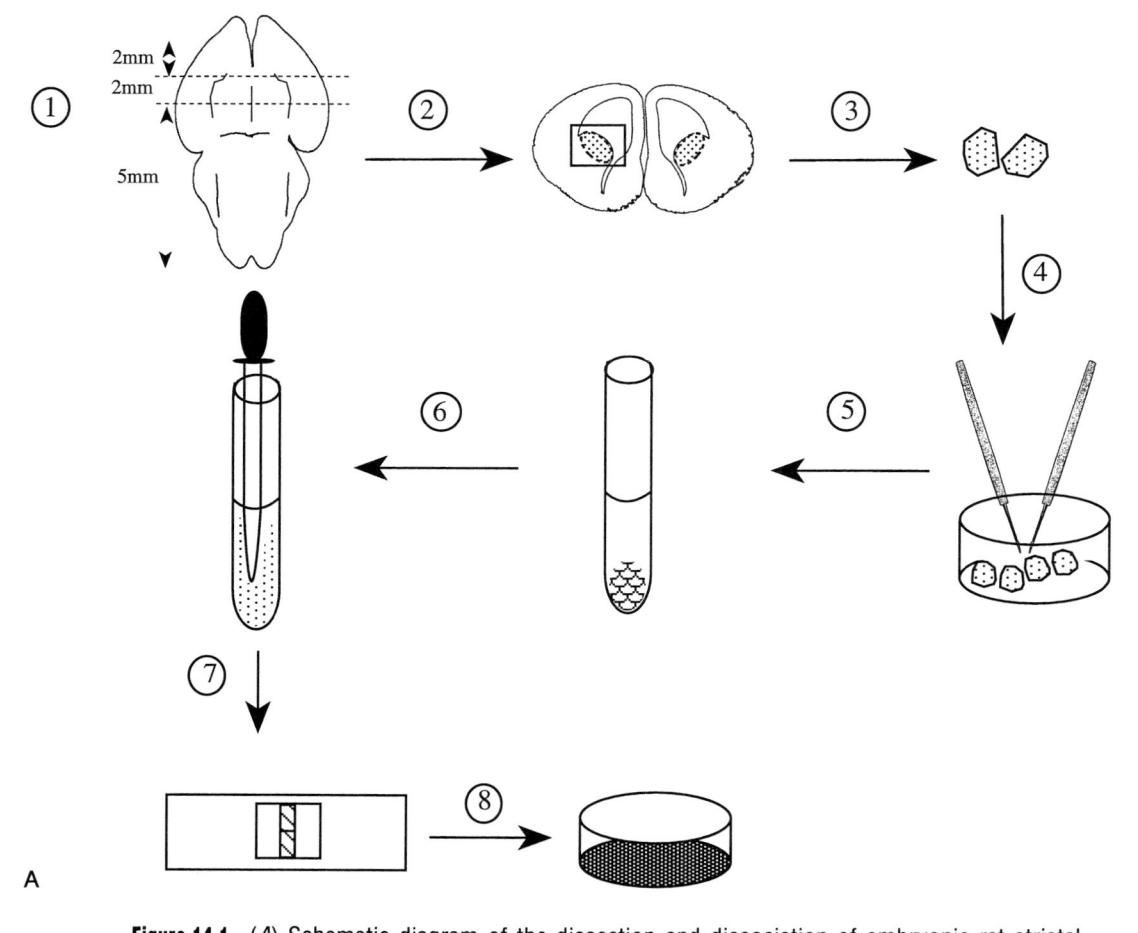

Figure 14.1 (*A*) Schematic diagram of the dissection and dissociation of embryonic rat striatal tissue. Step 1: With the brain ventral side up, a coronal section (approximately 2 mm thick) is cut. Step 2: The striatum (shaded area) is dissected from each brain slice. Step 3: Tissue pieces are transferred to a 60-mm Petri dish. Step 4: Micro-dissecting knives are used to mince the tissue into very small fragments. Step 5: Tissue fragments are treated enzymatically. Step 6: Tissue is dissociated mechanically by trituration with a fire-polished Pasteur pipette. Step 7: A hemacytometer is used to determine the total yield of cells. Step 8: The cell suspension is diluted and plated into 35-mm dishes at low density. (*B*) Photographic representation of striatal dissection. Step 1: The brain is placed with the ventral side facing up. Dashed lines show the outline of the two cuts that are made to yield an approximately 2-mm-thick tissue section. Step 2: Microscissors are used to cut through the brain at the level of the optic chiasm. Step 3: View of the brain following the first cut. Step 4: A second cut is made at the level of the midpoint of the hypothalamus. Step 5: The resulting tissue section shows the outline of the striatal tissue (dashed lines), which is carved out using microdissecting knives.

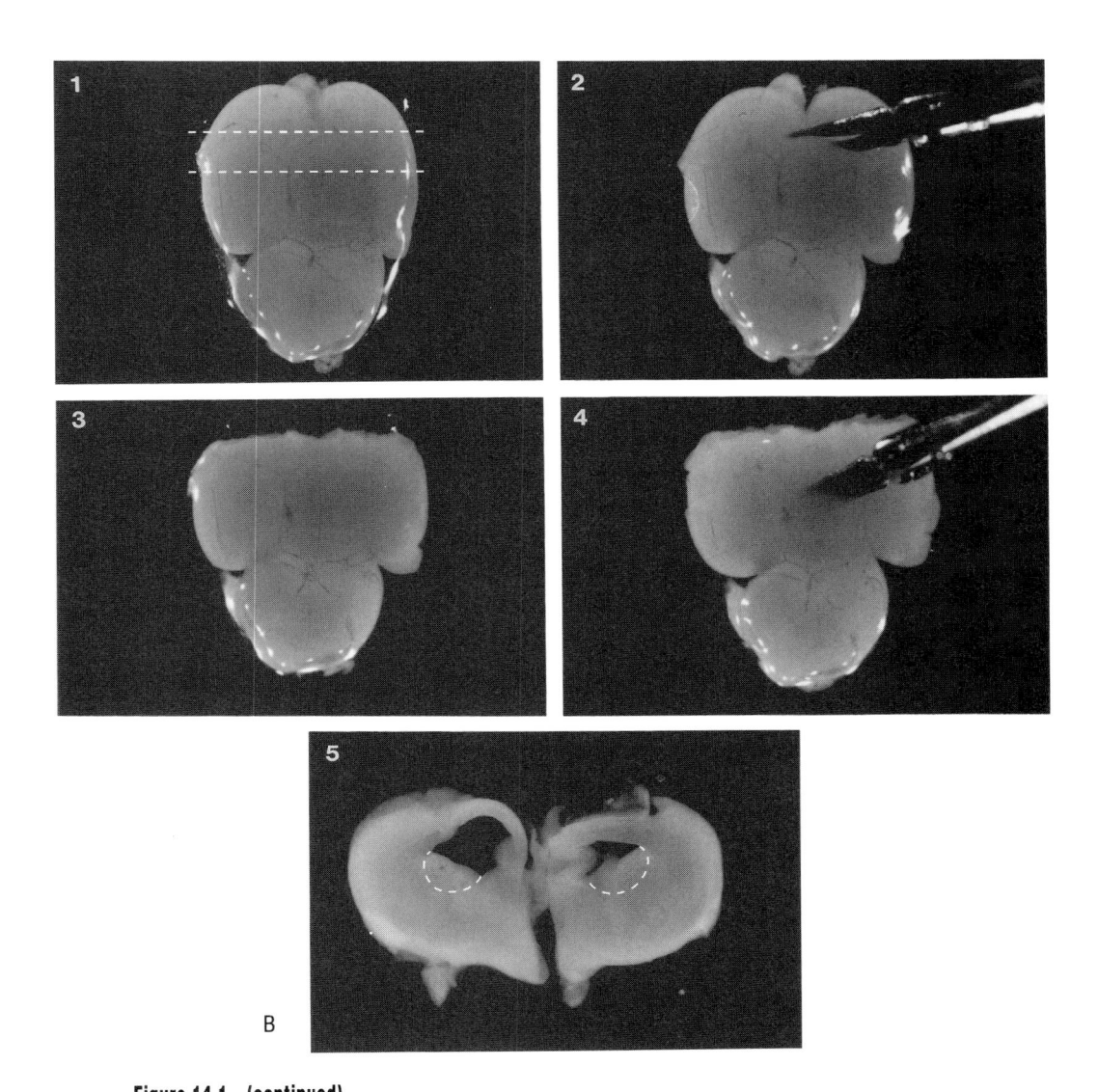

Figure 14.1 (continued)

the possibility that some pallidal tissue also may be included. Tissue fragments (see figure 14.1A, step 3) are transferred to a 60-mm Petri dish containing cold CMF-BSS. When the striata from all embryos have been collected, the pooled tissue fragments are minced into very small pieces (<1 mm) with the microdissecting knives (see figure 14.1A, step 4).

Dissociation and Plating

Once the striatal tissue has been finely minced, a Pasteur pipette is used to transfer the tissue fragments to a 15-ml conical tube. The tissue is allowed to settle, and the remaining medium is removed, again using a Pasteur pipette. CMF-BSS is added to bring the volume to 1.8 ml, followed by the addition of a freshly thawed 200 μl aliquot of a 2.5% trypsin solution (Worthington Biochemical Corp., Freehold, NJ, no. 34K780). The tissue fragments in trypsin are incubated for 10 min in a 37°C water bath, followed by the addition of 40 μl of a 10 mg/ml DNAse solution (type II, Sigma, no. D4527) for a further 10-min incubation (see figure 14.1A, step 5). Following enzymatic treatment, 8 ml of D-MEM/FCS is added to inhibit enzyme activity. Once the tissue fragments have settled, the medium is removed with a Pasteur pipette, and 1.5 ml of fresh D-MEM/FCS is added. Preparation of a cell suspension then is accomplished by trituration of the tissue through the bore of a fire-polished Pasteur pipette (see figure 14.1A, step 6). The use of fire-polished pipettes requires that the diameter of the pipette be reduced (to 0.5–1.0 mm) so as to allow gentle trituration without excessive shearing. Normally, we triturate approximately six times to obtain a dissociated cell suspension or until no obvious large pieces of tissue remain.

Cell yield is determined by using a hemacytometer to count cells that exclude trypan blue (see figure 14.1A, step 7). We add 10 μl of the cell suspension to a tube containing 40 μl of trypan blue (0.4%, Gibco BRL, no. 15250-020) and 50 μl of CMF-BSS, and 10 μl of this dilute cell suspension is added to each of two counting areas of the hemacytometer. Once the total number of viable cells has been determined, the cell suspension is diluted in SFM to achieve a plating density of 3×10^5 cells per 1.5 ml of medium, and this volume is added to each 35-mm tissue-culture plate (see figure 14.1A, step 8). Typically, we obtain 1 to 2×10^6 cells per embryo, with perhaps 90% cell viability. Depending on the number of embryos, 40 to 100 thirty-five-millimeter plates can be obtained from one litter. As normally we prepare a large number of plates on any

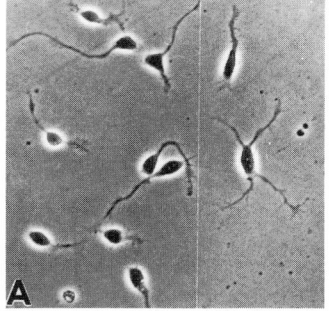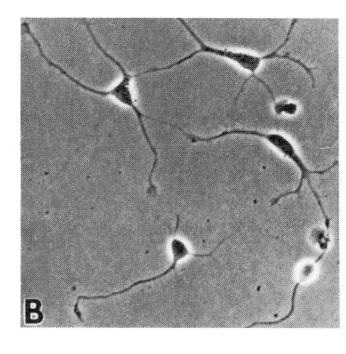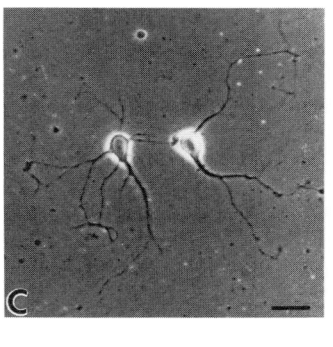

Figure 14.2 Appearance of striatal cell cultures. Phase-contrast photomicrographs showing low-density cultures at (A) 1, (B) 5, and (C) 8 days in vitro. Cells were plated at a density of 3×10^4 cells per square centimeter and maintained in serum-free medium throughout the culture period. Scale bar: 20 μm.

given culture day, we find it important to swirl the cell suspension gently several times during the course of plating to ensure even dispersion of cells. Cultures generally are not examined until at least 4 h after plating, to allow for optimal adhesion of cells to the substrate.

Maintenance of Striatal Cultures

Because the nature of the experiments in which we employ striatal cultures is short-term, it is not necessary to feed these cultures during the course of the 1-week culture period. Cultures simply are maintained in a 37°C/5% CO_2 incubator. When trophic factors are added to some cultures, we add a similar volume of vehicle (N2) alone to control cultures.

Appearance and Development of Cultures

Cultures are typically examined for the first time several hours after plating, so as not to disrupt the adherence process. By approximately 4 h after plating, most cells have adhered to the substrate, and neurons can be identified readily by their phase-bright appearance. At this time, some neurons have visible lamellipodia, whereas many other neurons already have begun to extend neuritic processes. By 1 day in vitro, neurite outgrowth is quite extensive (figure 14.2A), and arborization continues to become more elaborate throughout the course of the culture period (see figure 14.2B). By culture day 7 or 8 (see figure 14.2C), when most of our experiments are conducted, the total number of neurons has decreased

significantly from the number originally plated, thus permitting visualization of single cells at the light-microscopical level or by immunohistochemical means. Additionally, at 7 or 8 days in vitro, contamination by nonneuronal cells still is quite minimal (<5%).

What Can Go Wrong?

In general, we find that the methods herein described yield highly consistent and reproducible results. Nonetheless, as anyone familiar with primary neuronal culture knows, at times a culture preparation may yield less than optimal results. In such instances, one might consider several aspects of the culture preparation to trace the possible source of the problem.

Culture Substrate

Perhaps the most significant factor that influences the success of culture preparation is the choice of substrate (figure 14.3A,B). In cases wherein cells show poor adherence or limited neurite outgrowth, one should consider the possibility that an error occurred in substrate preparation, length of time of coating, or rinsing of the substrate. Commercial batches of polylysine and merosin should be prescreened for optimal adhesion.

Enzymatic Treatment

The period of exposure to proteolytic enzymes is critical to obtaining healthy cultures. Excessive exposure to trypsin or poor-quality trypsin may result in substandard cultures characterized by poor adherence to the substrate, limited neurite outgrowth, and reduced neuronal survival. If suboptimal cultures are obtained, one might consider preparation of fresh solutions or lengthening or shortening the enzymatic treatment time.

Mechanical Dissociation by Trituration

Following optimal enzymatic treatment, a few passes through the bore of a fire-polished Pasteur pipette are quite sufficient to dissociate the tissue pieces into a single-cell suspension. If this process is not achieved readily, excessive shearing will give rise to a low cell yield and poor viability. To prevent this result, the tryp-

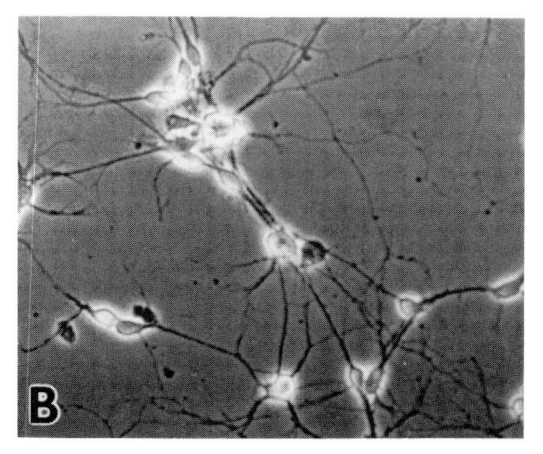

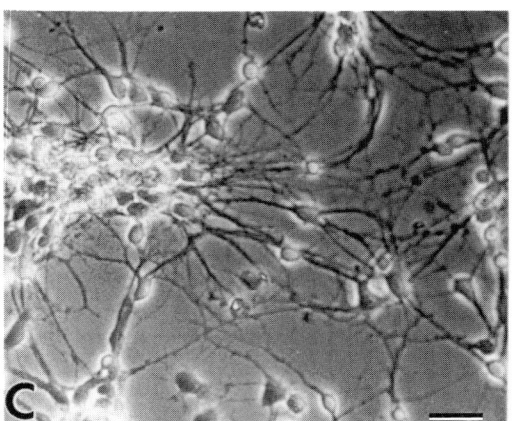

Figure 14.3 Examples of suboptimal cultures. Compared to cultures plated at low density on a substrate of polylysine and merosin (A), cultures plated on polylysine alone (B) appear to contain fewer neurons as well as cell clumps, whereas those plated at higher cell density (C) show a great degree of clumping and fasciculation. Scale bar: 40 µm.

sinization time may have to be increased, or a better lot of trypsin should be obtained

Cell-Plating Density

Cultures that are plated at a significantly higher density tend to display clumping of cell bodies and fasciculation of neurites over time (see figure 14.3C), which would certainly be problematic in experiments involving observations of the cells or their morphology. Cultures that are plated at a very low cell density and are not treated with exogenous growth factors may not sustain neuronal survival. Careful determination of cell yield and viability as well as frequent swirling of the cell suspension during plating are critical to ensuring optimal plating density.

Applications

We sought to develop a dissociated striatal culture system that would simplify examination of the biological responses of striatal neurons to neurotrophic factors by the use of cellular, biochemical and molecular approaches. Here we describe the application of this culture system to address several questions relevant to the biological effects of the neurotrophins.

Striatal Culture Expression of Functional Neurotrophin Receptors

To examine the expression of the genes encoding the neurotrophins and their receptors, the culture preparation that we have described was modified to include the use of large (60 mm) tissue-culture dishes in which cells were plated at a high density (3×10^6 cells per plate). These cultures were harvested for RNA extraction and were subjected to Northern blot analysis. This analysis revealed that cultured E17 striatal neurons express mRNA for *trk*B (the receptor for BDNF and NT-4/5 and, to a lesser extent, NT-3) and mRNA for *trk*C (the receptor for NT-3), but no detectable levels of mRNA for *trk*A (the receptor for NGF) or mRNA encoding the neurotrophins themselves (data not shown).

As a further means to assess the functional interaction of the neurotrophins with their cognate receptors in these cultures, we examined the ability of the neurotrophins to activate the immediate early gene c-*fos* (figure 14.4). We found that treatment with BDNF, NT-3 and NT-4/5, but not NGF, induced the expression of c-*fos*

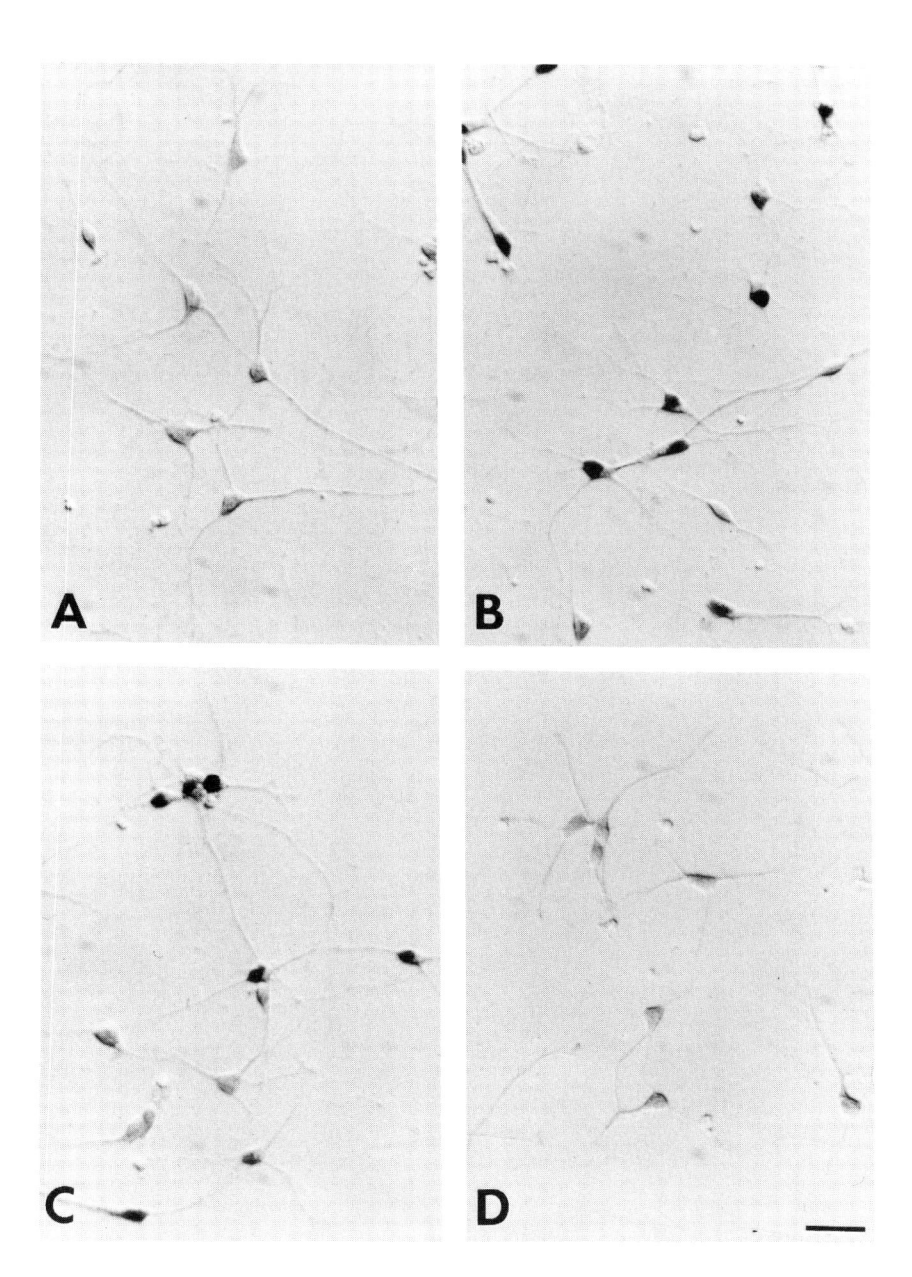

Figure 14.4 Immunohistochemical detection of c-*fos* protein. Following a 2-h stimulation with (*A*) vehicle, (*B*) BDNF, (*C*) NT-3, or (*D*) NGF, cells were stained for c-*fos* expression. Both BDNF and NT-3 treatment induce c-*fos* expression in approximately 40%–50% of all cells, whereas no c-*fos* expression is detected following stimulation with vehicle or NGF. Stimulation with NT-4/5 (not shown) results in c-*fos* expression similar to that seen following BDNF or NT-3 exposure. Scale bar: 20 μm.

Box 14.2 **Protocol for Immunohistochemical Detection of Intracellular Antigens**

Day 1

1. (For c-*fos* staining, incubate cultures with factors of interest for a predetermined period.) Wash cultures twice with phosphate-buffered saline (PBS).
2. Fix cultures with 4% paraformaldehyde for 30 min at room temperature.
3. For detection of neuron-specific enolase (NSE, Chemicon, no. AB 951), GABA (Sigma, no. A-2052), or c-*fos* (Oncogene Sciences, special order no. 2193031), incubate cultures with PBS containing 0.4% Triton X-100, 1% bovine serum albumin (BSA), and 4% normal goat serum (NGS) for 1–2 h at room temperature. When staining for calbindin (Sigma, no. C-8666), substitute normal horse serum (NHS) for NGS.
4. Incubate with primary antibody diluted in PBS containing 0.4% Triton X-100, 1% NGS, and 1% BSA (again substituting NHS for NGS when staining for calbindin) overnight at 4°C. We use anti-NSE at 1:1000, anti-GABA at 1:15,000, anti-c-*fos* at 1:30,000 and anti-calbindin at 1:5000. These dilutions were arrived at by trial and error. The experimenter should be prepared to test different batches of antibodies similarly.

Day 2

1. Wash three times (10 min each) with PBS containing 0.02% Triton X-100 and 0.25% BSA.
2. Incubate with secondary antibody [biotinylated goat anti-rabbit, 1:500, Vector Labs, Vectastain kit no. PK-4000 (for NSE, GABA, or c-*fos*) or biotinylated horse anti-mouse, 1:400 Vector Labs, Vectastain kit no. PK-4002 (for calbindin)] diluted in PBS containing 0.02% Triton X-100 and 1% BSA for 60 min at room temperature.
3. Rinse four times (15 min each) with PBS containing 0.25% BSA.
4. While rinsing, prepare avidin-biotin (ABC, Vector Labs, Vectastain kit) complex:

    20 µl A + 20 µl B/ml PBS + 1.0% BSA.

5. Immediately before use, dilute the ABC solution to 10 ml.
6. Incubate in ABC for 60 min at room temperature.
7. Rinse twice (10 min each) in PBS.
   For c-*fos* staining, rinse twice (10 min each) in acetate-imidazole buffer. For each 100 ml:

    77.5 ml distilled H_2O
    17.5 ml 1.0 M sodium acetate (pH 7.2)
    5.0 ml 0.2 M imidazole (pH 9.2)

    Adjust final pH to 7.2 with glacial acetic acid.
8. Develop with diaminobenzidine (10 mg/ml, Sigma, no. D-5905), for 2–10 min. Make up DAB in distilled H_2O, filter, and add 30 µl 1% H_2O_2 per 10 ml.

Box 14.2 (continued)

For c-fos staining, develop with diaminobenzidine-nickel sulfate solution
for 2–10 min. Add ingredients in given order. For each 10 ml:
7.92 ml distilled H_2O
1.25 ml 1.0 M sodium acetate
0.50 ml 0.2 M imidazole
263 mg nickel sulfate
300 µl DAB stock (10 mg/ml)

Filter and add 30 µl 1% H_2O_2.
9. For c-*fos* staining, rinse twice (10 min each) with acetate-imidazole buffer.
For all staining, finally rinse three times in PBS.

protein in approximately 40% to 50% of cultured striatal neurons, indicating the presence of functional neurotrophin receptors in these cultures.

Neurotrophin Promotion of the Survival of Striatal Neurons in Culture

Because cultures are plated at very low cell density and contain few glial cells, we have been able to combine cell count assays with immunohistochemistry at the end of a period of treatment with any of the neurotrophins (box 14.2). We have used immunohisto-chemical detection of neuron-specific enolase and cell count assays to determine that BDNF treatment results in a 40% increase in total neuron number at the end of a 7- to 8-day culture period (figure 14.5A). Similar assays revealed that the effects of the NT-3 or NT-4/5 on neuronal survival were slightly less than those of BDNF, whereas NGF did not affect survival. These types of cell count assays are facilitated by the fact that the base of the tissue-culture plates used has an embossed grid that allows systematic and unbiased cell counts to be made from only a limited area of the culture plate (see further).

Specific Neuronal Populations Wherein Survival and Differentiation are Promoted by the Neurotrophins

We used immunocytochemical methods and cell count assays to examine the effects of BDNF on neuronal expression of calbindin, a calcium-binding protein. We found that treatment of striatal cultures with BDNF upregulated the expression of calbindin by

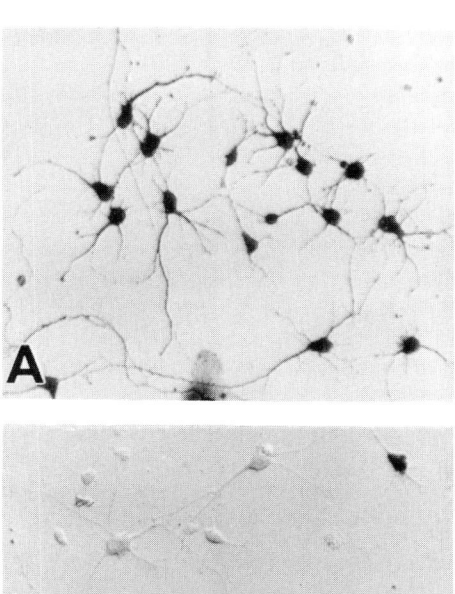

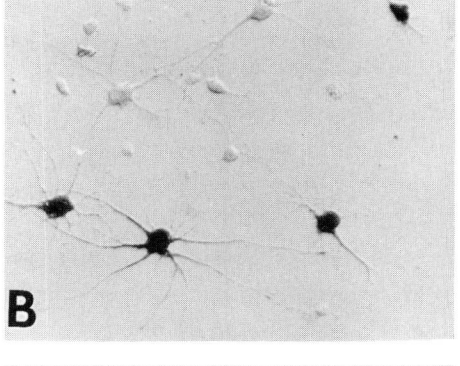

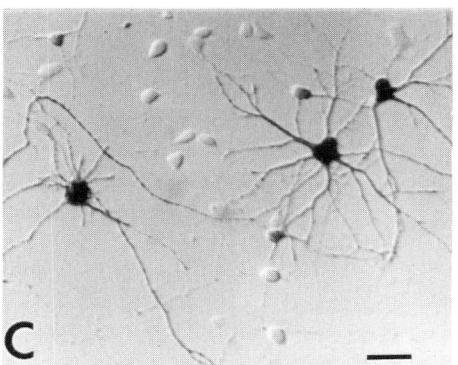

Figure 14.5 Immunohistochemical detection of striatal neurons and neuronal subpopulations. Detection of (*A*) neuron-specific enolase-, (*B*) calbindin-, and (*C*) GABA-immunoreactivity in striatal cultures after 8 days in vitro. Cultures were photographed with a 20× objective using Hoffman Modulation Contrast optics. Scale bar: 40 μm. (From R. Ventimiglia, P. E. Mather, B. E. Jones, R. M. Lindsay, The neurotrophins BDNF, NT-3 and NT-4/5 promote survival and morphological and biochemical differentiation of striatal neurons in vitro. Eur. J. Neurosci. 1995; 7: 213–222. Reproduced by permission of Oxford University Press.)

three- to five-fold (see figure 14.5B; Ventimiglia, Mather, et al., 1995). Our results suggest that BDNF may increase the calcium-buffering capacity of striatal neurons. This finding may have significance in that it has been suggested that the loss of calcium-buffering capacity associated with loss of calbindin may contribute to the pathogenesis of neurodegenerative diseases (Iacopino and Christakos, 1990).

Given that the largest neuronal subpopulation in the striatum is composed of the medium spiny projection neurons that use the neurotransmitter GABA, we were interested in assessing the responses of these neurons to the neurotrophins. Immunostaining of the striatal cultures with an antibody to GABA revealed that BDNF, NT-3, or NT-4/5 promote the survival or differentiation of striatal neurons expressing this phenotypical marker (Ventimiglia, Mather, et al., 1995; see figure 14.5C). As an additional measure of neurotrophin effects on striatal GABA neurons, we measured the high-affinity uptake of GABA (Tomozawa and Appel, 1986) in striatal cultures after 8 days of treatment with the neurotrophins. Compared to untreated cultures, treatment with BDNF, NT-3, or NT-4/5 produced a two- to three-fold increase in high-affinity GABA uptake, whereas NGF was without effect (Ventimiglia, Mather, et al., 1995). These results extended the finding that BDNF, NT-3, or NT-4/5 (but not NGF) promote the survival-differentiation of striatal GABA-immunoreactive neurons and additionally demonstrate the utility of this culture system in biochemical analyses.

The foregoing experiments lay the groundwork for the full characterization of this culture system. The extent to which interneurons are present in these cultures has not been evaluated but should be determined readily by the use of appropriate antibodies. We have not investigated the coexpression of GABA-immunoreactivity with specific neuropeptides that are known to be colocalized in vivo. We have, however, detected effects of the neurotrophins on expression of enkephalin, substance P, and dynorphin as measured by radioimmunoassay (not shown). Further work remains to be done to characterize fully the neuronal populations in this culture system.

Biological Responses Induced by the Neurotrophins

We observed a striking effect of neurotrophin treatment on the morphology of cultured striatal neurons that were GABA-immunoreactive (figure 14.6). Because methods that have been

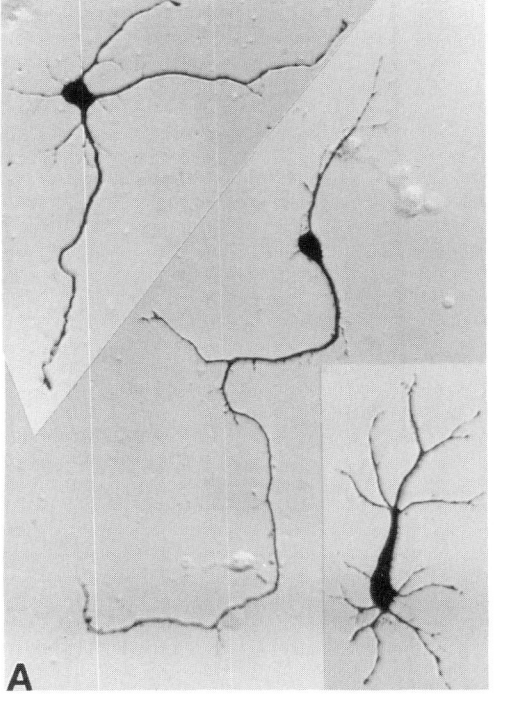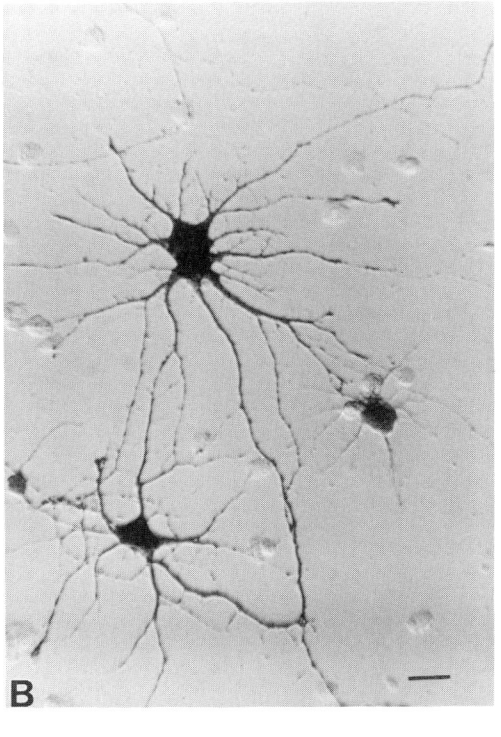

A B

Figure 14.6 BDNF promotes morphological differentiation of striatal GABAergic neurons. Striatal cultures that were maintained as controls or treated with BDNF for 8 days in vitro were processed for GABA immunoreactivity. (*A*) Composite of three GABA-immunoreactive neurons in untreated control cultures. (*B*) Representative GABA-immunoreactive neurons in a culture treated with BDNF. Note the enlarged cell bodies, increased number of branch points, and overall increase in dendritic arborization in the BDNF-treated neurons as compared to the untreated controls. Control and BDNF-treated cultures were photographed with a 40× objective using Hoffman Modulation Contrast optics. Scale bar: 20 μM.

used traditionally for quantitative morphometric analysis can be time-consuming and subjective, we developed a method for rapid, unbiased morphometric analysis of cultured neurons (Ventimiglia, Jones, et al., 1995) (figure 14.7). Whereas we used these methods to assess the effects of neurotrophic factors on the morphology of striatal neurons, the same method could be applied readily to study the effects of other soluble growth factors or extracellular matrix molecules. This method again takes advantage of the etched-grid culture dish and the low plating density that we employ. By applying this method to the morphometric analysis of GABA-immunoreactive striatal neurons, we determined that treatment with BDNF (and to a somewhat lesser extent NT-3 or NT-4/5)

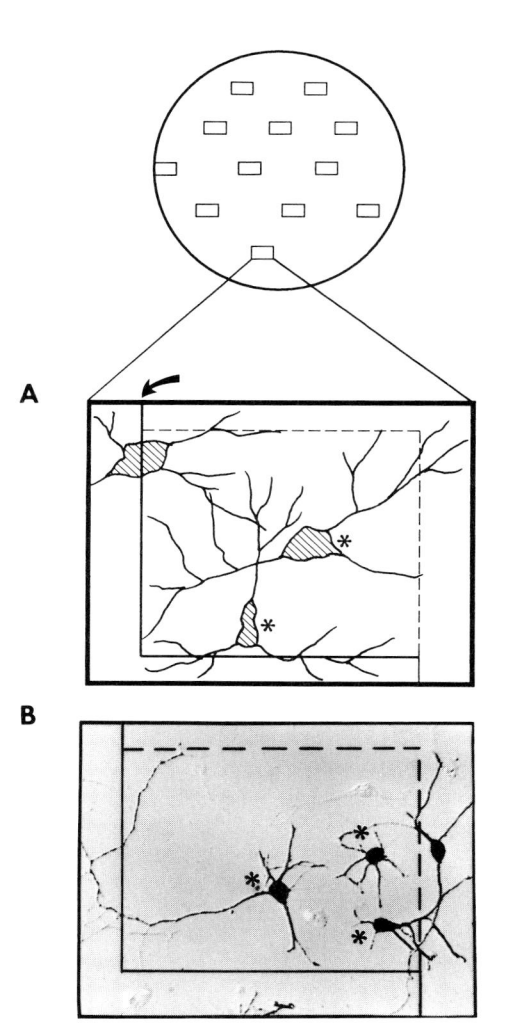

Figure 14.7 Diagrammatic representation of the systematic photographs and transparent counting frame used to perform quantitative morphometric analysis. Each small square
represents one photograph of the culture, which then was enlarged and analyzed.
(*A*) The enlarged diagram represents the photograph with the transparent counting
frame overlay. Note the full-drawn, solid-black exclusion edge (arrow). Two neurons
would be counted in this sample (asterisks). (*B*) Actual photograph of one area of
the culture plate with counting grid overlag. Three neurons would be counted in this
sample (∗). (Reproduced with permission from R. Ventimiglia, B. E. Jones, A. Moller,
A quantitative method for morphometric analysis in neuronal cell culture: unbiased
estimation of neuron area and number of branch points. J. Neurosci. Methods 1995;
57: 63–66.)

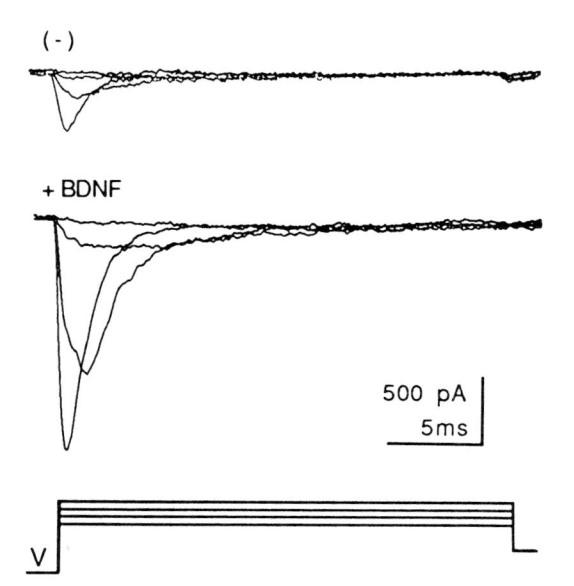

Figure 14.8 BDNF increases functional Na$^+$ channel expression in embryonic striatal neurons. Striatal neurons from E17 rat embryos were maintained in culture in the absence (−) or presence (+BDNF) of 50 ng/ml BDNF for 7 days before whole-cell patch clamp recordings were used to measure voltage-dependent Na$^+$ currents in response to changes in membrane potential (V). Superimposed current records illustrate the response to depolarizing pulses to −50, −40, −30, and −20 mV, from a holding potential of −80 mV and prepulse potential of 120 mV. Despite the increase in cell size after BDNF treatment (as indicated by measurements of cell membrane capacitance) the increase in peak Na$^+$ current amplitude in the BDNF-treated cell reflects an increase in Na$^+$ current *density*.

induced a nearly two-fold increase in cell body area and total area of neuritic arborization and an approximately three-fold increase in the number of dendritic branch points (Ventimiglia, Jones, et al., 1995).

The observed dramatic effects of BDNF on neuronal morphology, including increased dendritic branching, prompted us to investigate the functional consequences of neurotrophin treatment on the electrical properties of striatal neurons. Whole-cell patch clamp recordings, made from striatal cultures maintained for 1 week in the absence or presence of neurotrophins, revealed that BDNF treatment induced a significant increase in Na$^+$ current density (figure 14.8). These changes correlated with an increase in Na$^+$ channel gene expression as revealed by RNAse protection assays (Maue et al., 1995). Preliminary evidence suggests that the GABAergic neurons in the striatal cultures form functional synapses in culture (R. Maue, personal communication). Thus, this culture system facili-

tates studies that use the valuable combination of molecular and physiological approaches to assess the effects of neurotrophin treatment on neuronal function.

Conclusions

This chapter provides a detailed description of the preparation of low-density, serum-free cultures from embryonic rat striatum and its application to the study of the biological effects of neurotrophic factors. The methods that we have described may be applied to any region of interest in the nervous system. Additionally, the neurotrophic factors that we have employed in our studies now are available commercially. For those interested in investigating the responses of a particular population of neurons to neurotrophic factors, a good starting point would be the wealth of literature on the distribution of the neurotrophins, their receptors, and their effects on a wide range of cell types (for a review, see Lindsay et al., 1994).

In conducting the types of in vitro analyses that we have described, one must keep in mind the limitations of such a system. Afferent input to neurons, supporting glial cells, and other endogenous factors that are likely to influence the expression of various neuronal phenotypes in vivo are absent in a simplified culture system.

Though we acknowledge that any simplified in vitro system has inherent experimental limitations, that admission need not detract from the tremendous utility of developing well-designed cell culture paradigms. Our efforts in developing a reliable methodology to culture embryonic striatal neurons have facilitated greatly the identification of specific striatal neuronal populations wherein survival or differentiation is influenced by specific neurotrophic factors. Additionally, it has increased our understanding of the biological processes affected by the neurotrophins. In the long term, the identification of neuroprotective factors and elucidation of their mechanism(s) of action offer hope for understanding and preventing selective striatal cell death that occurs in such neurodegenerative diseases as Huntington's disease.

15 Cell Culture of Cholinergic and Cholinoceptive Neurons from the Medial Habenula

Raul Krauss and Gerald D. Fischbach

We are interested in cellular and molecular mechanisms involved in the formation and maintenance of synapses. Much of our work uses relatively sparse cell cultures of neurons dissociated from the central nervous system (CNS) and cultured together with their targets. Two major advantages of studying synapse formation in vitro are the accessibility of the cells for microscopy and electrophysiology and also the ability to control the extracellular environment. These advantages allow one to test whether specific differentiation and trophic factors can produce changes in protein and gene expression that influence synaptic function. The flexibility provided by cell culture is such that the cells can be visualized in a living state, from the earliest stages of their development until they attain a mature differentiated state.

The formation of cholinergic synapses between somatic motor neurons and skeletal muscle has been studied extensively. Initial attempts to enrich spinal cord cultures with motoneurons used the fact that motoneurons are among the largest cells present in the embryonic chick spinal cord. Dissociated spinal cord cells from 7-day chick embryos were separated according to size by 1-*g* velocity sedimentation. The cells in the large cell fractions contained perhaps seven times more choline acetyltransferase (ChAT) than did cells in the trailing fractions (Berg and Fischbach, 1978). Another approach took advantage of the observation that cholinergic neurons are among the first to withdraw from the mitotic cycle (Hamburger, 1948; Levi-Montalcini, 1950). Spinal cord cultures from 4-day-old chick embryos developed three times more ChAT than did 7-day-old cultures, and 50% of the large neurons innervated nearby myotubes (Berg and Fischbach, 1978). A more refined approach to identify motoneurons consists of retrograde labeling of motoneurons by injection of fluorescein-conjugated wheat germ agglutinin or Lucifer Yellow-wheat germ agglutinin into the hindlimbs of 5-day-old chick embryos. Neuronal cultures were prepared from spinal cords after waiting 16 h. The motoneurons could be visualized by fluorescence microscopy (Calof and Reichardt, 1984; O'Brien and

Fischbach, 1986a). Between 65% and 95% of the motoneurons survived the procedure. To purifty these motoneurons, dissociated ventral spinal cords were subjected to fluorescence-activated cell sorting, yielding more than 90% pure motoneurons (O'Brien and Fischbach, 1986a). A similar procedure using DiI retrograde labeling followed by fluorescence-activated cell sorting has been used in E14 rat embryos (Martinou et al, 1989). Finally, a different approach used size separation on a metrizamide cushion followed by panning with a monoclonal antibody that binds the p75 low-affinity nerve growth factor (NGF) receptor to purify E15 rat spinal cord motorneurons (Camu and Henderson, 1992). Motorneuron cultures such as these have been used to study synapse formation at neuromuscular junctions formed by cocultures with myotubes (Role et al., 1985) or with spinal cord interneurons (O'Brien and Fischbach, 1986b).

In recent years, interest has increased in the study of cholinergic neurotransmission in the CNS. Attention has been focused on nicotinic acetylcholine receptors (nAChRs), prompted mainly be the cloning of several members of the neuronal nicotinic receptor family. Different combinations of subunits may account for the rich diversity of nAChRs observed in peripheral and central neurons. Interest has been stimulated also by the social and clinical implications of the involvement of nicotinic cholinergic transmission in such degenerative diseases as Alzheimer's and Parkinson's and also in tobacco addiction. The advantages of nerve cell culture previously mentioned can facilitate the analysis of how the levels and distribution of various subunits might be regulated during development and in the mature brain.

The neurons from the medial habenular nucleus (MHb) represent an excellent system to study central cholinergic differentiation in culture. They have been shown to respond robustly to exogenous nicotinic ligands and have been proposed as a major site of action of nicotine in the CNS (McCormick and Prince, 1987). These cells can be distinguished both anatomically and in their functional connectivity from the neurons in the adjacent lateral habenular nucleus (LHb). They consist of a relatively homogeneous population of CNS neurons, about 10 μm in diameter (Tokunaga and Otani, 1978; Herkenham and Nauta, 1979), which are both cholinoceptive and cholinergic (Houser et al., 1983; Contestabile et al., 1987) and express many different nicotinic receptor subunits at high levels

(Wada et al., 1989). The connectivity of this nucleus is very simple and well-characterized. It receives only one major input through the stria medullaris, containing axons originating mainly in the medial septal nucleus, the supracomissural septum, and in the diagonal band of Broca (Gottesfeld and Jakobowitz, 1979; Herkenham and Nauta, 1979; Contestabile and Fonnum, 1983; Fonnum and Contestabile 1984; Woolf and Butcher, 1985). The output of the MHb is through the fasciculus retroflexus, which terminates in the interpeduncular nucleus (Herkenham and Nauta, 1979; Contestabile et al., 1987). To our knowledge, the presence of interneurons and of synaptic connections between neurons within the MHb has not been described. This well-defined connectivity is extremely useful (and rare in the CNS) because the input and the output can be lesioned independently prior to tissue dissociation, to study the effect of denervation or axotomy. Finally, in spite of its small size, the nucleus is relatively easy to dissect in rat embryos. Although the habenulo-interpeduncular system has a counterpart in avians, the MHb is not as large and discretely defined as it is in mammals.

Previous studies of mammalian MHb cells have been performed in acutely dissociated cells but not in cell culture (Mulle and Changeux, 1990; Mulle et al., 1992; Lester and Dani, 1995). We developed a protocol to culture cells from rat MHb both at high and low density. The high-density conditions were designed for molecular biology studies wherein a certain amount of RNA is needed for studies in gene expression. The low-density conditions, which are similar in other respects, are optimal for whole-cell recordings.

Rationale

Several parameters may affect the success of a new type of neuronal culture. To optimize the survival of MHb cultures we considered the age of the fetuses, the dissection and dissociation medium, different growth media, the need for serum, and the use of trophic factors.

Optimal Age for Dissection

It is generally thought that neuronal yield and survival are increased when the dissection is performed at an age close to the last

mitotic division of the cells to be cultured. The neurons in the MHb are born between embryonic day 16 (E16) and embryonic day 18 (E18) (Lenn and Bayer, 1986); therefore, we chose to dissect MHb from E18 rat brains. Although we have not compared systematically neuronal survival of MHb neurons dissected at different ages, a few experiments with cells dissociated from E19 embryos gave less optimal results. We have also prepared cultures of MHb neurons from neonatal rats, but the survival of the neurons was poor.

Substrate

Our first attempts at coating tissue-culture plates and glass coverslips with a mixture of polylysine and laminin were successful in providing a medium for the attachment of the cells and for neurite extension. We found it made no difference whether the two components were added as a mixture, or whether the plates were incubated first with polylysine, followed by laminin.

Dissection Medium

Routinely, we perform our dissections in the dissociation medium (DM) described in box 15.1. We have dissected also a few times in Hank's buffered saline solution (HBSS) but have obtained consistently better survival using DM. As a possible rationale, it has been suggested that the increase in the external K^+ concentration may prevent the rundown of the Na^+ and K^+ gradients. These conditions may decrease the activity of the Na/K ATPase pumps and effectively relieve the cell from a major source of metabolic stress and energy consumption. The use of kynurenic acid and magnesium blocks glutamate receptors and prevents glutamate-induced neurotoxicity. This protocol was essentially developed by Furshpan and Potter (1989) for the culture of hippocampal cells and is related to an idea originated by Bernard Katz to improve the survival of frog neuromuscular preparations in the cold (E. Furshpan, personal communication). The use of glucose to supply a source of energy, of oxygenation of the medium, and of ice to reduce the metabolic activity of the cells appear to become unnecessary (see also chapter 12). We perform the entire procedure at room temperature (with the exception of the enzymatic digestion at 37°C).

Box 15.1 Solutions

Dissociation Medium (10× DM stock solutions)

Final concentration (1×)	Stock solutions	Volume (ml) for 250 ml 10× DM
90 mM Na_2SO_4	2.0 M	112.5
30 mM K_2SO_4	0.75 M	100
5.8 mM $MgCl_2$	4.9 M	3
0.25 mM $CaCl_2$	0.1 M	6.25
1 mM HEPES	0.5 M	5

PROCEDURE

Prepare individual stock solutions, mix in the order indicated, add 5 ml phenol red stock (0.5%), adjust pH to 7.4 with ∼2.5 ml 0.1 N NaOH, complete to 250 ml. Sterilize with prewashed nylon filter (0.2 μm-pore). Store at 4°C. Note: Warm Na_2SO_4 and K_2SO_4 to dissolve. (Reagents are from Sigma.)

DM/Ky, Mg

To 45 ml DM add 5 ml Ky/Mg stock (10 mM kynurenate and 100 mM Mg^{2+}).

Ky/Mg Stock (10 mM kynurenate and 100 mM Mg^{2+})

To 250-ml flask add 190 ml H_2O, 1 ml phenol red stock, 1.75 ml 1 N NaOH, 378 mg kynurenic acid (Sigma, no. K-3375), and 2 ml 500 mM HEPES. Then sonicate to dissolve kynurenate and add 4.08 ml $MgCl_2$ (4.9 M). Make up to 200 ml. Add up to 1 ml 0.1 N NaOH for pH 7.4. Sterilize in prewashed nylon filter (0.2-μm pore).

Enzyme Solution (made fresh)

Add 9.6 ml DM/Ky, Mg to 4.5 mg cysteine-HCl (Sigma, no. C-1276). Neutralize with ∼0.26 ml 0.1 N NaOH. Add 100 units papain (Worthington, Freehold, NJ; no. 35S922), activate enzyme at 37°C 10–15 min, and filter in prewashed nylon (0.2-μm pore).

Trypsin Inhibitor (TI)

Add 9.6 ml DM/Ky, Mg to 100 mg TI (type II-0; Sigma no. T-9253), sonicate (if necessary), adjust pH (if necessary), and filter in prewashed nylon (0.2-μm pore).

DNAse 100×

1 mg/ml DNAse I (type II-S, Sigma no. D4527) in DM. Filter in prewashed nylon (0.2-μm pore) and store at −20°C.

Growth Medium (GM)

DMEM high-glucose (Gibco BRL, no. 11960-044)
4% fetal calf serum
1 × B27 supplements (Gibco BRL no. 17504-010)
2 mM L-Gln (1× Gibco BRL no. 25030-080)
1 × penicillin-streptomycin (Gibco BRL no. 15140-122; supplied at 100×)
1 mM sodium pyruvate (1× Gibco BRL no. 11360-013)

Serum-Free Medium (Prepare GM without fetal calf serum).

Growth Medium

A major factor in determining the success of a new type of neuronal culture is the choice of an optimal growth medium. We tested several variations in composition to optimize neuronal survival further, focusing mainly on the requirements for serum or supplements and the type of basal medium.

At present, we routinely plate the cells in Dulbecco's modified Eagle's medium (D-MEM) basal medium containing 4% fetal calf serum and B-27 supplements (Gibco, Gaithersburg, MD). Our first experiments showed that MHb neurons did not survive in D-MEM basal medium (containing pyruvate and antibiotics; see box 15.1, Solutions). Subsequently, the cells were grown in D-MEM plus a multivitamin and antioxidant supplement (B-27) or in D-MEM and fetal calf serum (FCS) and finally in D-MEM containing both serum and B-27. In each case, the cells were plated at an initial density of 580 cells per square millimeter in 24-well tissue-culture plates containing 0.5 ml medium per well. Survival was assessed by counting neurons every day for 5 days. As shown in figure 15.1A, the cells survive much better in the presence of both FCS and the B-27 supplements than they do with either one alone.

Very few cells can survive initially in the absence of serum. However, after a glial monolayer has reached confluence (about 5 days), serum no longer is required, and the cultures may be switched to serum-free medium. These defined medium conditions can be very useful for studies of the effect of growth factors. In some situations, it may even be a requirement because serum may mask their effect.

We also tested two different basal media on MHb neuronal survival: D-MEM and Neurobasal, a modification of D-MEM formulated to be used in conjunction with B-27, for the culture of hippocampal neurons (Brewer et al., 1993). Figure 15.1B shows that, in the presence of both FCS and B-27, MHb neuronal survival was significantly better in D-MEM. Under these conditions, nearly half the population of neurons initially plated died during the first 5 days. The remaining population can be maintained for longer periods without significant declines in the amount of surviving neurons.

It should be pointed out that the survival curves in figure 15.1A and B apply only to a given plating density. In fact, in these experiments, the cells were plated at a rather low density (580 cells/mm^2) to facilitate counting during a 5-day period. When the cells were plated at a higher density (i.e., in the cultures used for RNA analy-

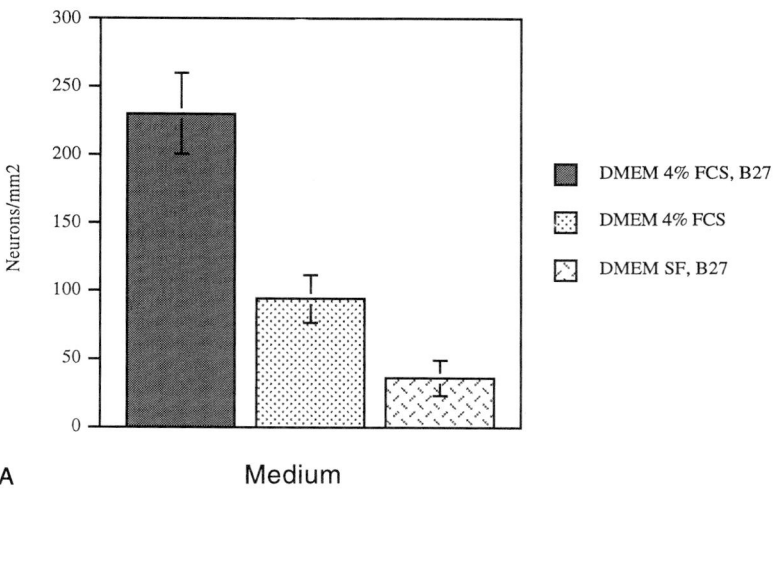

A

Medium

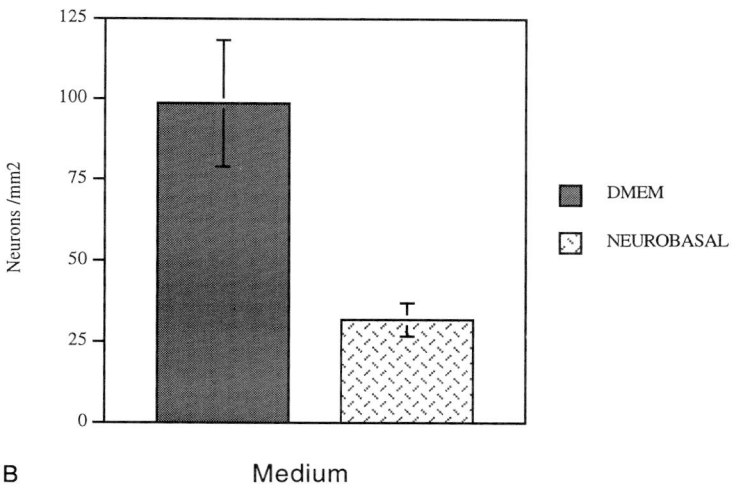

B

Medium

Figure 15.1 Optimization of the growth medium used in MHb cultures. (*A*) MHb neurons were counted after 5 days in culture in D-MEM medium with either 4% fetal calf serum (FCS), B-27 supplements, or a combination of the two. Better survival was obtained with a combination of 4% FCS and B-27 supplements. (*B*) Two different basal media, D-MEM and Neurobasal (Gibco) were tested on MHb neurons. Neurons were counted after 5 days in culture in medium containing both 4% FCS and B-27 supplements. Better survival was obtained when D-MEM was used as the basal medium.

sis, or for physiology wherein a small number of cells are plated at high density in the center of the coverslips), we did not detect any significant neuronal loss.

Growth and Differentiation Factors

Certain neuronal cell types require the presence of growth or trophic factors to survive in culture. A classic example is the need for NGF for the maintenance of sympathetic neurons of the superior cervical ganglion (Chun and Patterson, 1977). We examined whether several known trophic factors have an influence in the survival of MHb neurons in culture. Neurons were cultured for 5 days with NGF, brain-derived neurotrophic factor (BDNF), neurotrophin-3 (NT-3), and acetycholine receptor inducing activity (ARIA) in the presence (figure 15.2A) or absence (figure 15.2B) of FCS. Under these culture conditions, no further increase in neuronal survival was detected using any of these trophic factors.

Protocol for the Dissection and Culture of MHb Neurons

Preparations

ANIMALS

For our MHb dissection, we use E18 rat embryos (Sprague-Dawley) from either Taconic Farms or Charles River Laboratories (Wilmington, MA). Because the MHb is a small nucleus, the number of animals used to make cultures is greater than usually required for hippocampal or cortical cultures. The exact number depends on the type of assay intended. For biochemical assays (discussed later), where a larger amount of material is necessary, we usually process 2–4 pregnant rats with an average of 12 embryos each. This choice allows the plating of one to two 24-well tissue-culture plates. For physiology and immunocytochemistry, one litter usually is sufficient. The dissection takes approximately 1 h per litter.

SUBSTRATE

As discussed earlier, we have plated MHb neurons in a mixture of poly-D-lysine-laminin, with very good results. Prepare a stock solution of poly-D-lysine (Collaborative Research, no. 40210) 2 mg/

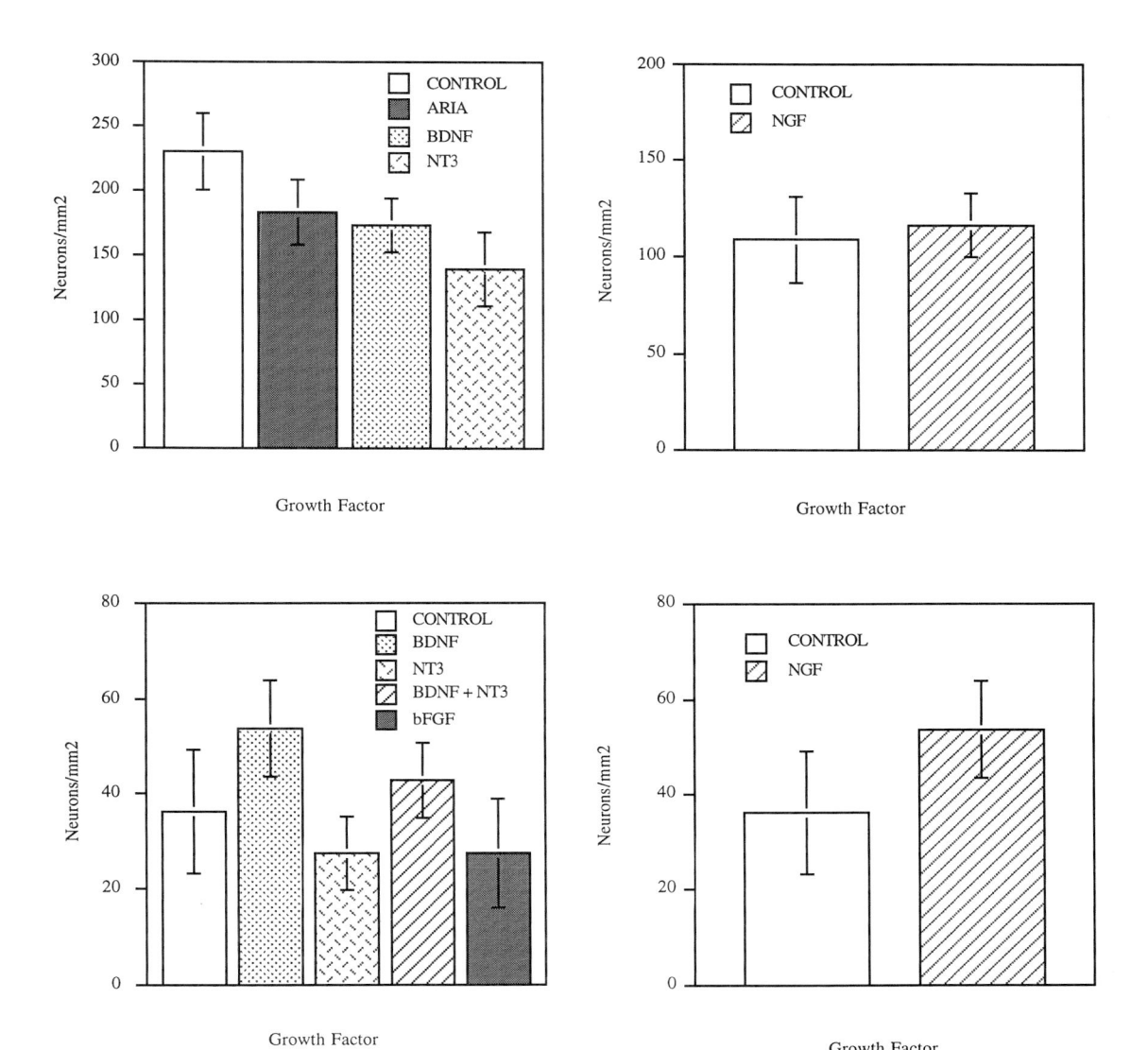

Figure 15.2 Effect of trophic factors on the survival of MHb neurons in culture. MHb neurons were counted after 5 days in culture in the presence of 100 ng/ml NGF; 50 ng/ml BDNF; 50 ng/ml NT-3; 10 ng/ml bFGF; or recombinant ARIA in COS cell-conditioned medium at a concentration that gave maximal response in a muscle nAChR incorporation assay, either in the presence (*A*) or absence (*B*) of serum. No improvement in survival was obtained with any of these factors in the culture medium.

ml (20×) in ddH$_2$O and sterilize by filtration. Laminin (Collaborative Research, Bedford MA, no. 40232) comes as a frozen solution containing 1 mg in variable amounts of 50 mM TRIS-HCl pH 7.4, 150 mM NaCl (always less than 1 ml). Bring the volume to 1 ml with ddH$_2$O, to make a 1 mg/ml stock solution (40×). For both solutions, make 200 to 300 µl sterile aliquots and keep them at −20°C.

For tissue culture plates, we coat with a sterile solution containing 0.1 mg/ml poly-D-lysine and 25 µg/ml laminin in ddH$_2$O and keep in a 37°C incubator overnight. We rinse the plates three times briefly, with sterile ddH$_2$O. The plates can be stored dried at room temperature for several weeks before use (David Cardozo, personal communication).

The protocol for coating sterile glass coverslips is the same as that for tissue-culture plates. First, clean the coverslips by storing them in 95% ethanol. Sterilize by flaming immediately before use. Coat as for tissue-culture plates, with 12-mm coverslips inside individual wells in a 24-multiwell tissue-culture plate. We have made attempts to improve the adhesion of the polylysine-laminin coat and of the cells, by etching the glass with 0.5 N NaOH for 3 to 5 h in 24-well plates, followed by extensive washing with ddH$_2$O. Sterilize the coverslips, before coating, with a 30 min UV-irradiation in a sterile hood. This etching procedure appears to improve cell adhesion in long-term cultures, but no difference appears between MHb cells grown on coverslips cleaned with ethanol or etched with NaOH in cultures younger than 8 to 10 days (Kristina Wietasch, personal communication).

As originally communicated by G. Banker and colleagues (and later corroborated by several laboratories), the source of the coverslips may affect neuronal survival, owing to the presence of impurities in the raw materials used to make the glass. We use Assistent-Brand high-quality borosilicate glass coverslips manufactured in Germany and sold by Carolina Biologicals (Burlington, NC).

SOLUTIONS AND CULTURE MEDIA
We perform the dissection in 1× DM prepared from a 10× stock (see box 15.1, Solutions). The MHbs are kept in DM plus kynurenate and magnesium (DM/Ky, Mg). As described previously, the ionic composition was designed to prevent the rundown of ionic gradients in the cells.

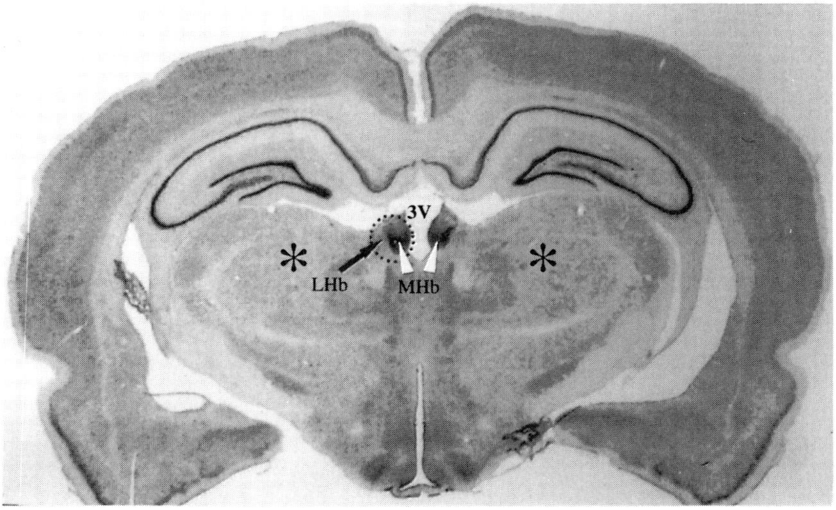

Figure 15.3 Coronal section at the level of the habenula. Section of an adult rat brain stained with thionin, a cell body stain. An equivalent section from an E18 embryo would look very similar. The dashed line shows the habenular nucleus, located in the dorsal part of the thalamus (asterisks). The lateral habenula (LHb) is indicated by the black arrow. The medial habenulae (MHb) correspond to the intensely stained cells shown by the white arrowheads at either side of the third ventricle (3V).

Our standard growth medium (GM) consists of D-MEM basal medium containing 4% FCS and the B27 supplement described by Brewer et al. (1993, see box 15.1). Frequently, we change to serum-free medium (see box 15.1) after the cells have grown in standard medium for 5 days (see later).

Cultures

DISSECTION OF FETAL MHB

The dissection of the MHb is relatively easy once the habenular complex is correctly identified visually. The habenular nucleus is a small structure, localized in the dorsal part of the thalamus, one on each side of the third ventricle (figure 15.3). The MHb consists of a tightly packed group of cells that can be readily distinguished from the LHb (see figure 15.3). The dissection is started by opening the skull, removing the brain, and placing it dorsal side up in DM. The instruments needed after this step are two no. 5 forceps and a scalpel with a no. 10 and a no. 15 blade.

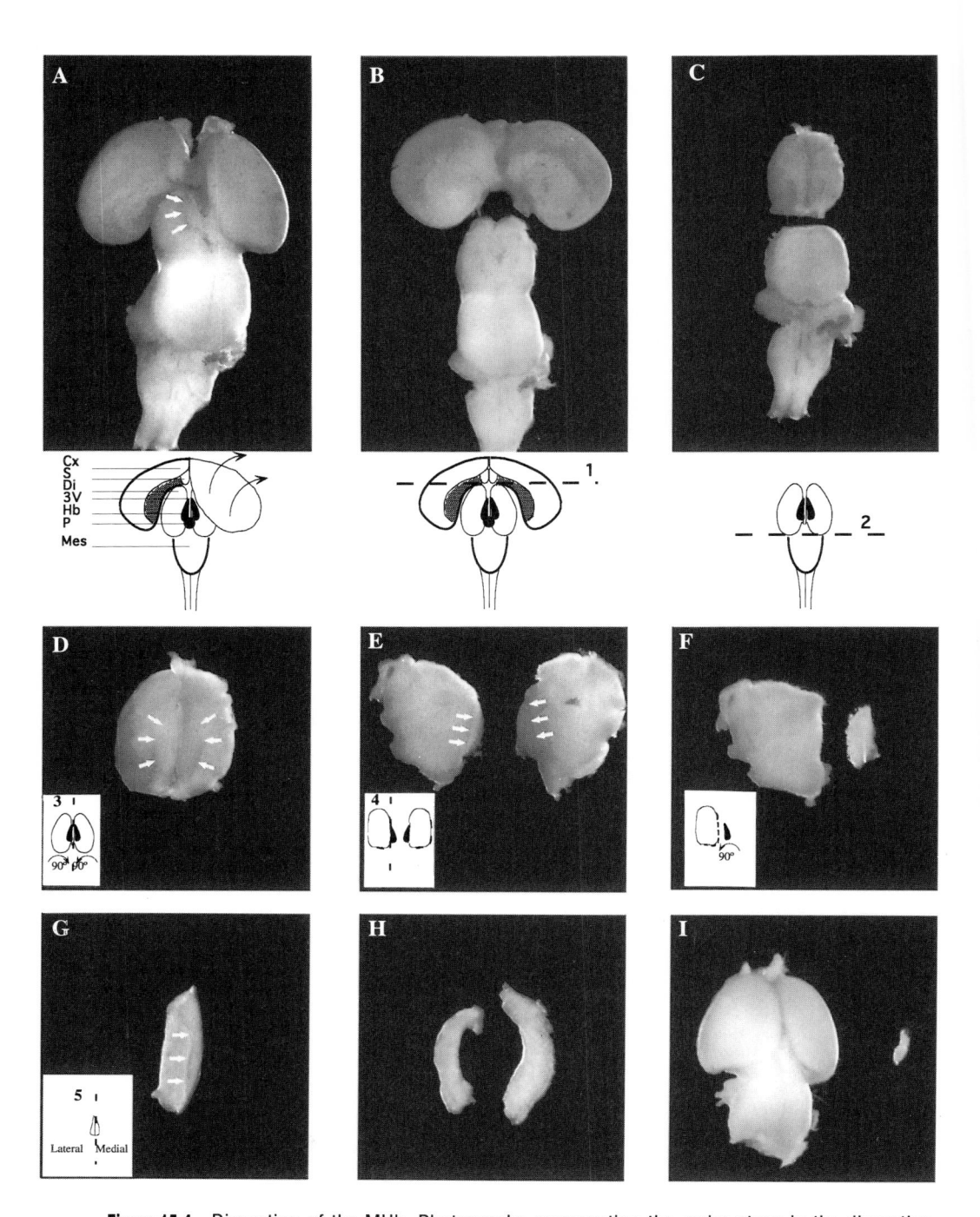

Figure 15.4 Dissection of the MHb. Photographs representing the major steps in the dissection procedure of a rat E18 brain (as seen through the dissecting microscope). The accompanying diagrams outline the major brain structures. The dashed lines represent the plane at which cuts need to be made. (*A*) Lift the cortex and move it anteriorly and to the side to expose the diencephalon. The arrows indicate the boundary of the

We recommend beginning with the following dissection procedure. Under a dissecting microscope, use the forceps to lift up the cortex (containing the hippocampus) from the diencephalon (containing the habenular nuclei). Start from the most caudal part and proceed until the entire diencephalon is exposed (figure 15.4A). Using the no. 10 scalpel blade, make a coronal cut between the diencephalon and the septum. The septum (with the cortex still attached) is discarded (see figure 15.4B, cut 1). Remove the pineal gland with a pair of forceps by lifting carefully and moving in a rostral direction. This process usually cleans the meninges present on top of the third ventricle and habenular region. At this stage, the third ventricle is exposed, and the habenular complex is visible as a pair of fusiform "swellings" along the dorsal wall of the ventricles. It may be necessary to clean the meninges around the LHb by peeling a small portion of it to the side. Make another coronal cut between the mesencephalon and the diencephalon and discard the mesencephalon (which will have the cerebellum plus brainstem attached; see figure 15.4C, cut 2). Separate the right and left diencephalon with a sagittal cut through the third ventricle in the anteroposterior axis (see figure 15.4D, cut 3). Turn over each half so that both lie flat on their medial side. A shallow groove, running in the anteroposterior axis, is visible near the dorsal side, delineating the border between the habenula and the thalamus (see figure 15.4E, arrows). With a pair of no. 5 forceps or a fine scalpel (a no. 15 blade), make a vertical cut along this groove to separate the habenula from the thalamus (see figure 15.4E, cut 4). At this stage, the habenular complex is isolated and is lying medial side down (see figure 15.4F).

habenula from the rest of the diencephalon. (*B*) Cut between septum and diencephalon (no. 1) and remove the pineal gland. (*C*) Make a second coronal cut to separate the diencephalon from the mesencephalon, cerebellum, and brainstem. (*D*) Isolated diencephalon showing the two habenular nuclei. Arrows indicate their boundaries. Make a third cut sagittally along the midline to separate left and right diencephalon. Turn each half 90 degrees onto its medial side (inset). (*E*) With each half lying on its medial side, separate the habenula from the thalamus (no. 4). Arrows indicate the boundary between the habenula and the thalamus. (*F*) After the habenula is isolated from thalamus, turn it on its ventral side (inset). (*G*) Cut (no. 5) along the membrane formed by the roof of the third ventricle (arrows) to separate MHb from LHb. (*H*) MHb on the right and LHb on the left side, after separation. (*I*) E18 rat brain with an isolated MHb on its right side for size comparison. Cx, cortex; Di, diencephalon; Hb, habenula; Mes, mesencephalon; P, pineal gland; S, septum; 3V, third ventricle.

It is very important to take care in remembering the orientation of the habenula so as to proceed to the next step, which is the separation of the medial and lateral halves. Turn the habenula to the side so that the thalamic side now faces down and the dorsal side faces up. A thin, short membrane (a remnant of the roof of the third ventricle) is usually visible on top along the midline (see figure 15.4G, arrows). Using that membrane as a reference, hold the habenula with forceps and with a small (no. 15) scalpel cut vertically along the midline in the anteroposterior axis to separate the medial from the lateral habenula (see figure 15.4G, cut 5). Transfer the piece corresponding to the MHb to a clean dish containing DM/Ky, Mg and collect the MHbs there until all the brains have been dissected.

The positioning of the brain in the dissecting dish is a matter of personal choice as long as the orientation of the habenula—in particular its medial and lateral sides—is always remembered. Our preference is to dissect two or three brains in parallel (in the same dish) until reaching the stage of dissecting the habenula. At this point, dissect the habenulae one by one and carefully align them on one side of the dish with their medial side pointing toward the left, taking great care not to disturb the liquid while dissecting the other brains. Then, cut to separate MHb from LHb sequentially and transfer the MHbs to a clean dish containing DM/Ky, Mg at room temperature until the end of the dissection.

We also have developed a faster, alternative protocol. However, this method should be attempted only after becoming completely familiar with the appearance of the relevant structures in brains dissected according to the procedure described earlier. Although this protocol saves a significant amount of time when many embryos are required, the brain is distorted in the procedure, making it difficult to recognize the habenula. The method takes advantage of the fact that the skull in the embryo is very soft and that both the skull and the skin are thin and transparent. This allows one to see the brain and cut a slice containing the habenula without first removing the brain from the skull.

Cut the head from the embryo and put it in a dry dish with its dorsal side up, the front held with forceps. Using a no. 10 scalpel blade, make a coronal cut at the posterior end of the sagittal fissure formed by the cerebral cortices (figure 15.5A, arrows), at the point where the posterior ends of the cerebral hemispheres cover the mesencephalon and form a lambdoid shape (see figure 15.5A, arrowhead; see also diagram in C). Still holding the head firmly, make

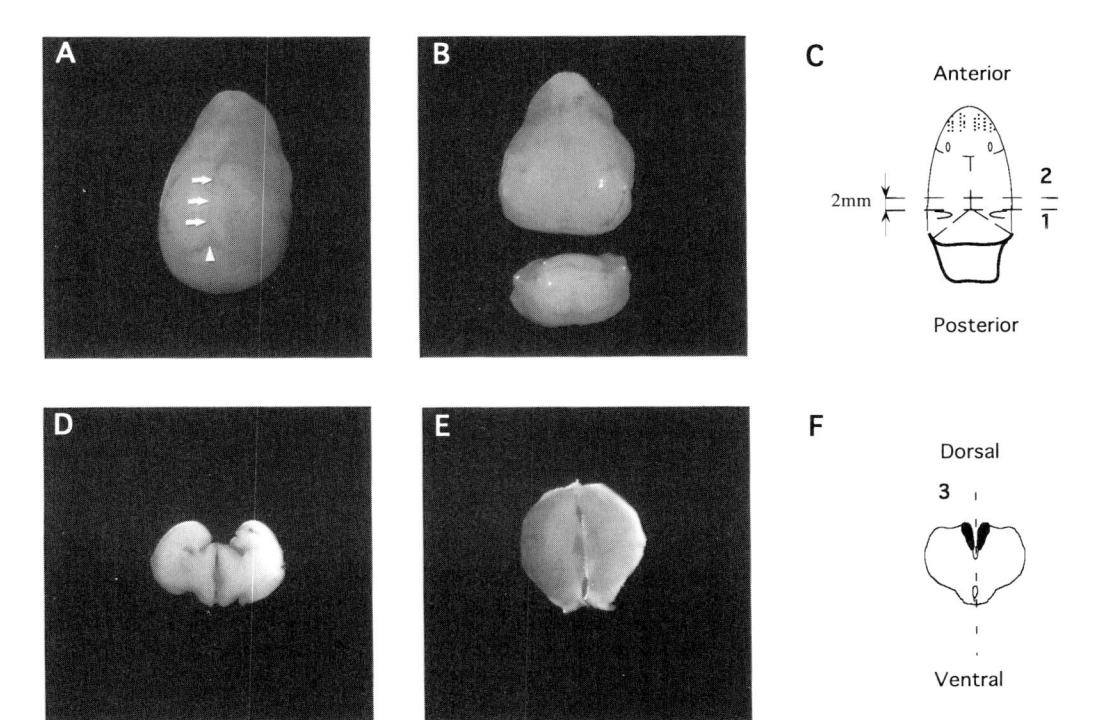

Figure 15.5 Alternative protocol. (*A*) Using a complete head, make a first coronal cut at the point indicated by the arrowhead (see diagram in figure 15.5C). Arrows indicate the sagittal fissure formed by the cerebral cortices. (*B*) With the forebrain still in the head, make a second coronal cut approximately 2 mm anterior to the first (see diagram in figure 15.5C). (*C*) Diagram of the head and the two cuts needed to isolate a brain slice containing the habenulae. (*D*) Turn the slice on its posterior side. After removing the surrounding skin and skull, remove the cortex. (*E*) With the slice still on its posterior side, make a cut through the midline to separate left and right diencephalon, as indicated in the diagram in (*F*) Continue the dissection from figure 15.4E.

another coronal cut at approximately 2 mm anterior to the first cut (see figure 15.5C). As the tissue is very soft, the cuts have to be made rapidly with a single sliding stroke; slow pressure on the blade will cause the tissue to collapse. Transfer the slice obtained in this manner to a dish containing DM and remove the surrounding skull and skin. These slices will contain the hypothalamus and the region of the thalamus containing the habenula (see figure 15.5D). With the slice lying on its posterior face, remove the cortex (see figure 15.5E). Then make a midsagittal cut through the third ventricle (see figure 15.5F) and continue the dissection as described in the main protocol. Frequently, because of the opening made in the skull by the first cut, the complete forebrain will come

Box 15.2   Digestion and Trituration Protocol

1. Incubate MHbs in 2–3 ml enzyme solution 30 min at 37°C. Agitate gently four or five times during the incubation period.
2. Rinse with 2 ml DM/Ky, Mg.
3. Rinse with 2 ml DM/Ky, Mg containing 20 µl of 100× DNAse. Incubate 4–5 min until the MHbs disaggregate completely.
4. Rinse with 2 ml DM/Ky, Mg.
5. Incubate 5 min in 2 ml TI.
6. Rinse once with 2.5 ml TI and triturate, in TI, *gently*, with 2-ml plastic pipette approximately 50 times. (As an option, if tissue remains, remove cells, add 2.5 ml TI, triturate again, and pool the two solutions.)
7. Centrifuge 6 min in IEC clinical centrifuge at 1000 rpm followed by 2 min at 1500 rpm.
8. Remove the supernatant, containing dead cells and debris, and resuspend gently in 2 ml GM.
9. Count, dilute with GM to the appropriate cell density, and plate.

out of the cranium on making the second cut. This is not an inconvenience; the brain still is removed much faster this way. In fact, some investigators may prefer to do this intentionally instead of obtaining a slice.

DISSOCIATION OF TISSUE AND CULTURE CONDITIONS
After dissection, transfer the MHb to a 15-ml conical tube with a Pasteur pipette. The pipette should be wetted previously to prevent small pieces of tissue from sticking to the glass. See box 15.2 for summary of digestion and trituration protocol. After waiting a few seconds for the fragments to settle at the bottom, remove the supernatant and incubate the cells in 2.5 ml of papain solution at 37°C for 30 min. Resuspend the tissue by gentle agitation of the tube four or five times during that period.

Carefully remove the supernatant and discard. Rinse the fragments with 2.0 ml of DM/Ky, Mg at room temperature. After the tissue settles to the bottom, rinse the fragments with 2 ml DM/Ky, Mg containing 20 µl of 100× DNAse (see box 15.1). The DNAse is used to disaggregate the MHb fragments, which tend to clump due to DNA released by lysed cells. This action interferes with the subsequent trituration and separation of the cells. However, we found that including the enzyme at this washing stage makes it unnecessary to introduce it during the trituration itself. Incubate 4 to 5 min at room temperature until the MHbs disaggregate com-

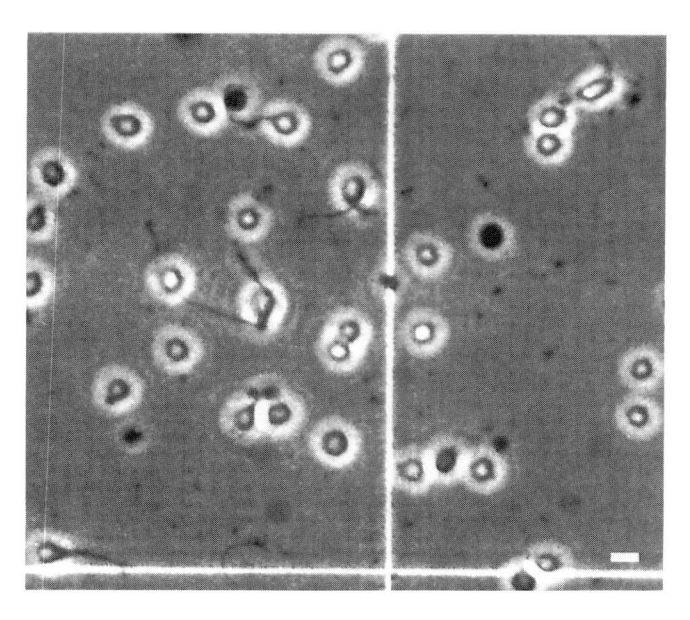

Figure 15.6 Freshly dissociated neurons from the MHb. E18 MHb were dissected and digested in papain as described in the protocol. After gentle trituration, a sample was counted in a hemocytometer. The photograph taken through the hemocytometer shows cells of a uniform size, many of them having processes still attached. Scale bar: 10 µm.

pletely. This condition can be checked by gentle agitation; the pieces of tissue should move freely in the solution. Rinse again with 2 ml DM/Ky, Mg, remove the supernatant, and incubate 5 min at room temperature in 2 ml trypsin inhibitor (TI). Change the supernatant for another 2.5 ml of TI and triturate, gently, with a pre-wetted 2-ml plastic serological pipette (Falcon no. 7507), moving the solution up and down approximately 50 times with the aid of a rubber bulb. If tissue remains, the supernatant containing the cells may be removed, adding 2.5 ml TI to the remaining tissue and triturating again, pooling the two supernatants. Careful trituration is very important to achieve good survival of the cultures. The up-and-down strokes must be gentle but firm, or the tissue will not disaggregate. If the procedure has been performed correctly, no aggregates will remain, and most cells will have short processes still attached to the cell bodies (figure 15.6). We discourage the use of a flame-constricted Pasteur pipette because the turbulence usually is too harsh. The goal is to achieve as much dissociation as possible by enzymatic action rather than by mechanical shearing forces.

After trituration, centrifuge the cells 6 min in an IEC (International Equipment Co, Needham Heights, MA) clinical centrifuge

at 1000 rpm followed by 2 min at 1500 rpm. Most of the debris and dead cells float on the surface. Carefully remove the supernatant, starting from the top and moving down with the pipette until reaching the cells. Resuspend the cells gently in 2 ml GM. Count a small aliquot (20 µl) in a hemocytometer, dilute with GM to the appropriate cell density, and plate. Although it is small, the MHb is tightly packed with small neurons. Our usual yield is some 120,000 cells per MHb (or ~250,000 per animal), so a four-litter dissection typically will yield approximately 1.2×10^7 cells.

PLATING DENSITY

The survival of the cultures is affected by cell density. We found that neurons plated at 400,000 to 1,000,000 cells per well in 0.5 ml medium in 24-well tissue-culture plates (diameter, 15 mm per well) can survive for up to 8 weeks in a 10% CO_2 incubator at 37°C. These cultures usually are used for the extraction of total RNA to be analyzed by Northern blotting.

For physiology or microscopy, fewer cells are required. In these experiments, visualization is improved by plating at a lower cell density and on glass coverslips held in 24 multiwell tissue-culture plates. Bring the cells to a density of 1,000,000 cells per milliliter in GM. Carefully deposit a 70-µl aliquot (70,000 cells) in a drop in the center of each 12-mm coverslip. Transfer the plates to a 10% CO_2 incubator at 37°C, using care to minimize agitation so that the cells settle in the center of the coverslips. After 1 to 1.5 h, gently increase the volume in each well to 0.5 ml with GM, using care not to disturb the cells.

FEEDING

Usually, we feed the cells once a week, replacing only half the medium. We do so to allow the accumulation of factors that are produced by the cells themselves and act in an autocrine or paracrine fashion. Replacing only half the medium also minimizes mechanical disturbances and the chance of transient drying of the cells. Nutrients and medium evaporation are not limiting, so we also have had good survival with no feeding at all for 4 weeks!

In some circumstances, it may be desirable to grow the cells in the absence of serum. One obvious situation would be to assay polypeptide growth factors. We found that dissociated MHb neurons can survive in serum-free medium for long periods. It is essential, however, to grow the cells in complete medium for 4 to 5 days to

allow glial cells to proliferate and form a feeder layer before switching to serum-free conditions. Glial cells do not proliferate as rapidly in serum-free medium. This might be an advantage, because it will stop the glial cells from taking over the cultures; however, long-term survival may be affected.

DESCRIPTION OF CULTURES

Freshly dissociated MHb neurons appear small ($\sim 10\,\mu m$), homogeneous, and phase-bright. Very short neurites can be seen by 1 day after plating and are clearly visible by 2 days. A small number of floating dead cells ($\sim 10\%$) and debris may occur at this stage, but they do not increase over time. The processes become longer and more elaborate by the third day of culture. Large, flat cells, which presumably are glial, start to be visible between 1 and 2 days after plating. They increase in number with time and, by day 5, they usually form a confluent monolayer, with many neurons growing on top. At this time, most of the cellular debris present in the first few days has disappeared. After several days, the neurons are rounder and more fusiform than they are polygonal and multipolar (figure 15.7). In some neurons, thick tapering processes (probably corresponding to dendrites) can be observed, although we have not attempted a more detailed characterization of cell polarity. If neurons survive for 5 days, usually they can be maintained for several weeks.

Troubleshooting

In general, this system has given us very little trouble. Once the dissection, the trituration, and the growth medium were optimized, the cultures have been very reproducible.

Occasionally, a large number of cells may die during the first 3 or 4 days. We have attributed the problem to three possible sources. The first one is the serum. All batches of serum need to be tested for toxicity, even after heat inactivation. Commonly, different batches of serum will present differences in the way they affect neuronal survival, and some batches actually may be toxic. The growth medium itself is quite stable. We have used medium kept at 4°C for up to a month without any significant difference in yield or survival. The second source seems to be related to the quality of the trituration. As was mentioned earlier, the trituration must be very gentle; for that reason, we use a 2-ml plastic serological pipette instead

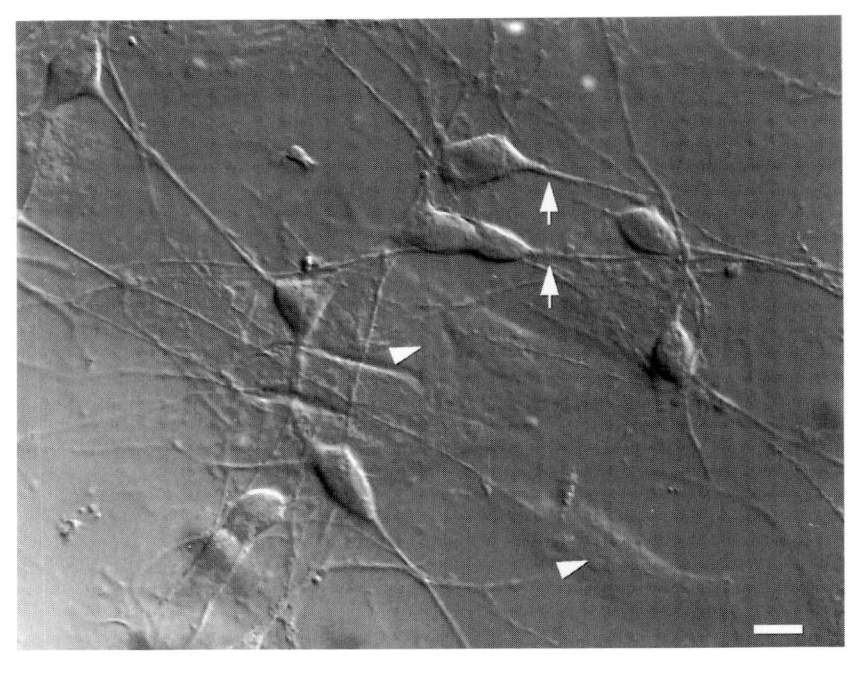

Figure 15.7 MHb neurons after 5 days in culture. MHb neurons were cultured as described in the protocol. The cells were plated on poly-D-lysine-laminin-coated coverslips and maintained in culture for 5 days in growth medium. The picture was taken under Nomarski optics. Neurons are growing on top of a layer of glial cells (arrowheads). The arrows indicate tapering processes, presumably dendritic, coming from MHb neurons. Many processes originating from neurons outside the field of view can also be seen. Scale bar: 10 μm.

of a Pasteur pipette. We also recommend that papain be prepared fresh for each dissection. After the enzyme is in solution for more than 2 or 3 days, harsher trituration conditions are needed to disrupt the tissue. Usually, this condition can be diagnosed on discovery of a large amount of cellular debris that tends to accumulate in the center of the wells. The third cause of early neuronal death seems to be related to the age of the fetuses. If animals older than E18 are used, sometimes the yield of surviving neurons is compromised. The use of older animals also appears to compromise long-term survival, even if the cultures look healthy during the first week.

Occasionally, approximately 7 days after plating, when the glial cell layer already has formed, some of the cultures peel off the glass or even from tissue-culture plastic. We assume that this reaction is due to poor substrate adhesion, because it happens only in some

(but not all) of the wells of a multiwell plate. Should it happen consistently with glass coverslips, an alternative is to etch them with 0.1 N NaOH as described.

We have also observed a certain difficulty in maintaining the cells when they are plated at low density (<600 cells/mm^2). When cells are needed for electrophysiological recordings, we usually plate them in a dot in the center of the coverslip as described. An alternative, which we have not yet explored, is the use of MHb- or glial-conditioned medium.

When all else fails, the best thing to do is to start again, preparing fresh medium.

Applications

These cultures can be used in studies of regulation of expression of nAChR subunit genes and proteins. Neuronal nAChRs are made up of several subunits. A total of eight α and three non-α, or β, subunits have been identified by molecular cloning (Boulter et al., 1986, 1987, 1990; Goldman et al., 1987; Nef et al., 1988; Wada et al., 1988; Deneris et al., 1989; Duvoisin et al., 1989; Couturier 1990a,b). In situ hybridization studies have shown that the nAChR subunits have a distinct and sometimes overlapping distribution (Wada et al., 1989). It is likely that different combinations of subunits can generate pharmacologically and physiologically distinct types of receptors (Boulter et al., 1987; Wada et al., 1988; Duvoisin et al., 1989; Couturier, 1990a,b). MHb cultures could also be used to study the physiology and pharmacology of different types of CNS nAChRs and to correlate that information with their subunit composition. Because these neurons are both cholinoceptive and cholinergic, they could be used as a CNS model to study the formation and maintenance of cholinergic synapses.

We have used this system to study the effect of ARIA, a differentiation factor that is isolated from the CNS and promotes the synthesis of nicotinic AChRs in muscle (Jessell et al., 1979; Usdin and Fischbach, 1986; Falls et al., 1993). We wanted to determine the potential role of ARIA in the regulation of neuronal nicotinic receptors in the CNS. We decided to study that regulation at the level of gene expression by looking at the levels of mRNA—and at the level of the receptors—by recording whole-cell nicotinic currents.

We have determined already that the ARIA receptor, a member of the epidermal growth factor receptor family of tyrosine kinases, can

Days in culture   2   3   5   L6
ARIA   - + - + - +   - +

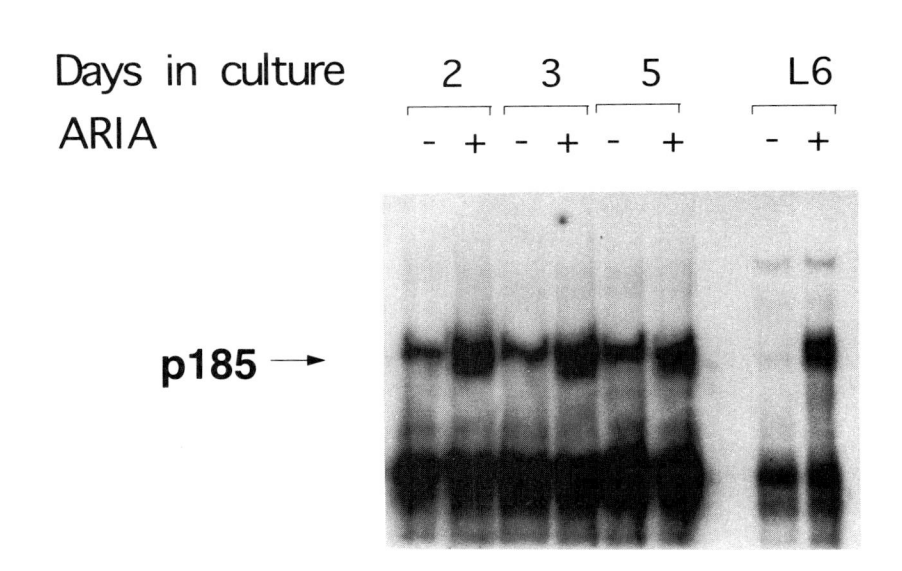

p185 →

Figure 15.8 Activation of the ARIA receptor in MHb cultures. MHb neurons were cultured as described for 2, 3, and 5 days. At the times indicated, the cells were treated with ARIA
for 45 min. The cells were dissolved in Laemmli sample buffer, and equal aliquots
were subjected to PAGE followed by Western blot analysis using a monoclonal antibody against phosphotyrosine. A band at approximately 185 kDa, corresponding to
the ARIA receptor, is labeled specifically on treatment with ARIA. The two lanes on
the right show the effect of ARIA treatment of the L6 muscle cell line, as control.

be activated in MHb cultures. After ARIA treatment for 45 min, a
band of ∼185 kDa is phosphorylated on tyrosines. As shown in
figure 15.8, the cells respond to this factor at 2, 3, and 5 days of
culture. There is a constitutively phosphorylated protein with a
slightly higher M_r. than the broad band visible in the treated cells,
and probably is unrelated to the ARIA receptor.

In situ hybridization studies indicate the presence of several
nAChR subunits in the MHb (Wada et al., 1989). We determined
the expression of nAChR subunits in our MHb cultures by Northern
blotting.

Our protocol is as follows: RNA from 400,000 to 1,000,000 cells
per well (following a variation of the acid guanidinium thio-
cyanate-phenol protocol of Chomczynski and Sacchi, 1987) using
1 ml of Ultraspec solution (BIOTECX, Houston, TX) for each well of
a 24-well plate. We follow the instructions of the manufacturer,
with the exception of adding 1 µl of 20 mg/ml molecular biology
grade glycogen (Boehringer Mannheim GmbH, Cat. no. 901 393) to
the aqueous phase, as a carrier, before the addition of isopropanol.
Precipitate the RNA overnight at −20°C to increase the yield of

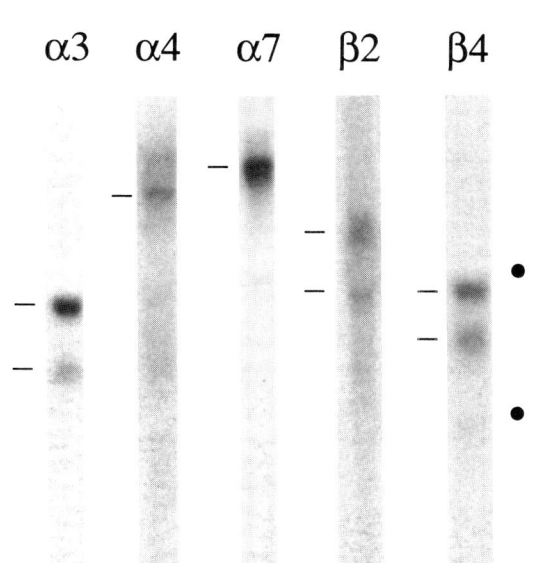

Figure 15.9 nAChR subunits are expressed in MHb cultures. MHb neurons were cultured for 5 days. Three µg of total RNA were analyzed by Northern blotting using probes specific to the 3′ untranslated region of nAChR subunits α3, α4, α7, β2, and β4, as indicated in the figure. (cDNAs kindly provided by Dr. Jim Boulter.) The dots on the right indicate the position of the 28s and 18s rRNA bands. Northern blots were prepared and hybridized essentially as described in Rosen et al. (1990). Hybridization was performed at 42°C for 18 h. Final high-stringency wash was 45 min at 45°–50°C in 0.1× SSC, 0.1% SDS.

total RNA. Typically, we obtain 4 to 8 µg of total RNA per well. Electrophorese 3 µg of total RNA in a 1.3% agarose gel containing 2.2 M formaldehyde as recommended by Rosen et al. (1990). Instead of making a thin gel by surface tension, as in Rosen et al. (1990), we calculate the amount of agarose solution required to make a 4-mm-thick gel in a standard horizontal electrophoresis gel box. This variation produces gels of approximately the same thickness as a surface-tension gel but facilitates the procedure. Blot onto positively charged nylon membrane (Magnagraph 0.45 µ; MSI, Westboro, MA, Cat. no. NJOHY45OF5) by capillary transfer using 10× SSC.

We determined that nAChR subunits are expressed abundantly in MHb cultures. Figure 15.9 shows a Northern blot prepared from rat MHb cultures, probed for nAChR α3, α4, α7, β2, and β4. More than one transcript size is evident in each case. The presence of multiple transcripts of these subunits has been described by Boulter et al. (1990) in PC12 cells and may represent differences in the length of the untranslated regions or alternatively spliced

forms. We could not detect the α2 and α5 mRNAs in our cell cultures. This repertoire is similar to that described in the MHb by in situ hybridization (Goldman et al., 1987; Wada et al., 1989). The variety of nAChR subunits in the MHb, therefore, is present also in the cultures, making this a system suitable for studies of the regulation as well as the physiology and pharmacology of nAChRs in the CNS.

16 The Cerebellum: Purification and Coculture of Identified Cell Populations

Mary Elizabeth Hatten, Wei-Qiang Gao, Mary E. Morrison, and
Carol A. Mason

Development of the Cerebellar Cortex; A Model for Cortical Histogenesis

For more than a century, the cerebellar cortex has been a focal point for studies about the development of the brain. Ramón y Cajal (1888) first illustrated the five principal cells of the cerebellum and heralded the unusual two-step migration of the granule neuron across the surface of the anlage and inward along the Bergmann glial fiber system (figure 16.1). This former phase, formation of a displaced germinal zone (which Cajal called the external germinal layer [EGL], provided a means of expansion of the pool of granule neurons into the largest single cell population in brain (Miale and Sidman, 1961; Altman and Bayer, 1985a,b). Indeed, by some accounts (Kandel et al., 1991), as many granule cells are found in the cerebellum as there are neurons in the cortex! This fact, along with the detailed knowledge of the other principal cell type—the Purkinje cell—and the circuitry that underlies the region, makes the cerebellum accessible to cellular analysis.

Cultures of Cerebellar Cells Provide Assays for Specific Steps in Cerebellar Development

Over the last decade, we have developed methods to purify the cell populations of the developing cerebellum and to culture them either in isolation or in combination with the other classes of cells. The general hypothesis underlying these methods is that isolation of specific cell populations will reveal the mechanisms that regulate the developmental processes of any given cell. The small size and incredible abundance of the granule neuron make it the easiest cell to obtain in large numbers. The identity of purified cells can be confirmed by cell-marker expression and by ultrastructural analysis. These methods render possible the isolation of other cell populations for studies of the major steps in cerebellar histogenesis: generation of specific classes of neural cells, precursor cell proliferation in specialized zones, directed cell migration along glial fibers, formation of neuronal layers, synaptogenesis, and the formation of functional neuronal circuits. Among these processes, our

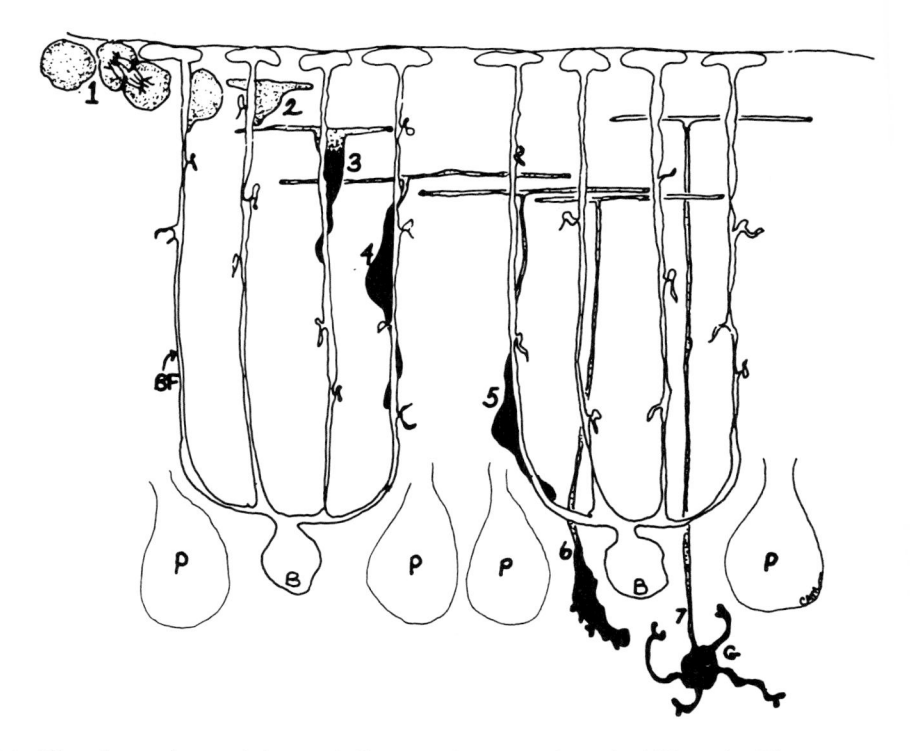

Figure 16.1 Migration pathway of the cerebellar granule neuron from the EGL to the IGL.

own interests have focused on development of culture systems that provide assays for the role of local signals, including cell-cell interactions and positional information (reviewed in Hatten and Heintz, 1995).

As is the case for cellular histogenesis, the program of synaptogenesis in the cerebellum also is well-studied (Mason, 1984, 1986, 1990; Chedotal, 1992). The cerebellum is a region of choice for many of these studies because, in addition to simplicity of cell classes, two types of extra-cerebellar afferents, climbing and mossy fibers, innervate cerebellar target cells: Purkinje and granule neurons, respectively (Palay, 1974). Detailed anatomical studies allow the design of culture experiments on a time frame and scale that approximate processes so well-documented in classic studies. Thus, in vitro methods allow a systematic search for mechanisms that regulate the formation and maintenance of specific axon-target cell interactions.

Another benefit of working with cerebellar cell populations is the availability of genetic perturbations of cerebellar development and the ability to recombine these mutant cells with wild types. As

postulated by Hatten and Sidman (1978), this approach is particularly important in defining extrinsic factors that regulate cerebellar development. Recombining purified wild-type and mutant granule cells from the neurological mutant *weaver* has unveiled the cellular mechanisms regulating granule cell development (Hatten et al., 1986; Gao et al., 1992; Gao and Hatten, 1993; Kofuji et al., 1996). The ability to purify either wild-type or mutant granule cells, subsequently to label the purified cells, and to transplant them into a wild-type environment in vivo has permitted studies of migration and the acquisition of mature neuronal phenotype. Finally, recombining purified Purkinje cells with purified granule cells or astroglia has revealed that granule cells, the presynaptic afferent of Purkinje cells in vivo, are potent regulators of Purkinje cell survival and differentiation in vitro (Baptista et al., 1994), and also has opened the door to investigating the molecular contributions of the granule neuron in a systematic manner (Morrison and Mason, 1998). Recently, the production of a wide range of targeted gene disruptions has allowed further examination of the role of selected gene families in cerebellar development. Clearly, this will be a forefront of future experiments.

In addition to the wealth of correlative information on the timing and specificity of interactions in vivo and in vitro, the use of molecular probes of specific cell markers with patterns of expression restricted to one cerebellar cell type allows resolution of the interactions leading to the differentiation of the granule cells and Purkinje cells. In mastering the methods needed to culture identified cerebellar cell populations, one also provides an experimental approach to preparing RNA or DNA from isolated cell populations for Northern or Southern analysis or to preparing cDNA libraries from either the vast granule cell population or the small Purkinje cell population. Such an approach has yielded more than 100 markers for granule cell and Purkinje cell development (Hatten and Heintz, 1995).

In this chapter, we focus on methods for the culture and analysis of primary cerebellar cells. The isolation procedures we describe can be used also to harvest specific classes of cells for use in generation of cell lines. Infection of granule cells with retroviral constructs containing oncogenes (or other constructs) can be achieved easily in reaggregate cultures, owing to the extensive proliferation of the cells in that particular culture setting (Gao and Hatten, 1994). Infection of the astroglial cells likewise is an easy process, as they

too proliferate under the culture conditions we describe. Purkinje cells present a greater challenge, but emerging methods for the production of cDNA libraries from single cells and for infection with adenoviral constructs suggest that these approaches will be available soon for Purkinje cells. The present review offers an important feature of these experiments: the ability to start with an identified cell population.

Though we focus our comments on local inductive signals that regulate gene expression and cell behaviors critical for cell positioning and cellular organization of the developing cerebellar cortex, the application of the methods we have developed to the analysis of ion channels also is important. From the use of cell lines already generated (e.g., B6 granule cell line; see Gao and Hatten, 1994) or cell lines produced by short-term immortalization and screening for cells that express ion channels of interest, the use of cell purification approaches is powerful. This finding has been realized in our recent study on the action of the mutant *weaver* GIRK2 potassium channel in granule cell development (Kofuji et al., 1996). Neurophysiological studies of granule cells purified from wild-type and *weaver* neurological mice, in combination with expression and physiology studies in oocytes, allowed elucidation of the molecular action of the weaver gene in granule cell development.

Purification of the Cell Classes of the Developing Cerebellar Cortex

The Granule Cell

A number of general classes of experiments can be performed with granule cells. Because granule cells are small and have a large nucleus, they have the highest density of all the cell types in the cerebellum and can be separated into a 95% pure "small cell fraction" in a two-step density gradient. The "large cell fraction" resulting from the gradient contains the rest of the glial cells, Purkinje cells, and large interneurons (e.g., basket and Golgi cells). For studies on the steps in granule cell development, progenitor cells can be purified at ages when neurogenesis, migration, assembly into the internal granule cell layer, or interaction with ingrowing afferent axons occur. To dissect any of these events further, the culture conditions can be modified to assay the developmental step under study.

As an example to study mechanisms of neurogenesis within the EGL, the cells are cultured as cellular reaggregates prior to cell migration and formation of the mature cerebral cortex (figure 16.2A and color plate 7). In this setting, the high frequency of cell-cell interactions among the precursor cells replicates the dynamic of interactions within the EGL. As discussed in the section General Methological Strategies, reaggregates form under conditions wherein the cells are plated at high density on an untreated culture surface. The relatively higher cell-cell adhesion between the cells, as compared with cell-substrate adhesion, generates the reaggregates. Once formed (24–36 h), these reaggregates can be assayed for proliferative capacity by adding bromodeoxyuridine (BrdU) or other measures of DNA synthesis or can be transferred to a substratum that supports neurite formation for assays of neural differentiation. Cell viability is high in the reaggregate setting.

Although the reaggregates are easily prepared and the cells tend to thrive within them, they are not suitable for quantitation of cellular behavior on a per-cell basis. To meet that aim, we modify the setting slightly by plating the purified EGL cells at a high density on a culture substratum, forming a dense monolayer or "carpet" (figure 16.3B and color plate 8). Thereafter, we label a small aliquot of the cells with a lipophilic dye, such as PKH-26 or any other marker, plate the labeled cells onto the carpet of unlabeled cells, and monitor the differentiation of labeled cells. When fluorescent labeling is used, the labeled subpopulation stands in contrast to the "invisible" carpet underneath (see figure 16.3A). Thus, one can provide a setting with high-frequency contacts, yet visualize the behavior of individual neurons. Moreover, one can quantify features of those neurons easily with microscopy.

For studies of neuron-glial interactions, especially of neuronal migration along glial fibers, a different strategy is used. In these experiments, we harvest the small cell fraction and plate it on a coated substratum (see figure 16.2B). The high ratio of neurons to glia induces the elongated glial profiles seen to support migration in vitro. Details of migration assays can be found in Fishell and Hatten (1991) and in Fishman and Hatten (1993). As a follow-up to our migration studies, Rivas and Hatten (1995) examined the organization of the neuronal cytoskeleton during migration, a specialized form of cell motility along glial fibers (figure 16.4). Understanding the molecular cues that initiate migration and axon formation also requires examination of the cellular trafficking of

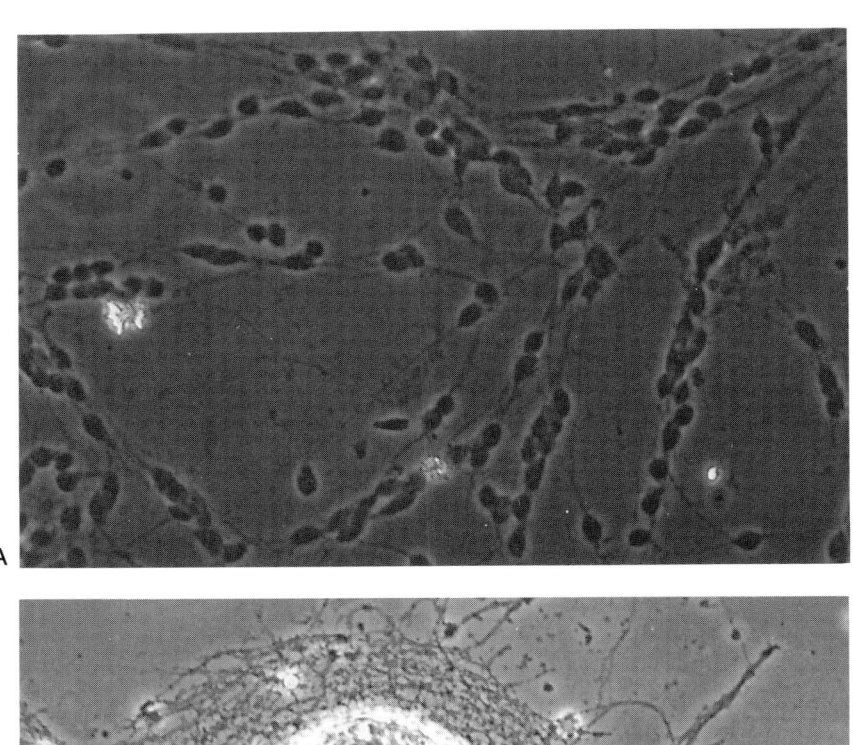

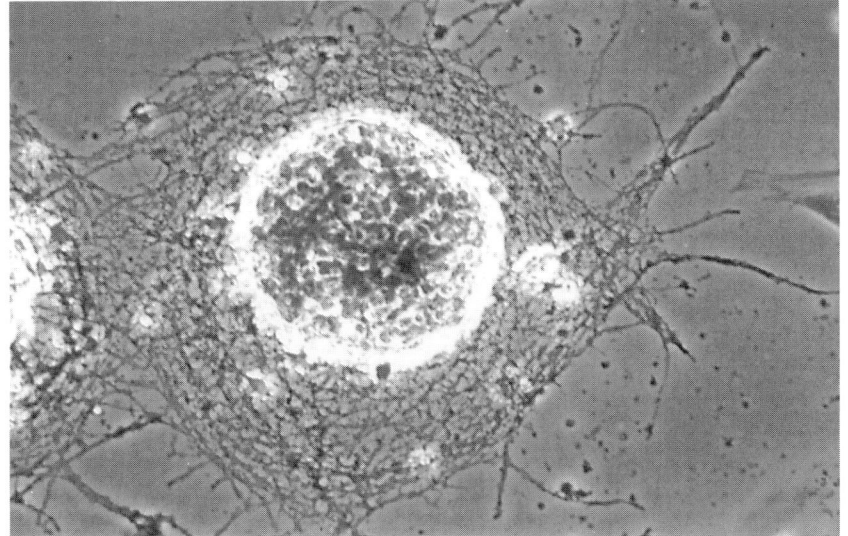

Figure 16.2 Granule neurons in culture. (*A*) Reaggregates plated on coated substrate (1000 cells per microliter); note the "halo" of neurites after 24 h. Scale bar: 100 μm. (*B*) Low-density culture on coated substrate (100 cells per microliter) after 24 h. Scale bar: 100 μm. See plate 7 for color version.

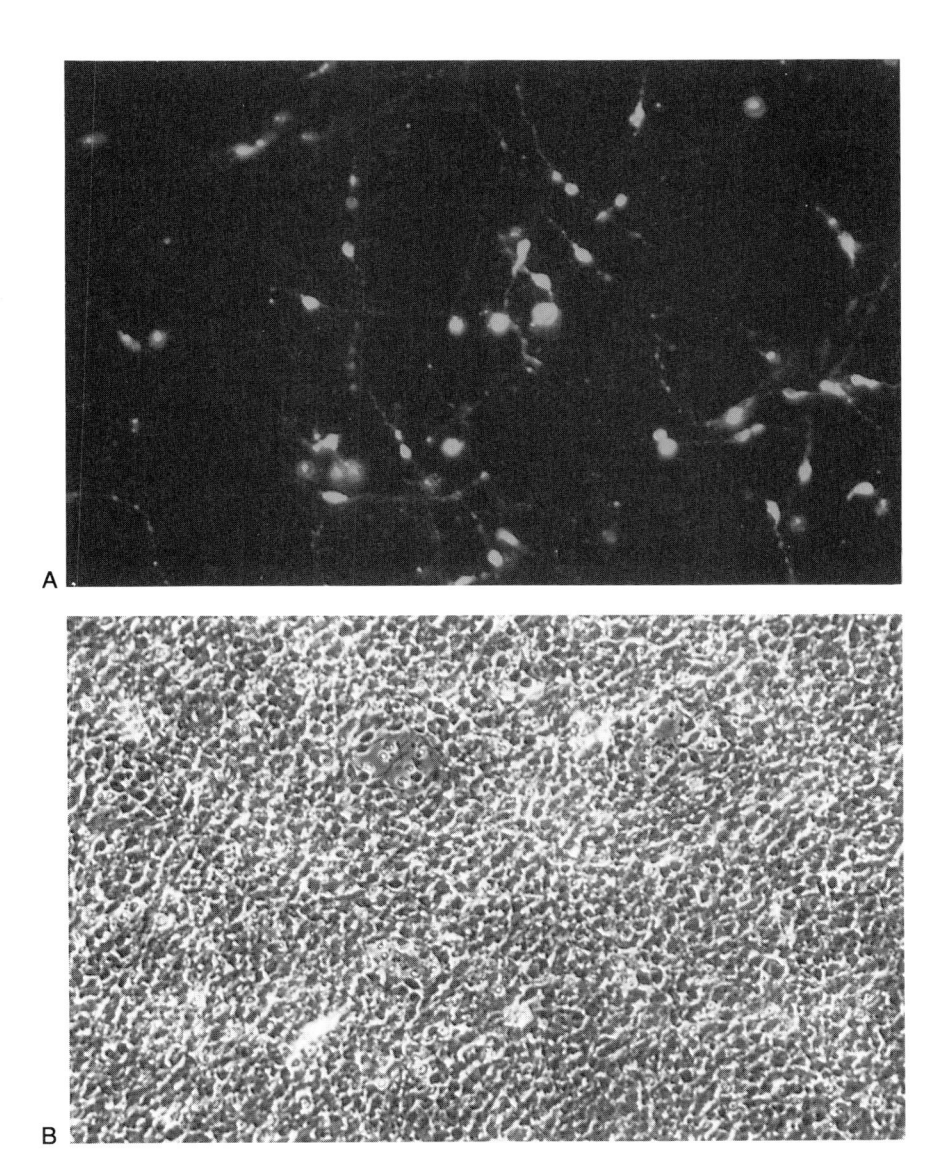

Figure 16.3 Labeled granule neuron subpopulations visible against unlabeled cells. (*A*) PKH-26-labeled granule neurons. Scale bar: 100 μm. (*B*) Unlabeled "carpet" (4000 cells per microliter) of granule neurons. Scale bar: 100 μm. See plate 8 for color version.

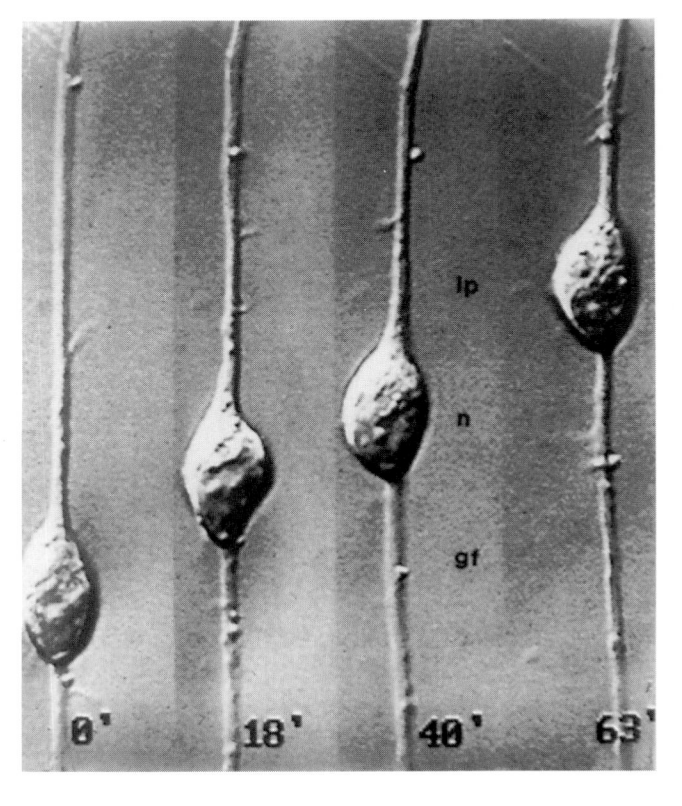

Figure 16.4   Neurons migrate along astroglial fibers in vitro. Time elapsed (min) in real time. 1p, leading process; n, cell body of migrating neuron; gf, glial fiber.

molecules that establish the polarity of both the migrating cell (Powell et al., 1997) and of cells undergoing dendrite formation. The microculture system is well-suited to assays of peptide and membrane trafficking during migration and process formation, as large numbers of cells can be harvested for parallel biochemical or molecular biological assays.

Recombining purified wild-type and mutant granule cells from the neurological mutant *weaver* has unveiled the cellular mechanisms regulating granule cell development (Hatten et al., 1986; Gao et al., 1992; Gao and Hatten, 1993; Kofuji et al., 1996). The ability to purify granule cells, subsequently to label the purified cells, and to transplant them in vivo has permitted studies of migration and the acquisition of mature neuronal phenotype.

Another feature of granule cell development is the interaction with target cells, the Purkinje cells, and with ingrowing afferent

axons—the mossy fibers—assayed by recombining select cell partners in vitro, such as purified granule cells with pontine mossy fiber explants. These experiments have revealed mechanisms of afferent growth regulation by target cells, in particular, the role of NMDA receptors in this process (Baird et al., 1992a,b, 1996). Moreover, by purifying cells from older cerebella, we found that this "stop signal" weakens after approximately postnatal day 10 (P10) (Zhang and Mason, 1998). Finally, recombining purified Purkinje cells with purified granule cells has revealed that granule cells, the presynaptic afferent of Purkinje cells in vivo, are potent regulators of Purkinje cell survival and differentiation in vitro (Baptista et al., 1994).

Other combinations clearly are possible and the flexibility of the system, labeling cells with dyes, retroviral marking, gene transfer, or species mixing (rat and mouse) all offer experimental approaches to other steps in development. The emerging power of molecular markers for specific stages of development and for methods to assay ion channel expression and function will broaden the base of these assays.

The Purkinje Cell

For more than a century, the distinctive morphology of the Purkinje cell and its pattern of interactions with cerebellar interneurons have attracted widespread study. Isolation of this important class of neuron has been exceedingly difficult, owing to the small number (100,000 in the mouse) and the fragile nature of these cells in culture. Whereas the granule cell offers an abundant yield after a two-step purification scheme, more elaborate strategies are necessary to harvest Purkinje cells and support their differentiation in vitro.

The removal of the larger population of the granule cells provides an approach to purifying the Purkinje cell. The balance of the cell population consists of the interneurons (basket, stellate, and Golgi II cells), neurons of the deep nuclei (targets of Purkinje cells), and astroglia. The purification of Purkinje cells relies on knowledge of the spectrum of cell-surface antigens expressed by their precursors at early phases of differentiation. A first immuno-panning step eliminates unwanted neuronal and glial precursors that express G_{D3} on their surface. As studies had shown that Thy-1 was prominent on the Purkinje cell, we pursued an approach to

isolate the Purkinje cell by positive selection in a second immuno-panning step with anti-Thy-1 (Charlton et al., 1983, Baptista et al., 1994).

A second factor in developing a strategy to isolate a rarer popu-lation is to determine the time frame during normal development when immature cells are most abundant. This period generally is the phase just prior to terminal differentiation, a phase that pre-cedes loss by cell death. In the case of the Purkinje cell, maximal cell numbers are seen in the late embryonic period, just prior to the vast expansion of the granule cell precursor population and ini-tiation of synaptogenesis. For our culture experiments, therefore, we use cerebellar tissue harvested between embryonic day 18 (E18) and P0 to isolate young Purkinje cells.

Of all the cell types in the mammalian brain, the Purkinje cell is among the most widely studied. After birth, Purkinje cells develop a characteristic, highly branched dendritic tree in a stereotyped series of developmental stages (figure 16.5C and color plate 9). In midgestation, Purkinje cells have smooth cell bodies and a few smooth processes; at this time, climbing fibers contact the Purkinje soma but have not arborized. Neonatally, the simple processes of the Purkinje cells disappear, and many thin processes appear around the soma, which is contacted by a nest of climbing-fiber terminals. Later, apical dendrites emerge, and climbing fibers grow along the developing Purkinje dendrites, as parallel fibers from the granule cells extend at right angles to the Purkinje dendrites. As Purkinje cell dendrites reach terminal differentiation, climbing and parallel fibers contact specific sets of dendritic spines (reviewed in Baptista et al., 1994).

The close timing of Purkinje cell differentiation relative to climbing- and parallel-fiber growth suggests a role for afferent innervation in dendritic differentiation, long hypothesized from analyses of experimental or genetic ablations of cerebellar afferents (e.g. Altman, 1972; Rakic, 1975; Sotelo, 1975; Privat, 1976). This work suggested that parallel fibers play a more significant role in Purkinje cell dendrite induction than do climbing fibers.

Culture of isolated Purkinje cells offers several experimental approaches that are not possible with slice preparations. First, one can examine the extent of extrinsic, local factors that the young Purkinje cell requires to develop its characteristic patterns of gene expression and arborization. This development is achieved by sys-tematic adding back of the other cellular and axonal components of

the system, the input neurons (the granule cells), incoming axons (olivary and pontine axons), and astroglial cells from the region of origin of the cell under study. Such an approach has yielded new insights into Purkinje cell development, especially regarding the importance of cell-cell and axon–target cell interactions to Purkinje cell differentiation. These in vitro preparations are just beginning to be used for gene expression studies and for physiological studies. Future work obviously will combine the in vitro methods outlined here with molecular biological approaches, either by transfection of selected genes into purified Purkinje cells or by the isolation of Purkinje cells from animals with targeted gene disruptions.

The recent development of a protocol for purification of Purkinje cells to 80% to 90% homogeneity (Baptista et al., 1994), along with the ability to purify cerebellar granule neurons (Hatten, 1985), (1) verified that the granule neuron is a potent regulator of Purkinje dendritic development, and (2) opened the door to more stringent tests of factors affecting Purkinje cell dendritic development (Morrison and Mason, 1998). Purified Purkinje cells cultured alone never develop nature dendrites, whereas Purkinje cells cocultured with purified granule neurons undergo full dendritic development (Baptista et al., 1994).

Pontine Explants

How afferent axons recognize their target cells and stop growing once they encounter them is a central issue in neural development. The ability to purify granule neurons, a major target neuron in the cerebellar cortex, has produced an experimental culture system by which to analyze the regulation of afferent extension by target cells.

A major extracerebellar afferent is the mossy-fiber system, arising from a number of brainstem and spinal cord sources. The basilar pontine nuclei comprise one such source, and are accessible and visible on the bottom of the brain. Explants of the pontine nuclei can be cocultured on beds or next to fields of purified granule neurons. Neurite length and growth cone behavior then can be monitored.

In contrast to neurite growth on astroglia, which is abundant and rapid, outgrowth of pontine explants on granule neurons is reduced greatly, as mossy fiber growth cones stop extending when they meet a granule cell. These findings led us to propose that the granule neuron presents a "stop-growing" signal to its afferents (Baird

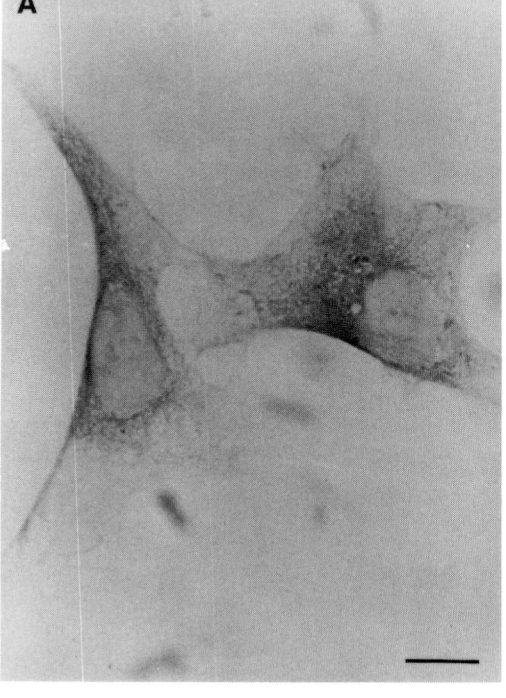

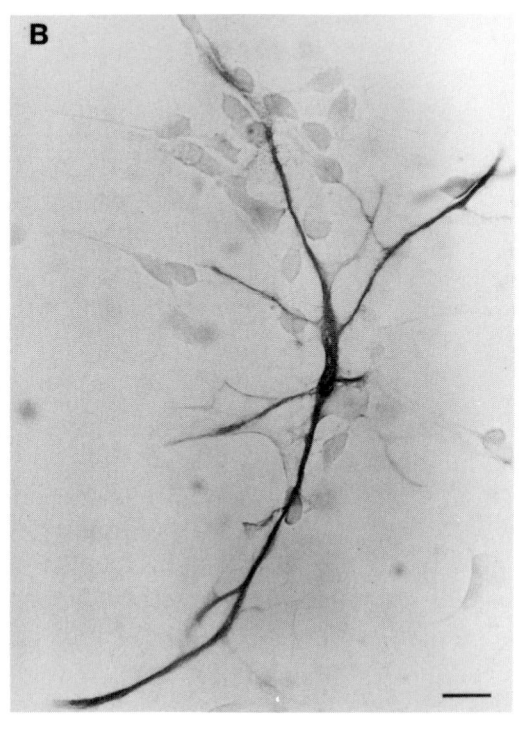

Figure 16.5 Astroglial and Purkinje cells in culture. (*A*) Purified astroglia. Scale bar: 20 μm. (*B*) Astroglia cultured in association with granule neurons. Scale bar: 20 μm. (*C*) Purkinje cell cultured on neurites of granule cell reaggregates, 21 days in vitro. Note stalked spines on highly differentiated dendrites (arrow). See plate 9 for color version.

et al., 1992a,b). Preparation of pontine explants is relatively simple, but there are a number of considerations for and indications of successful growth. First, in mouse, we have observed abundant outgrowth when explants are taken from P0 mice, the age during which pontine afferents have grown toward and enter the cerebellum (Zhang and Mason, 1998). Pontine explants taken after postnatal day 2 (P2) do not grow very well. Second, the pons will not grow at all in serum-containing medium, nor will it extend neurites well on polylysine alone, but neurites will grow on polylysine with laminin. Third, on substrate alone, pontine neurites are abundant and fasciculated, often displaying clockwise or counterclockwise curvature, whereas on cellular monolayers, pontine neurites are less fasciculated. Finally, to distinguish the pontine explant neurites against the cellular background of granule or other

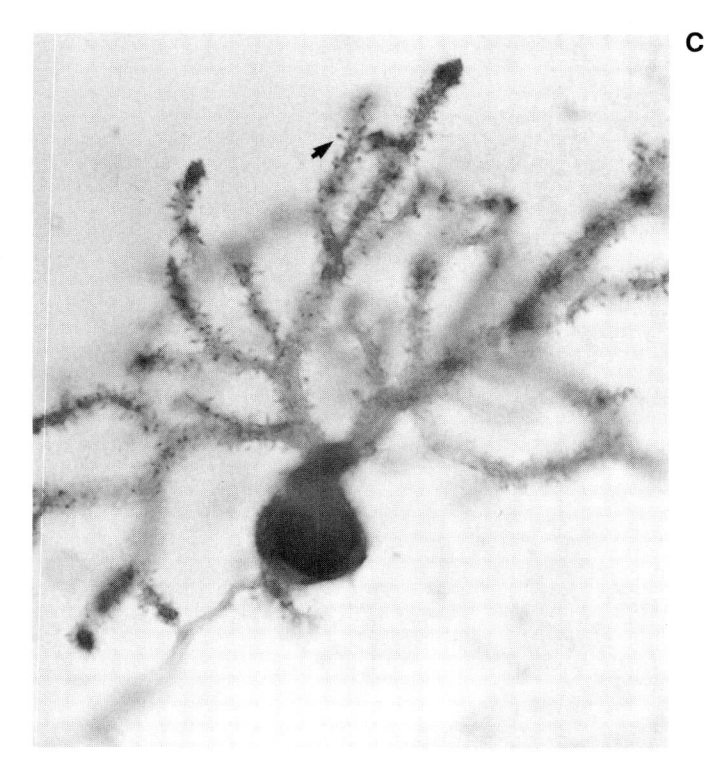

C

Figure 16.5 (continued)

cells, a mouse neuron-specific monoclonal antibody (M6) can be used (C. Lagenauer, University of Pittsburgh).

The other major extracerebellar afferent system, the climbing fibers from the inferior olivary nuclei, have been quite difficult to grow using the foregoing approaches and rationales, but methods are being developed to this end (Baird, personal communication).

The Astroglial Cell

Purified astroglia can be obtained from the large cell fraction of the Percoll gradient in either of the granule or Purkinje preparations, for analysis of astroglial differentiation or for glial support of neuronal migration, neurite growth, and dendritic differentiation. Large yields of radial glia and astrocytes also can be harvested and purified from embryonic and early postnatal cortex and hippocampus by using this general rationale. Studies of glial cells in isolation from neurons have revealed several basic principles of

their development and physiology. In comparison with cerebellar neurons, glial cells rely on interactions with neurons to sustain a program of differentiation. In the absence of neurons, the glial cells fail to extend processes and enter the cell cycle, undergoing active proliferation. Addition of neurons arrests glial proliferation if the cell cycles are synchronized by standard methods, including leucine or methionine starvation over a 24-h period (Hatten, 1985).

The isolation of glial cells has led to important insights into the factors that control their proliferative capacity and differentiation (see figure 16.5A,B). This is especially relevant to tumor formation and regeneration events in injured mature brain. Studies by Hunter (Hunter and Hatten, 1995) indicate, for example, that the development of the astroglial cell, in contrast to the neurons, is bidirectional, with mature cells able to revert to an immature phenotype after addition of a neuron-derived protein (RF60). Work is underway to purify a novel peptide factor that controls glial progression from radial glial forms in the embryonic brain to astrocytes in the mature brain. Cloning of this factor clearly will enhance our ability to culture mature glia and test their interactions with neurons or axons. Other studies have shown the importance of peptide growth factors, primarily platelet-derived growth factor, to glial survival and development.

General Methodological Strategies

The first step toward mastery of the more complex cell separations and recombinations desirable for so many experiments is simply to generate healthy cultures of the total cerebellar cell population. This process allows the experimenter to become familiar with methods needed to harvest a viable cell population and to test media, sera, and other components of the culture system. The cultures we have developed are "micro" cultures: they are prepared in a small volume. In our experience, culturing CNS cells in a small volume improves viability and differentiation of the cells. The age of the tissue from which the cells are obtained also is a critical factor in the culture approach. A general rule is to obtain cells from the developmental period of interest. This rule is compromised by the available numbers and viability of cells at different ages. The optimal ages for granule cell cultures are postnatal days 6 to 8, a time when all the cerebellar cell types are present in vivo. Purkinje cells should be harvested at E18 through P1, before the granule cell

population has expanded and while the Purkinje cells can be purified on the basis of their differential expression of cell-surface
antigens.

In preparing cerebellar cultures, two competing factors must be
managed. First, the aim will be to get the cells safely into culture as
quickly as possible (30 min is optimal). However, care must be used
during the separation of the cells into a single-cell suspension—the
trituration step—not to break or damage the cells. This is accom-
modated best by fire-polishing the Pasteur pipette used to triturate
the cells, selecting pipettes allowing clear visualization through the
polished "hole." When the pipette tip has too small an opening, the
pressure on the cells reduces their viability. Moreover, in triturating the cells, a slow up-and-down motion at the speed of a child's
"see saw" on the playground should be used. This phase is the
most critical of the culture preparation.

In preparing a single-cell suspension from intact tissue, the four
most important issues are the buffer (see further), the purity of the
proteolytic enzymes, a gentle trituration of the cells with a fire-
polished Pasteur pipette, and a time that minimizes manipulation
of the cells. The purity of the enzymes used to digest the tissue is
especially critical. One can use either trypsin or papain, and the
inclusion of DNase in these solutions ensures digestion of any DNA
that might be released by damaged or dying cells.

After the preparation of a single-cell suspension of viable cells,
the density at which the cells are plated becomes the next critical
issue. For cerebellar cells, a range between 500 and 1000 cells per
microliter is optimal. Plating the cells at high densities gives maximal cell survival. It is advisable to assay the plating efficiency of
your cultures, a measure of the percentage of viable cells. This task
is accomplished by counting the number of trypan blue–negative,
viable cells in the plating suspension, counting the number of live
cells in the culture after 24 h in vitro, and dividing the number
of live cells in culture by the total number of viable cells plated
(adjusting for the volume used). Once mastered, the methods we
describe should generate cultures with a plating efficiency well
above 90%.

CULTURE VESSELS
Our culture methods have been developed for small volumes, to
accommodate the often tiny cell populations available in the
embryonic cerebellum and to maximize cell survival. To culture

the extremely small number of granule cells harvested from the early embryonic cerebellar anlage (Hatten and Sidman, 1978), we used a culture dish commonly used in immunological assays, namely Terasaki wells. These culture dishes have 60 microwells, each of which contain 12 to 15 µl of medium. With small cell populations, Terasaki wells are the most practical tool for testing a wide variety of cell densities, media, sera, and the like with a single cell preparation. They are perfect also for plating at single-cell densities. Like other tissue-culture plasticware, these dishes can be coated with poly-D-lysine (PLYS) or other desirable substrates to improve cell adhesion and neurite production (Hatten and Sidman, 1978).

A second general approach is to make a microwell in a larger culture dish. This structure is achieved by drilling a hole in the large dish and affixing a glass coverslip at the site of the previously drilled hole, creating a well with a volume of 20 to 40 µl. This method, first introduced by Mary Bunge (Bunge et al., 1965), has been in use in our laboratories for two decades. The use of a glass coverslip as a "false bottom" allows oil-immersion microscopy and high-resolution imaging of the behavior of the cells during cell migration, neurite extension, or axon-target interactions (Edmondson and Hatten, 1987; Gregory et al., 1988; Mason et al., 1988; Fishell et al., 1993; Baird et al., 1994; Rivas and Hatten, 1995). For these cultures, we use a 50-mm bacteriological dish. The latter offers three advantages: First, the lid snaps shut, preventing evaporation of the medium (when three drops of water are placed around the culture well); second, this dish has three knobs, which allows precise alignment of the dish for viewing cultures at multiple time points; and third, the dish is shallow, facilitating certain types of microscopy. The coverslips can be removed with a razor blade at the conclusion of any experiment, processed through xylene by standard methods to remove the Vaseline paraffin sealing medium, flipped, and mounted permanently on a glass microscope slide. This last feature allows convenient storage of cultures or marker staining for future reference.

The third and easiest approach is to use Lab-Tek chamber slides. This system is a commercial adaptation of the microculture dish, with plastic chambers mounted on a glass microscope slide via a synthetic, nontoxic "gasket." Two drawbacks to these slides are the relatively larger volume of 200 to 300 µl needed (not an issue with

granule cells or glial cells) and the danger that washing the cultures will remove the cells, as a high surface tension generally exists across the meniscus of the medium. Medium always should be removed and added by slow pipetting along the sides of the wells. This system is ideal for immunostaining or in situ hybridization analyses. Small volumes of antibodies or probes are used and, at the conclusion of the procedure, the plastic chambers are removed by a gentle pulling motion. Afterward, the gasket can be removed with forceps, and a coverslip can be applied for permanent storage of the experiment. Equally, 4-, 8-, or 16-well chamber slides can be used.

CULTURE SUBSTRATES

Three culture substrates are used in our cultures; all act to neutralize the negative charge on commercially available culture dishes or glass. The most popular choice has been polylysine (PLYS) (see Letourneau, 1975). We use the D-isomer to minimize digestion of the substrate by the cells. A range of concentrations of PLYS is effective (100–500 µg/ml), and polymers with molecular weights greater than 3×10^5 have proved to work best. Even PLYS obtained from our preferred vendors varies in quality; hence, every new lot must be tested for each cell culture type. Once an effective lot has been chosen, the main concern is the shelf-life of the PLYS solution. In preparing the solution fresh for each culture, low concentrations can be used. If the solution is kept for 2 to 5 days, the polylysine will deposit on the walls of the bottle before it is used to treat the culture dishes; thus, higher concentrations are necessary for routine use. To apply the substrate, simply place a small volume of the solution in the dishes and incubate at 35°C for a period ranging from 30 min to overnight. Ensure that the excess PLYS is washed off with several changes of water, not buffer, and allow the surface to air-dry in the laminar flow hood just prior to use.

Another substrate option is Matrigel, a solubilized basement membrane preparation available with or without added growth factors. Matrigel should be thawed slowly on ice, and the stock solution never should be allowed to warm to room temperature, or else it will harden. We dilute the stock to 250 µg/ml (1 : 50) in CMF-PBS and coat the culture dish for several hours at 35°C. The dishes then are rinsed three times with CMF-PBS. The dishes should not be allowed to dry; best results are obtained when Matrigel-coated dishes are used immediately.

Cultures of pontine explants require coating glass surfaces with laminin and with PLYS. As for the PLYS, each lot of laminin must be tested with the particular cell types or explants to be used in the actual experiment. The appropriate concentration of laminin can vary from lot to lot, but 20 µg/ml is a good starting point. Our usual combination involves coating the culture surface first with 500 µg/ml PLYS as described, followed by 20 µg/ml laminin for 45 min at 35°C. Storage of the laminin solution at 4°C will lower slowly the concentration available for the tissue-culture surface.

CULTURE MEDIA

In harvesting the cells from intact tissue, we use a variation of Tyrode's solution, a buffer that contains high concentrations of glucose (Trenker and Sidman, 1978). High amounts (6–8 mM) of glucose help to increase the viability of the cells. During dissociation, a CMF version of Tyrode's solution is used; hence, our term for this version of Tyrode's buffer: *CMF-PBS*. Other simple buffers work well with cerebellar cells, including Ringer's solution, modified to contain proper amounts of sodium and potassium for mammalian cells and supplemented with glucose (as described) to a concentration of 6 to 8 mM.

In choosing a cell culture medium for the suspension of cerebellar cells, we have always used the least enriched media, such as basal medium Eagle (BME). Serum is helpful, because it arrests the action of the proteolytic agents used to dissociate the cells and because it contains lipids that support membrane expansion (e.g., neurite outgrowth). At the same time, serum contains factors that can affect the outcome of experiments and promote the growth of unwanted contaminating cell populations. The latter usually are glial cells or (possibly) fibroblastlike cells in cases where the meninges were not removed properly.

Among sera, horse serum contains the lowest concentration of peptide growth factors that stimulate glial growth. In addition, horse serum rarely contains lipids that are common to bovine sera which can be toxic to the cells. All serum first must be heat-inactivated by raising its temperature to 55°C for 30 min prior to use in culture medium. The most important step taken in assuring the reproducibility of experiments is to obtain and to test a number of lots of serum from a supplier. Test the lots to see which one promotes high viability, then buy a large amount of that lot number!

For many experiments, generally those wherein the effect of other proteins—growth factors, antibodies, receptors, and the like—are being assayed, serum cannot be included in the medium in the major phase of the culture period. For those cases, a serum-free medium is necessary. However, maximal cell viability is obtained when the cells are plated first in serum overnight and then changed to serum-free medium. In our experience, lipid-free bovine serum albumin (BSA) can be substituted for serum in BME to bring the protein concentration to approximately 5 to 8 µg/ml as per serum-containing media. It is important to use lipid-free BSA to avoid variation in the effects on the cells.

Another key factor required by the cells is fresh glutamine. Degradation of glutamine, either during storage on the shelf or in the cultures, is a primary cause of low viability. Glutamine should be stored in frozen aliquots to ensure that it is fresh, and media should not be stored more that 5 days prior to use, once the glutamine has been added. Similarly, medium should be changed every 3 to 5 days, primarily to refresh the glutamine supply.

SOURCE OF CELLS FOR CULTURE

In most cases, rat cells survive the conditions of tissue disruption and culture at much higher rates than do mouse cells. If general cultures are the aim, start with rat cells. We obtain Sprague-Dawley rats from Zivic Miller (Portersville, PA). Some rat supply houses have a problem with Kilham rat virus, a parvovirus that causes cerebellar hypoplasia but otherwise presents no obvious clinical symptoms. If a different supplier is chosen, ensure that the serological test results for Kilham rat virus are available. For ages, the day of birth is considered postnatal day 1 (Altman and Bayer, 1985a,b).

The rationale for using mouse cells is the potential for genetic experiments, using either naturally occurring neurological mutants or animals with targeted gene disruptions. We obtain C57BL/6J mice from Jackson Laboratories (Bar Harbor, ME), and we maintain a pathogen-free breeding colony on site to provide large numbers of timed pregnancies. C57Bl/6J is the mouse strain of choice for cerebellar studies because so much is known about the anatomy and development of this strain. For mice, we designate the day of vaginal plugging as E0 and the day of birth P0.

In cases where it is desirable to mix cells of different ages or sources, one can simply mix rat and mouse cells in a common

culture, using species-specific antibodies, such as M6, to distinguish the cells (Baird et al., 1992a). In interspecies cultures, no apparent differences are found between the survival or differentiation of rat neurons or glial cells and those derived from mice.

Getting Started

Cultures of whole cerebellum, or "mixed" cultures, should be attempted prior to the purification of specific cell types. Examining cultures of whole cerebellum, in which all the cerebellar cell types are present, will allow the experimentor to become familiar with the general features of cell development in vitro. As described, factors such as the age and composition of the culture medium, the choice of substrates, and the dissociation technique can affect the quality of cerebellar cultures and should be tested by preparing cultures of mixed cerebellar cells. Mixed cultures can be prepared from any animal age, embryonic through postnatal.

A final reason to perform mixed cultures before trying purified cultures is to develop a technique for rapid yet clean cerebellar dissections. Even investigators accustomed to working with fresh tissue may have some difficulty removing all the meninges from the cerebellum. One should practice dissecting cerebella of the appropriate age until each complete dissection takes 3 to 5 min. The most viable cultures are those in which the cells were harvested very quickly, yet handled gently.

The best ways to ensure the preparation of a good-quality culture are threefold. First, the culture should be free of large "flat" fibroblastic cells. These cells generally are derived from the meninges and soon will overgrow a culture of neurons and glial cells. Second, the neurons plated should have a round, phase-bright appearance when viewed under the microscope. Healthy cells have smooth contours, both around the cell soma and along the length of the processes. "Ragged" edges to the cells or varicosities along the length of the processes are signs of ill health. In addition, vacuoles within the cells often precede cell death. If the number of flat cells is low (less than 1%), the glial cells are well-differentiated, and lots of phase-bright neurons bearing neurites are visible, a successful culture has been accomplished.

The final step in ensuring the quality of the cultures is to perform the cell-plating efficiency assays with trypan blue (as described).

A plating efficiency above 85% is a good start. With continued practice, this number routinely will exceed 95%.

Mastering the methods needed to produce heathly neurons that bear long processes in vitro and cultures with negligible numbers of nonneural cells readies one to try the cell separation methods. They are not more difficult, just more time-consuming. The same themes will ensure success: getting the cells prepared as quickly as possible, keeping track of the plating efficiency, and handling the cells gently enough (no air bubbles, no rough centrifugations, etc.) to keep them intact. Again, a major feature of our culture approaches that aids in high viability is keeping glucose levels up in the 6 to 8 mM range during cell preparations. This high sugar content keeps the osmolarity high enough to help the cells to seal leaks that occur during the disruption of the tissue and preparation of single cells.

Always remember that valuable cell relationships are disrupted when the cells are brought into culture, whether it be among precursors or among cells and their synaptic partners. Respecting this by treating the cells gently and giving them such factors as serum and high glucose to help them to survive the shock of removal from their normal environment helps them to recuperate quickly, generating neurites and forming connections that will sustain their survival in culture.

In retrospect, making a good culture of purified cells, although more time-consuming and at a glance perhaps daunting, is not more difficult than a good mixed culture. The basics are the key: gentle trituration of the cells, use of high-quality enzymes for dissociation, addition of serum to stop the enzymatic processes, and providing a microculture environment that can be conditioned rapidly with factors made by the cells, to help them to help themselves survive and prosper.

In carrying out the cell separations, pay close attention to the details we provide. They all are important. Do not take shortcuts, but also do not delay as you go through the procedures. Remember that the cells are in shock between the time of tissue disruption and the time at which the incubator doors close. Follow the methods precisely until obtaining cultures that look like the ones we illustrate. Be patient. We find that newcomers to the laboratory often require a month or more to master the methods even with experienced people all around them. The best teacher is experience. We

always recommend that newcomers to the lab simply do the methods every day until they come naturally.

Culture Protocols

Cerebellar Cell Cultures

The optimal ages for cultures of the total cerebellar cell population are P5 to P7, but Purkinje cell survival in these cultures is optimal if cells are dissociated from neonatal cerebellum. Dissociation of P6 mouse tissue by the protocols given yields 5.0 to 6.0×10^6 cells per cerebellum, whereas P0 will yield 1.5 to 2.0×10^6 cells per cerebellum. We have provided a protocol for five cerebella.

DISSECTION

1.a. Spray 70% ethanol over tools after they are washed. Wrap all instruments and sterilize either by autoclaving or by dry heat (60°C overnight).

b. Administer deep anesthesia by placing the early postnatal rat or murine pups on ice (4°C) for 10 to 20 min.

c. Decapitate the animals with large, surgical scissors and place the head in a sterile Petri dish. Remove the brain by making two incisions along the lateral surface, holding the snout in large forceps.

d. Remove the skull by inserting fine scissor edges gently under the skull along the lateral aspect. Pull the skull off with Dumont fine forceps (no. 4 or no. 3c) and remove the brain to a drop of ice-cold CMF-PBS in a Petri dish.

e. Using fine forceps or fine (no. 11) scalpel blades, amputate the cerebellum across its base, severing the connections coursing through the cerebellar peduncles. Transfer the tissue to another drop of CMF-PBS, being careful to keep the tissue moist. For all subsequent steps, keep the Petri dishes and tubes containing the tissue on ice, whenever possible. Chilling the tissue retards the action of proteolytic enzymes.

f. With indirect illumination, remove the meninges, a veil-like covering, from the surface of the cerebellum. Use care to remove as much of this tissue as possible, teasing apart the cerebellar lobes in older pups to achieve this. In younger animals (P0–P3), the meninges are easier to remove, often coming free as a single piece of translucent tissue.

g. Mince the tissue into small chunks with either the fine forceps or scalpel blades in a "scissorlike" motion. Remove the minced tissue to a tube for cell dissociation with a fire-polished Pasteur pipet.

h. Collect the intact tissue in a 15-ml polypropylene conical tube also filled with CMF-PBS and place on ice. Polypropylene is favored, as cells do not adhere readily to its surface.

SINGLE-CELL SUSPENSION

2. Replace the CMF-PBS with 1 ml of trypsin-DNase solution and let stand at room temperature for 5 min.

3. Remove the trypsin-DNase solution and add 1 ml of DNase.

4. Triturate with a series of three sequentially smaller-bore, fire-polished, 9-inch Pasteur pipettes until a single-cell suspension is obtained. The first pipette should have an orifice approximately the same size as an unpolished pipette; the third should be sealed nearly completely. Use care to draw the cells up and down in a gentle, slow motion, never allowing air bubbles in the fluid. Bubbles are especially troublesome, as the high surface tension lyses the cells. As single cells are generated, the suspension becomes progressively more opaque. In general, 12 to 15 "strokes" in each pipette should be sufficient to generate a suspension. Small clumps of tissue will always appear and are difficult to break down; these should be abandoned. Stopping the trituration before all the cells are suspended helps to ensure that the cells harvested are intact, healthy cells.

5. Centrifuge the cells. In centrifuging the cells, use the slowest possible effective speed. Higher speeds damage the cells. We spin our cells at $700 \times g$, $4°C$, for 5 min. A number of different table-top centrifuges can be used (IEC, Beckman, Sorvall).

6. Resuspend the cells in 2 ml of CMF-PBS and 0.5 ml of DNase by the same gentle trituration motion used to make the suspension. It is important to keep the cells cold ($4°C$) through all these steps to minimize proteolytic damage.

7. To remove large clumps from the single-cell suspension, two methods are used. The simplest is to let the suspension stand for 20 to 30 s, during which time large aggregates settle to the bottom of the tube. Also, the cells can be passed through a 33-μm nylon mesh held in a "Swinney filter" better to ensure the removal of cell aggregates.

8. Spin the cells at $700 \times g$, $4°C$, for 5 min.

9. Resuspend the cell pellet in 1 ml serum-containing medium plus 50 µl of DNase.

10. Count the cells with a hemocytometer.

11. Plate on Lab-Tek wells at a density of 500 to 1500 cells per microliter. (Optimal volume is 200–300 µl; well diameter is approximately 6 mm.)

12. Change to serum-free medium on the next day. If the intent is to test various additions to the medium, allow the cells to attach to the wells for 60 to 90 min in the incubator and change to the desired medium on the day of the preparation. These cultures can be maintained for up to 21 days, with medium changes every 3 to 4 days.

Granule Neuron Cultures

Although cell suspensions can be prepared from mice or rats at any time in the first postnatal week, P5 to P6 animals tend to generate the highest yield of viable granule cells ($1-2 \times 10^6$ granule cells per animal). The cell yield drops considerably in use of cells purified at P8 to P10. For these older preparations, the tissue should be minced prior to proteolysis, and the time of digestion should be lengthened.

SEPARATION OF GRANULE NEURONS FROM GLIAL AND OTHER LARGE CELLS

Follow the cerebellar cell culture protocol from step 1 through step 7. To separate a purified population of granule cells, take the filtered, 2.5-ml cell suspension and load it onto a Percoll gradient (described later). As mentioned, the low bouyant density of granule cells allows clean separation from other classes of cerebellar neurons, which are lighter. In good preparations, the two cell layers will be sharply defined. The upper layer is the "large cell fraction" containing Purkinje cells, interneurons, and glial cells, whereas the lower layer is the "small cell fraction" enriched in granule neurons (figure 16.6). As the gradient is run, keep in mind the fact that Percoll can be toxic if the cells stand in the solution.

PREPARATION OF THE PERCOLL GRADIENT

8. Steps 1 through 7 are identical to those for cerebellar cell cultures. To prepare the gradient, first add 10 ml of 35% Percoll to a 50-ml

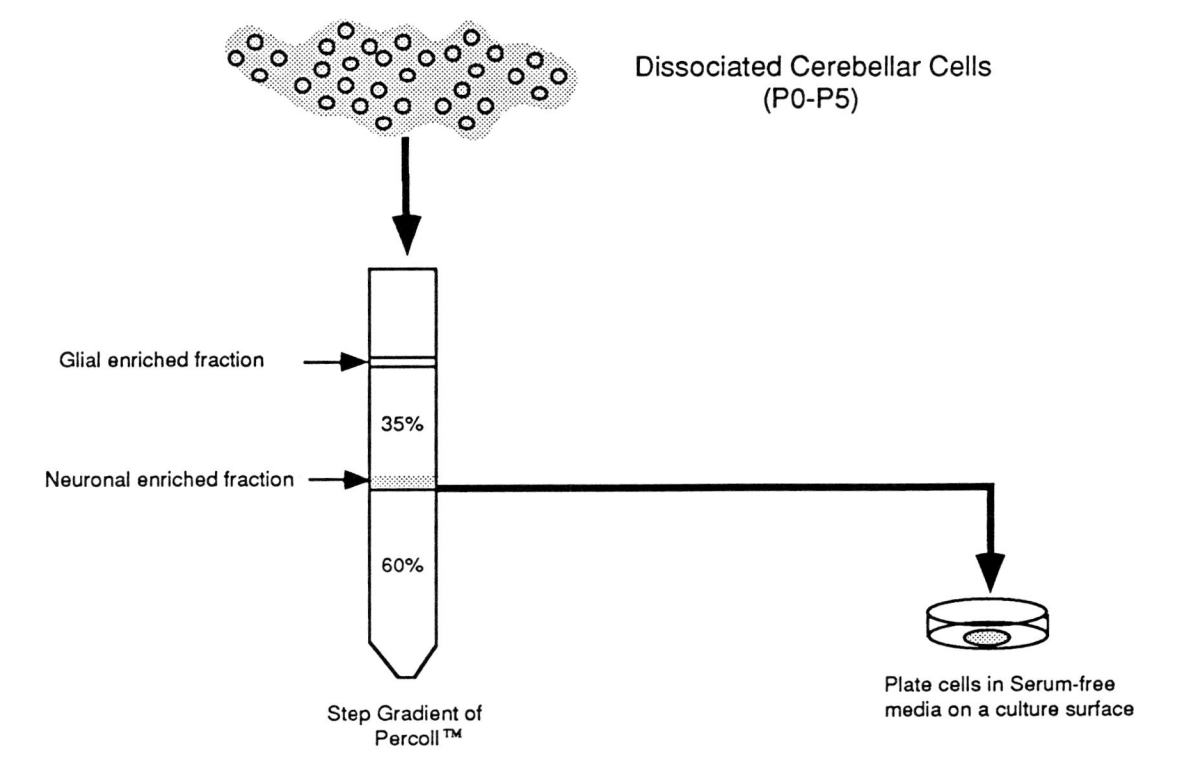

Dissociated Cerebellar Cells
(P0-P5)

Glial enriched fraction

35%

Neuronal enriched fraction

60%

Step Gradient of
Percoll™

Plate cells in Serum-free
media on a culture surface

Figure 16.6 Scheme for the purification of granule neurons, and preparation of astroglial curture. P0, postnatal day 0; P5, postnatal day 5.

polystyrene conical tube. (Polystyrene is best here, as it is clearer than polypropylene, making it easier to see the separated cell fractions). Fill a 10-ml syringe with 60% Percoll, place it needle down into the conical tube, and slowly expell the 60% Percoll to form a layer beneath the 35% Percoll. The most critical aspect of a clean separation of granule neurons is the generation of a sharp step gradient. It is monitored easily by adding a dye (a drop of trypan blue) to one of the solutions, generally the 60% solution, so that you can see the interface between the two steps of Percoll. If the line across the "step" is not crystal clear, discard the gradient and make a new one.

9. Load the cell suspension by pipetting it carefully down the side of the conical tube, onto the 35% Percoll.

10. Centrifuge the cells into the gradient. Spin at 2000 × g for 10 min. *Leave the brake off for this step!* Optimal results are obtained in a refrigerated centrifuge.

11. Remove the gradients very carefully, so as not to disrupt the layers. When viewed against a light or a dark background, two cell layers will be apparent, one at the top of the Percoll and the other, the granule neurons, at the 60% and 35% Percoll step interface. If a "string" of cells is evident all down the tube, discard the preparation.

12. Holding the tube at a very slight angle, remove the two cell layers, using a new Pasteur pipette for each layer.

13. Quickly add the granule neurons to a 50-ml tube filled with ice-cold CMF-PBS to dilute the remaining Percoll.

14. Centrifuge the cells at $800 \times g$, 4°C, for 5 min.

15. Resuspend the pellet in 2 ml granule cell culture medium plus 50 μl DNase.

PREPLATING THE GRANULE CELL FRACTION

The granule cell fraction can be purified further by preplating steps based on the cell's rapid adhesion to culture substrate. To remove any glial cells, we "preplate" the cells on a conventional plastic Petri dish coated with a low concentration of the substrate PLYS (50–100 μg/ml for 1 h) for 30 to 40 min at 35°C. For ensured purity, this step can be repeated. Because glial cells attach to such culture substrates much faster and stronger than do neurons, the neurons can be harvested in the culture medium and transferred to another coated dish.

Without preplating steps, the granule cell fraction after Percoll gradient separation contains approximately 95% of granule cells. After two to three preplatings in granule cell medium, a higher than 99% purity of granule cells can be achieved according to immuno-cytochemical, cytological, and ultrastructural criteria. Preplating cells in granule cell medium also allows cells to recover from enzymatic digestion and mechanical dissociation. After the last preplating step, transfer the cells into a polypropylene tube, tritu-rate slightly to ensure an even suspension of cells, and count the cells with a hemocytometer. Purified granule cells can be used immediately. Three types of cultures are described: monolayers, reaggregates, and collagen gels.

MONOLAYER CULTURES

The purified granule cells can be plated also on a PLYS substrate as a monolayer. At a density of 500 or more cells per microliter in serum-free medium, granule cells grow well, extend neurites, and

survive for up to 7 to 10 days. At low density (<50 cells per microliter), survival of granule cells is poor. Most cells die within days. However, addition of growth factors, such as neurotrophin 4/5 or BDNF, enhances the survival of granule cells (Gao et al., 1995). Therefore, though low-density culture is good for survival assay, the high-density culture allows for maintaining the culture for a longer time for many other purposes, including electrophysiological, biochemical, immunocytochemical, morphological, and molecular biological studies.

REAGGREGATE CULTURES

When granule cells are plated in granule cell medium (with serum) at high density (1000 cells per microliter) in untreated Lab-Tek slide wells, they form reaggregates instead of attaching to the culture dish (Gao et al., 1992). Immature granule cells in the reaggregates continue to proliferate. Thus, granule cell reaggregates mimic the germinal zone of the developing brain wherein neuronal progenitors are compacted highly and are in direct contact. Once the reaggregates are transferred to a culture substrate (e.g., PLYS), many cells rapidly undergo differentiation, as evidenced by neurite formation. Therefore, one can compare the proliferating reaggregate cultures with differentiating cultures (either reaggregates grown on a substrate or dissociated monolayer cell cultures) to assay neuronal proliferation and differentiation.

To facilitate the reaggregation of the cells, gently shake the culture well a few times after plating. Aspirate half the medium and add more fresh medium on the second day. Cells can form good reaggregates after 2 days in untreated wells or plates in granule cell medium. Remove the reaggregates into tubes containing granule cell medium and spin down the reaggregates very gently at a speed of $200 \times g$. Gently aspirate the medium and resuspend the reaggregates in medium, then plate them in serum-free medium on a PLYS substrate as a monolayer culture or in a collagen gel as a three-dimensional culture. Neurite outgrowth should be evident within a day or two after reaggregates are transferred to a substrate. The extent of neurite growth is assayed by measuring the distance from the edge of the reaggregate to the perimeter of the halo of neurites (Gao et al, 1991).

THREE-DIMENSIONAL COLLAGEN MATRIX CULTURES

Granule cells can be cultured also in three-dimensional collagen matrix at high density (1000 cells per microliter). Two advantages

characterize this type of culture: One can visualize the radial projection of neurites extended by the reaggregates in three dimensions rather than in two, and one can position granule reaggregates accurately with other developing tissue or at various distances to study cell-cell interactions between the two types of tissues.

Rat tail collagen (type 1, 3.76 mg/ml formulated in 0.02 N acetic acid) is mixed with 10× BME medium and 2% sodium bicarbonate in a ratio of 9:1:1 and is placed on ice just before use (Gao et al., 1991). Suspend the purified granule cells or reaggregates in the collagen and pipette 25 to 50 µl of the collagen containing the cells to the bottom of a Lab-Tek well or a 35-mm dish. If coculture is carried out, position the reaggregates with the cocultured tissue closely (either in direct contact or not) using fine forceps or a fine glass probe under a dissecting microscope. Then place the culture in an incubator (5% CO_2) at 37°C for 5 to 10 min until collagen is gelled. Add 200 to 300 µl (for Lab-Tek) or 2 ml (for a 35-mm dish) of serum-free medium to the dish to cover the collagen matrix. The culture medium is changed every other day thereafter. The collagen gel can be fixed in 4% paraformaldehyde (in 0.1 M PO_4 buffer, pH 7.4) prior to immunocytochemical staining with cellular antigen markers.

DYE LABELING OF GRANULE CELLS

To study the role of cell-cell interactions in neuronal proliferation and differentiation, purified granule neurons can be prelabeled with a lipophilic dye, PKH-26, before mixing and coculturing with other unlabeled cells (Alder et al, 1996).

1. Wash the purified granule cells in CMF-PBS and pellet the cells.
2. Resuspend the cell pellet in 0.5 ml of diluent solution and mix with 0.5 ml of 2 µM PKH (provided by the manufacturer). Let this mixture stand for 5 minutes at RT.
3. Stop the reaction by adding 1 ml of serum for 1 min.
4. Dilute the cells with 10 ml of CMF-PBS.
5. Wash two to three times in granule cell medium by sedimentation at 700 × g.
6. Count the dye-labeled cells.

Now one can coculture dye-labeled granule neurons with other unlabeled cells as described (Gao et al., 1992). This process allows visualization of how labeled granule cells proliferate or differentiate in an environment that mimics the germinal zone of developing brain.

TRANSPLANTATION OF PURIFIED GRANULE CELLS INTO
DEVELOPING BRAIN

To provide a parallel in vivo system, purified granule cells can be
prelabeled with two different fluorescent markers and implanted
back into the developing brain. The combination of two fluorescent
markers, fluorescent microbeads (Lumafluor lnc.; see Katz, 1984)
(1:400 dilution in culture medium, 1 h) and PKH-26 (labeling cells
with the beads in the culture plate and washing before labeling
the cells with aforementioned PKH-26) provides a control for dye
transfer after cell implantation.

Wash the labeled cells several times and suspend in Leibowitz
L-15 medium plus 9 mg/ml glucose. Approximately 2.5×10^4 cells
per microliter can be implanted into the developing cerebellum
(Gao and Hatten, 1993) or other regions of the brain, such as the
hippocampus, by injection with the use of a Hamilton syringe
mounted vertically in a stereotaxic device. Prior to injection, the
animals can be anesthetized and immobilized by placing them at
4°C or on ice for 1 to 2 min. Lower the needle gently through a
small incision in the skin to a position just beneath the meninges.
Inject approximately 1 µl of cell suspension slowly at each site,
remove the syringe, rinse the skin with CMF-PBS, and pat it dry
before you seal it with Vetbond. Warm the animal and return it to
the litter for 1 to 7 days. After various survival times, anesthetize
the animals with nembutal prior to perfusion with 4% paraformaldehyde in 0.1 M phosphate buffer (pH 7.4). Remove the cerebella by dissection, postfix in the same fixative, wash in PBS, and
embed in 3% agarose gel. Serial sections (90–100 µm) can be cut
with a vibratome, and labeled cells can be visualized with a confocal or an epifluorescence microscope. Studies in our laboratories
have indicated that implanted granule cells can become integrated
into developing cerebellum and follow each of the developmental
steps of host cells, including extension of parallel fibers, migration
along Bergmann glial cells, positioning in the internal granule
layer, and establishment of dendrite arborization (Gao and Hatten,
1994).

MOLECULAR STUDIES OF PURIFIED GRANULE CELLS

Once granule cells have been purified, they are amenable to molecular studies. For example, RNA may be isolated from granule
cells and then subjected to either Northern analysis or reverse
transcriptase–polymerase chain reaction analysis to detect and
quantitate the level of transcription of a particular gene of interest.

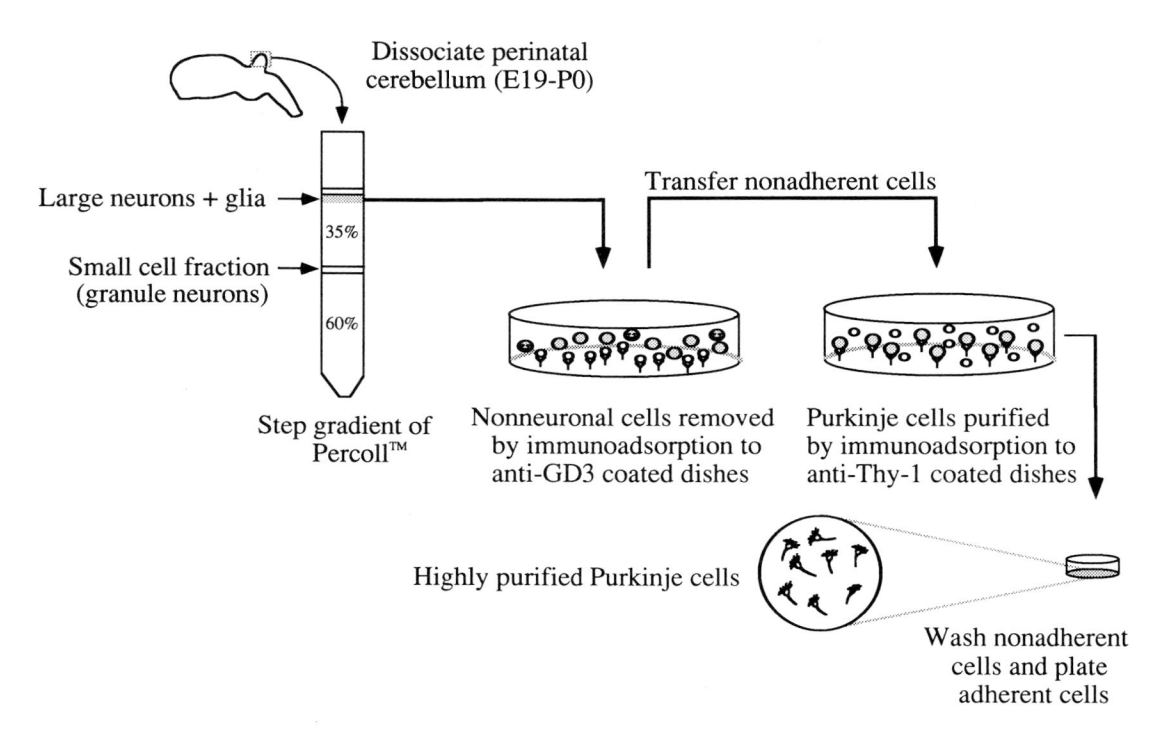

Figure 16.7 Scheme for the purification of Purkinje cells.

In brief, cells can be prepared, pelleted, and stored at −80°C until enough cells are collected for RNA preparation. Roughly 10 to 30 µg of RNA can be obtained from 5 to 10×10^6 granule cells when RNA is prepared by standard methods. The glial fraction of the granule cell preparation also can be subjected to a similar analysis (Zheng, et al., 1996).

Purkinje Cell Cultures

The Purkinje cell purification begins with the same procedure used to harvest granule neurons, with the modification of a more gentle papain dissociation and "negative" and positive immunopanning steps to get rid of unwanted precursors and to enrich for Purkinje cells, respectively, in the large cell fraction. The first few times Purkinje cell purification experiments are performed, it is a good idea to save a small aliquot of the cells (perhaps 5% of the total volume) from each step and plate them separately to permit following the fate of the Purkinje cells (figures 16.7, 16.8). After allowing these aliquots to attach to the microwells for at least 1 h, fix and

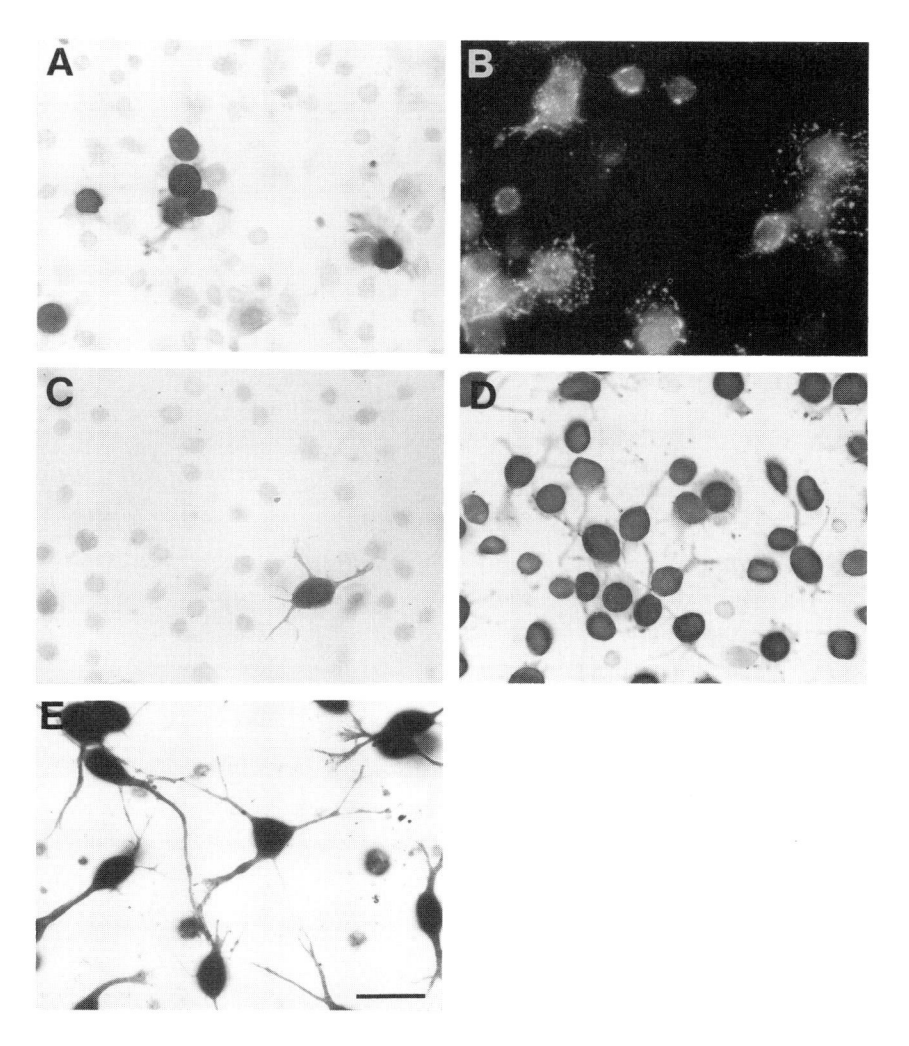

Figure 16.8 Composition of different cell fractions during the Purkinje cell purification procedure. Numbers refer to steps in the Purkinje cell protocol at which cells were plated (if in tubes), or steps at which cells were fixed on plates and subsequently immunostained. (*A*) Step 10. After dissociation, Purkinje cells are 5%–10% of total cell population. (*B*) Step 16. Large cell fraction from Percoll gradient, containing Purkinje cells (20%). Many other non-Purkinje G_{D3}-postitive contaminating cells (precursors, glia) still are present. (*C*) Step 19. On the first immunopanning dish coated with anti-G_{D3}, adherent cells include few calbindin-positive Purkinje cells but many unlabeled cells. (*D*) Step 20. An almost pure population of calbindin-positive Purkinje cells have adhered to the anti-Thy-1 dishes. (*E*) Purified Purkinje cells in culture for 1 day are viable and have short, multiple processes. (*A, C, D, E*) Purkinje cells visualized by labeling with calbindin-D_{28K} antibody. (*B*) Non-Purkinje cells visualized with antibodies to the surface ganglioside G_{D3}. Cultures were maintained in vitro for 3 h (*A–D*) or 1 day (*E*). Scale bar: 20 µm.

immunostain them by using anticalbindin D_{28k}, a Purkinje cell–specific marker within the cerebellum (Christakos et al., 1989). This technique will allow pinpointing the source of any problems with purification.

Only perinatal animals (P0–P1) can be used in this protocol. Expression of the Thy-1 marker used to select Purkinje cells in the final, positive imunopanning step is too low before E18 to P0 to be used for successful panning but increases in other cerebellar cells in older pups, giving a narrow time window during which Thy-1 is a usable marker for Purkinje cell purification. Moreover, expression of the G_{D3} marker that is used in the negative immunopanning step to remove glial cells and immature neurons decreases in older pups. Other combinations of negative and positive markers probably could be chosen to allow purification of Purkinje cells from other ages of animals, but our laboratories have not yet conducted these kinds of experiments. Our protocol was devised for 21 to 24 P0 to P1 mice; the procedure is the same for mice and rats (also used perinatally), but the form of anti-Thy-1 used for mice (Thy-1.2) differs from that used for rats (Thy-1.1) (Charlton et al, 1983).

GROWTH OF R24 CELLS FOR PREPARATION OF G_{D3} ANTIBODY
R24 hybridoma cells are obtained commercialy from ATCC as frozen aliquots. For R24 production, thaw the vial of cells and remove to a 15-ml conical tube containing 10 ml of ice-cold growth medium (348 ml RPMI 1640, 40 ml fetal bovine serum, 4 ml MEM nonessential amino acids, 4 ml penicillin-streptomycin, and 4 ml L-glutamine, adjusted to pH 7.6, filter-sterilized, and stored at 4°C). Mix gently and spin 5 min at $700 \times g$. Resuspend cells in 10 ml warmed medium, split into two 6-cm tissue-culture dishes, and incubate at 37°C overnight. In 1 to 2 days, spin down cells and resuspend cells from each dish in 10 ml prewarmed medium, count, and transfer to 75-cm^2 tissue-culture flasks to expand, maintaining cells at 5×10^5 cells per milliliter in flasks, with caps kept loose.

For supernatant production, grow enough hybridoma cells to seed the desired final volume of G_{D3} supernatant at a minimum of 1 to 2×10^5 cells per milliliter. Spin down the cells, resuspend in the same medium as earlier, and allow them to grow for approximately 5 days. Collect the supernatant, spin at $2000 \times g$ for 10 min to pellet cells and debris, and aliquot the supernatant. Store aliquots at or below −20°C.

Functional testing of each batch is critical! After each Purkinje preparation, fix the anti-G_{D3} dishes with 4% paraformaldehyde and imunostain with anti-calbindin D_{28k} and some with anti-GFAP antibody. A positive outcome would be maximum glial fibrillary acidic protein–positive cells with very few calbindin-positive cells on the anti-G_{D3} dishes (figure 16.8).

DAY 1: COAT DISHES

1. Place 3 ml of 50 mM Tris-HCl, pH 9.5, in each of eight 60-mm Petri dishes. Swirl the dishes to distribute the solution evenly. Also, for each anti-G_{D3} dish (make four), add 24 µl (60 µg) of goat anti-mouse IgG (final concentration approximately 20 µg/ml). For mice, for each anti-Thy-1.2 dish (make four), add 8 µl (8 µg) of anti-Thy-1.2 antibodies. For rats, for each anti-Thy-1.1 dish (make four), add 60 µg of goat anti–mouse IgM. This primary antibody is necessary for efficient adherence of Thy-1.1 to the plates for good panning. Incubate all dishes and wells at 4°C overnight.
2. Coat microwells with PLYS (500 µg/ml) and incubate at 4°C overnight.
3. If the intent is to coculture Purkinje and granule neurons, purify the granule neurons from P4 mice the day before the Purkinje purification, as described. Plate granule cells in serum-free medium at 1000–1500 cells per microliter per Lab-Tek well (200 µl total volume).

DAY 2

1. At the beginning of day 2 (the procedures should take some 8 h), wash the anti-G_{D3} dishes with 3 to 4 ml of sterile, filtered phosphate-buffered saline (PBS) three times, leaving the dishes moist. Replace the PBS with 5 ml of undiluted anti-G_{D3} supernatant per plate. Incubate at room temperature (RT).
2. For rat Purkinje cells, wash the goat anti–mouse IgM plates with PBS as for the G_{D3} dishes and replace the PBS with 3 ml of 50 mM Tris-Cl, pH 9.5, containing 8 µg of anti-Thy-1.1. (For mouse, use anti-Thy-1.2). Incubate at RT.
3. Warm 50 ml CMF-PBS, BME, and BME with BSA to RT.
4. Before dissection, prepare the papain solution at RT. Papain is used instead of trypsin because it is less likely to strip Thy-1 from the cell surface. For 5 ml of solution, combine 5 ml of Earle's solution with EDTA and NaHCO$_3$, 150 µl of DNase solution (0.5 mg/ml), and 60 µl of papain (26 units/mg = 31.43 mg/ml). The final concentration of papain is 10 units/ml.

Approximately 10 min before use, add 1.2 mg of L-cysteine (solid) per 5 ml of papain solution. This 10-min incubation with a reducing agent activates the papain (note light orange color). Acrodisc-filter the papain solution into a 6-cm Petri dish.

Dissection and Dissociation

5. Dissect out cerebella, clean off meninges, and collect into ice-cold CMF-PBS. Transfer to a Petri dish and cut each cerebellum into two or three pieces.

6. Transfer tissue pieces into the dish with the papain solution by using a plastic pipette (with as little CMF-PBS as you can manage) and move into a 35.5°C incubator for 45 to 60 min. During this time, wash the Lab-Tek well three times with distilled water, and dry in a laminar flow hood.

7. Transfer tissue to a 15-ml conical tube. Remove papain solution and add 2 to 3 ml medium, supplemented with horse serum (HS).

8. Triturate with three fire-polished Pasteur pipettes, as for mixed cultures and granule cells. Spin the dissociate for 30 s at $700 \times g$. Remove the supernatant to another tube. Add another 1 ml of HS medium and 100 µl of DNase to the pellet and triturate again.

9. Repeat step 8 three or four times. Spin the combined supernatants 3 min at $700 \times g$.

10. Resuspend the cells in 2 ml of CMF-PBS (RT) plus 100 µl of DNase for each Percoll gradient. Use five or six mice (4–5 rats) per gradient.

Separation of Cells by Percoll Gradients

11. Prepare the Percoll gradients in 50-ml conical centrifuge tubes as described earlier for granule neuron purification.

12. Centrifuge the gradients at $2000 \times g$ for 10 min. *Leave the brake off*!

13. While the Percoll gradients are spinning, wash the anti-G_{D3} dishes three times with 3 ml each of PBS and leave them in BME with 0.2% BSA in the incubator for 20 min to 1 h.

14. Holding the gradients up to a point-light source (a fiberoptic dissecting light works well), remove the cell suspension–35% interface with a fire-polished Pasteur pipette. The Purkinje and glial cells should be visible as a white haze against the blue Percoll. (Note: If only purified Purkinje cells are desired, only the 35% gradient is needed. Overlay cell suspension onto the 35% layer; the cells accumulate at the interface with the 35% layer.)

15. Quickly add the cells to a 50-ml tube filled with ice-cold CMF-PBS to dilute the Percoll.

16. Centrifuge the cells at $700 \times g$ for 5 min.

Immunopanning

17. Resuspend the cells in 1 ml BME plus a few drops of DNase. Mix well and add BME minus BSA to a total of 8 ml (2 ml per panning dish). Remove the BME + BSA from the panning dish. Transfer 2 ml of cells to each anti-G_{D3} panning dish. Wash out the cell tube with 4 ml of BME (1 ml per panning dish) and transfer 1 ml to each panning dish. Shake to mix. Place in incubator for 45 to 60 min.

18. Meanwhile, wash the anti-Thy-1 panning dishes three times with 3 to 4 ml of PBS and incubate with BME + BSA for 20 to 60 min. Warm the remaining CMF-PBS to 37°C.

19. After the anti-G_{D3} panning-binding step, harvest the nonadherent cells by tapping the edge of the culture dish gently against the side of the bench and suck off the medium. Remove the BME + BSA from the anti-Thy-1 dishes and transfer the 3 ml of cell suspension to an anti-Thy-1 dish. Place in incubator for 45 min; 5% to 10% of the cells should remain adherent to the G_{D3} dishes; this corresponds to some 150 cells per 10× field.

20. To remove the Thy-1-nonadherent cells, wash the panning dishes five to eight times with 3 to 5 ml of warm CMF-PBS. Light tapping after the second and fifth washes will help to detach loose cells and debris.

21. To remove the Thy-1-adherent cells, incubate dishes with 2.5 ml of trypsin-EDTA for 10 min at 37°C. To facilitate cell detachment, gently aspirate and expel the trypsin-EDTA solution against most of the dish bottom surface eight to ten times per dish, using a polished Pasteur pipette.

22. Collect the trypsin-EDTA with cells and add 1 to 3 ml HS medium.

23. Spin the cells for 8 min at $850 \times g$. Resuspend in 50 µl of DNase and 0.5 to 1.0 ml of serum-free medium.

Plating

24. Count the cells and plate at 1500 cells per microliter (200 µl total volume) in Lab-Tek wells coated with PLYS and washed three times with sterile distilled water (dH$_2$O). If added to granule neurons, cells can be plated at one-tenth this density.

25. Change medium the next day and every 3 to 4 days thereafter. *Exception*: If the intent is to add exogenous factors to the medium,

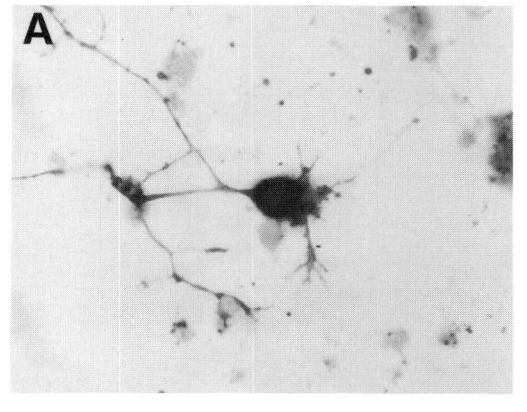
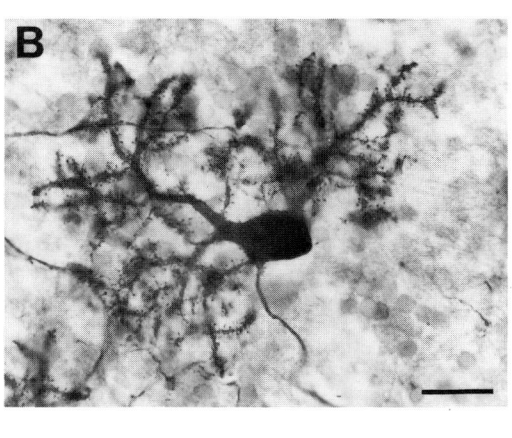

Figure 16.9 Purkinje cells in culture, 21 days in vitro. (*A*) Purified Purkinje cells cultured alone extend axons but do not extend mature dendrites. (*B*) Purified Purkinje cells cocultured with purified granule neurons elaborate dendrites with spines. Scale bar: 20 μm.

plate the cells in a minimal volume (e.g., 100 μl) and allow the cells to attach to the substrate for 60 to 90 min, checking with an inverted microscope to ensure that all cells are adhering. Remove all but 40 μl of the medium once the cells have attached and replace with the desired, supplemented medium. Change medium every 3 to 4 days thereafter. Our yield is 20,000 to 25,000 cells per pup.

Purkinje cell differentiation can be checked by fixing and immunostaining a test well with anti-calbindin D_{28k} to visualize dendrites, as described in Baptista et al. (1994) and in figures 16.8 and 16.9.

Pontine Explant Cultures

Coat a culture vessel (usually Lab-Tek chamber slides) with 500 mg/ml PLYS overnight at 4°C. Wash the wells two or three times with dH_2O and coat with 20 mg/ml laminin in CMF-PBS for 1.5 to 2 hours at room temperature. Wash two or three times with CMF-PBS, keeping the wells moist at all times, and plate the explants on the coated wells.

1. Remove the P0 brain gently from the skull, as described.
2. Transfer the brain into ice-cold CMF-PBS in a Petri dish. With the dorsal side down, remove the meninges overlying the pons. Turn

the brain upright and cut the brain and brainstem sagittally with a microscalpel.

3. The pontine nucleus can be seen clearly as a small bump at the ventrorostral curve of the brainstem. Excise the pontine nucleus from the brainstem and transfer it into a second plastic dish with CMF-PBS.

4. Dice each pontine nucleus half into small explants 100 to 300 μm in diameter with a microscalpel (Roboz no. 37-7545).

5. Wash explants three times with CMF-PBS to remove debris.

6. Wash them three times with serum-free medium and transfer into a medium-filled coated well by barely touching the surface of the medium with the pipette tip, gently expelling the explants. Place in incubator for 1 to 2 h to allow explants to attach to the substrate before adding other cells. If cocultured cells are plated in a special configuration (e.g., on a half-dish; see Baird et al., 1992a), add explants after plating the cells.

Astroglial cultures

Astroglial cells are obtained from cerebellar tissue harvested from C57BL/6J mice or Sprague-Dawley rats at P3 to P6. The tissue is prepared and processed as for the granule cell purification, including the preplating step. The Percoll gradient separation is performed, and the cells adhering to the low-concentration PLYS plates (50–100 μg/ml) from the preplating step (as originally described by Hatten, 1985) are maintained in serum-containing medium in 60-mm PLYS-coated (described earlier) bacteriological plastic Petri dishes for 2 to 4 days. After 1 day in vitro, the dishes are washed twice with CMF-PBS to remove remaining neurons, then are kept in serum-containing medium to allow astroglial proliferation and to induce further neuronal detachment (Gilad et al., 1990).

Astroglia that have been cultured as described 2 to 4 days and upward to 3 months are harvested with trypsin and replated at the desired density in glass coverslip or Lab-Tek wells. The culture surface is treated with PLYS (50 or 500 μg/ml) or PLYS followed by laminin (20 μg/ml, 45 min at 35.5°C). Initial plating is carried out in glial cell medium containing 10% horse serum. After several hours or 1 day (especially if neurons are added), the medium is exchanged for serum-free medium. (Note: Compared to freshly harvested astroglia, astroglia that have been maintained for more than

5 days may change properties that are relevant to growth support of certain cell interactions (see Wang et al., 1994).

Astroglial cells are the only cell population that we culture in larger dishes, expanding them into 35-mm dishes or 100-mm dishes. These cultures must be monitored carefully for contamination (bacteria, yeast) as their slow growth rate requires several weeks to produce large cell populations. Glial proliferation can be increased by addition of basic-fibroblast growth factor or platelet-derived growth factor to the cultures. Fetal bovine serum is rich in these factors, offering a reasonable alternative to costly peptide growth factor additives. Unlike neurons, glial cells can be transferred by typical trypsinization protocols. This possibility provides an approach to recombining purified glial cells with neurons harvested at later times. In general, we maintain a "stock" of primary glial cells for use in recombination experiments.

Appendix

Recipes

Before starting the experiments, prepare the following solutions and media. Filter all the solutions and media with 0.2-μm-pore-size filter units and store them at 4°C unless otherwise specified.

BME stock solution: Per 100 ml : 86 ml dH$_2$O; 10 ml Earle's balanced salt solution, 10× (Gibco); 1 ml BME amino acids; 1 ml BME vitamins; 2 ml 1M NaHCO$_3$; pH to 7.2 to 7.4.

BME with BSA: Dissolve 100 mg BSA in 50 ml BME stock.

BME without BSA: Add 1 ml 30% glucose to 49 ml BME stock.

CMF-PBS (Tyrode's): Per liter: 8 g NaCl; 0.30 g KCl; 2 g glucose; 0.50 g NaH$_2$PO$_4$ · H$_2$O; 0.25 g KH$_2$PO$_4$; 2 ml 2% stock NaHCO$_3$; 0.5 ml 0.5% phenol red solution; pH to 7.4.

4× CMF-PBS-EDTA: For 1 liter: 32 g NaCl; 1.2 g KCl, 2 g glucose; 2 g NaH$_2$PO$_4$ · H$_2$O; 1 g KH$_2$PO$_4$; 8 ml 2% NaHCO$_3$; 10 ml 1-M EDTA; pH 8.0.

DNase solution: Per 200 ml : 100 mg DNase; 197.7 ml BME; 2.26 ml 30% glucose; store at −20°C.

Earle's solution with EDTA and NaHCO$_3$: For 200 ml : 20 ml 10× Earle's salts; 170 ml dH$_2$O; 5.2 ml 1M NaHCO$_3$; 3.1 ml 30% glucose; 2 ml 50-mM EDTA.

Granule cell medium: Per 100 ml : 81.5 ml BME stock solution; 1.5 ml 30% glucose; 1 ml penicillin-streptomycin; 1 ml L-glutamine; 10 ml horse serum; 5 ml fetal bovine serum (*heat-inactivated serum only*); pH to 7.4.

Glial cell medium: Per 100 ml : 85 ml BME stock solution; 1.5 ml 30% glucose; 1 ml penicillin-streptomycin; 1 ml L-glutamine; 10 ml horse serum (*heat-inactivated serum only*); pH to 7.4.

4% Parafomaldehyde in 0.1M phosphate buffer: Make 8% paraformaldehyde in dH$_2$O by heating to 60°C while stirring; do not exceed 60°C. Add drops of 10 N NaOH until solution becomes clear (usually 1–4 drops per 100 ml). Cool to RT. Aliquot and store at −20°C. Add equal volumes of 0.2-M Sorensen's phosphate buffer and 8% paraformaldehyde to make 4% paraformaldehyde in phosphate buffer.

PBS: Per liter: 8 g NaCl; 0.2 g KCl, 0.23 g NaH$_2$PO$_4 \cdot$H$_2$O; 1.15 g NaH$_2$PO$_4$; pH to 7.3.

Percoll stock solution: Sigma P-1644 Percoll comes as a liquid. To each liter of Percoll, add about 6.5 ml 1N HCl over a 3 to 4 h period, to a final pH of 7.4. Adding HCl too fast will cause the Percoll to aggregate.

35% Percoll For 100 ml : 35 ml Percoll; 25 ml 4× CMF-PBS-EDTA; 40 ml dH$_2$O.

60% Percoll For 100 ml : 60 ml Percoll; 25 ml 4× CMF-PBS-EDTA; 15 ml dH$_2$O; four drops of 4% trypan blue to aid in 35% to 60% Percoll layer visualization later.

Poly-D-lysine: Dissolve at 500 µg/ml in dH$_2$O. Store aliquots at −20°C.

Purkinje cell serum-containing medium: Per 25 ml : 21 ml BME stock solution; 1.2 ml 10% glucose; 50 µl penicillin-streptomycin; 250 µl L-glutamine; 2.5 ml horse serum (*heat-inactivated serum only*); pH to 7.4

Serum-free medium (granule neurons/glia): Per 50 ml : 46.2 ml DMEM, 0.5 ml 100× L-glutamine; 0.5 ml 100× penicillin-streptomycin; 0.8 ml 30% glucose; 1 ml 50× B-27 supplement, 1 ml 100× N2 supplement; pH to 7.4.

Serum-free medium (Purkinje cells): Per 50 ml : 46.5 ml BME stock; 0.5 ml L-glutamine; 2.4 ml 10% glucose; 100 µl 100× penicillin-streptomycin; 0.5 g BSA (fraction V; Sigma A-9418); 0.5 ml serum-free supplement (Sigma I-1884); pH to 7.4.

0.2 M Sorensen's phosphate buffer: Make 0.2 M monobasic phosphate stock solution (27.59 g/L NaH$_2$PO$_4 \cdot$ H$_2$O). Make 0.2 M dibasic

phosphate stock solution (28.39 g/L NaHPO$_4$). Add one part monobasic to four parts dibasic for 0.2-M Sorensen's buffer; pH 7.2 to 7.3.
Tris buffer, 50 mM: Dissolve 302.5 mg Tris base in 50 ml dH$_2$O; pH to 9.5 with 1 N HCl.
Trypsin-DNase solution: Per 100 ml : 1 g trypsin; 100 mg DNase; 99.4 ml CMF-PBS; 22.5 mg MgSO$_4$ · 7H$_2$O; 0.6 ml 1 N NaOH; store at −20°C.

Supplier Index

Trypsin	Worthington (Freehold, NJ)
DNase	Worthington
Trypsin-EDTA	Gibco (Gaithersburg, MD)
Basal medium Eagle's (BME)	Gibco
Dulbecco's modified Eagle's medium (DMEM)	Gibco
Fetal bovine serum	Gibco
Horse serum	Gibco
Serum-free supplements	Sigma (St. Louis, MO)
Bovine serum albumin	Sigma
Poly-D-lysine	Sigma
PKH-26 Cell Linker Kit	Sigma
Matrigel	Collaborative Biomedical Products (Franklin Lakes, NJ)
Laminin	Collaborative Biomedical Products
Rat tail collagen	Collaborative Biomedical Products
Swinney filter holders	Fisher (Pittsburgh, PA)
LabTek chamber slides	Nunc (Naperville, IL)
Vetbond	Henry Schein (Port Washington, NY)
Anti-Thy-1.2 antibodies	Boehringer-Mannheim (Indianapolis, IN)
Anti-Thy-1.1 antibodies	Sigma
Anti-calbindin (D$_{28k}$)	SWant (Bellinzona, Switzerland)
FITC secondary antibodies	Cappel (Durham, NC)
Fluorescent microbeads	Molecular Probes (Eugene, OR)
Surgical instruments	Roboz (Rockville, MD)
R24 cell line	ATCC (Bethesda, MD)

Acknowledgments

Many people in our laboratories contributed to the methods described herein. We especially thank Ann Francois, James Edmond-

son, Urs Gasser, Gord Fishell, Carlos Baptista, Douglas Baird, Kim Hunter, Lena Hofer, Li-Chong Wang, Stan Ward, Xiao-Lin Liu, Chen Zheng, and Qin Zhang. We are especially indebted to Christine Gallagher and Janet Alder for their expert editing of this manuscript. Supported by NIH grants NS 15429 (MEH), NS 16951 (CAM), National Research Service Award Fellowship (NS098 64 MEM) and P01-NS 30532 (MEH).

Authors' note: The methods reported here represent updated or expanded versions of previously published protocols. Where short forms of methods are given, more detail can be found in the original publication as referenced.

17 Organotypic Slice Cultures of Neural Tissue

*Beat H. Gähwiler, Scott M. Thompson, R. Anne McKinney,
Dominique Debanne, and Richard T. Robertson*

*"Tissue culture" is an art which has flourished under false pre-
tenses ... In the absence of the many factors which maintain tissue
and organ structure, migrating and growing cells tend to arrange
themselves in sheets, in radiating strands, or haphazardly. Thus,
they no longer represent a tissue, but are in fact cell colonies or cell
cultures.*
—J. H. Hanks, 1955

Two methods for culturing slices currently are available: the roller
tube technique and the membrane technique. Both methods can
use the same culture media, and essentially the same techniques
are used for the preparation of the slices. They differ, however,
with respect to the techniques by which the cultures are embedded
and maintained. The basic principle of the roller tube technique
consists of attaching slices of any brain region onto glass coverslips
and incubating them in rotating tissue-culture tubes for several
weeks. The slow rotation results in a periodic alteration of the gas-
liquid interface to which the cultures are exposed; that is, the cultures sometimes are immersed, sometimes only covered by a film
of medium. This process not only facilitates gas and medium ex-
changes but leads to considerable thinning, thus allowing identified cells to be observed in living, unstained tissue after some 2
weeks in vitro.

Tissue slices also can be placed on porous, transparent membranes and maintained at the interface between air and the culture
medium. These membrane cultures do not thin to the same degree
as that seen with roller-tube cultures and may be more useful for
studies in which three-dimensional organization is important (e.g.,
electron microscopic analysis or electrophysiological recording of
compound potentials and population spikes). Slice cultures produced by either technique retain the basic structural and connective organization of their tissue of origin; thus, they are termed
organotypic or *histotypic*.

Historical Background

The roller-tube technique originated in the late 1940s when Hogue (Hogue, 1947) and later Costero and Pomerat (Costero and Pomerat, 1951) started to grow neural tissue in roller tubes on glass coverslips. During the last 15 years, the technique has undergone major changes and developments. First, the introduction of plastic labware has changed incubation techniques and cultivation procedures considerably. Second, slicing techniques that were used for the preparation of acute slices—in particular mechanical tissue choppers and vibratomes—were adapted for use with tissue cultures (Gähwiler, 1984c). Third, methods were developed to grow organotypic cultures in chemically defined culture media (Annis et al., 1990; Wray et al., 1991). Fourth, the development of techniques for coculturing tissue derived from different anatomical regions has greatly extended the potential of organotypic cultures for developmental and physiological studies (Gähwiler and Hefti, 1984; Gähwiler and Brown, 1985a).

Organotypic cultures have been prepared by several other approaches that differ mainly in the way the tissue is incubated: in Maximow double-coverslip assemblies (Maximow, 1925), in perfusion chambers (Rose, 1954), or in Petri dishes Beach et al., 1982; (Romijn et al., 1988). The Maximow technique (Crain, 1976); Toran-Allerand, 1990) yields organized tissue cultures that remain—even after prolonged cultivation periods—several cell layers thick. These cultures attain a high degree of differentiation and can be observed easily without removal from the culture assembly. They are, however, not easily accessible and not well-suited for those electrophysiological recording techniques requiring access to individual neurons.

Rationale for Using Organotypic Slice Cultures

Over the years, we have attempted to develop an in vitro preparation that ideally fulfills the following criteria: (1) The tissue should remain organotypically organized; (2) it should be accessible for experimental manipulations; (3) it should contain neurons displaying a high degree of cellular differentiation; and (4) it should permit studies of the development and characteristics of axonal connectivities within and between different brain areas. We briefly review each of these criteria and present some examples of each.

Tissue Organization

Maintenance of histotypic organization clearly is a major benefit of this technique. Of practical benefit, organotypicity allows the experimenters to identify the region or cell group of interest and also maintains local circuitry and neuron-glial relationships. During the preparation of slice cultures, utmost care is taken to dissect the tissue as carefully as possible to avoid damage that would disrupt its histotypic architecture. The degree of organotypic organization varies with the age of the donor animals and the type of tissue that is cultured. Tissue taken from younger animals generally shows greater alteration of its histotypic organization than does tissue taken from older animals. Further, during long cultivation periods, slice cultures may show some reorganization as evidenced by analysis of synaptic rearrangements. The vast majority of nerve cells are found to innervate their normal target cells. However, because of the loss of normal afferent projections and target areas, the intrinsic neuronal connections reorganize themselves to a certain extent and take over some additional synaptic sites (Zimmer and Gähwiler, 1984, 1987; Frotscher and Gähwiler, 1988).

Accessibility

The great popularity of culture methods draws to a large degree on the following principles: Culturing provides a much greater degree of control over the biochemical milieu of the tissue than what occurs in vivo, living nerve cells can be observed directly under the microscope, and important cellular and developmental processes can be studied under well-controlled experimental conditions. Therefore, it is considered a great advantage that slice cultures thin to quasi-monolayer thickness, facilitating both direct exposure to experimental reagents and direct microscopic observation of living cells with contrast-enhancing optics (Gähwiler, 1984a,c; 1988). Morphologically identified neurons then can be studied with a variety of methods, including patch clamp and optical recording techniques (Llano et al., 1988; Gähwiler and Llano, 1989; Audinat et al., 1990).

Athough diffusion barriers for drugs and other chemical agents are weaker than in the thicker Maximow-type cultures or in acute slices, untreated slice cultures (without irradiation and antimitotics) eventually become ensheathed by a thin layer of membranes of

nonneuronal cells. This membrane sheath covering can markedly impede the penetration of substances in the living culture and even of histochemical or immunocytochemical reagents after culture fixation.

Thin organotypic slice cultures are suited optimally for the application of sophisticated recording techniques, such as optical monitoring of membrane potentials and of cytosolic calcium dynamics (Knöpfel et al., 1990b,c). This potential is illustrated by a study in which single-electrode voltage-clamp and microfluorometric recording techniques were applied to evaluate whether changes in cytosolic free Ca^{2+} concentrations are involved in the blockade of Ca^{2+}-activated potassium currents by muscarinic and noradrenergic agonists (Knöpfel et al., 1990a). It is expected that the combination of electrophysiological and microfluorometric recording techniques will open up powerful new ways to study dendritic information processing and properties of synaptically organized neuronal networks.

Cellular Differentiation

For cultivation, neural tissue usually is removed from the natural environment during early phases of development. At this stage, some neurons still may be being generated, while others have only started to extend dendritic and axonal processes. Differentiation is likely to depend on a number of factors, such as the presence of chemical mediators and the cellular microenvironment to which the neurons are exposed. A large number of studies have demonstrated that nerve cells continue to differentiate and mature in slice cultures. Indeed, a recent study of development of single cerebral cortical neurons (Annis et al., 1993) demonstrated remarkable parallels in morphological and physiological aspects of development in slice cultures and in situ.

Why such a high degree of neuronal differentiation can be attained with slice cultures is not altogether clear. Any factors released by remote afferent fibers are, of course, absent, because these fibers are cut during preparation of the slice. However, the neurons are embedded in a microenvironment that seems to resemble closely the natural one. Analysis of hippocampal and cerebral cortical cultures by immunohistochemical and dye injection techniques has revealed that all major neuronal and glial cell types are present (Gähwiler,

1984a; Caeser et al., 1989; Streit et al., 1989; Annis et al., 1990, 1993). The age of the donor animals also appears to be critical in differentiation and maturation. For example, some studies suggest that if cerebellar tissue is derived from 8- to 11-day-old postnatal rats, cells do not continue to mature beyond the level attained at the time of explantation (Jaeger et al., 1988; Kapoor et al., 1988). Therefore, we use 0- to 1-day-old rats for the cultivation of cerebellar tissue (Gähwiler, 1984c). For hippocampal tissue, the optimal age appears to be 6 to 7 days postnatally.

Axonal Connectivity

Normal local axonal circuitry within the slice is maintained during culturing and, as noted, some reorganization sometimes occurs and results in abnormal connectivity. However, long extrinsic afferent and efferent fibers are severed during the slicing procedure, and distal segments rapidly degenerate during the first few days in vitro. In an attempt to establish an in vitro analog of axonal connectivities between brain areas, we have cocultured slices derived from brain regions anatomically remote but interconnected in situ. Further, the use of large single tissue slices that contain both the cells of origin and the terminal fields of a particular pathway can be used to study developent and target selectivity (Baratta et al., 1996). Such approaches can provide powerful models for studying aspects of the development and function of neuronal projections.

Cocultures have been instrumental in elucidating mechanisms involved in synaptic transmission. This is illustrated by the example of septohippocampal cocultures (Gähwiler and Hefti, 1984), wherein fibers originating in the septum establish functional synaptic connections with hippocampal target neurons. Electrical stimulation of septal tissue has been shown to induce in hippocampal pyramidal cells a slow muscarinic excitation that lasts up to several minutes and is mediated by a reduction in both a voltage-dependent and a Ca^{2+}-dependent potassium conductance (Gähwiler and Brown, 1985b; Gähwiler et al., 1989).

Cocultured slices differ in many respects from preparations in which neurons dissociated from different brain areas are mixed together and cocultured. The latter preparations are well-suited for some studies (e.g., certain aspects of trophic interactions), but electrophysiological experiments are restricted by the difficulties

encountered with identification and selective stimulation of neurons derived from the origin of the projection and from the target region.

Protocol for Preparing Organotypic Slice Cultures

General Techniques

One of the main advantages of this technique[1] is that tissue slices can be studied in culture for several weeks. However, longevity of the cultures can be achieved only by ensuring that all work for preparing and maintaining the cultures is done in a sterile environment and that all tools for preparing the cultures are clean and sterile. Use of a laminar flow hood or dedicated sterile room and continual observation of sterile technique are recommended strongly to keep the cultures uncontaminated. All surgical tools and any instrument that will come into contact with the tissue must be sterilized, either by heat or gas methods. An ethanol lamp is useful for continual resterilization (flaming) of surgical tools to insure that they remain uncontaminated during the culturing process. In our experience, careful use of sterile technique makes the addition of antibiotics to the cultures unnecessary.

Culture Medium

A variety of media have been used in tissue culture work, as evidenced in other contributions to this volume. Culture medium provides essential nutrients to the growing cultures; thus, the preparation and composition of the medium is of critical importance for producing consistently good quality cultures. Essentially, two types of culture media have been used: serum-based and serum-free defined media. For much of our work, we have chosen to use a serum-based medium for several reasons. First, the inclusion of serum provides an effective buffer for the medium, thus allowing the culturing process to take place without the need to control carbon dioxide concentration in the incubator. Second, serum contains a variety of poorly characterized nutrients, growth factors, and hormones that promote health and growth of the cultured tissue. Third, serum-based medium is simple to prepare and maintain.

As used in our laboratories, serum-based medium consists of a solution of basic nutrients, most of which are available from Gibco (Gaithersburg, MD). The ingredients include Eagle's basal medium without glutamine [with either Earle's (Gibco no. 21010) or Hank's (no. 11370) salts], a balanced salt solution (BSS), with either Earle's [(no. 24010) or Hank's (no. 24020) salts], and horse (Gibco no. 16050) or calf serum in concentrations of 10% to 30%. Typically, we use 25% horse serum. Phenol red is included in the basal medium and the BSS as an indicator of the pH of the medium. We prepare the medium in quantities of 100 ml by the following recipe: 50 ml basal medium (Eagle's), 25 ml BSS, either Earle's or Hank's, and 25 ml horse serum. The serum must be screened for mycoplasma to reduce the chances of contamination of the cultures; the recommended serum is screened by Gibco. Serum is stored at $-20°C$ and is thawed at room temperature. Complement is inactivated by heating the serum in a water bath at 56°C for 30 min before using. Basal medium should be purchased without glutamine and stored at 4°C. The BSS with Earle's salts contains more bicarbonate than that with Hank's salts and will offer more buffering capacity against the greater carbon dioxide produced by larger cultures.

In addition to the foregoing major ingredients, we supplement the medium with glucose (Sigma Chemical) and glutamine (Gibco). To 100 ml of medium, we add 1 ml of a 50% solution of glucose and 0.5 ml of 200 mM L-glutamine. Both glucose and glutamine are prepared in water and added to the medium through a sterilizing filter.

An advantage of serum-based media—that it contains uncharacterized factors that promote growth and maintenance of neural tissue—also is a disadvantage. Studies that attempt to characterize the molecular factors that regulate various aspects of neural development and deafferentation require the use of a chemically defined medium. Several authors have presented descriptions of serum-free media (e.g., Romijn et al., 1988; Annis et al., 1990; Robertson et al., 1991; Wray et al. 1991). Although defined media offer the clear advantage that everything provided exogenously to the culture is identified, neurons and glial cells intrinsic to the culture likely secrete a variety of factors that are unknown; thus, no medium is "defined" fully after it is added to the cultures.

Because the medium in the culture tubes is changed frequently, it is critically important to ensure that the medium is maintained sterile. It is prudent periodically to place 1 ml of medium in a

culture tube in the incubator to check for growth of contaminating organisms.

Choice of Animals

Tissue from a variety of animals can be used for culturing. Most of our experience has been with infant rats and mice. The best age of animals for culturing may vary from region to region and should be determined empirically. In general, use of early postnatal animals (0–6 days) results in good-quality cultures. In some cases, tissue from fetuses is preferred (e.g., for the dorsal thalamus).

Dissections

It is imperative that the dissections proceed quickly, to reduce the length of time between animal sacrifice and separation and exposure of cut tissue slices to BSS or medium. Any prolonged delays will result in deterioration of the tissue and consequent reduction in quality of the cultures. A reasonable goal in the dissection is to have cut slices separated in less than 5 to 10 min after animal sacrifice. With reason, some believe that placing the animal in an ice bath prior to sacrifice (to cool the brain and slow metabolic processes) may result in better-quality slices, particularly if the dissections are lengthy. Further, the dissection solutions should be cold, and the entire procedure should be performed over ice. It also is recommended strongly that practice dissections be undertaken and that the dissected block of tissue be processed histologically to verify that the desired region of tissue has indeed been collected.

Animals are decapitated by a quick scissor cut at the level of the foramen magnum. Small dissecting scissors are used to cut through the skull horizontally on both sides at a level just above the ears. The dorsal part of the skull then can be removed, using either the scissors or a pair of forceps. The technique for removal of the brain will vary somewhat, depending on the particular brain region that will be cultured. In general, a small spatula (approximately 4×150 mm, available from dental supply companies) is used to cut the cranial nerves and to ease the brain out of the cranium and into a large drop of glucose-enriched (6.5 g/L) cooled Gey's BSS (Gibco no. 14260) in a sterile Petri dish. Note that Gey's BSS is available for "tubes" and "slides." The latter must be used for the dissection, as it has a lower bicarbonate concentration and maintains a phys-

iological pH in air. The brain then is viewed under a dissecting microscope and is dissected by using razor blade knives and fine forceps. Care must be exercised to use only very gentle handling of the tissues and to ensure that the tissue is kept moist at all times. An excessively high air flow in the laminar hood can cause the tissue to dry quickly. Because of the need to keep the time between sacrifice and placement of the slices in BSS to minimum, it is best to dissect only one region from each brain. The particular procedures for dissection will, of course, vary with the desired region, and readers should refer to discussions of particular dissection procedures (e.g., Robertson et al., 1989).

Razor blade knives (e.g. from G. Martin, Tuttlingen, Germany or from Fine Science Tools, North Vancouver, Canada) are used to isolate the brain region of interest. All cuts should be made quickly and cleanly, to avoid damaging the tissue. The ideal size of the block of tissue will vary with the goals of the study. In general, the block of tissue should be kept small to facilitate handling but still large enough to contain all desired components of the targeted region. Meninges and major blood vessels are removed from the tissue quickly and carefully by using fine forceps. Removal of meninges facilitates the task of cutting the block of tissue and separating the slices. These steps will require some practice to ensure that the desired block of tissue can be dissected with a minimum of damage.

Tissue Slicing

Several means of slicing the tissue block can be used. With some practice, slices of tissue can be prepared by hand, using knives made from razor blades or scalpels. However, slices of more consistent thickness require the use of a commercially available tissue chopper or vibrating microtome. The vibratome is useful for particularly large blocks of tissue, but a tissue chopper is used more commonly for smaller pieces. All surfaces of the slicing apparatus that come in contact with the tissue are sterilized with 70% ethanol.

In using a tissue chopper, the block of tissue is transferred onto a sterilized plastic sheet (Aclar, Allied Chemical International Inc.; or Plastoscreen 250, Mühlebach Inc., Brugg, Switzerland) and placed on the stage of the chopper, with a flat surface down and the desired plane of section parallel to the plane of the razor blade. If necessary, a small drop of plasma with thrombin will hold the

tissue in place during sectioning. The thickness of the slices can vary from about 200 to 700 μm; we recommend about 400 μm. Of course, thinner sections are more fragile and may contain fewer undamaged cells; thicker sections are easier to handle but may allow insufficient diffusion of oxygen and nutrients to the center of the slice and may not thin as well. The tissue block is chopped continuously, allowing the cut slices to accumulate like slices of a loaf of bread. It is helpful to keep the blade of the tissue chopper moist to prevent slices of tissue from sticking to the blade. The block of tissue must be kept moist at all times. If chopped within 5 min, drying usually is not a problem. If necessary, a drop of Gey's BSS can be added.

The plastic sheet with tissue slices is transferred into Gey's BSS in a sterile Petri dish. Under a dissecting microscope, two spatulas are used to remove the slices gently, one by one, from the front of the block. The slices should be separated as quickly and gently as possible to get them immersed in the Gey's BSS. Prolonged delays in separating the slices cause them to stick together. Sections can be trimmed further with razor blade knives to remove unwanted or damaged tissue. Again, all cuts should be made cleanly. Slices of some 3 to 4 mm square appear to be maximal. Larger slices are very difficult to handle and perhaps not as satisfactorily cut with a tissue chopper.

The use of a vibrating microtome is especially useful for cutting larger pieces of tissue. The block of tissue is prepared with a flat surface parallel to the desired plane of section; this flat surface is attached to the cutting stage of the vibrating microtome with Superglue. Slices are cut at 300 to 400 μm and collected in cooled Gey's solution or culture medium.

It is essential to check the quality of the slices closely under the microscope and to choose for culturing only those slices that are free from visible damage (i.e., cuts or folds). This is an important "quality control" check point. The slices then are transferred to a Petri dish and stored in Gey's BSS or culture medium. In some cases, it is important to maintain the slices in serial order, so slices can be placed in 6 to 10 small drops of BSS arranged at the perimeter of the Petri dish. Sections may be stored in BSS at 4°C for several hours before embedding on coverglasses; storing the cut slices may allow cut membranes to close and also permit diffusion of released proteolytic enzymes and excitatory amino acids away from the tissue.

At this stage, the cultures can be subjected to ionizing radiation to reduce proliferation of nonneuronal cells. For this purpose, a Petri dish containing freshly cut slices in Gey's BSS is exposed to 800 to 1200 rads delivered continuously for perhaps 5–10 min from a therapeutic x-ray machine.

Preparations of Slice Cultures: Roller Tube Cultures

GENERAL PROCEDURES
Slices of tissue will be mounted onto glass coverslips. Coverslips should be purchased from a reputable source (Gold Seal, Clay Adams; or Vitromed, Basel, Switzerland) and received precleaned. Coverslips need to be small enough to fit into the culture tubes but large enough to hold the cultures and be manipulated easily. A size of 12 × 24 mm works with 16-mm culture tubes. Even though "precleaned" coverglasses are used, all coverglasses should be cleaned additionally in ethanol, washed thoroughly in very clean water, placed again in ethanol, and dried quickly before sterilization at 200°C for 2 h. The use of soap or detergents should be avoided.

The method of attaching slices of tissue to the coverslips is very important. The means of attachment must be strong enough to withstand the continual rolling action and should be a substrate conducive to growth of the cultures. Two techniques are in common use: the plasma clot and the collagen gel techniques.

PLASMA CLOT
Chicken plasma is available from several commercial sources, either frozen or lyophilized. We have obtained consistently good results with plasma from Cocalico Biologicals (Reamstown, PA). It is prepared according to the directions on the package, then centrifuged at 2500 × g at 4°C for 30 min to sediment any fibrin that may be in the plasma. This procedure produces a working solution for embedding the sections. Thrombin for clotting the plasma also is commercially available. Thrombin (purchased from Merck, no. 12374) can be reconstituted in sterile water or Gey's BSS and can be centrifuged along with the plasma. A working solution of 150 NIH units per milliliter in Gey's BSS is sterile-filtered. This solution can be stored in frozen aliquots. The exact concentration of the thrombin solution may vary slightly and should be determined empirically. We have had variable results with some commercially

available plasma (see Troubleshooting) and, in some cases, have prepared plasma ourselves (Paul, 1965). Adult chickens are bled by cardiac puncture using sterile technique. Heparin is added (at the lowest concentration that prevents clotting, usually 0.25 mg/ml) and whole blood is centrifuged at 2500 rpm at 4°C. The supernatant plasma then is removed and stored at −20°C.

Sterilized coverglasses are arranged in a sterile disposable dish, with a drop of 30 μl plasma in the center of each coverslip. Under a dissecting microscope, a fine spatula is used to place one tissue slice (or more than one if making cocultures) in the center of each drop. The spatula is used to spread the plasma over the surface of the coverslip. A drop of 30 μl thrombin is added to each coverslip and mixed thoroughly with the plasma and thrombin. The plasma and thrombin must be mixed well, and the tissue slices must be repositioned quickly, as the plasma will cover the tissue and start clotting within 10 to 30 s. Single slices should be placed approximately in the center of the coverslip; cocultures should be separated from each other by 1 to 3 mm. It is helpful to keep a written record of type of sections, orientation, and any notable features for each coverslip. The coverslips with cultures should be kept horizontal in a Petri dish for several minutes so that the plasma will coagulate well before placing the cultures in the culture tubes. The coagulated plasma should have the consistency of a thick jelly so that it could be cut with a knife (after about 5 min).

Cultures then are placed in screwtop culture tubes. We use either round-bottomed (Nunc, no. 146183) or diagonal-flat bottomed (Nunc, no. 156758) culture tubes (16 × 110 mm). These tubes are an appropriate size to hold the coverslips and also fit into a standard tube holder on the roller drum. Culture medium then is added to the tubes, some 1 ml for the round-bottomed tubes or 750 μl for the diagonal-flat bottomed tubes. These volumes will allow the cultures to be immersed in medium during half a rotation and be out of the medium during the other half rotation. Culture tubes with cultures then are placed in a roller drum (New Brunswick Scientific Co., model TC1 or TC2) in an incubator or laboratory oven at 35° to 36°C and rotated at 10 rph. Serum-based media obviate the need to control carbon dioxide levels or humidity.

COLLAGEN-COATED COVERSLIPS

An alternative technique is to coat the coverslips with collagen. Collagen can be obtained from commercial sources (e.g., Upstate

Biotechnology Inc., Lake Placid, NY), but we prefer to produce our own by dialyzing rat tail collagen (Bornstein, 1958). Coating with collagen is a two-stage process, involving first coating with poly-lysine and second with collagen (Bornstein, 1958). We have used either poly-D-lysine (Sigma, no. P7280; MW range, 30,000–70,000) or poly-L-lysine; both are effective. The polylysine facilitates attachment of collagen on the coverslip. Polylysine is prepared as a solution of 25 µg/ml in distilled sterile water; coverslips are dipped briefly in the solution and allowed to dry. About 60 to 80 µl of the dialyzed rat tail collagen is spread on the coverglass, then exposed to ammonia vapor by placing them in a covered Petri dish containing a few drops of concentrated ammonia. After 5 to 10 min, excess ammonia is removed, and the collagen is conditioned by placing the coverslips in Hank's BSS for at last 2 h. Coated coverslips can be stored in tissue-culture medium for up to 2 weeks prior to use. Slices of tissue are placed on the moist collagen and arranged in the preferred orientation. Cultures on coverslips then are placed in culture tubes with 750 µl of medium. These culture tubes are placed in the incubator and allowed to rest horizontally without rotating for 24 h. This time allows the tissue slices to attach to the collagen. Culture tubes then are placed in the roller drum and are handled in a manner similar to that for cultures attached by the plasma clot technique.

Preparation of Cultures on Membranes

Procedures for culturing slices on membranes are taken from the description by Stoppini et al. (1991). Their technique is remarkably straight-forward and relatively simple. Of course, it avoids the necessity of attaching the slice to a coverslip so that it can withstand the continual rotations in the roller drum.

The "membranes" used for culturing are commercially available; we have experience with two types. Most of our work has been performed with the membranes supplied by Millipore (the Milli-cell, 30-mm culture plate insert with 0.4-µm pore; Millipore Corp., Bedford, MA; catalog no. PICM 030 50). The membranes are 30-mm sheets attached to the bottom of a round polystyrene body that measures some 10 mm high by 30 mm across. Although these membrane inserts are designed for use with standard six-well tissue-culture plates, we have obtained better results by placing the inserts in a 15-mm × 100-mm Petri dish. We believe the improved success

is due to greater movement and exchange of the culture medium while cultures are rocking (see later). The polystyrene body is designed to keep the insert membrane 1 mm above the chamber in which it is placed.

We have additional (although limited) experience with the Transwell cell-culture chambers supplied by Costar (the Transwell-COL, 24.5-mm insert with 0.4-μm pore; Costar, Cambridge, MA, cat. no. 3425). The Costar system is intended for use with the Costar six-well culture dishes (cat. no. 3406), which are designed to hold tissue slightly above the bottom of the well.

The membranes can be purchased with collagen or other extra-cellular matrix coating or can be coated by the user with any of several extracellular matrix substances or even a layer of glial cells. We routinely do not coat our membranes in preparation for slice cultures. Both types of membranes are transparent as long as they are wet, allowing observation of living (or fixed) tissue with bright-field or phase-contrast optics.

Slices of tissue are prepared as described. For single cultures, each slice is placed alone on a culture insert by using a smoothly polished spatula bent at 90 degrees. For cocultures, two (or more) slices are placed on the membrane insert and separated by 1 to 2 mm. Excess medium around the slice is removed by aspiration, and a small drop (20 μl) of medium is placed on the slice so that it is covered by a thin film of medium. Too much medium on or around the slices will interfere with their attaching to the membrane. Four membranes, with cultures, are placed into a sterile Petri dish containing 7 ml of medium. We use either the serum-based medium described or the EOL-1 defined medium developed by Annis et al. (1990). The cultures are held in a 36°C incubator with 5% CO_2 for 24 h to allow the cultures to attach to the membranes. Following the attachment period, the Petri dishes containing the cultures are placed on a rocking platform (Red Rocker; Hoefer Instr., San Francisco, CA) and allowed to rock gently for the remainder of the culture period. Culture medium is changed every 2 to 3 days.

Membrane cultures thin during the culture period but not to the degree seen in roller-tube cultures. In our experience, much of the thinning occurs during the first few days in culture, probably re-sulting primarily from removal of damaged tissue at the cut tissue surfaces. After 2 to 3 days, the slices maintain a thickness of some

100 µm for the duration of the culture period. We have had success with a variety of sizes of tissue slices, including slices of entire forebrain hemispheres (Baratta et al., 1996).

Living cultures grown on membranes can be analyzed and processed by many of the same procedures commonly used for roller-tube cultures. Because the membrane supporting the culture can interfere with optics, some special considerations are in order. In particular, membranes remain transparent only while they are hydrated. Membrane cultures can be fixed with aldehydes or other fixatives while attached to the membranes. If dehydration is important, cultures must be removed carefully from the membrane. After fixation, cultures can be processed for morphological analyses while still attached to the membranes or they can be teased gently off the membranes with a camel's hair brush and processed like individual slices of tissue cut by standard techniques. We examine these cultures routinely under bright-field, phase-contrast, or fluorescence microscopy. These cultures can be also used for physiological studies.

Care and Maintenance

Healthy cultures will metabolize the culture medium and will have to be fed with new medium once or twice per week. As the medium is metabolized by a healthy culture, it becomes more acidic, and the phenol red in the medium turns from a pinkish red to a salmon-pink color. Feeding of the cultures always should occur under a laminar flow hood using sterile procedures. Only a few cultures should be removed from the incubator at one time. The technique is simply to pour out or aspirate the old medium into a beaker and to add an appropriate volume of new medium. It may be a good idea to replace only a portion of the medium at any time, so that any trophic factors produced by resident neurons or glial cells are not removed totally. Round-bottomed tubes take a bit more medium (about 750 µl–1 ml) than do flat-bottomed tubes (about 400–500 µl) and Petri dishes take several milliliters. Exact volume should be determined empirically. The cultures survive for several weeks to months in vitro. To reduce the number of nonneuronal cells, antimitotic drugs (cytosine arabinoside, uridine, and fluorodeoxyuridine, 10^{-6}–10^{-7} M each; Sigma) usually are added for 24 h approximately 4 to 5 days after the cultures were started.

Characterization of Organotypic Slice Cultures

A defining feature of slice cultures is that they retain much of the organization one observes in the same tissue in situ. Anatomically, this organization is expressed in the cytoarchitectures of cell populations, the morphology of single cells, the patterns of connections formed, and the transmitter phenotypes. Physiologically, the organotypic organization is manifested in the neurons' repertoire of voltage-dependent ionic conductances, neurotransmitter receptors, and second-messenger systems. We present three examples of the culture technique. These examples typify both the roller-tube and the membrane techniques. Either technique can be effective using the same tissue source; again, the major difference in results from the two techniques appears to be in the thickness of the cultures.

Hippocampus

The characteristic lamellar cytoarchitecture of the hippocampus—consisting of the pyramidal cell subfield and the fascia dentata—is readily apparent in both living unstained cultures and in histologically prepared cultures (figure 17.1C). As a general principle, it appears that the degree of tissue organization in the final culture is dependent to a large extent on the maturity of the tissue at the time of explantation. For example, within the hippocampus, cell division is completed for the pyramidal cells by birth, whereas dentate granule cells continue to divide up to 2 weeks after birth, particularly in the medial, or free, blade (Bayer, 1980). As a result, we often observe that the medial blade of the dentate in our hippocampal cultures is considerably less well-defined than is the lateral blade (Zimmer and Gähwiler, 1984). In addition, the morphology of individual granule cells in the medial blade is somewhat more variable than those in the lateral blade (Zafirov et al., 1994). Injections of dye into individual cells in either region demonstrate that, although the neurons are relatively primitive at the time of explantation, after 2 weeks in vitro, they have become differentiated into the mature morphological structure, both in terms of dendritic branching patterns and of ultrastructural features. For example, pyramidal cells in area CA3 exhibit a large ascending primary apical dendrite with numerous secondary and higher-order branches and many radially oriented basal dendrites (figure 17.1C). Granule cells, by contrast, extend two or more primary dendrites from only one pole of the cell body. In addition, both pyramidal and granule cell

dendrites are richly endowed with spines (see figure 17.2 and color plate 10) that can be seen under the electron microscope to contain asymmetrical synaptic contacts. As in situ, the spines on the proximal portion of the apical dendrite of CA3 cells may be enlarged even further and may be specialized at the sites of termination of the granule cell axons (Frotscher and Gähwiler, 1988). Other morphological cell types (i.e., bipolar, multipolar, and aspiny cells), corresponding to local circuit neurons, are revealed with immunohistochemical stains directed against transmitter-related markers, such as γ-aminobutyric acid (GABA), tyrosine hydroxylase, acetylcholinesterase, somatostatin, and others.

Axonal elaboration occurs largely after the time of explantation for hippocampal slice cultures, yet proceeds according to patterns and principles established in situ (Zimmer and Gähwiler, 1984). Granule cell axons (i.e., the mossy fibers) extend into a narrow region of the proximal portion of stratum radiatum in area CA3, as shown in Timm's stained material. In hippocampal slice cultures, as in situ, these axons never extend beyond the CA1-CA3 border. By the use of cocultures of the fascia dentata with either isolated CA1 or CA3 subfields, it was possible to show that only rarely and in the absence of CA3 cells would mossy fibers innervate the CA1 region, suggesting that complex signals regulating the synaptogenic abilities of mossy fiber axons persist in these cultures (Zimmer and Gähwiler, 1987). Interestingly, granule cell axons typically produce a supragranular axon collateral in culture, similar to the phenomena observed in situ following partial deafferentation of the dentate gyrus. Presumably, this sprouting fills vacant synaptic territory created by the loss of afferents from the entorhinal cortex (Zimmer and Gähwiler, 1984). In addition, CA3 axons in culture can be shown to give rise to local axon collaterals within the CA3 region and to project to the apical and basilar dendrites of the CA1 region. The distribution of CA1 cell axons is not yet known but is likely to be somewhat different from the intact tissue by virtue of a lack of their normal remote targets.

Many neurons expressing unique neurotransmitter phenotypes do not become fully mature until after the time of explantation. Interneurons that use the inhibitory transmitter GABA, for example, mature several weeks after birth (Seress and Ribak, 1988). Using anti-GABA antibodies, we have shown (Streit et al., 1989) that GABA-immunoreactive neurons in hippocampal slice cultures exhibit a variety of appropriately located nonpyramidal morphologies

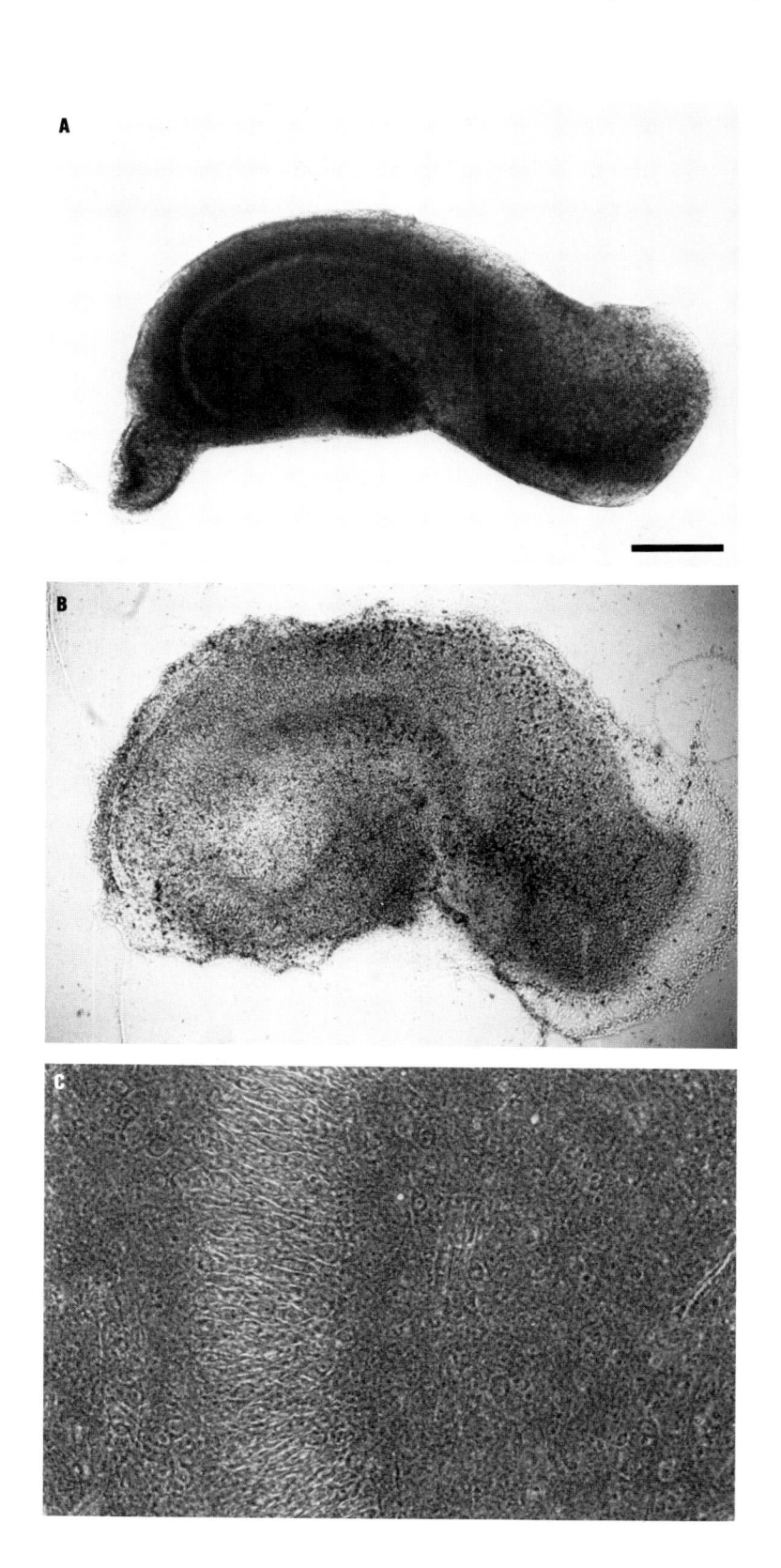

and that these cells form inhibitory synapses primarily with the soma and proximal dendrites of pyramidal cells (figure 17.3), as they do in situ. Although not quantified, the ratio of GABAergic cells to pyramidal cells appears to be qualitatively similar to the ratio from in situ material and clearly more typical than are some dissociated cell cultures (Hoch and Dingledine, 1986). Furthermore, prominent inhibitory postsynaptic potentials are elicited readily with local stimulation and can be abolished by blocking postsynaptic GABA$_A$ receptors with the selective antagonist bicuculline (see figure 17.3). When inhibitory postsynaptic potentials have been abolished, paroxysmal depolarization shifts (analogous to interictal epileptiform discharges) are evoked in response to local stimulation or occur spontaneously (Scanziani et al., 1994). These events occur synchronously throughout the local population of cells in a stereotypical manner, reflecting the collective properties of a specifically organized neuronal network (Traub and Wong, 1982). Convulsant induced discharge in dissociated hippocampal cell cultures appears significantly different from that in acutely prepared slices or slice cultures, presumably as a result of their relatively disorganized patterns of connections.

Basal Forebrain Cholinergic System

Basal forebrain cholinergic neurons (including the cholinergic neurons of the medial septum) have been demonstrated to grow quite well in tissue slice cultures (Gähwiler et al., 1987; Distler and Robertson, 1992, 1993). Much of the work has been done examining growth of cholinergic (AChE-positive) axons from the basal forebrain into cerebral cortex using coculture preparations. These studies have demonstrated remarkable growth during the culture

Figure 17.1 Hippocampal slice cultures, live and unstained. (*A*) Hippocampal slice obtained from a 5-day-old rat pup viewed with bright-field illumination after 1 day in vitro. Note the presence of well-defined pyramidal and granule cell layers. (*B*) Another hippocampal slice culture after 4 days in vitro. Note that the culture has already thinned considerably and that nonneuronal cells have migrated away from the margins of the slice. It still is possible to observe a cell body layer. The dark round cells are macrophages, which tend to decrease in number after 10 to 14 days in vitro. (*C*) Hippocampal slice culture after 11 days in vitro viewed with phase-contrast optics. Although the culture has not thinned completely at this age, now it is possible to discern in stratum pyramidale individual neurons with dark cytoplasm, a large clear nucleus, and a bright outline in phase contrast. Scale bar: 600 μm (*A, B*); 100 μm (*C*).

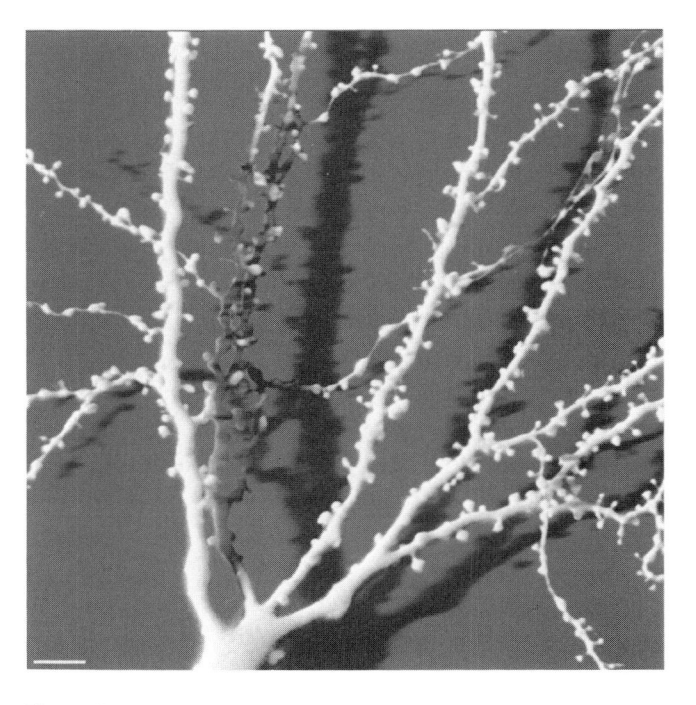

Figure 17.2 Three-dimensional, pseudocolored reconstruction of the apical dendritic tree of a Lucifer yellow–filled CA3 pyramidal cell in a hippocampal slice culture (from 100 confocal optical sections). Scale bar: 5 μm. See plate 10 for color version.

period, and cholinergic afferents to cortex display morphological features at both the light and electron microscopic levels that are similar to what is seen in vivo (Distler and Robertson, 1992, 1993). We have studied basal forebrain-cortical cocultures using both the roller-tube and the membrane techniques. Although the cultures prepared by the roller-tube technique thin to a greater degree than do those in the membrane cultures, we have not detected consistent differences between cultures prepared by the two methods.

This basal forebrain cholinergic system also is conducive to studies employing large single-slice cultures that contain the basal forebrain and the cerebral cortex within the same slice of tissue (Baratta et al., 1996). Brains of neonatal rats (postnatal day 0 to postnatal day 5) are sectioned with a vibrating microtome. As illustrated in figure 17.4A, major anatomical landmarks can be seen easily in freshly cut and unstained slices. This clarity allows accurate selection of appropriate slices for culturing. These slices are maintained on membranes for periods of at least several weeks, while maintaining their histotypic organization (see figure 17.4B).

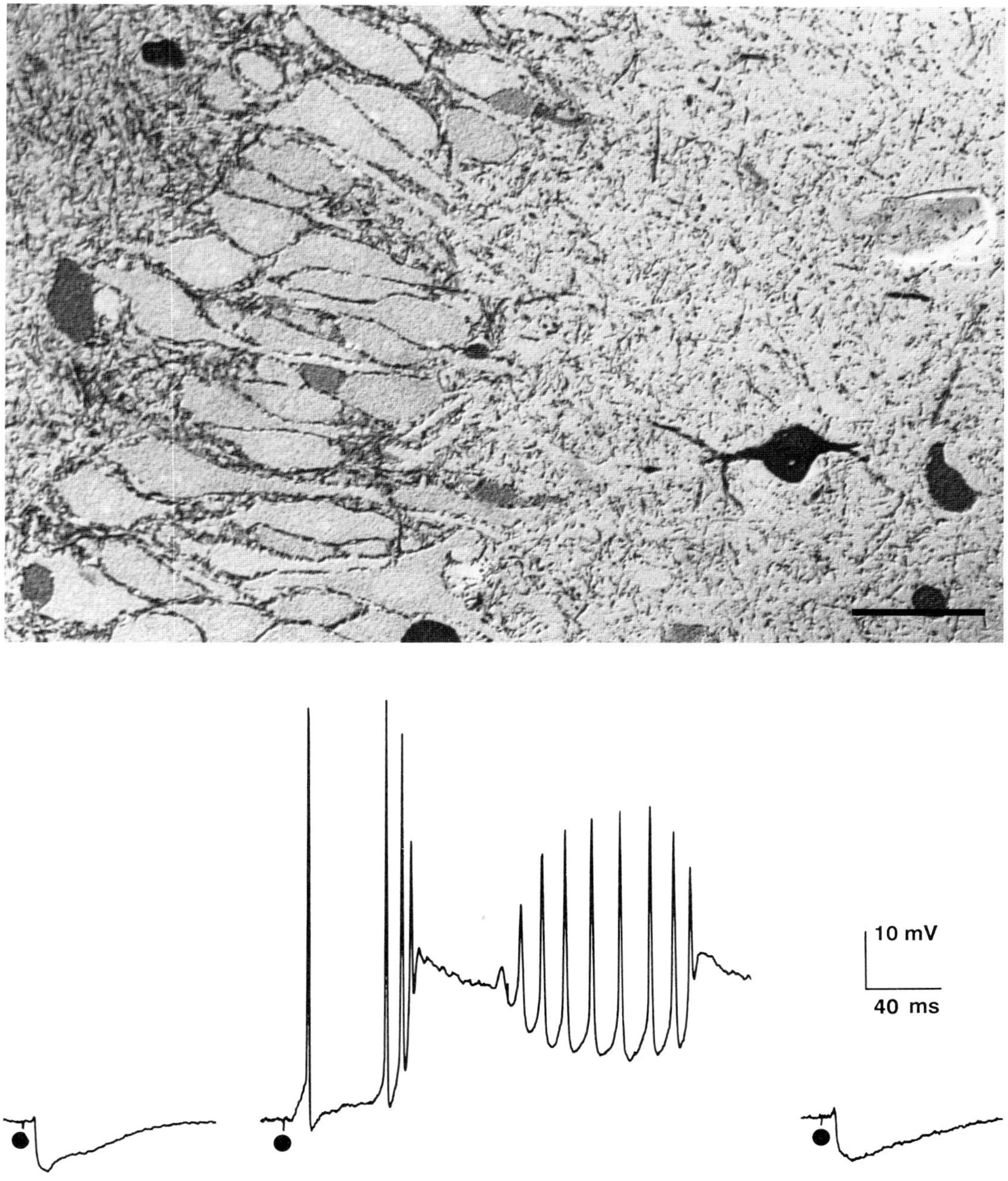

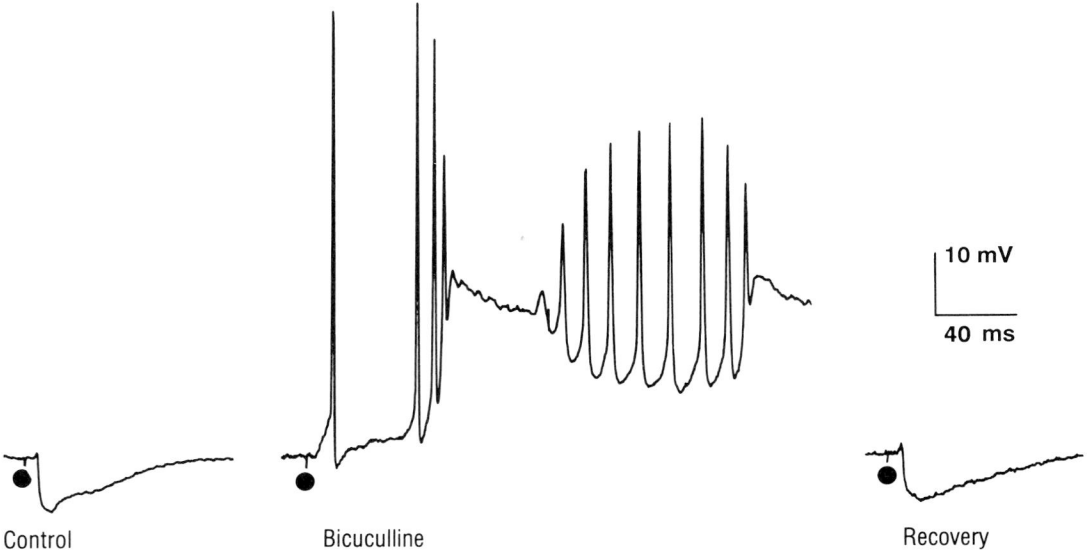

Figure 17.3 GABA in hippocampal slice cultures. (Top) Thin section of a hippocampal slice culture after 20 days in vitro, which has been stained with a monoclonal antibody against GABA (mAb 3A12). Note the presence of densely stained puncta surrounding the outlines of pyramidal cell somata and the presence of immunoreactive non-pyramidal cells in stratum radiatum and at the borders of stratum pyramidale. Scale bar: 50 μm. (Bottom) Synaptic responses recorded intracellularly from a CA3 pyramidal cell and evoked with stimulation of the mossy-fiber pathway. In control solution, a prominent hyperpolarizing inhibitory postsynaptic potential (IPSP), indirectly evoked, is observed. Bath-application of 10 μM bicuculline abolishes the IPSP, and stimulation now results in a paroxysmal depolarization shift. After washout of bicuculline, the IPSP recovers.

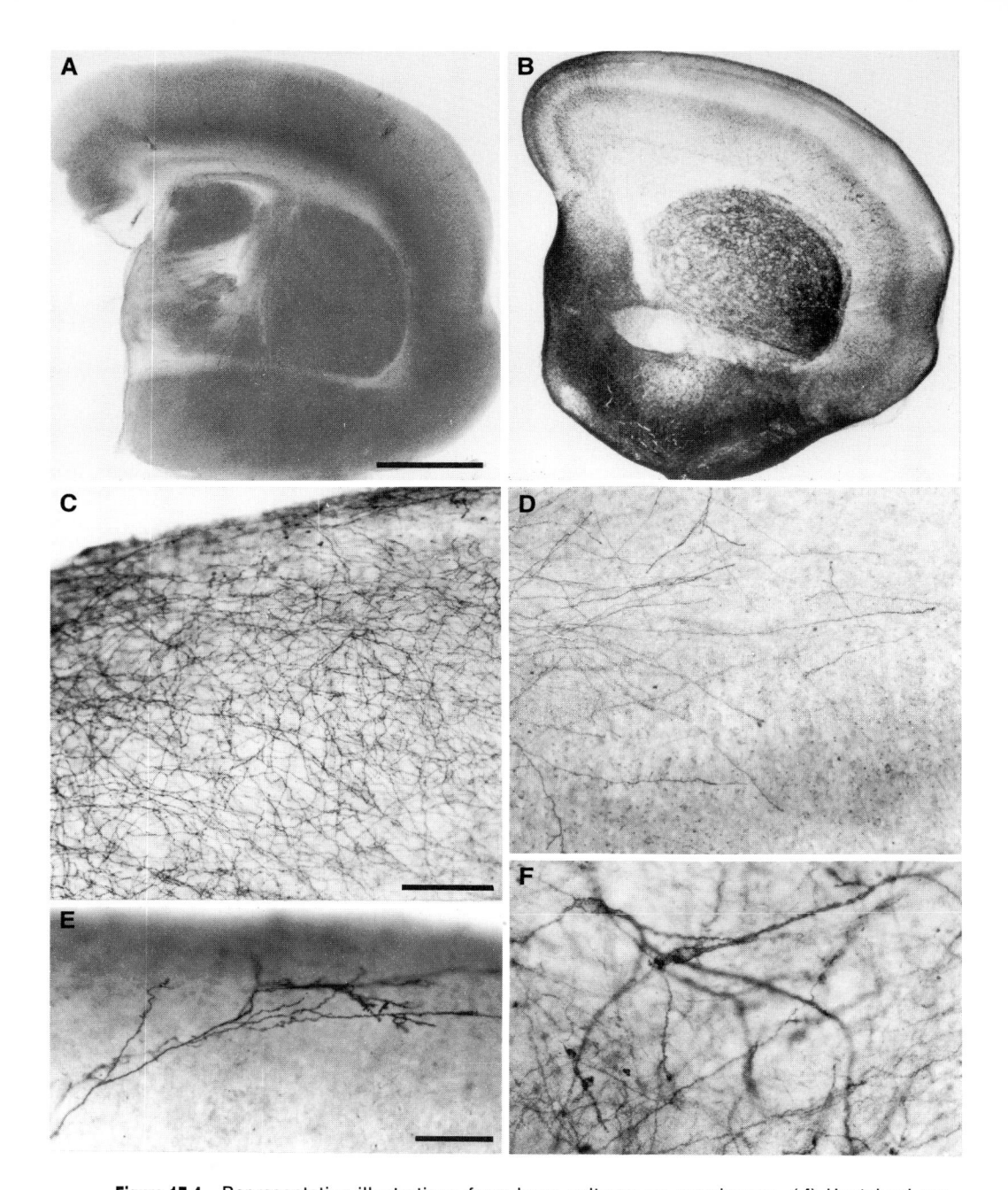

Figure 17.4 Representative illustrations from large cultures on membranes. (*A*) Unstained section of freshly cut forebrain showing major anatomical features useful for selecting slices for culturing. (*B*) AChE-stained culture after 14 days in culture; note the organotypic organization. (*C*) AChE-stained basal forebrain axons in lateral cortex. (*D*) AChE-stained axons in cingulate cortex. (*E*) High magnification of an AChE-stained axon branching in the molecular layer of lateral cortex. (*F*) AChE-stained multipolar neuron in basal forebrain.

The basal forebrain cholinergic neurons display remarkable development and differentiation in these cultures, as detected by both AChE histochemistry and by choline acetyltransferase immunocytochemistry. Cholinergic neurons in basal forebrain display mostly multipolar morphologies (see figure 17.4F), although some bipolar neurons also are seen. These neurons send out AChE-positive axons that grow into the cerebral cortex by two routes. The larger group of fibers travels laterally, along the ventral and lateral border of the striatum, before turning dorsally to innervate much of lateral cortex, and another group of axons courses dorsally from the septum to reach medial cortex (see figure 17.4E). These axons then continue to grow dorsally and laterally to innervate much of the cortex.

The growth of axons from basal forebrain to lateral and medial regions of cortex occurs in vitro. Although some basal forebrain axons have reached cortex by the age at which we prepared the cultures, our studies of normal tissue have revealed no evidence for direct connections between basal forebrain and lateral or medial cortex at that time. However, at least some of basal forebrain neurons that were axotomized during the preparation of the slice cultures survive and likely grow new axons in culture. Basal forebrain neurons can be retrogradely labeled by fluorescent-labeled microspheres in newborn animals, and these fluorescently labeled neurons survive in slice cultures (Baratta et al., 1994).

Cerebellum

Cerebellar cultures from newborn rats thin during the first 2 weeks in vitro, from the original 400 µm into a monolayer preparation. After 10 to 15 days in vitro, living Purkinje cells are characterized by a large soma and a dark cytoplasm (viewed with phase-contrast microscopy) (figure 17.5, top). Purkinje cells no longer align in single rows but cluster to form foliumlike structures, mainly at the periphery of the cultures. In contrast, the deep cerebellar nuclei form distinct groups of densely packed cells, located near the base of the culture (see figure 17.5, bottom).

Purkinje cells continue to differentiate in vitro but do not develop the full dendritic arborization characteristic of adult Purkinje cells in situ, probably because of the unusual course of parallel fibers in these two-dimensional cultures (Blank and Seil, 1982). Despite this unusual morphology of Purkinje cells, the basic circuitry of the

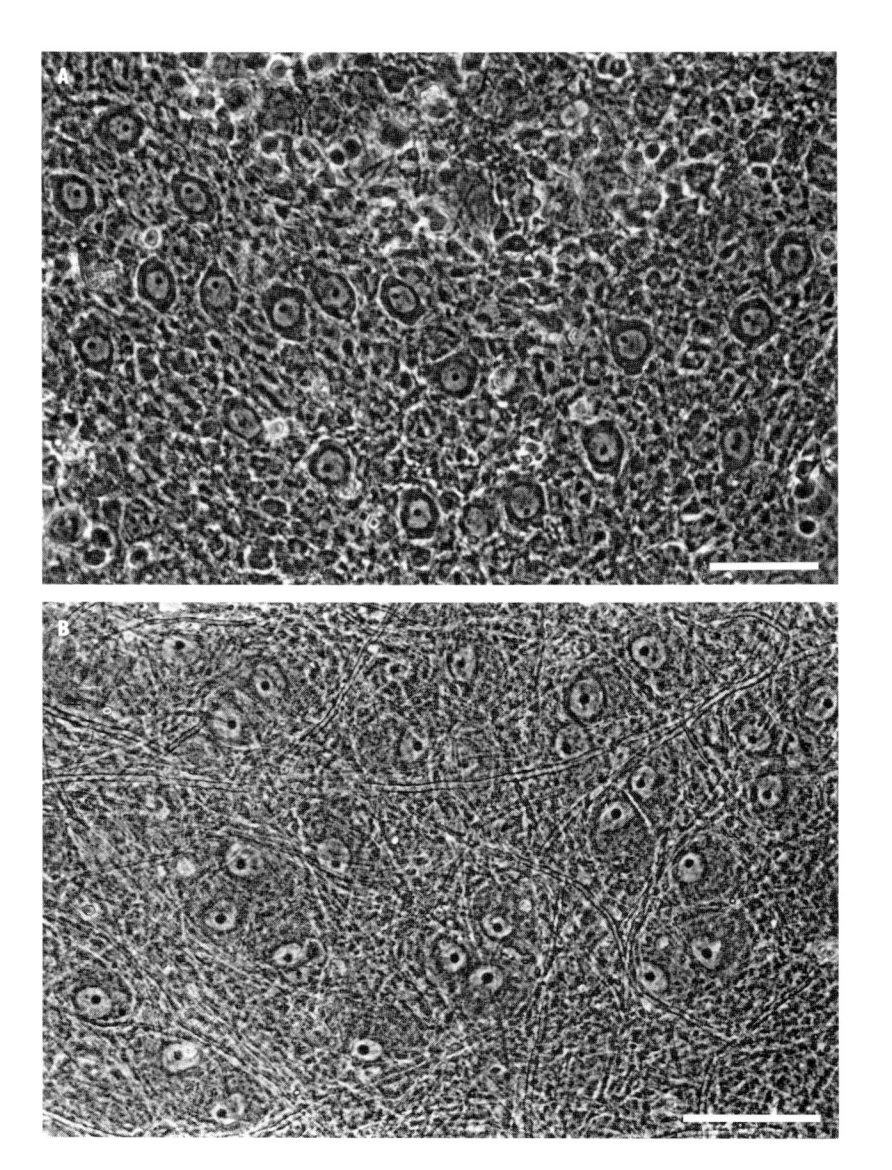

Figure 17.5 Living cerebellar neurons viewed with phase-contrast optics. (*A*) Purkinje cells after 28 days in vitro. (*B*) Neurons of the deep cerebellar nuclei after 24 days in vitro. Scale bar: 50 μm (*A*); 60 μm (*B*).

cerebellum is well-preserved in slice cultures. Immunocytochemical staining of cerebellar cultures with antibodies raised against the Ca^{2+}-binding protein calbindin results in specific labeling of Purkinje cells. Furthermore, the axons of labeled Purkinje cells can be shown to project to the deep cerebellar nuclei (Audinat et al., 1990; Gähwiler and Knöpfel, 1990; Llano et al., 1992; Mouginot and Gähwiler, 1994). Purkinje cell axons become myelinated during the second week in vitro and, with phase-contrast optics, can be seen to surround the neurons of the deep cerebellar nuclei (see figure 17.5, bottom). Although the axons of granule cells no longer form a well-defined parallel fiber pathway, it is possible to elicit graded synaptic responses in Purkinje cells with local electrical stimulation (Audinat et al., 1990). As for parallel fiber stimulation in situ, pharmacological antagonists of non-NMDA receptors abolish these local synaptic responses, whereas NMDA antagonists have no effect (Audinat et al., 1990).

Projections from the inferior olivary complex to the cerebellum can be prepared with cocultures of a slice containing the inferior olive from 3-day-old rats together with a cerebellar slice. Within the first 2 weeks in vitro, olivary fibers bridge the gap between the two explants and grow into the cerebellum to innervate cerebellar neurons. In extracellular (Gähwiler, 1978) and intracellular (Knöpfel et al., 1990b) recordings, we observed that olivary stimulation results in the generation of complex responses in Purkinje cells, closely resembling the characteristic climbing-fiber responses recorded in situ or in acute cerebellar slices. In contrast to the effects of local electrical stimulation, the climbing-fiber response in Purkinje cells is not graded but is all-or-none at threshold (Knöpfel et al., 1990b).

Troubleshooting

Getting Started

The decision to develop the slice-culture technique in your laboratory is not one to be made lightly. Preparation of these cultures is perhaps more difficult than are conventional cell-culture methods, and there may be no one down the hall who is using the technique and to whom you can turn for help. Considerable expenditure of

time, effort, and money can be expected before you can gaze contentedly at your first perfect organotypic monolayer. Nevertheless, with practice and attention to detail you will succeed; there are no secret tricks. Furthermore, once the technique is running, it tends to be consistent, or at least as consistent as you are. The following suggestions may be of help.

1. To ensure success with minimal delay and frustration, we suggest attempting to follow the foregoing recipe as closely as possible, including the recommended suppliers of media, plasticware, and so on. For example, all plastic test tubes have different permeabilites to carbon dioxide. The Nunc tubes we recommend are particularly low in permeability, thus preventing rapid diffusion of metabolically released carbon dioxide out of the tubes and preserving the proper pH of the medium.

2. Start with hippocampus, cerebral cortex, or cerebellum as a reference point before attempting to culture the brain region of interest. These structures are large and relatively easy to identify and dissect (even in neonatal animals) and have proved especially robust and reliable. In addition, the hippocampus has a well-defined cell-body layer that can prove useful in assessing the health of the tissue after a few days in vitro (see figure 17.1B).

3. Keep things as simple as possible at first. While this is perhaps not optimal, the fewer steps involved at the beginning, the fewer opportunities for things to go wrong. Do not bother with x-irradiation or antimitotics. Attempt to get the slices cut, embedded, and in the incubator as quickly as possible. Do not try to get too many slices from one brain.

Dissection

Perhaps the most difficult task for the novice is the dissection step. This is particularly true for those with no previous experience in dissecting living material or neonatal animals. If you have previously made acute slices or dissociated cell cultures, for example, it is likely that few problems will be to encountered here and you can be reasonably confident that your slices were alive at the time they were inserted in the incubator (see later). On the other hand, we recommend that absolute beginners get extensive practice at dissecting before attempting their first cultures. It is also recommended that you start with animals of an age around 2 weeks after

birth before moving to 1- to 6-day-old pups. In younger animals with smaller, less mature brains, the tissue is extremely soft and fragile, making it more difficult to handle. This advice also holds for people who have experience in dissecting adult brains only. Of course, too much emphasis on speed of dissection may compromise the quality of dissection. Both should be optimized; however, as long as the tissue remains moist, careful gentle handling of the material is probably most critical. The tissue should be kept chilled during dissection and separation of sections.

Attachment

Two substrates have been used successfully to allow the slices to attach: chicken plasma and collagen. Collagen offers the advantage of providing a somewhat defined matrix, which may be desirable for developmental experiments. It is, however, relatively time-consuming to prepare and, if insufficiently thick, may fail to keep the slices attached to the coverslips adequately. Unfortunately, some commercial supplies of chicken plasma have been detrimental to the health of cultures. One problem seems to be that different suppliers use different types and quantities of anticoagulants during the manufacturing procedure. We recommend the chicken plasma sold by Cocalico (Reamstown, PA), which has proved quite reliable in our experience.

Occasionally, slices become detached from the coverslip during the first day or two in the incubator. First, ensure that the plasma is clotted firmly, (i.e., that an adequate amount of thrombin was used and the final volumes of the plasma and thrombin solutions used on each slice were nearly the same). Second, be sure that you have not used an excess of plasma and thrombin. Paradoxically, a thin clot holds better than a thick one. Slices sometimes do not adhere to the membranes; this problem appears to stem from too much medium on the membrane. The tissue slice should be at the interface of the medium and the membrane, not immersed in medium atop the membrane.

Why did they die?

The blessed few will have their first batch of cultures thrive from the beginning. More likely, at some point you will be faced with an incubator full of dead cultures. Unfortunately, autopsies are rarely

informative; nevertheless, often it is possible to identify the cause of death and to remedy it. First, and easier to solve, is a problem that arises at some point after you have had some successful cultures. The problem most likely results from a change or inconsistency in your technique. Check first for new batches of supplies, different suppliers, media ingredients, expiration dates on ingredients, variations in washing procedures, and so forth. It is best to try a new lot of medium before the old, proven lot is used up. In this way, any deficiencies in the new lot can be assessed by using the old lot as a reference. Likewise, never change two variables of the procedure at the same time. Whenever an attempt is made to change the usual technique, it is recommended that a number of cultures be prepared using the old technique at the same time to serve as a control. Variability exists between individual cultures and between sets of slices from individual animals. Therefore, it is recommended that a sufficient number of cultures (at least 10) be used as a control group, preferably including slices taken from more than one animal. Even with the utmost care and consistency, at times the quality of the cultures will deteriorate for reasons that never will be determined, and often they will improve spontaneously for no apparent reason—*deus ex machina.*

A more important problem, one perhaps more difficult to solve, concerns methods for determining the health of cultures while they still are living. We recommend starting with hippocampus, because it has a well-defined cell body layer that is visible with any kind of optics and even with the naked eye. The cell body layer of a healthy culture will be more translucent than the surrounding tissue (see figure 17.1C). (Cultures can be viewed with phase-contrast microscopy through the flat-bottom tubes or while on membranes in Petri dishes, or representative cultures can be removed from the culture container, although this may result in loss of sterility.) Hippocampal cultures typically lose a visible cell body layer if they are dead. Note that often all the nerve cells in a culture will be dead, but the irrepressible glial and ependymal cells will almost always survive. It takes a very large mistake to have a culture in which not even glial cells are alive. It should be possible to discern individual nerve cells in living cultures as early as 4 to 7 days in vitro (see figure 17.1B). After approximately 2 weeks in vitro, neurons typically have a dark cytoplasm and a bright outline under phase-contrast optics (see figure 17.1C). The nucleus is large, fairly clear, and

contains a prominent small, very dark nucleolus. (Processes are not visible without intracellular injection of dyes or staining). Clear pathological signs of cellular atrophy are swelling of somata, inclusion of lipid droplets, and a pale cytoplasm. Because of the greater thickness of membrane cultures, individual nerve cells usually are not visible.

The first step is to attempt to identify the point at which the cultures died. Were they dead from the start, or did they die gradually in the incubator? Two clues to look for are the presence of a visible cell body layer, as described, and the pH of the culture medium. Typically, the medium starts off slightly alkaline, then, as metabolic carbon dioxide production increases, the pH shifts toward acidity. The healthier the culture, the more robust and rapid this acidification. In general, if all the cultures are dying gradually in the incubator, suspect a problem with the medium. However, if even one culture among many survives perfectly, the culture medium must be adequate. Be sure that the amount of medium in the test tubes or Petri dishes is sufficient. Check the temperature of the incubator; beware of inhomogeneities. The motor of the roller drum can generate considerable heat. Slices that are handled too roughly often result in cultures with incomplete or partial cell body layers. Infected cultures are immediately recognizable by a cloudy, acidified medium and almost always result from accidental contamination of instruments and solutions during dissection.

Alternatively, if the cultures lose a visible cell body layer after the first 1 or 2 days in the incubator and never show any evidence of an acidic pH shift, probably they are dead or dying from the start. Of course, be sure you have not made any errors in following the procedures described above. Then, the first suspect should be the dissection process itself, especially for those with little experience with this procedure. Unfortunately, it is relatively difficult to assess the viability of the slices. If you have experience or can get experienced help, it is possible to test the slices physiologically in an acute-slice chamber or by isolating individual cells acutely via the method of Kay and Wong (1986). The second likely cause of dead cultures is problems with the handling and storage of cultures subsequent to slicing. Check the pH of the Gey's BSS used in dissecting and holding the slices. Potential sources of problems also include using insufficiently cleaned or toxic coverslips or using contaminated water or alcohol to clean the coverslips or instruments. These problems can only be solved empirically.

Applications

The basic protocol presented in this chapter can be used for the cultivation of tissue from almost any part of the nervous system and from different species (Gähwiler, 1981a). The results can vary, however, and depend both on the age of the donor animals and the anatomical origin of the tissue. In tissue from very young animals, cells tend to migrate, and the original cytoarchitecture may become partly distorted. Survival of neurons, on the other hand, is greatly reduced in tissue derived from older animals. As a compromise, early postnatal animals are commonly used for the organotypic cultivation of brain slices. In our own hands, tissues of rat hippocampus, cerebral cortex, septum, cerebellum, and hypothalamus, (Gähwiler, 1984c; Wray et al., 1988; Distler and Robertson, 1992; Annis et al., 1993) have provided the most consistent results and yielded quasimonolayer cultures that remain organotypically organized. Tissue from midbrain (Gähwiler, 1978; Knöpfel et al., 1989), and spinal cord (Braschler et al., 1989; Delfs et al., 1989) also is well-suited for the slice-culture approach, although the tissue (in particular spinal cord tissue) sometimes remains one to four cell layers thick even following prolonged cultivation periods. Finally, this cultivation procedure has been applied for the cultivation of peripheral nervous tissue (Braschler et al., 1989) and for endocrine cells (Gähwiler, 1984b).

Organotypic slice cultures can be used to address a wide range of issues related to the development and function of the nervous system, as described. The types of anatomical and neurochemical experiments performed with these cultures to date require little in the way of specialized techniques or apparatus, and methodologies established for other preparations probably may be adapted with minor modification.

Morphological Experiments

The introduction of confocal laser-scanning microscopy has provided the neurobiologist with a powerful tool with which to visualize nervous tissue within intact specimens. The major advantage of confocal microscopy over conventional imaging systems is the possibility to section intact specimens optically, thus eliminating structures that are out of the plane of focus. The combination of the confocal technique with microinjection of low-molecular-weight

hydrophilic probes provides excellent visibility of neuronal structures. One problem facing physiologists is obtaining good physiological recordings and also recovering well-labeled cells afterward. Numerous new dyes and intracellular tracers have appeared recently, but many are nonfixable or result in recording electrodes with high electrical resistance.

Lucifer yellow has been a favored tracer for many years because it can be visualized directly by excitation at 488 nm with a mercury lamp and it can be fixed with aldehyde fixatives (Stewart, 1978). In practice, we have found Lucifer yellow to be excellent for the visualization of spine morphology but to diffuse too slowly for visualization of the axonal arborization. The tip of sharp microelectrodes is filled with an aqueous 4% Lucifer yellow (lithium salt) solution and back-filled with 1 M potassium methylsulfate (pH = 8). Lucifer yellow can be injected into well-impaled cells with hyperpolarizing current pulses. Unfortunately, however, the dye does increase the resistance and noise level of the electrodes. The cells can be observed during the filling procedure; however, excessive light exposure can lead to necrosis of the cell or "blebbing" of processes. Satisfactorily filled cells are placed immediately in Bouin's fixative overnight at 4°C. Fixed cultures are washed in deionized water for 30 min (three times) and immediately are mounted in Fluorostab, AMF2 (Bio-Science Products, Emmenbrücke, Switzerland). This permanent mounting medium contains antifading agents and does not require dehydration, which otherwise reduces fluorescence.

In our laboratories, we visualize dendrites and dendritic spines by using either a Zeiss LSM 410 or a BioRad MR600 confocal laser-scanning microscope. Best resolution is obtained with a 100 × 1.4-NA plan-apochromat oil-immersion lens and an analog zoom factor of three (see figure 17.2). The external argon ion laser (Omnichrome series 43), pretuned to 488 nm, is used to excite the Lucifer yellow. A long-pass 570-nm filter, a dichroic beam splitter of 488/543 nm, and a pinhole size of 15 are used for imaging. Optical slices are made at 0.15-μm intervals, and each image is averaged to improve the signal-to-noise ratio. Images are transferred to a Silicon Graphics Indigo2 workstation and are processed by using Imaris software (Bitplane AG, Zurich, Switzerland) to produce a three-dimensional simulated-fluorescence, projected image. Confocal images permit the structure of the spines to be seen more clearly then with conventional microscopy.

For the study of axonal morphology, both biocytin (Horikawa and Armstrong, 1988) and neurobiotin (Kita and Armstrong, 1991) have proved to be preferable to Lucifer yellow, although spine morphology is somewhat inferior. Neurobiotin has a slightly lower molecular weight than does biocytin. In addition, neurobiotin only enters cells when depolarizing current is injected. This offers the advantage that the quality of the electrophysiological recording can be evaluated before filling the cell, so that many cells can be impaled within a circumscribed region of the tissue without labeling. In addition, both tracers can be detected with avidins or streptavidins that have been conjugated with either fluorescent labels or horseradish peroxidase, permitting intracellular labeling to be combined with immunocytochemical or electron-microscopic techniques. A disadvantage of biocytin and neurobiotin is that they cannot be visualized while filling.

Biocytin-filled cells are fixed in 4% paraformaldehyde in 0.1 M phosphate buffer (pH 7.4) at 4°C for 12 h, then are washed in 0.1 M phosphate buffer containing 0.1% bovine serum albumin (BSA) for 2 h. BSA prevents the nonspecific binding of the avidin fluorochrome. Cultures then are treated with 0.4% Triton X-100, a detergent that enhances the penetration of the avidin conjugates into the tissue, in phosphate buffer containing BSA for 2 h at room temperature. The Triton X is removed by washing (three times) in phosphate buffer and BSA for 30 min, followed by incubation in the avidin conjugate of choice. For Neuralite-Texas Red (Molecular Probes, Portland, OR) we use a 1:500 dilution for 2 h at 4°C; other conjugates may differ in dilution and incubation time. Following an overnight wash to remove nonspecific fluorescence, the cultures are mounted permanently with Fluorostab.

If biocytin is to be observed with avidin horseradish peroxidase, cultures should be fixed in 0.1 M phosphate buffer with 4% paraformaldehyde and 0.1% glutaraldehyde. We have used the ABC kit (Vector Labs, Burlingame, CA) successfully. Glutaraldehyde must be omitted for fluorescence imaging because it increases background fluorescence.

Double labeling of cell pairs can be performed with injection of Lucifer yellow into postsynaptic cells, for visualization of spines, and biocytin into the presynaptic cell, for visualization of the axon (see figure 17.6 and color plate 11). The biocytin cell can be labeled with any avidin-fluorochrome conjugate excited at a wavelength different from that of Lucifer yellow. Cultures injected with the two

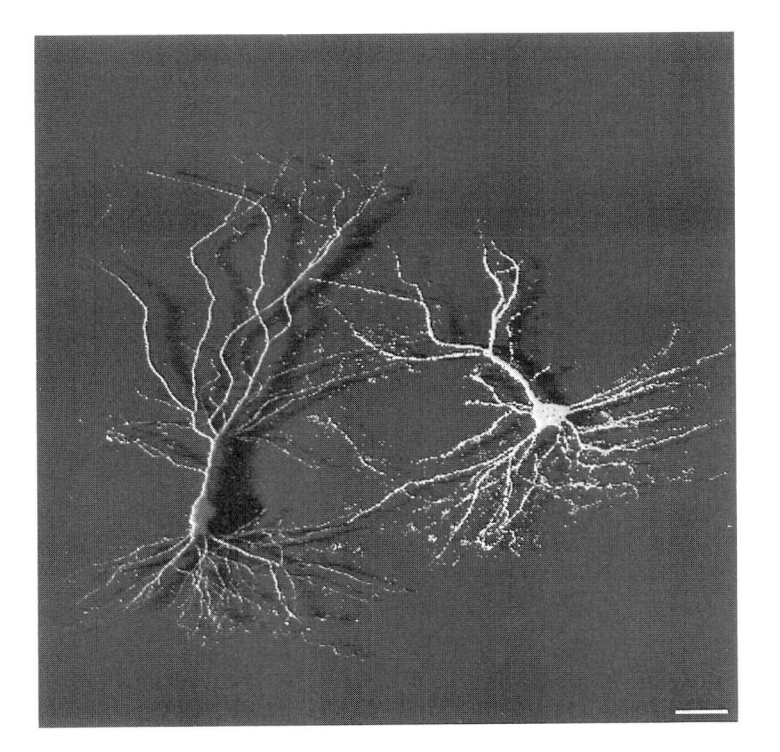

40 mV

0.1 mV

20 ms

Figure 17.6 Three-dimensional pseudocolored reconstruction of a CA3 pyramidal cell pair, filled with Lucifer yellow (green) and biocytin (red, labeled with avidin Texas red). Image was prepared from 38 optical slices (1-μm thick) by using a 20 × 0.5–NA plan neofluor lens. The biocytin-filled cell was not as well filled—hence the flatter appearance. The axon of the biocytin-filled cell formed a synapse with the Lucifer yellow–filled cell, as could be observed electrophysiological (above) and with higher magnification (not shown). Scale bar: 60 μm. See plate 11 for color version.

tracers are fixed with 4% paraformaldehyde in 0.1 M phosphate buffer and treated as described for biocytin. Several investigators have processed slice cultures for immunocytochemistry (e.g., Wray et al., 1988; 1991; Caeser et al., 1989; Knöpfel et al., 1989; Streit et al., 1989; Annis et al., 1990; Gähwiler et al., 1990; Distler and Robertson, 1993). The slice cultures, as noted, can be treated similarly to a tissue slice, although membrane cultures typically should be resectioned on a cryostat (Baratta et al., 1996). The major impediment is the penetration of reagents through the glial cell membranes that typically cover the cultures. Freeze-thaw methods or addition of higher strengths of detergent often are needed for good results. Detailed protocols for the application of in situ hybridization methods to organotypic slice cultures recently have been published (Gerfin-Moser and Monyer, 1994).

Physiological Experiments

For physiological experiments, cultures are transferred to a recording chamber mounted on an inverted microscope, which ideally is equipped with phase-contrast or differential interference–contrast optics. Epifluorescence attachments are a useful option as well. The cultures can be perfused continuously with balanced solutions—typically we use Hank's- or Tyrode's-based solutions—and will remain alive in the chamber for 8 or more hours. A description of the recording chamber and microscope arrangements is given in Gähwiler and Knöpfel (1990). Because of the proximity of the cells in the monolayer to the bathing solution, we find it unnecessary to provide additional oxygenation. Also, the concentration of bicarbonate in the solution is fairly low so that physiological pH, as monitored with phenol red, is maintained in room air (see Audinat et al., 1990, or Debanne et al., 1995, for typical BSS compositions).

The accessibility of the cells in the monolayer to the bathing solution is a tremendous advantage in electrophysiological experiments. Pharmacological agonists and antagonists can be bath-applied at known concentrations and reach steady-state concentrations within 1 to 2 min. In addition, use of relatively low-resistance micropipettes for intracellular recording of neuronal activity facilitates application of single-electrode voltage-clamp recording techniques. Another microelectrode filled with 2 M NaCl and having a resistance of about 4 MΩ can be positioned at an appropriate location within the culture to activate defined axonal pathways selectively.

Monopolar anodal currents of low intensity (5–50 µA) and brief duration (100 µs) should be used, because excess stimulation can induce lasting epileptiform discharge or spreading depression.

Organotypic slice cultures offer the additional advantage of allowing application of the patch-clamp technique to record membrane currents from morphologically identified neurons. Furthermore, the mechanical stability of the seal formed between the patch pipette and the neuronal membrane allows use of fast-perfusion systems for rapid applications of drugs at known concentrations. Though it is not necessary to clean the cultures enzymatically or mechanically, we have observed that a thin layer of presumed glial processes often covers the neuronal surface, impeding seal formation. Therefore, we routinely use cultures that were irradiated or treated with antimitotics to reduce the number of glial cells. Nomarski optics are helpful in choosing neurons that have a relatively clean surface. Thinner cultures seem to contain more neurons that are free of glial overgrowth. Nevertheless, we routinely attempt to patch cells within the culture, not those lying directly on the surface. The patch pipette, typically around 3 to 4 MΩ for whole-cell or 3 to 10 MΩ for cell-attached recording, is inserted into the tissue while maintaining strong positive pressure. In the best cases, overlying tissue can be seen to be blown away as the pipette approaches the cell to be recorded. It should be noted that forming high-resistance giga-ohm seals with cells in these cultures probably is not as easy as with low-density dissociated-cell cultures. Furthermore, not all series of cultures are equally easy to work with (in our experience). Nevertheless, high-quality recordings can be obtained at a reasonable rate.

A final advantage to using slice cultures is that the connectivity between pairs of cells is considerably higher than that typically observed in ex vivo hippocampal slices, in which a very high proportion of the axons are severed during the preparation of the slices. In practice, we have found that an action potential in a given CA3 pyramidal cell will elicit a monosynaptic excitatory post-synaptic potential in >50% of simultaneously recorded CA3 and CA1 pyramidal cells in slice cultures (Debanne et al., 1995), compared to <6% in ex vivo slices (e.g., Sayer et al., 1990). Nevertheless, the properties of the unitary connections in the slice cultures appear virtually identical to those seen in ex vivo slices. For example, unitary excitatory postsynaptic potentials between CA3 pyramidal cells have an amplitude of perhaps 1 mV in both

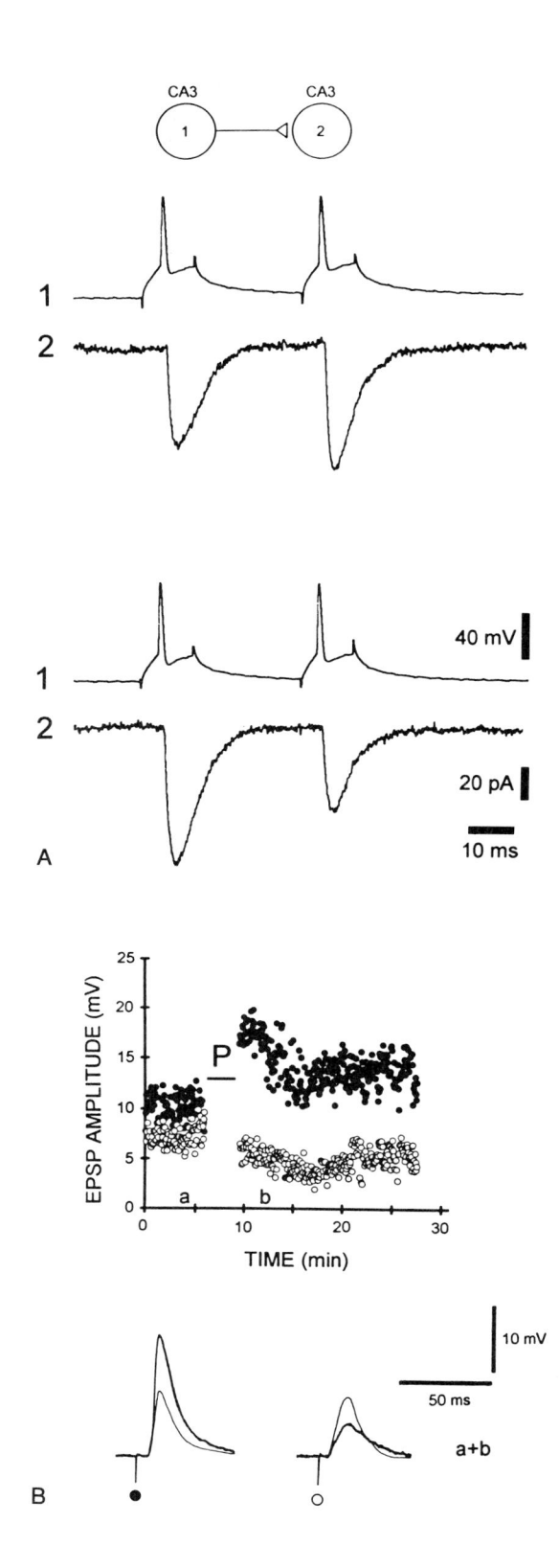

slice cultures and acute slices. We have used such cell-pair recordings to address the mechanisms underlying short-term plasticity in the form of paired-pulse facilitation and paired-pulse depression, which are readily obtained, depending on the experimental conditions (figure 17.7a).

An additional feature of hippocampal slice cultures is that they display several forms of synaptic plasticity that appear identical to those described in ex vivo slices. We have observed that long-term potentiation can be induced with tetanic stimulation of either Schaffer collateral inputs to area CA1 or recurrent collateral inputs to CA3 pyramidal cells and by synchronous pairing of presynaptic stimuli with postsynaptic depolarization via an intracellular microelectrode (Debanne et al., 1994) (figure 17.7b). We also have obtained long-term depression with either maintained stimulation at moderate frequencies—so-called homosynaptic depression—or by asynchronously pairing synaptic stimulation and postsynaptic depolarization (figure 17.7b)—so-called associative depression (Debanne et al., 1994). Both forms of long-term synaptic plasticity are blocked by either NMDA receptor antagonists or chelators of intracellular calcium (Debanne et al., 1994), as described in ex vivo hippocampal slices.

Conclusion

The highly developed cellular and synaptic differentiation obtained in organotypic cultures thus offers unique advantages for the study

Figure 17.7 Synaptic plasticity in hippocampal slice cultures. (*A*) Paired recordings from two monosynaptically coupled CA3 pyramidal cells. Two action potentials in cell 1, triggered with depolarizing current injection from the intracellular microelectrode, elicit excitatory postsynaptic currents (EPSCs) in the whole-cell voltage-clamped postsynaptic cell 2. If the pair of action potentials is triggered when release probability is low, the amplitude of the second EPSC is smaller than is the first (upper traces). If the pair of action potentials is triggered when release probability is high, the amplitude of the second EPSC is larger than is the first (lower traces). (*B*) The amplitude of excitatory postsynaptic potentials (EPSPs) in a CA1 pyramidal cell evoked by extracellular stimulation of two inputs is plotted as a function of time. After control values were obtained, depolarizing current pulses were injected repeatedly into the cell via the intracellular recording electrode (at time indicated by *P*). A long-lasting potentiation of the EPSP amplitude was seen for the input stimulated synchronously with the depolarizing pulses, whereas the input stimulated with a delay of 800 ms from the end of the depolarizing pulse exhibited long-term depression (for details, see Debanne et al., 1994). Representative EPSPs taken from the times indicated by "a" (thinner trace) and "b" (thicker trace) in the graph are shown superimposed below.

of structure and function in the central nervous system. A whole spectrum of electrophysiological and optical recording techniques —ranging from single-channel recordings to network analysis—can be applied to study the activity of nerve cells identified on the basis of morphological criteria. Moreover, the slice-culture approach (and in particular the cocultivation of tissue from different brain areas) offers opportunities to investigate basic mechanisms underlying the role of trophic and tropic substances, the specificity of axonal fiber growth, and recognition of target sites.

Acknowledgments

We greatly appreciate the technical assistance of Roland Dürr, Lucette Heeb, Lotty Rietschin, Roland Schöb, and Elizabeth Vollenweider, and of Casey M. Annis, Janie Baratta, and Dun H. Ha. Work was supported by the Swiss National Science Foundation, the Dr. Eric Slack-Gyr Foundation, and the United States National Institutes of Health (grant NS 30109).

Note

1. A video training film is available from the Brain Research Institute in Zürich. (From Prof. Beat Gähwiler, Brain Research Institute, University of Zürich, Switzerland.)

Mark Noble and Margot Mayer-Pröschel

Interest in the biology of the glial cells of the central nervous system (CNS) has increased enormously in the last two decades, as ever greater numbers of neurobiologists have come to regard these cells as something more than the packing material surrounding the neurons of the brain and spinal cord. This increased interest is at it should be, for how could the cells that represent 90% to 95% of the cells of the CNS be anything other than fascinating in their biology and of critical importance in their function?

This chapter discusses a variety of approaches to studying the glial cells of the CNS. The focus will be on the cells of the rat CNS, but protocols similar to those provided have been used also to study cells derived from mice and from humans. The only attempt at being comprehensive has been in respect to techniques from our own laboratory, as the number of techniques now used to study the biology of glial cells easily would fill a volume in itself. Protocols are grouped according to broad subject matter, with an initial set (Protocol sections I and II) devoted to the topics of tissue-culture media, substrates, and immunofluorescence.

Astrocytes

The Multifunctional Astrocyte

To prepare purified astrocytes and astrocyte-conditioned medium, see Protocol Section III. Our first cell of concern is the astrocyte. Astrocytes occupy a central role in the formation, maintenance, and repair of the CNS. Unlike oligodendrocytes, which have the single and highly specialized function of myelinating the white-matter tracts of the CNS, astrocytes have been proposed to have a large number of different functions depending on their spatial and temporal location in the CNS. For example, astrocytes and radial glial cells provide a cellular scaffold for the migration of newly formed neurons out of the ventricular zones of the developing CNS

(Rakic, 1988; Gasser and Hatten, 1990a,b). Astrocytes have been demonstrated also to provide an excellent substrate for the outgrowth of central and peripheral neurons in vitro (Noble et al., 1984; Fallon, 1985) and have been suggested to act as a substrate for the extension of neurites in vivo during development and injury in neonatal animals (Silver et al., 1982; Smith et al., 1986 a). Astrocytes also have been shown to modulate the migration, proliferation, and differentiation of both perinatal and adult forms of the oligodendrocyte type-2 astrocyte (O-2A) progenitor cell in vitro (as discussed later; Noble and Murray, 1984; Raff et al., 1985; Temple and Raff, 1985; 1986; Small et al., 1987; Wolswijk and Noble, 1989; Wolswijk et al., 1991).

In addition to promoting the migration and maturation of both neurons and oligodendrocyte precursor cells, certain specialized populations of astrocytes or radial glial cells may form transient barriers to either neurite extension or to the migration of O-2A progenitor cells. For example, neurite extension has been suggested to be prevented at specific times during development by astrocytes and radial glial cells in the roof plate, in the midline of the optic tectum (Snow et al., 1990), and in the developing barrel fields of the somatosensory cortex (Crossin et al., 1989; Steindler et al., 1989; Steindler et al., 1990). Furthermore, a specialized population of astrocytes in the lamina cribrosa of the optic nerve has been suggested to prevent to migration of O-2A progenitor cells from the optic nerve into the retina (ffrench-Constant et al., 1988).

Astrocytes also play a central role in CNS response to injury. The period after penetrating mechanical injury to the CNS is characterized by clearance of debris from the lesion by macrophages and astrocytes and the establishment of an array of hypertrophied astrocytes and fibroblasts—termed a *glial scar*—that serves to seal the lesion site (Reier et al., 1983). Astrocytes have been shown to proliferate in certain circumstances at sites of CNS injury (Latov et al., 1979, Takamiya et al., 1988; see also Shafit-Zagardo et al., 1988, and Hatten et al., 1991) and to increase greatly their expression of glial fibrillary acidic protein (GFAP), such elevated expression often extending into the hemisphere contralateral to the lesion. The astrocytes involved in this response to penetrating injury, characterized by their GFAP immunoreactivity and hypertrophied morphology, have been termed *reactive astrocytes* (Bignami and Dahl, 1976; Reier et al., 1983; Barrett et al., 1984; Mathewson and Berry, 1985; Miller et al., 1986).

A marked difference is seen in the abilities of neurons to grow through sites of CNS injury in neonatal and adult animals. Astrocytes in the region of neonatal CNS lesions appear to permit axonal growth through or around the lesion, whereas a corresponding injury in adult animals is characterized by a complete lack of axonal growth through the lesion (Reier et al., 1983; Barrett et al., 1984; Smith et al., 1986; Carlstedt et al., 1987; Liuzzi and Lasek, 1987). It has been possible to study the age-dependent failure of astrocytes to support neurite outgrowth in a number of in vitro systems. Astrocytes isolated from injured regions of the adult CNS are far less able to support the growth of central and peripheral neurons in vitro than are those from neonatal animals (Geisert and Stewart, 1991). Furthermore, maintenance of monolayer or three-dimensional astrocyte cultures in vitro also results in a time-dependent decrease in the ability of these cultures to support neurite outgrowth (Fawcett et al., 1989; Smith et al., 1990). The apparent age-dependent ability of astrocytes to support neuronal regeneration in vivo and in vitro is accompanied by a decrease in the intrinsic ability of a given neuronal population to regenerate with age, whether in intracerebral grafts (Björklund and Stenevi, 1984), in intraocular grafts (Seiger and Olson, 1977), or in three-dimensional astrocyte cultures (Fawcett et al., 1989; reviewed in Fawcett, 1992).

Still another function of astrocytes is in induction of the blood-brain barrier, the specialized vascular-associated structure necessary to maintain constancy in the CNS environment. It has been known for some years that capillaries that enter the CNS develop permeability properties different from those in the periphery, and these permeability properties appear to be induced by interaction of the endothelial cells with astrocytes. In recent years, it has even become possible to generate blood-brain barriers in vitro by coculturing endothelial cells with astrocytes in appropriate conditions (Rubin et al., 1991; Wolburg et al., 1994).

Astrocyte Purification
One of the first critical steps in the study of astrocytes is to prepare purified cultures of these cells. In our laboratories, we have achieved this by modifying the methods first introduced by McCarthy and deVellis(1980) to reliably obtain cultures composed of >98% astrocytes. Such cultures consist of astrocytes of the type-1 phenotype,

and it is astrocytes of such a phenotype that have been characterized most extensively. (The name *type-1 astrocytes* obviously implies the existence of other kinds of astrocytes that also can be studied. These "other" astrocytes are called *type-2 astrocytes*, and they are discussed in more detail later.)

Once purified astrocytes are available, they can be used readily for studying the ability of their surfaces to promote neuronal growth or to induce division or differentiation of neural progenitor cells just by plating the cells of interest on top of the astrocyte monolayers. Alternatively, the astrocytes can be used as a source of conditioned medium to study the effects of soluble factors produced by the astrocytes. These focuses of attention reflect our experimental biases and do not address the many areas in which astrocytes themselves are the focus of study. An excellent introduction to the study of astrocytes as distinct entities is offered by Levison and McCarthy (1991).

Studies on Glial Progenitor Cells: The O-2A Lineage

One of the important challenges in developmental biology is to decipher general principles that may underly the formation of all the many tissues of the body. This challenge contains many distinct components, of which an important one is the deciphering of the rules that govern the behavior of precursor cells that eventually will give rise to the many cell types of the organism. This component itself can be separated into the study of precursor cells with extremely broad developmental potential and those that operate under a more restricted lineage specification.

Within the CNS, the precursor cell population that has been studied most extensively is one with a restricted lineage potential. These precursor cells, first identified in the optic nerves of perinatal rats (Raff et al., 1983a,b,c), give rise in vitro to two mature glial cell populations: oligodendrocytes and type-2 astrocytes. Oligodendrocytic differentiation of these cells, which are called *O-2A progenitor cells*, occurred when progenitors were grown in chemically-defined medium and did not require the presence of inducing factors. In contrast, astrocytic differentiation required the presence of appropriate inducing factors, at least one of which is found in fetal sera of a number of different species (Raff et al., 1983a,b,c). Fortunately for the development of this field, it is possible to obtain large numbers of O-2A progenitors simply by dis-

sociating the optic nerves of the 7-day-old rats. In such cultures, grown in chemically defined medium, the percentage of O-2A lineage cells in the culture can be as high as 50%, and only a minority of these will have differentiated into oligodendrocytes in vivo at this age. Thus, it is possible to generate cultures useful for a great many types of experiments without requiring the use of sophisticated techniques, although certainly cell purification is crucial in many experiments (as discussed later). By working in the optic nerve, one has the additional advantage that the tissue itself contains no intrinsic neurons. As all the axons that run through the optic nerve have their cell bodies located somewhere else, a simple dissection of this nature immediately eliminates contamination from this nonglial cell type. The optic nerve, however, should not be considered as composed wholly of glial cells. Contaminating meningeal tissues can largely be removed by simply stripping away this thin sheet of cells that covers the outside of the nerve trunk. The endothelial cells and other cell types that contribute to the blood vessels within the nerve, as well as microglia, will be present also in these heterogeneous cultures. The degree to which any given cell type contributes to the final culture depends on the age of the animal and on the culture conditions. Endothelial cells will not grow well on polycation-coated surfaces, for example. Type-1 astrocytes are a major contributor to cultures derived from newborn animals but not to cultures derived from 7-day-old rats. Astrocytes will proliferate, however, if cultures are grown in serum-containing medium rather than in the chemically-defined medium normally used to study O-2A progenitor cell and oligodendrocyte biology.

It should be pointed out at this stage that identification of all the stages of differentiation in the O-2A lineage, as well as recognition of other cell types, is carried out by staining with cell-type specific antibodies, as detailed in our protocols later. Oligodendrocytes, the cells that produce myelin in the CNS, are of particular interest, as these are the cells that are destroyed in such conditions as the autoimmune disease of multiple sclerosis. Type-2 astrocytes, in contrast, remain a problem for the neurobiologist, for it is not yet clear when and where such cells might occur in vivo (Fulton et al., 1991). Some believe that the O-2A progenitor cell should be called simply an *oligodendrocyte precursor cell* (e.g., Skoff and Knapp, 1991), whereas others use the O-2A lineage terminology. Being believers that differentiation pathways that occur in vitro also are used in vivo, we use the latter terminology. That this decision may be

warranted is supported by the results of a variety of experiments in which O-2A progenitor cell lines have been implanted in demyelinating lesions of the rat spinal cord and have been found to produce both oligodendrocytes and astrocytes in vivo (reviewed in Franklin and Blakemore, 1995). Nonetheless, in vivo properties of the astrocytes derived from O-2A progenitor cells remain unknown. Moreover, it is still unclear why astrocytes can be generated from at least two distinct lineages or whether still other lineages exist and also can give rise to astrocytes. (For preparation of *perinatal* O-2A progenitor cells, see protocol section IV.)

Initial studies on oligodendrocytic differentiation of O-2A progenitors isolated from optic nerves of perinatal rats presented the paradox that the cells we were studying were isolated at a time of maximal division of this lineage in vivo (Skoff et al., 1976a,b), yet cells did not divide in tissue culture. Resolution of this paradox began with the discovery that cortical astrocytes promoted O-2A progenitor division in vitro (Noble and Murray, 1984). The astrocytes used in these studies expressed a phenotype like that of type-1 astrocytes of the optic nerve, which are the first identifiable glial cells to appear in the nerve (Miller et al., 1985). The similarity of these two populations led us to suggest that these astrocytes were responsible for supplying the mitogen(s) required to keep O-2A progenitors in division. Moreover, populations of O-2A progenitors grown in the presence of purified cortical astrocytes were capable of undergoing extended division while also continuing to generate more oligodendrocytes (Noble and Murray, 1984), a pattern of behavior like that occurring in vivo. Thus, the failure of O-2A progenitors to divide in our initial in vitro studies was due to the lack of necessary mitogens, which appeared to be supplied by another glial cell type.

The effects of purified cortical astrocytes and of type-1 astrocytes from the optic nerve on O-2A progenitor division in vitro appear to be mediated by platelet-derived growth factor (PDGF; Noble et al., 1988; Raff et al., 1988; Pringle et al., 1989; Gard and Pfeiffer, 1990). O-2A progenitors exposed to either PDGF or astrocyte-conditioned medium exhibited a bipolar morphology, migrated extensively (with an average migration rate of $21.4 + 1.6\,\mu\text{m/h}$), and divided with an average cell-cycle length of 18 h (Small et al., 1987). PDGF also was as potent as type-1 astrocytes at promoting the correctly timed differentiation in vitro of embryonic O-2A progenitors into oligodendrocytes (Raff et al., 1988). Moreover, antibodies to PDGF blocked

the mitogenic effect of type-1 astrocytes on embryonic O-2A progenitor cells, causing these cells to cease division and to differentiate prematurely even when growing on monolayers of type-1 astrocytes.

The Question of Timing

One of the questions of great interest in developmental studies is that of developmental timing. Understanding the mechanisms underlying the appropriately timed generation of the various cell types of the body has been studied extensively in the O-2A lineage.

It was observed more than a decade ago that cortical astrocytes could promote the correctly timed differentiation in vitro of O-2A progenitors isolated from optic nerves of embryonic rats (Raff et al., 1985). In these experiments, O-2A progenitor cultures were prepared from optic nerves of embryos of various ages and were grown on astrocyte monolayers. The number of days that elapsed before the first appearance of oligodendrocytes in these cultures was correlated precisely with the embryonic age from which the cells were isolated, such that cells from younger animals went through a longer period of cell division before generating their first oligodendrocytes. Moreover, regardless of the age from which the cells were isolated, the first oligodendrocytes appeared in vitro at a time corresponding to the time at which they would have appeared in vivo.

The control of timing in oligodendrocyte development continues to be a topic of considerable interest, but opinions vary considerably on how timing is controlled and how many timing mechanisms exist and on other related matters. As discussion of the concerns in this arena would take considerable additional space, the reader is referred to four papers that we feel to be particularly crucial: Barres et al., 1994; Bögler and Noble, 1994; Ibarolla et al., 1996, and Zhang and Miller, 1996.

Studies on O-2A Progenitor Division, Differentiation, and Survival

O-2A progenitors also can express a variety of developmental programs other than the one elicited by exposure to PDGF (Bögler et al., 1990). For example, O-2A^{perinatal} progenitors induced to divide by basic fibroblast growth factor (bFGF) were multipolar and showed little migratory behavior. In addition, cells induced to divide by bFGF had a cell-cycle length of 45 ± 12 h, in contrast with the $18 \pm$

4 h cell-cycle length elicited by exposure to PDGF. These results indicate that PDGF and bFGF function in the O-2A lineage as modulators of differentiation as well as functioning as promoters of cell division. PDGF and bFGF also differ in their effects on oligodendrocytes themselves, in that only bFGF is able to promote division of these cells (Eccleston and Silberberg, 1985; Saneto and DeVellis, 1985; Bögler et al., 1990). Moreover, bFGF can inhibit the differentiation of purified O-2A[perinatal] progenitors (McKinnon et al., 1990; Mayer and Noble, 1992), an inhibition that can be overridden by a factor (or factors) secreted by astrocytes (Mayer and Noble, 1992) and also by ciliary neurotrophic factor (CNTF) and leukemia-inhibitory factor (LIF; Mayer et al., 1994). An ever-increasing number of factors modulate the differentiation of O-2A progenitor cells, including also members of the neurotrophin family (Barres et al., 1994; Cohen et al., 1996; Ibarolla et al., 1996).

Precursor Cell Expansion by Cooperating Growth Factors

One of the most surprising and intriguing results to emerge from studies on mitogenic modulation of O-2A progenitor cell division and differentiation was the discovery that O-2A progenitors exposed simultaneously to PDGF and bFGF continued to divide without differentiating into oligodendrocytes (Bögler et al., 1990). For example, cultures of optic nerves of 19-day-old rat embryos began to generate oligodendrocytes after 2 days when established in the presence of PDGF alone (Raff et al., 1988; Bögler et al., 1990), yet remained oligodendrocyte-free even after 10 days of growth in the presence of PDGF + bFGF (Bögler et al., 1990). Further experimentation has demonstrated that O-2A[perinatal] progenitors can be grown continually for at least many weeks in vitro as long as cells are exposed continuously to both these mitogens. This effect is not unique to the combination of PDGF and bFGF, and growth of these cells in the presence of PDGF + neurotrophin 3 (NT-3) in chemically defined medium lacking thyroid hormone has similar effects.

It is clear that the ability to generate expanded precursor cell populations allows one to consider realistically the challenge of repairing damaged tissues by precursor cell transplantation, for it is this manipulation that allows one to grow large quantities of primary precursor cell populations without requiring the generation of cell lines. Demonstration of remyelination by transplanted O-2A progenitor cells has been carried out by several groups. In our

studies, we found that highly enriched populations of O-2A^{perinatal} progenitors expanded in vitro for 3 weeks were able to remyelinate >90% of the denuded axons in a lesion site after transplantation (Groves et al., 1993). That such transplantation is associated with the restoration of normal conduction then was demonstrated by the subsequent studies of Utzschneider et al. (1994).

The O-2A^{adult} Progenitor

To attempt to gain insights into the cellular mechanisms under-lying repair of demyelinated lesions in the adult animal, we also initiated studies on O-2A progenitors of the adult CNS. In our initial studies, which again were focused on the rat optic nerve, we found that O-2A progenitors isolated from adult animals differed from their perinatal counterparts in several ways. The biology of the adult-derived cells was so distinctive as to warrant a different name, thus leading us to adapt the terminology O-2A^{adult} and O-2A^{perinatal} progenitors (although, in publications concerned solely with the cells derived from perinatal animals, we use the term *O-2A progenitor cell* to denote the perinatal cells). O-2A^{adult} progeni-tors have a unipolar morphology in vitro (Wolswijk and Noble, 1989), whereas O-2A^{perinatal} progenitors usually are bipolar (Small et al., 1987; Wolswijk and Noble, 1989). In addition, O-2A^{adult} pro-genitors have a longer average cell-cycle time in vitro than do O-2A^{perinatal} progenitors (65 $\pm$ 18 h vs. 18 $\pm$ 4 h; Noble et al., 1988; Wolswijk and Noble, 1989), migrate more slowly (4.3 $\pm$ 0.7 μm/h vs. 21.4 $\pm$ 1.6 μm/h; Small et al., 1987; Wolswijk and Noble, 1989), and take longer to differentiate (5 days vs. 2 days for 50% differ-entiation; Wolswijk and Noble, 1989). Furthermore, O-2A^{adult} pro-genitors stimulated to divide by type-1 astrocytes are O4$^+$, whereas dividing O-2A^{perinatal} progenitors are O4$^-$ (Wolswijk and Noble, 1989; I. Sommer and M. Noble, unpublished observations).

Before a brief review of some of the discoveries made in respect to O-2A^{adult} progenitor cells, perhaps it is worth noting first that the study of these cells is not a trivial undertaking. The yield of cells from a single adult optic nerve is some 1500 cells, thus offering far too few cells to quantify by using a hemocytometer. A larger cell yield can be obtained by isolating cells from the adult spinal cord, and these cells appear to have the same characteristics of the O-2A^{adult} progenitor cells of the optic nerve (Engel and Wolswijk, 1996). Thus, groups interested in studying the biology of these cells

are undertaking a challenging effort. Nonetheless, the opportunity to study an adult-specific precursor cell population offers more than ample rewards to make such efforts well worthwhile.

The discovery of an adult-specific glial precursor population raised a series of questions addressed in our subsequent studies. These questions were: (1) When do O-2A^{adult} progenitors first appear; (2) what is the developmental origin of these cells; (3) how is a population of O-2A progenitors maintained in the optic nerve of adult animals; and (4) what are the molecular mechanisms responsible for the differences in behavior between O-2A^{perinatal} progenitors and O-2A^{adult} progenitors?

O-2A^{adult} progenitorlike cells can be identified in rat optic nerve cultures from as early as 7 days after birth, whereas such cells do not appear to be present in optic nerve cultures isolated from newborn animals (Wolswijk et al., 1990). O-2A^{adult} progenitors become the dominant progenitor population in the optic nerve by 1 month after birth. However, replacement of the *perinatal* progenitor population by the *adult* occurs gradually, and both O-2A^{perinatal} and O-2A^{adult} progenitors can be isolated from optic nerves during the period between 7 days and 1 month after birth.

The source of O-2A^{adult} progenitors during development appears to be a subpopulation of O-2A^{perinatal} progenitors (Wren et al., 1992). This hypothesis is supported by time-lapse microcinematographic observations of cultures of dividing progenitors isolated from optic nerves of 3-week-old rats. In these experiments, we observed families of cells in which the founder member expressed characteristics of O-2A^{perinatal} progenitors and initially gave rise to further cells with the characteristics of O-2A^{perinatal} progenitors (i.e., bipolar morphology, rapid rates of migration and division), but subsequent progeny in the family expressed the characteristics of O-2A^{adult} progenitors (i.e., unipolar morphology, slow rates of division and migration). In addition, continued passaging of *perinatal* progenitors on monolayers of purified cortical astrocytes was associated with the generation of *adult* progenitorlike cells and loss of *perinatal* progenitorlike cells, a transition superficially similar to that which appears to occur in vivo (Wolswijk et al., 1990).

In contrast to the events thought to be involved in the initial appearance of O-2A^{adult} progenitors, we think that maintenance of these cells in the adult optic nerve may be the result of asymmetric division and differentiation of O-2A^{adult} progenitors themselves

(Wren et al., 1992). Analysis of the composition of individual colonies derived from O-2A^{adult} progenitors, grown at clonal densities, indicates that these cells can produce colonies containing both oligodendrocytes and dividing progenitor cells. Such a colony composition is strikingly different from that observed in colonies derived from O-2A^{perinatal} progenitor cells grown in the same conditions, suggesting that the signals that induce differentiation of all members of clones derived from perinatal progenitors exert lesser effects on the adult-derived cells.

The apparent predilection of O-2A^{adult} progenitors to undergo asymmetric division and differentiation is consistent with the hypothesis that these cells are stem cells (Wren et al., 1992). O-2A^{adult} progenitors also express other properties of stem cells, such as long cell-cycle times (Wolswijk and Noble, 1989; Wolswijk et al., 1991; Wren et al., 1992). The composition of clonal colonies of O-2A^{adult} progenitors growing in vitro on purified cortical astrocytes for 25 days also suggests that some of these cells may be able to exist in a near quiescent state, with cell-cycle lengths in excess of 150 h, without differentiating (Wren et al., 1992). Moreover, O-2A^{adult} progenitors seem to be capable of undergoing prolonged self-renewal, at least in vitro (Wren et al., 1992). Finally, these cells have the important quality of being maintained in the optic nerve throughout life (Wolswijk and Noble, 1989; Wolswijk et al., 1990). Thus, at this stage of our research, we suggest that it is most appropriate to regard O-2A^{adult} progenitors as stem cells (i.e., that these cells are capable of functioning as a self-renewing population throughout life) and to regard O-2A^{perinatal} progenitors as true progenitor cells (i.e., cells which are programmed to differentiate within a limited time-span).

The derivation of O-2A^{adult} progenitors from O-2A^{perinatal} progenitors has interesting implications in respect to the possible developmental origin of stem-cell populations. The results of our studies suggest that precursor cells with properties appropriate for early development can give rise not only to terminally differentiated end-stage cells but also to a second generation of precursors with properties appropriate for later developmental periods (see discussions in Wolswijk and Noble, 1989; Noble et al., 1991). In the O-2A lineage, it is this second group of precursors that represents the self-renewing stem cells. Whether the ancestral relationship between stem cells and prestem cells in other lineages is similar to that seen in the O-2A lineage is not yet known.

We have begun only recently to investigate the molecular mechanisms that allow O-2A^{perinatal} and O-2A^{adult} progenitors to express their different behaviors, and we know very little about the physiological alterations that underly the differences between these cells. We have seen that O-2A^{perinatal} and O-2A^{adult} progenitors express their characteristic properties when grown on the same monolayer of purified cortical astrocytes (Wolswijk et al., 1990). We have found also that both types of progenitors can be isolated from optic nerves of perinatal rats of between 7 days and 1 month old, suggesting that these populations also coexist in vivo. Moreover, we found that the specific properties of O-2A^{adult} progenitors are elicited by growth in the presence of PDGF (Wolswijk et al., 1991), just as exposure of O-2A^{perinatal} progenitor cells to PDGF is associated with expression of the specific properties that characterize these cells (Noble et al., 1988). Thus, these two cell types respond to a single signaling molecule by expressing different behaviors. Taken together, these results indicate that the differences between the O-2A^{adult} and O-2A^{perinatal} progenitors are intrinsic to the cells themselves and are not likely to be due to, for example, changes in the microenvironments found in the perinatal versus adult CNS or due to responsiveness to different growth factors found within the same environment.

It is clear also that the genetic mechanisms that underlie the expression of the O-2A^{perinatal} progenitor cell phenotype are not inactivated irreversibly in O-2A^{adult} progenitors. Exposure of *adult* progenitor cells to the combination of PDGF + bFGF causes a transient expression of a bipolar phenotype in association with rapid cell division and migration (Wolswijk and Noble, 1992). We have proposed that this reexpression of properties, such as those of O-2A^{perinatal} progenitor cells, may be relevant to the repair of demyelinating damage in the CNS.

The Oligodendrocyte as a Model System for the Study of Cell Death

Though it might become of considerable importance to be able to repair damaged tissues by transplantation of precursor cells, one also would like to be able to prevent the cell damage that might have led to the necessity for such intervention and to prevent any chronic degenerative processes that might lead to subsequent destruction of the transplanted cells. Thus, as a part of our general interests in tissue repair, we have been particularly interested in

the identification of means of preventing the death of oligodendrocytes.

In analyzing compounds that protect cells against death, we have found it experimentally useful to distinguish between death caused by exposure to toxic stimuli (i.e., death by murder) and that caused by exposure to suboptimal amounts of necessary trophic factors (i.e., death by neglect). These terms are used primarily to define two distinct experimental paradigms but also may have relevance for intervention in particular physiological processes. For example, apoptotic cell death occurring during normal development has been suggested to be due to insufficient quantitities of necessary trophic factors in the immediate environment (Raff, 1992). Consistent with such suggestions, it is known that experimental supplementation of trophic factors during early development can prevent such cell death in a variety of tissues (E. M. Johnson et al., 1986; Barde, 1989; Barres et al., 1992; Koseki et al., 1992; Coles et al., 1993). In contrast, cell death that follows injury more generally appears to be due to the local release of cytotoxic stimuli. It seems less likely that supplementation of trophic factors will be sufficient generally to protect cells against such death, although some promising in vitro results have been obtained in this regard (Schubert et al., 1992; Louis et al., 1993; Maiese et al., 1993).

Oligodendrocyte cell death is interesting because of the severe clinical consequences of destruction of these cells. Of particular clinical concern is the death of oligodendrocytes associated with demyelination in multiple sclerosis (MS) and in the periventricular white-matter injury thought to underly spastic motor and cognitive deficits frequently seen in premature infants (Dambska et all, 1989; van de Boor et al., 1989; Leviton and Paneth, 1990; Matthews, 1991; Oka et al., 1993). In both instances, it has been suggested that cytotoxic stimuli are the cause of oligodendrocyte death, thus providing a contrasting paradigm with the apoptosis of oligodendrocytes that occurs, for example, during development of the rat optic nerve; rather than being due to the appearance of cytotoxic factors, this latter cell death appears to be due to the presence of inadequate amounts of trophic factors to support all the oligodendrocytes present in this tissue (Barres et al., 1992; Raff et al., 1993).

The death of oligodendrocytes in premature infants recently has been suggested to be due to glutamate exposure, which is toxic for these cells in vitro (Oka et al., 1993). Unlike the more commonly studied receptor-mediated cell death induced by glutamate (Choi

and Rothman, 1990; Meldrum and Garthwaite, 1990), it appears that glutamate toxicity for oligodendrocytes is mediated by uptake of glutamate via a low-affinity uptake system that can operate as an exchange mechanism with intracellular cystine (Kessler et al., 1987; Zaczek et al., 1987; Oka et al., 1993). Glutamate uptake by oligodendrocytes is associated with a reduction in intracellular cystine levels (Oka et al., 1993). Then follows a fall in levels of intracellular glutathione, a metabolic product of cystine that is important in the control of cellular redox state and in protecting cells against damage associated with oxidative stress (Meister and Anderson, 1983; Taniguchi et al., 1989).

Glutamate-mediated death has not been invoked as a cause of oligodendrocyte death in MS patients, but one of the compounds of interest in this disease may cause death also by oxidative stress. This compound is tumour necrosis factor–alpha (TNF-α), one of the major cytokines involved in the generation of an inflammatory response. TNF-α has been reported to kill oligodendrocytes in vitro and has been found also to be present in MS lesions (Hofman et al., 1986; Selmaj and Raine, 1988; Merrill, 1991; Selmaj et al., 1991; Louis et al., 1993). If oligodendrocytes can be killed directly by TNF-α, such a vulnerability could contribute to the pathogenesis of MS lesions without requiring the presence of a specific immune response directed against myelin. Moreover, oligodendrocyte vulnerability to damage from TNF-α also could exacerbate damage caused by specific immune responses in MS patients. It has been suggested that the cytotoxic effects of TNF-α (on cells other that oligodendrocytes) are mediated through reactive oxidiative intermediates (Wong et al., 1989; Schulze-Osthoff et al., 1992, 1993).

N-acetyl-L-cysteine Protection Against Death Induced by TNF-α and by Glutamate

Our studies on cell death have been focused on the particular goal of identifying molecules of potential therapeutic utility. Our initial studies were founded on observations that N-acetyl-L-cysteine (NAC) was a potent inhibitor of TNF-α-stimulated expression of genes involved in the control of human immunodeficiency virus latency (Lioy et al., 1993; Mihm et al., 1991; Roederer et al., 1990, 1991, 1992; Staal et al., 1990).

As expected from the protective effect previously reported for cystine and cysteine (Oka et al., 1993), NAC protected oligodendrocytes against glutamate-induced cell death (Mayer and Noble,

1994). Glutamate was cytotoxic for purified oligodendrocytes within 24 h at concentrations ranging from 10 µM to 2 mM. Cultures exposed to 100 µM or 200 µM glutamate for 24 h showed a 50% reduction in the number of live oligodendrocytes, and cultures exposed to 2 mM glutamate showed a >85% reduction in cell number. In contrast, cultures exposed to up to 200 µM glutamate in the presence of 1 mM NAC did not show any reduction in the numbers of live oligodendrocytes, and cultures exposed to 2 mM glutamate + 1 mM NAC exhibited only a slight fall in cell number. NAC also protected oligodendrocytes against cell death induced by exposure to 20 ng/ml TNF-α, a dose that yielded a plateau killing of 50% to 60% of unprotected oligodendrocytes over 3 days. Significant protection against TNF-α-mediated killing was conferred by 0.1 mM NAC, and complete protection was afforded by 1 mM NAC.

How NAC and Ciliary Neurotrophic Factor Act in Synergy to Protect Oligodendrocytes from Death Induced by TNF-α

The first indication that our studies on NAC were leading to unexpected discoveries came from examining the ability of NAC to interact with ciliary neurotrophic factor (CNTF) to protect oligodendrocytes against killing by TNF-α. While we were conducting studies on the ability of CNTF to promote the generation, maturation, and survival of oligodendrocytes (Mayer et al., 1994), Louis et al., (1993) reported that oligodendrocytes could be rescued from the lethal effects of TNF-α by CNTF. Therefore, we began also to study the effects of CNTF in our own experimental systems. Although in our own subsequent experiments CNTF never protected oligodendrocytes as well as even 0.1 mM NAC, even at CNTF doses of up to 50 ng/ml, we did find a striking synergy between these compounds (Mayer and Noble, 1994). For example, we found that cultures exposed to 0.5 ng/ml CNTF + 0.01 mM or 0.1 mM NAC contained significantly more live oligodendrocytes than did those exposed to NAC alone or to 0.5 ng/ml CNTF alone (which had no significant effect on survival). At higher doses of CNTF, the combined effect of the two compounds appeared to be additive.

NAC Enhancement of Oligodendrocyte and Neuron Survival in Paradigms of Apoptosis Associated with Exposure to Suboptimal Amounts of Trophic Factors

The observations that CNTF is a survival factor for oligodendrocytes (Barres et al., 1993; Louis et al., 1993; Mayer et al., 1994)

and the synergistic interactions that we observed between CNTF and NAC in protecting oligodendrocytes against death induced by TNF-α led us to investigate possible contributions of NAC to cell survival in circumstances of growth factor withdrawal (Mayer and Noble, 1994). It is well-known that cells die not only from injury but also from apoptosis if they are not exposed to adequate amounts of appropriate trophic factors (E. M. Johnson et al., 1986; Barde, 1989; Barres et al., 1992, 1993; Koseki et al., 1992; Raff, 1992; Coles et al., 1993). In an effort to examine the protective effect of NAC against this form of cell death, NAC was added to cultures of spinal ganglion neurons exposed to suboptimal doses of nerve growth factor (the appropriate trophic factor for 70%–85% of these neurons; Gorin and Johnson, 1979; E. M. Johnson et al., 1980, 1986; Barde, 1989; Carroll et al., 1992; Ruit et al., 1992) or to oligodendrocytes exposed to suboptimal doses of CNTF or insulinlike growth factor (IGF-1); Barres et al., 1992; Louis et al., 1993; Mayer et al., 1994).

We observed (Mayer and Noble, 1994) dramatic effects of NAC on cell survival in cultures of spinal ganglion neurons derived from day-16 rat embryos and exposed to suboptimal doses of NGF. Cultures exposed to NAC plus either 1 or 10 ng/ml NGF contained 300% to 1000% more neurons than those exposed to NGF alone. Analysis of DNA synthesis by bromodeoxyuridine (BrdU) incorporation (Gratzner, 1982) confirmed that this increase in neuronal number was not due to cell division, strongly implicating differential cell death as the reason for the difference.

Exposure of oligodendrocytes to NAC also enhanced markedly the extent of survival obtained with suboptimal quantities of known trophic factors, although NAC was not by itself sufficient to rescue cells from death associated with growth factor deprivation (Mayer and Noble, 1994). Cultures of pure oligodendrocytes treated with any dose of CNTF examined—and most doses of IGF-1—contained significantly more live oligodendrocytes if cultures were exposed also to 1 mM NAC. Particularly interesting was that the presence of NAC in cultures exposed to doses of CNTF or IGF-1 that by themselves had little or no effect on cell survival was now associated with the presence of significant numbers of live oligodendrocytes.

To determine whether other compounds with antioxidant activity could also cooperate with known trophic factors synergistically to promote cell survival, we examined the effects of 0.5 ng/ml CNTF

on oligodendrocyte survival when applied together with vitamin C or Trolox. Although neither of these antioxidants had any effect when applied by themselves, the addition of either compound together with 0.5 ng/ml of CNTF now resulted in significant levels of oligodendrocyte survival.

Possible Avenues of Interest in Regard to NAC

The multiple effects of NAC that we have discovered have several novel aspects. It had been known previously that antioxidants such as cysteine and dithioerythritol can promote the survival of chondrocytes (which produce autocrine survival signals) in low-density cultures (Bruckner et al., 1989; Tschan et al., 1990; Ishizaki et al., 1994). It is not known whether such effects are related to the well-studied requirements of lymphocytes for glutathione if they are to function normally (Fishman et al., 1981; Dröge et al., 1983; Hamilos and Wedner, 1985; Fidelus and Tsan, 1986; Fidelus et al., 1987; Fidelus, 1988; Hamilos et al., 1989; Merrill, 1991; Eylar et al., 1993; Suthanthiran et al., 1990). More specifically relevant to our own experiments, it had not been reported previously that antioxidants can alter the dose-response curve to receptor tyrosine kinase or gp130 family receptor agonists as promoters of cell survival.

Our studies on NAC appear to offer the first demonstration of a reagent of potential use as a pharmaceutical that can synergize with established trophic factors to prevent death induced both by cytotoxic stimuli and by exposure to suboptimal amounts of trophic factors. It was surprising to identify a single molecule that offered such a range of beneficial effects.

The spectrum of protective activity offered by NAC renders this molecule particularly interesting. In future research, it will be important to determine the mechanism(s) by which NAC causes the effects we observed. At present, two major known modes of action exist for this compound, both of them related to antioxidant activity. NAC is an effective scavenger of free radicals and also is one of several compounds that can be used to augment intracellular levels of glutathione (Meister et al., 1986; Burgunder et al., 1989; Aruoma et al., 1989; Taniguchi et al., 1989; Staal et al., 1990). Both these activities may contribute to the ability of NAC to protect oligodendrocytes against death induced by TNF-α or glutamate exposure.

In regard to the mode of action of NAC, it is important to note that it is one of several compounds the can be used to augment

intracellular levels of glutathione, the major scavenger of reactive oxidative intermediates (ROI) present in all eukaryotic forms of life (Anker and Smilkstein, 1994; Smilkstein et al., 1988; Aruoma et al., 1989; Burgunder et al., 1989). Glutathione generally is required to protect cells against damage by oxidants and is able to reduce and thereby detoxify these potentially damaging chemical species. NAC enters cells readily and replenishes the intracellular cysteine required to produce glutathione, thus leading to an increase in glutathione levels. NAC also reacts directly with ROI, thus protecting cells against these toxic compounds. This twofold action of NAC places this compound in a class wholly different from other ROI scavengers (such as superoxide dismutase, catalase, ascorbate, α-tocopherol) that do not enhance cellular production of glutathione.

In contrast to the possible mode of action of NAC in protecting oligodendrocytes against death induced by exposure to toxic stimuli, the role of NAC in promoting cell survival in conditions of trophic factor deprivation is considerably more enigmatic. It is possible that the synergistic interactions between NAC and receptor tyrosine kinase or RawTK agonists are due to an NAC-induced increase in intracellular glutathione levels, but it seems likely that the real mechanisms are far more complex and interesting.

Protocol Section I: General Reagents and Methods

Preparing Reagents

Three general rules for working with cells of the O-2A lineage (and other CNS lineages) will save a great deal of wasted effort.

1. For all indications wherein water is to be used in making up reagents, use only tissue-culture-grade water. Even small amounts of impurities can kill O-2A progenitor cells. One example of suitable water is available from Gibco BRL Gaithersburg, MD (filtered, endotoxin-screened, cell-culture-grade, cat. no. 15230-162)

2. In all cases wherein a solution is to be filtered, it is essential to prewash the filter with 5 to 10 ml of double-distilled water, Dulbecco's modified (D-MEM), L-15, Eagle's medium, phosphate-buffered saline (PBS), or some similar solution before filtering the material that will be applied to cells. The wash step removes detergent that is applied to these filters as a wetting agent, and the material in the wash step (and the tube in which it is collected) is discarded.

3. Do not use HEPES-containing medium for dissections or cell preparations. The exposure of O-2A progenitor cells to HEPES will reduce cell viability dramatically. Instead, use L-15 (Gibco BRL 11415) or other media that do not require HEPES to maintain their pH when exposed to air.

Chemically Defined Medium (D-MEM-BS)

O-2A progenitor cells must be grown in chemically defined medium, as fetal serum will induce these cells to differentiate into type-2 astrocytes. For serious problems in growing cells, usually it is possible to improve survival by addition of 0.25% to 0.5% fetal calf serum (FCS) without altering differentiation, but we try not to use any serum at all.

To make D-MEM-BS, mix together the following ingredients (Bottenstein and Sato, 1979):

D-MEM (Gibco BRL no. 11995-065) plus 25 µg/ml gentamicin (Gibco BRL no. 15750-011)	469 ml
Insulin (preprepared, see following protocol)	10 ml
Transferrin (preprepared, see following protocol)	5 ml
Glutamine (preprepared, see protocol)	5 ml

Also needed is the addition of 11 ml of the following mixture:

First make up the following components:

*   200 ml PBS + 0.72 ml bovine serum albumin (BSA) path-o-cyte 4 (ICN Biochemicals, St. Louis, MO, Pentex)
*   200 ml H_2O + 322 mg putrescine (Sigma no. P-7505)
*   20 ml ethanol (EtOH) + 8.0 mg thyroxine (T_4, Sigma no. T-2501)
*   20 ml EtOH + 6.74 mg triiodothyronine (T_3, Sigma no. T-2752)

Combine the preceding four solutions and add 2 ml each of the following:

*   20 ml EtOH + 12.46 mg progesterone (Sigma no. P-0130)
*   20 ml H_2O + 7.74 mg selenium (Sigma no. S-1382)

This mixture will yield a total volume of 444 ml, which must be filtered through a 0.22-µm filter, aliquoted in 11-ml aliquots in sterile tubes, and stored at −20°C.

Note: Use 95% EtOH instead of absolute EtOH, as many formulations of the latter contain low levels of toxic benzene impurities.

Note: For some experiments, it is necessary to use D-MEM-BS that is free of thyroid hormones. To make up the D-MEM-BS mixture for these experiments, simply leave out the T_3 and T_4. Add instead corresponding amounts of EtOH to the mixture, to avoid altering other aspects of the composition.

TRANSFERRIN
Concentration of stock solution: 10 mg/ml transferrin (Sigma no. T-2252) in double-distilled water.

1. Use 2 g for 200 ml of chemically defined medium.
2. Filter the solution.
3. Store at −20°C in 5-ml aliquots.

INSULIN
Concentration of stock solution: 0.5 mg/ml insulin (Sigma no. I-5500) in 10 mM HCl.

1. Use 200 mg for 400 ml of final volume.
2. Predilute 200 mg insulin in 100 ml H_2O and add HCl (1 N/ca. 10 ml) until insulin is dissolved.
3. Filter through 0.22-μm filter.
4. Add sterile water to a final volume of 400 ml.
5. Store at −20°C in 10-ml aliquots.

Enzymes

To dissociate primary tissues and to remove cells from flasks, have ready the enzymes listed in the following sections.

TRYPSIN
Concentration of stock solution = 0.25% (Sigma no. T-8253) in D-MEM.

1. Make 50 ml trypsin solution at 2.5 mg/ml. As the trypsin powder does not dissolve completely, spin down in a pre-cooled centrifuge at 4000 rpm for 5 min before filtering through a 0.22-μm filter. Always wear gloves when handling trypsin, as getting it on your skin may cause irritation.
2. Aliquot in 1- and 2-ml volumes in bijous (for non-Europeans, these are 5- to 7-ml sterile tubes with screw-on caps).

3. Place bijous immediately on dry ice to freeze solution before it autodegrades.
4. Store at $-20°C$.
5. Defrost just before use.

COLLAGENASE

Final concentration of stock solution: 1.33% collagenase (Worthington, cat. no. 4188) in L-15.

1. Make a 13.3 mg/ml solution in L-15. This mixture will form a murky suspension.
2. Spin out big lumps at 4000 rpm for 10 min. Although this leads to differences in specific activity between batches, we have no reason (thus far) to believe that it is a major problem.
3. Filter through a 0.45-μm filter.
4. Store at $-20°C$ in 1- and 2-ml aliquots.
5. Defrost just before use.

SOYBEAN TRYPSIN INHIBITOR-DNASE SOLUTION

1. Make a solution of 0.52 mg/ml soybean trypsin inhibitor (Sigma no. T-9777, 5200 units/ml), 0.04 mg/ml bovine pancreas DNase (Sigma no. D-4263), and 3.0 mg/ml BSA (Sigma no. A-2153) in D-MEM or L-15.
2. Stir for 15 min to aid solubilization.
3. Filter through 0.22-μm filter.
4. Store in 1-, 2-, and 4-ml aliquots at $-20°C$.

ETHYLENEDIAMINETETRAACETIC ACID SOLUTION
Dissolve sodium ethylenediaminetetraacetic acid (Sigma EDS) in calcium- and magnesium-free (CMF) D-MEM or CMF L-15. Store at $4°C$ after filtering.

Preparation of Substrates for Promoting Cell Growth

You also need to decide whether you're going to grow cells on glass coverslips or on tissue-culture plastic. Cells tend to grow better on plastic but are easy to stain for immunofluorescence analysis when grown on glass coverslips. The simplest coatings to use are poly-lysine or polyornithine, which will cause cells to stick to a coated surface through electrostatic interactions. As far as we can tell,

there is no significant difference between using polylysine or poly-ornithine or between using the D or L forms of either. Poly-L-lysine (PLL) is used as an example.

PREPARATION OF STERILE COVERSLIPS

1. Wash coverslips several times with 95% EtOH.
2. Wash with sterile tissue-culture-grade water and leave to dry, or wash in a similar way and dry-heat sterilize.

We are concerned, but not yet convinced, that different coverslips from different manufacturers may have different properties as regards cell growth, even after coating by polycations. If cultures are growing well on plastic but not on glass, consider changing glass suppliers.

PLL
Concentration of stock solution = 13.3 µg/ml (Sigma no. P-1274).

1. Make up at 4 mg/ml in stock solution in sterile water.
2. Filter through 0.22-µm filter.
3. Aliquot 100 µl in sterile Eppendorf tubes and label.
4. Prior to use, thaw and dilute 100 µl in 30 ml water.
5. Coat coverslips in wells or in dishes. Coat by flooding sterile coverslips with dilute PLL solution and allow to coat for at least 60 min before use. Before using, wash twice with tissue-culture-grade water. If the intent is to plate cells in a small volume of medium in a droplet on a coverslip, the surface must be dried in air before applying cells.

Note: Coating of tissue-culture plastics may be used to generate more uniform results between experiments. We have had unfortunate experiences with tissue-culture plastics in which particular lots have not been coated correctly in the factory. Coating with PLL can compensate for such between-batch variations in plastics quality.

Preparation of Growth Factors

Cells do not survive in D-MEM alone. The insulin in D-MEM-BS provides one of the necessary survival signals for O-2A lineage cells, possibly through stimulation of IGF-I receptors. Other growth factors of importance in studying the O-2A lineage include PDGF, bFGF, CNTF, LIF, and IGF-1. All are made up in the same manner:

1. Make up growth factors in L-15 medium containing 5% vol/vol Path-o-Cyte BSA.
2. Always filter the medium *before* adding it to the growth factor (which will come as a sterile powder). Dissolve factor in an appropriate volume of medium, normally at 10 µg/ml.
3. Aliquot the solution in small containers in volumes of 10, 20, 50, and 100 µl per container, and so on. The volumes used should be chosen to yield enough growth factor for a single experiment without having a great deal left over.
4. Seal containers, label them with the volume contained, and store at −20° or −70°C as indicated for the specific growth factor.

Note: The source of growth factors can make significant differences in experimental outcome. Wherever possible, we compare growth factors from at least two sources. At present, we purchase the "core" growth factors from PeproTech Inc., Princeton, NJ (CNTF, 450−50; bFGF, 100−183; IGF-1, 100−11; LIF, 300−05; NT-3, 450−03, 100−13A) or from Promega (TNF-α, G5241).

Preparation of NAC

The use of NAC to promote cell survival and enhance response to receptor tyrosine kinase agonists is discussed in Mayer and Noble (1994). To make up NAC, follow this recipe:

Stock concentration = 100 mM in D-MEM.

1. To make a total of 5 ml of stock, take 81.5 mg (= 16.3 mg/ml) of NAC purchased from Sigma (no. A-8199). It is critical to smell the NAC when opening its container for the first time. Any sulphurous (rotten egg−like) smell given off would indicate that the NAC is oxidized and should be thrown away.
2. Centrally important to the success of these experiment is the manner in which NAC is made up. This compound is highly acidic and also is hydrolyzed rapidly in basic solution. Thus, the pH must be titred for application of NAC to cells, but the titration must be carried out with an NaOH solution no more concentrated than 1 N. We have found that it is preferable to prepare a concentrated solution of NAC (100 mM) in D-MEM and to use the phenol red pH indicator contained in the D-MEM as an indicator of when the solution is suitable for use. Start by adding 4 ml of D-MEM to enough NAC to make up 5 ml. On addition of 1 N NaOH dropwise to such a solution agitated by a stir bar, one can see the color

change during the titration process. Take time in adjusting the pH so as not to hydrolyze the NAC. At the moment that a stable salmon-orange color is achieved, stop the titration. Make up the final volume to 5 ml with more D-MEM. The stock solution of NAC then is filtered and frozen in small aliquots. In monitoring color, check that pH is not above 7.0 during freezing and thawing; if it is, throw it away and start again.

If D-MEM, cannot be used, use a good pH meter and tissue-culture-grade water. Once NAC is thawed, use it immediately. Throw away unused material.

Protocol Section II. Immunofluorescence Analysis

Solution Preparation

HANK'S STAINING MEDIUM
Once your cells are growing, you may wish to analyze them by immunofluorescence microscopy. To do this you will need a staining solution, which is made up as follows:

1. Fill 1-L flask with either one pack of prebalanced Hank's balanced salts without sodium bicarbonate (Imperial Lab no. 3-0322-31) or 9.9 g/L Hank's powder.
2. Add 4.76 g/L HEPES, free acid (Sigma no. H-3375) and 5.20 g/L HEPES, sodium salt (Sigma no. H-7006).
3. Add 940 ml water and dissolve components.
4. Add 5 ml 10% Na azide to prevent bacterial growth.
5. Add 50 ml donor calf serum.
6. Store at 4°C.

PARAFORMALDEHYDE (4%) SOLUTION
Dissolve 4 g of paraformaldehyde (powder) in 10 ml water by adding 100 μl 1-M NaOH and heating to 60°C. Cool slightly and add 10 ml of 10× PBS. Bring to 100 ml with H_2O and adjust pH to 7 to 7.6 using HCl. Make up fresh before use.

ANTIFADE (DABCO)
Fluorescein fading is an enormous annoyance, and an unnecessary one. To prevent fluorescein from fading, make up a solution of

2.5% 1,4-diazabicyclo[2.2.2] octane (DABCO) (Sigma no. D-2522). Dissolve 200 mg in 10 ml glycerol by heating to 37°C. Store at 4°C wrapped in foil.

Although some laboratories use paraphenylenediamine (PPD) as an antifading reagent, we recommend against this. PPD is highly toxic, whereas DABCO is relatively inert.

Indirect Immunofluorescence Analysis

The various CNS cell types are identified with a number of different antibodies, and the binding of these antibodies is visualized with three different fluorochromes. When cells are immunolabeled only with antibodies (Abs) that recognize intracellular antigens, the cells can be fixed immediately in methanol for 10 min at −20°C.

Many antibodies are used to study glial cells. The primary ones we use are: mouse IgM monoclonal antibody (mAb) A2B5 (which binds to tetrasialogangliosides and other antigens; Eisenbarth et al., 1979); mouse IgM mAb 04 (which binds to sulfatide and another oligodendrocyte antigen; Sommer and Schachner, 1981); mouse IgG3 mAb anti-galactocerebroside (GalC; Ranscht et al., 1982); mouse IgG1 mAB anti-bromodeoxyuridine (BrdU, which is incorporated into DNA during S phase; Gratzner, 1982); and rabbit polyclonal anti-GFAP, a specific marker of astrocytes; Bignami et al., 1972). The anti-GFAP is purchased, usually from Sigma (no. G-9269), and the anti-BrdU is obtained from Sigma (no. B-2531). Other antibodies can be purchased from various suppliers or obtained from the American Tissue Culture Collection or from the authors of the primary papers describing them. Generally, we purchase our secondary, fluorochrome-conjugated antibodies from Southern Biotechnology, Inc., although many suitable suppliers of such antibodies exist. In testing them, make sure to test for cross-reaction with antibodies of other classes. The working dilution of the fluorochrome-conjugated antibodies should be at least 1:100.

A very important rule is never to let the coverslips, or other surfaces on which you might grow cells, dry out during the staining procedures. Drying will cause a great deal of nonspecific staining and make subsequent analyses uninterpretable.

1. Place coverslips with the cells of interest on platforms and fix the cells in 4% paraformaldehyde in PBS. A platform can be made by cutting off the top of an Eppendorf tube (or using the cap of a small

centrifuge tube) and gluing it to the surface of a 100-mm Petri dish. Regardless of the materials used to build this chamber (and usually they are jury-rigged out of readily available materials), the goal is that the surface on which the coverslip rests is large enough to hold the coverslip, yet small enough so that its outer diameter is less than that of the coverslip itself; otherwise the liquid on top of the coverslip will, with high probability, be drawn off onto the surface of the platform, thus leading to drying of the coverslip.

2. For staining surface antigens, incubate cells in 50 µl of the primary Ab solution for 20 to 30 min at room temperature in a humidified chamber. These chambers can be made simply by taking a 100-mm Petri dish or any other structure that appeals to your sense of design and gluing platforms (see the preceding description) to the surface that is associated with a shorter side wall (for ease of lifting the coverslips). The chambers are humidified simply by taking a piece of tissue paper, rolling it up into a tube, wetting it, and packing it against the wall of the chamber. Then, as long as you remember to put the lid on, the coverslips will not dry out.

In using an Ab to a surface molecule and an Ab to an intracellular antigen, first immunolabel the cultures with the antibody to the cell-surface molecule(s), then with the antibody to the intracellular antigens (after fixation for 10 min in methanol at −20°C).

An important tip for handling coverslips is to buy a good pair of watchmaker's forceps (e.g., from Shandon Lipshaw, Pittsburgh, PA). These are sufficiently well-made so that heavy pressure is not required to hold the coverslip firmly, an important consideration as the coverslips are so fragile that pressing on them with a standard forceps often will shatter them.

A second important tip concerns the lifting of coverslips from the tray or Petri dish in which they are growing prior to staining. The best tool we have found for this purpose is a large syringe needle (18- or 21- gauge). Press the sharp tip against a hard surface to bend it back at a right angle (bending it back in this way perhaps a millimeter or less). This lifting fork can be inserted under the glass coverslips to lift them sufficiently to grip them with the watchmaker's forceps. We strongly recommend trying this a few times before conducting a critical experiment, as most people break quite a few coverslips in learning this simple procedure.

3. Rinse coverslips several times in Hank's staining solution.
4. Visualize the binding of the primary Abs with fluorescein isothiocyanate (FITC)- or tetramethylrhodamine isothiocyanate (TRITC)-

conjugated second Abs (for example, purchased from Southern Biotechnology Associates Inc., Birmingham, AL). If a third color is needed, incubate cells after the primary antibody with biotin-conjugated second Abs (Southern Biotechnology) followed by coumarin (AMCA)-labeled streptavidin (Molecular Probes Inc., Eugene, OR).

5. After the immunolabeling, place coverslips face down on a drop of DABCO-containing glycerol (see the foregoing), remove excess fluid, and seal coverslip with clear nail varnish.

6. Examine cultures on a microscope using transmission-phase-contrast and epiilluminated fluorescence optics, the latter with filters optimized for distinguishing between FITC, TRITC, and AMCA emission.

Note: If the primary Abs were produced in different species or are of different subclasses, cultures can be incubated simultaneously with more than one primary Ab followed by class-specific or species-specific second layers. If antibodies of the same subclass are used, use either directly conjugated primary Abs or use an indirect sequential labeling protocol to find the overlap. In the latter case, immunolabel two sets of duplicate coverslips; label one set with primary Ab X followed by TRITC-labeled secondary Abs, primary antibody Y, and FITC-labeled secondary Abs; label the other set with primary Ab Y followed by TRITC-labeled secondary Abs, primary antibody X, and FITC-labeled secondary Abs. In the first set of coverslips, the $Y + X -$ cells are labeled with FITC but not with TRITC. In the second set, the $X + Y -$ cells are labeled with FITC but not with TRITC. The proportion of cells that are $X + Y +$ can be determined by subtracting from 100% the proportion of cells that are $X + Y - (x\%)$ and the proportion of cells that are $Y + X - (y\%)$ (100% $- x\% - y\%$).

BrdU Labeling of Cells and Anti-BrdU Staining

1. Add BrdU to cells to a final concentration of 10 µM.
2. Allow cells to continue their in vitro growth for 4 h (for rapidly dividing cells), 8 h (for cells with intermediate cell-cycle lengths), or overnight (for slowly dividing cells).
3. Stain as usual for surface antibodies.
4. Fix cells with ice-cold methanol for 15 min at −20°C.
5. Stain cells as usual with intracellular antibodies.

6. Add to each coverslip 30 µl 0.2% paraformaldehyde and incubate 60 s. Do *not* exceed the recommended incubation time or it will be difficult to obtain reproducible results.
7. Wash coverslips.
8. Add 30 µl 0.07 M NaOH and incubate for 7 min.
9. Wash coverslips.
10. Add 30 µl anti-BrdU monoclonal antibody (1:100) and incubate for 20 min.
11. Wash coverslips.
12. Add 30 µl anti-IgG$_1$-RITC or FITC (1:100) and incubate for 20 min.
13. Before sealing all coverslips, check whether stain has worked. Repeat if unsuccessful. If successful, seal coverslips.

Protocol Section III. Preparation of Astrocytes and Astrocyte-Conditioned Medium

Multiple strategies have been developed for purification of cells, and each of them has its intrinsic merits. In general, our bias has been toward purification strategies that can be carried out readily in most laboratories. Thus, generally we do not use flourescence-activated cell sorting for cell purification, although we have used this technique on some occasions (Barnett et al. 1993). Because of the extensive cell loss that occurs with such sorting, we prefer to use immunopanning procedures in dealing with the low cell numbers encountered in working on the optic nerve. Our immunopanning strategy for O-2A progenitor cells is described in this chapter, and we routinely obtain purities of >99% by using these methods.

As a general comment, we never study O-2A progenitor cells or oligodendrocytes prepared by the shake-and-isolate procedures originally described by McCarthy and DeVellis (1980), in which brain-derived cultures are grown for 7 to 10 days in vitro in medium containing 10% FCS after which the surface growing cells are removed by overnight shaking on a rotary platform. Even though this technique is used routinely, we remain concerned that growth of cells in serum-containing medium followed by removal by overnight shaking may not resemble closely environments encountered by these cells during the course of normal development. In addition, we have found that if we take five flasks of cells prepared at the same time from the same dissection and compare the composition of the population enriched for oligodendrocytes and O-2A progenitor cells, the flask-to-flask variability is enormous. Just

in a simple comparison of this nature, we have seen cultures that are 90% O-2A lineage cells and cultures that are 50% O-2A lineage cells, with contributions from astrocytes and microglial cells or macrophages making up the remainder of the culture. Anyone using these techniques is well-advised to use some manner of immunopurification procedures after shaking, so as at least to insure a high level of enrichment for cells of interest. It is our experience, however, that similar (or greater) numbers of O-2A lineage cells can be obtained by immunopurifying cells directly from corpus callosum or even from whole brain. However, note that we do use for many purposes a modification of the astrocyte purification protocols described by McCarthy and DeVellis (1980). We would prefer to use immunopurification also to isolate our astrocytes directly from brain, but the surface markers presently available have not allowed us to achieve a degree of purity sufficient to allow clean experiments to be conducted.

The surest way to grow successful O-2A progenitor cells and neurons and oligodendrocytes is to grow them on monolayers of type-1 astrocytes or in medium conditioned by purified type-1 astrocytes. Astrocyte cultures are prepared as outlined in the following sections.

The Founding Culture

1. Dissect cortex from newborn or 1-day old rats, place into L-15 medium, and remove meningeal tissues, hippocampus, caudate, and other internal structures to leave the cortical sheets.
2. Mince cortical tissue into small pieces with a scalpel.
3. Transfer with a pipette to 250 µl of collagenase stock solution (1.33% in L-15) for every 1 ml of L-15 (or D-MEM). Use 1 to 1.5 ml of total solution volume per two rat brains.
4. Incubate for 30 min at 37°C.
5. Centrifuge for 5 min at 1000 rpm (approximately $230 \times g$) or for 1 min at 3000 rpm (approximately $2,000 \times g$).
6. Remove supernatant.
7. Resuspend in a solution of CMF EDTA-containing solution, mixed with trypsin stock solution. The ratio to use is between 1:4 and 1:10 trypsin stock:EDTA solution, with the exact ratio depending on the strength of the trypsin. Basically, if dissociation is good but viability is poor, try reducing the trypsin concentration.

8. Add 300 μl of soybean trypsin inhibitor and DNase solution for 5 min.

9. Centrifuge as described.

10. Remove supernatant and add 500 μl of D-MEM-BS.

11. Triturate into a cell suspension, beginning with gentle passage through a 5-ml pipette and continuing (if necessary) to an 18-gauge needle. (In general, the tissue will be dissociated sufficiently by 10 passages up and down a 5-ml pipette).

    Note: Do not pass air bubbles through the medium when triturating. Each air bubble will kill many cells. Be gentle!

12. Transfer to tissue-culture flasks containing D-MEM supplemented with 10% FCS. Use a density of about 2×10^6 cells per 25-cm² flask. This usually works out to 1 brain per 25-cm² flask or 2 to 3 per 75-cm² flask. The volume of medium used is 5 ml per 25-cm² flask and 10 ml per 75- or 80-cm² flask. Cultures are maintained in a humidified incubator at 37° to 37.5°C, with carbon dioxide content of between 5% and 10%. (Normally, we use 7.5%.)

13. Replace medium at the end of day 1 and on each third day.

14. At 7 to 10 days, a confluent culture should result.

15. When culture is confluent, seal lid firmly, wrap with parafilm, and tape to a rotary platform. Set platform to rotate at a speed just below that at which foaming of the medium will occur. Let shake overnight, making sure that cells are not exposed to light (as this will kill them). It is best to carry out this step at 37°C in an incubated rotary platform or in a 37°C room.

16. Remove supernatant and replace it with fresh D-MEM-FCS.

17. Add 200 μl of 1 mM cytosine arabinoside/10 ml medium and put cells in incubator for 48 h. The cytosine arabinoside is added to kill off dividing cells (such as meningeal contaminants, O-2A progenitors, and microglial cells). The astrocytes are spared, as they are not dividing in these confluent cultures.

18. Change medium to fresh D-MEM-FCS and leave cells to recover for 24 h.

19. Repeat steps (17 and 18) to deplete further any remaining dividing cells.

This procedure yields cultures of approximately 98% type-1 astrocytes. These cultures can be enriched further by using complement-mediated killing to remove any remaining O-2A progenitor cells and by the use of irradiation to prevent the generation of new progenitor cells from A2B5-negative pre-O-2A progenitor

cells. Cultures at this level of purity are satisfactory for many types of experiments, such as being used as growth substrates for neurons or as sources of conditioned medium. If the intent is to grow O-2A progenitor cells directly on the astrocytes, with certainty that all the O-2A progenitor cells studied are derived from the added cells, the irradiation and complement killing are necessary. In such experiments, it is essential to examine control cultures of astrocytes (to which no new cells have been added) to ensure that the cells being studied are not derived from residual cells present at a low frequency in the astrocyte population.

Complement Kill to Remove O-2A Progenitor cells, Type-2 Astrocytes, and Oligodendrocytes

1. Wash monolayer with several mls of EDTA-containing CMF medium, then incubate with EDTA-containing CMF medium (10 ml for 75-cm^2 flasks) for 5 min at 37°C.
2. Add trypsin solution at 1:20 and leave at 37°C for 5 min.
3. Add 1 ml of soy bean trypsin inhibitor-DNase solution and tap cells loose.
4. Pipette cells gently up and down several times and place in a 15-ml centrifuge tube.
5. Centrifuge at 3000 rpm (approximately 2000 × g) for 5 min.
6. Add together complement (1:10 dilution of rabbit or guinea pig complement) and add one-third final volume of A2B5 and one-third final volume monoclonal antibody supernatant, together with medium to make up the final volume (final volume, 1–2 ml). Filter the mixture (and do not forget to prewash the filter). We always test the complement on cultures that are not crucial, as occasional batches of complement are extremely toxic.
7. Tap side of centrifuge tube to loosen cells and add 1 to 2 ml of the complement-antibody mixture to cells.
8. Resuspend cells in the complement-antibody mixture and leave at 37°C for 30 min.
9. To wash cells, top off tube with D-MEM-FCS and centrifuge for 10 min at 1000 rpm (approximately 230 × g). Resuspend cells in desired medium for replating, although the best monlayers are obtained with D-MEM-FCS. Plate cells at densities of 750,000 per 25-cm^2 flask; 200,000 per slide flask; 20,000 to 40,000 per coverslip, in volumes of 5 ml, 1.5 ml, and 0.5 ml, respectively. Generally, this

technique will yield astrocyte monolayers wherein the astrocytes are sufficiently flat to allow excellent visualization of any cells (e.g., O-2A progenitor cells, neurons) plated on the cell surface.

10. Leave cells for 1 day in D-MEM-FCS to settle. Monitor on the microscope. Often, cells have formed a confluent monolayer within 24 h. Cultures then are fed according to the needs of harvesting conditioned medium later or according to the needs of individual experiments.

To Make Conditioned Medium

1. After cells have settled for 1 day, wash flask twice with D-MEM-BS. Add 5 ml fresh D-MEM-BS per 25-cm^2 flask and 10 ml for 75-cm^2 flask. Leave medium to condition for 48 h.

2. Collect conditioned medium and replace with D-MEM-BS for a second 48-h collection.

3. If conditioned medium is to be used within 24 h, it can be stored at 4°C in the dark (as light will break down ingredients in the medium; for example, breaking glutamine down to yield ammonia and the neurotoxic agent glutamate). In making material for storage, store in 10 to 20-ml aliquots. If material is prepared carefully, it will not require filtering after thawing. You should, however, centrifuge the thawed aliquot (3000 rpm, 5 min) before use, as it frequently will contain precipitated proteins after thawing.

4. To promote O-2A progenitor cell division, use conditioned medium in a 50:50 mixture with fresh D-MEM-BS. We have found that cells respond better if the medium is allowed to adjust to proper temperature and pH in the incubator before applying to cells.

5. In general, we do not put astrocytes through more than two conditioning cycles without giving them a rest in D-MEM-FCS for 24 to 28 h. The serum concentration in this mixture can be dropped to 5%.

For Pure Astrocyte Monolayers Rather than Conditioned Medium

1. Go back to the last step of the complement-killing section, wherein cells have been allowed to settle in D-MEM-FCS for 24 h.

2. Irradiate at 2000 rad (20 grays). This is done routinely by placing cultures in whatever radiation source is available locally. In irradiating cells in flasks, remember to seal them tightly. In irradiating

monolayers on coverslips, seal the tray with parafilm so that the pH of the medium is maintained as well as possible. The irradiation will kill off pre-O-2A progenitors and leave >99.5% pure mono-layers.

3. Replace medium immediately after irradiation with medium of choice (usually D-MEM-BS for plating cells on the astrocytes).

4. Allow monolayers to grow for 24 h before adding cells, thus giving the fresh medium a chance to be conditioned by the astrocyte monolayer.

Protocol Section IV. O-2A^{perinatal} Progenitor Cells

Almost all the initial experiments on O-2A progenitor cells were carried out with preparations of perinatal rat optic nerve. Dissection of this tissue from 7-day-old rat pups yields cultures highly enriched in O-2A progenitor cells. The techniques used for the optic nerve can be adapted for any other region of the CNS except for the olfactory bulb (which contains a separate glial population of olfactory nerve–ensheathing cells [Barnett et al., 1993]).

Mixed Cultures

1. Dissect optic nerves or other regions of the CNS from which O-2A progenitor cells will be purified. Remove meningeal tissues as much as possible by stripping them away.

2. Mince tissue into small pieces with a scalpel and incubate in 1.3% collagenase for 30 min at 37°C. The total volume at this step should be 1 ml for optic nerves from 20 to 40 rat pups. (We rarely dissect fewer than 10 pups at a time, as the cell yield is too low.)

3. Add one-fourth the total volume in trypsin solution and leave for 15 min at 37°C.

4. For nerves derived from rats older than 5 days postbirth, add an additional trypsin incubation. Spin down tissue chunks for 1 min at 3000 rpm and resuspend in a fresh trypsin solution for a further 15 min at 37°C.

5. Let tissue chunks settle, or spin at 3000 rpm for 1 min. Add to this cell suspension 1 to 2 ml of soybean trypsin inhibitor–DNase solution. Leave for 5 min. Spin cells as described and resuspend in 1 ml D-MEM-BS and triturate through fine needles. *This is a critical stage in this preparation.* Start with a 19-g needle attached to a 1-ml

plastic hypoallergenic syringe and take the tissue through gently once or twice, being careful to avoid introducing air bubbles into the fluid. Take only some 80% of the volume into the needle at a time, to avoid accidentally pulling the syringe plunger out too far, thus compromising sterility. Proceed to three or four passes through a 23-g needle. Allow the chunks to settle out, then, with extreme care, remove the top 500 to 700 μl of the volume and place in a separate bijou. This is done because the cells that already have been dissociated from the tissue will only be damaged by further trituration, and there is no reason to subject them to such treatment. Add 300 to 500 μl of D-MEM-BS, then take 6 to 10 passes through a 27-g needle. This must be done with extreme gentleness, for being too rough will reduce the cell yield greatly. If visible chunks of tissue remain, again allow the chunks to settle and remove the top 300 μl and add them to the other dissociated cells. Then take the remaining tissue through 6 to 10 passes through a 27-g needle, mix all the dissociated cell preparations together, and determine the total cell number with a hemocytometer. To judge whether handling has been sufficiently gentle, examine a drop of cell suspension under the microscope. If cells can be found readily with interesting looking processes attached to them, consider it a good job. If cells all look round, you have either been too rough or have dissected the spleen by mistake.

Note: If you are making a special formulation of D-MEM-BS for your experiments, you may need to dissociate cells in this special formulation as well.

6. The suspension of cells then is topped up to give the volume required for plating. This amount varies with different experiments although, for growth on glass coverslips, we tend to use 2000 to 4000 cells plated in a 25-μl drop. In general, it is best to plate cells in the minimum possible volume, then to feed to the final volume after the cells have had 30 min to attach to their substrate.

a. Do not spin the cells down, as many of them will be lost by introducing such a step.

b. The yield that can be expected is 50,000 cells per optic nerve from a 7-day-old rat pup, of which >50% seem to be O-2A lineage cells. If you isolate cells from optic nerves of younger animals, the yield of O-2A progenitor cells is reduced because they are proportionally less well-represented in the optic nerve. A higher cell number can be obtained by using O4 Ab to positively select cells from the entire brain (with the olfactory bulbs removed). Again, the total number of

cells obtained is higher if 7-day-old rat pups are used, but useful numbers of cells can be obtained from younger animals.

7. Cells are grown in a humidified incubator at 37.5°C. Generally, we use 7.5% CO_2 but have grown cells successfully at CO_2 concentrations from 5% to 10%.

Within 24 h, cultures should contain clearly viable cells with a variety of morphologies. O-2A progenitor cells are bipolar, with an elliptical cell body and two long processes (sometimes one) that may be several times the length of the cell body. Oligodendrocyte cell bodies are rounder, and these cells make many processes generally extended symmetrically around the cell body. Mixed cultures also contain type-1 astrocytes, which are much flatter in appearance than are the O-2A lineage cells. Type-2 astrocytes have a small cell body and long thin processes symmetrically arranged around the cell body. If cultures are particularly good, healthy O-2A progenitor cells may be visible within a few hours after plating. If cultures at 24 h do not contain O-2A progenitor cells, it is unlikely that they will recover.

If you are having problems growing cells, there are a number of matters to check. To check general viability of the preparation, plate the optic nerve cells on monolayers of purified type-1 astrocytes at densities of 5- to 10,000 cells per 13-mm coverslip. If these cultures do not contain viable O-2A progenitor cells, there is something wrong with your preparation. For example, you may have added too much trypsin or triturated too harshly. It is also possible that one of the reagents contains a toxic impurity. It is exceptionally annoying when this happens, as it means screening through every reagent separately. Fortunately, in 15 years of working with these cells, this has only happened to us twice.

If O-2A progenitor cells grow well on type-1 astrocytes but not on plastic or coverslips, something may be wrong with the materials. Sometimes it is of value to switch from polylysine to polyornithine (even though there is no apparent reason why this should make a difference). We also have had toxic batches of plastics. For example, early on in the course of this work, we had a period of several months during which our experiments were working perfectly but, in the laboratory of Martin Raff (University College London, UK), the O-2A progenitor cultures were dying. Fortunately, at that time we were within a few blocks of each other and could trade reagents easily to identify the problem (which turned out to be a batch of 24-

well trays that were actually toxic). So, in the face of problems, it may be worth growing cells in or on plastics (or coverslips) from different suppliers.

If cells grow well but all turn into oligodendrocytes in the presence of PDGF (for example), it may be that the problem is a batch of growth factor that has a poor specific activity; we have had batches wherein the specific activity was one-tenth of the expected value. In such a case, try increasing the growth factor concentration tenfold or testing growth factors from another supplier. If the growth factor has a lower-than-advertised activity and is not inducing O-2A progenitor cell division at expected concentrations (5 ng/ml for PDGF and bFGF), call the supplier. In our experience, suppliers have been willing to replace, at no cost, cytokine batches that have low activity.

In general, we don't expect people to generate good cultures until they have made several attempts (although there has been no shortage of people who get everything working from the very first effort). So, if the first attempts don't work, don't give up.

Purification of O-2A Progenitor Cells

The procedure for purification of O-2A progenitor cells is a modification of the method of Wysocki and Sato (1978), as adapted to glial cell purification by Barres et al. (1993) and modified again in our laboratory (Mayer et al., 1994; Mayer and Noble, 1994). It is called *immunopurification* or *panning*. The procedure is based on using a negative selection procedure first to remove unwanted cells (e.g., astrocytes, meningeal cells, oligodendrocytes, and microglial cells or macrophages), then on using a positive selection step to purify the O-2A progenitor cells themselves.

To purify O-2A progenitor cells, three Abs are needed: the Ran-2 Ab (Bartlett et al., 1980), which binds to type-1 astrocytes and meningeal cells; antigalactocerebroside (GalC) Ab (Ranscht et al., 1982a), which binds to oligodendrocytes; and either the A2B5 Ab (Eisenbarth et al., 1979) or the O4 Ab (Sommer and Schachner, 1981). The first two Abs are used for negative selection, and one of the last two is used for positive selection of O-2A progenitor cells. The advantage of the A2B5 Ab is that it labels O-2A progenitor cells early in their development; the disadvantage is that it is an O-2A lineage–specific marker only in the optic nerve. The O4 Ab is completely O-2A lineage–specific for all regions of the CNS, with

the exception of the olfactory bulb (wherein it labels olfactory nerve–ensheathing cells; Barnett et al., 1993), but it begins to label O-2A progenitor cells only at a stage slightly later than that labeled by the A2B5 Ab.

PREPARATION OF PANNING DISHES

1. Incubate 100-mm tissue-culture plastic Petri dishes (Nunclon) overnight with anti-IgG (H + L) for panning Abs of any of the IgG classes or with anti-IgM for panning Abs of the IgM class. Ran-2 and anti-GalC are both IgGs; both A2B5 and O4 are IgMs. The anti-Ig Abs are prepared in 50 mM Tris, pH 9.5, at a concentration of 1 mg/ml, and 10 ml is added to each plate. Solutions can be reused up to five times before they are depleted significantly. The monoclonal antibodies are added, in our hands, as hybridoma supernatants. The protein concentration of the supernatant is 2.5 μg/ml for anti-Ran-2 and anti-GalC Abs and 5 μg/ml for the A2B5 Ab. Note, however, that this concentration may vary in different labs. If panning is not working, refer to the troubleshooting comments at the end of this protocol; it may be necessary to alter Ab concentrations.

2. Prior to use of the panning dishes, wash them three times with D-MEM. Then incubate them with 10 ml of the cell type–specific Ab for at least 1 hour at 37°C in the incubator. If the cell type–specific monoclonal Ab has not been prepared in serum-free chemically defined medium, it is necessary to add BSA as a carrier protein. It is critical in this protocol that the cell type–specific antibodies not be prepared in the presence of 10% serum and that the hybridoma supernatants have been harvested in a serum-free medium.

3. Immediately prior to adding cells, wash again three times with D-MEM.

PREPARATION OF CELLS

1. At this point, you realize that you should have read the entire protocol before starting, because now you learn that while the panning plates were being washed, tissue was also being enzymatically treated.

2. Dissect optic nerves or other regions of the CNS from which O-2A progenitor cells will be purified. Remove meningeal tissues as much as possible by stripping them away.

3. Mince tissue into small pieces with a scalpel and incubate in 1.3% collagenase for 30 min at 37°C.

4. Spin tissue down for 5 min at 1000 rpm, then for 1 min at 3000 rpm, and resuspend in 30 units/ml of activated papain (Worthington Biochemical Corporation, LSO 3127). Papain is used because it is a gentler digestive enzyme than is trypsin, leaving intact protein epitopes that are destroyed by trypsinization. The papain is activated by dissolving it in D-MEM in a 37°C water bath and adding (grain by grain) HCl-cysteine until the pH is acidic. Then the solution is neutralized with sodium hydroxide, using the pH indicator in the D-MEM to indicate the correct pH. Filter this mixture directly onto the cells, first making sure to wash the filter with 5 to 10 ml of D-MEM or tissue-culture-grade water. Many filters contain a small amount of detergent as a wetting agent, and this will kill the O-2A progenitor cells.

   Note: You can use this enzymatic mix to prepare mixed cultures but you cannot use trypsin if you are going to pan cells as the anti-Ran-2 Ab used to select against astrocytes and meningeal cells recognizes a protein sensitive to trypsinization.

5. Allow the tissue chunks to incubate for 1 h at 37°C in the papain solution.

6. Add to this cell suspension 0.04 mg/ml of bovine pancreatic DNase, also made up in D-MEM. Leave for 5 min. Spin cells as described, resuspend in 1 ml D-MEM-BS, and triturate through fine needles. As for the preparation of mixed cultures, *this is a critical stage in this preparation*, and the foregoing comments also are applicable here. Start with 19-g needles and take the tissue through gently once or twice, being careful to avoid introducing air bubbles into the fluid. Proceed to three or four gentle passes through a 23-g needle, then six to ten gentle passes through a 27-g needle.

7. The suspension of cells then is topped up to 5 ml and added to the first panning dish, which is Ran-2 for negative selection against astrocytes and meningeal cells.

8. Leave for 20 min at 37°C and gently shake the plate from time to time.

9. Take away the supernatant and add this supernatant to the second negative selection plate (anti-GalC). In addition, wash the Ran-2 plate with 1 ml of D-MEM-BS and add these cells to the second dish.

10. Incubate again for 20 min, gently shaking the plate again from time to time.

11. Remove the supernatant, which is now highly enriched (by virtue of negative selection) for O-2A lineage cells and add to the third A2B5 or O4 dish. This time, do not wash the plate, as the oligodendrocytes come off too easily.

12. After 20 min, again with gentle shaking of the plate from time to time, discard the supernatant, as the O-2A progenitor cells have now stuck to the plate. Wash with 2 ml of D-MEM-BS and discard this wash.

13. Add 1 ml of D-MEM-BS and gently scrape off the cells with a cell scraper (also known in some countries as a *policeman*, for reasons unknown to us). We use a disposable cell scraper (Costar cat. no. 3010, sterile). Do not use trypsin to remove the cells, as this leads to a decrease in cell viability. Check whether all cells have been removed from the plate, put the medium into a bijou, and count a representative droplet of the cells on a hemocytometer.

a. Do not spin the cells down or all of them will be lost.

b. The yield that can be expected is 2×10^5 pure O-2A progenitor cells from an initial 2×10^6 mixed cells from optic nerves dissected from twenty 7-day-old rat pups. In isolating cells from optic nerves of younger animals, the yield of O-2A progenitor cells is reduced, because they are proportionally less well-represented in the optic nerve. A higher cell number can be obtained by using O4 antibody to positively select cells from the entire brain (with the olfactory bulbs removed). Again, the total number of cells obtained is higher if 7-day-old rat pups are used, but useful numbers of cells can be obtained from younger animals.

TROUBLESHOOTING

If cells are not sticking to the panning dishes, the most likely problem is that the antibody concentrations are too low. Another possible reason is that nonspecific sites have not been saturated completely during the BSA step. In either case, increase the concentration of antibody or BSA, respectively. Another possible problem might be that cells are dead after scraping them off. The most likely explanation for this is that you used too much force or you used the wrong scraper. Another possibility is that the procedure has taken too long, in which case add PDGF and NAC after the collagenase step. This also helps to prevent cells from differentiating prematurely. If, at the end of the panning procedure, viable cells remain but are not pure, it may be that antibody concen-

trations are too low on the dishes used for negative selection. As for growth of O-2A progenitor cells, panning may not work the first time, but persistence should lead to success.

Growth of O-2A Progenitor Cells and Oligodendrocytes

The manner in which cells are grown depends on the experimental questions to be asked. As most of our experimentation is conducted in such a manner as to observe clearly the behavior of single cells and their progeny, most of our methods are specialized for low-density culture. This approach is the most demanding way in which to grow cells, and these techniques work perfectly well with higher-density cultures.

Three general methods enable one to grow progenitor cells as purified populations. One method allows expansion of progenitor populations, the second allows analysis of the behavior of clones undergoing both expansion and differentiation, and the third generates pure populations of oligodendrocytes or type-2 astrocytes.

In all cases, barring the generation of type-2 astrocytes, cells are grown in D-MEM-BS on PLL-coated glass coverslips, slide flasks, tissue-culture flasks, and the like. To generate type-2 astrocytes, in contrast, cells simply are grown in D-MEM containing 10% FCS (D-MEM-FCS).

EXPANSION OF PURE POPULATIONS OF O-2A PROGENITOR CELLS

To expand pure populations of O-2A progenitors, two different growth conditions can be used. Both of these conditions promote the continuous division of O-2A progenitor cells while preventing the generation of oligodendrocytes.

1. Cells can be exposed to 10 ng/ml PDGF + 10 ng/ml bFGF while growing in D-MEM-BS. Fresh growth factors need to be added at least every other day, and preferably every day. In general, it is best to feed cultures by replacing only half of the medium at any feeding; this replacement of medium should be carried out every other day. This method, originally described in Bögler et al. (1990), has been used to generate expanded populations of O-2A progenitor cells that are capable of forming oligodendrocytes and remyelinating demyelinated axons in experimental lesions in vivo (Groves et al., 1993). It is striking, however, that cells grown in this way

change with time in culture and eventually become unable to respond to PDGF when applied in the absence of bFGF. Our interpretation of these results is that the biological clock that appears to limit the mitotic lifespan of O-2A progenitor cells dividing in response to PDGF continues to measure elapsed time even when differentiation is blocked by the presence of both mitogens (Bögler and Noble, 1994; see also Ibarolla et al., 1996).

2. A second way to expand O-2A progenitor populations is to grow them in the presence of 10 ng/ml PDGF + 5 ng/ml NT-3 in chemically-defined medium containing no thyroid hormone. It appears at present that cells grown in this manner are able to maintain a rapid rate of division for a longer period than are cells grown in the presence of PDGF + bFGF. Little is known, however, about the ability of these cells to function normally in vivo following transplantation.

GROWTH OF O-2A PROGENITORS ON ASTROCYTE MONOLAYERS
To study differentiation in a manner that may be related to events in vivo, O-2A progenitors can be grown on monolayers of purified cortical astrocytes, in the presence of astrocyte-conditioned medium (Noble and Murray, 1984), or in medium supplemented with 10 ng/ml of PDGF (a potent O-2A progenitor mitogen secreted by purified cortical astrocytes; Noble et al., 1988; Raff et al., 1988; Richardson et al., 1988). Embryonic O-2A progenitor cells grown in this manner generate oligodendrocytes with a timing similar to that which occurs in vivo (Raff et al., 1985, 1988). In general, it is critical in these experiments that fresh PDGF be added every day, although in extremely-low-density cultures, it is possible to add fresh PDGF every other day. If cultures are being grown in astrocyte-conditioned medium (but not in the presence of astrocytes), we also refeed every day.

PURE CULTURES OF OLIGODENDROCYTES
To generate pure cultures of oligodendrocytes, it is only necessary to deprive O-2A progenitor cells of mitogen while they are growing in chemically-defined medium. Then they will differentiate into oligodendrocytes within 3 days. It is important to note, however, that if they have been grown in the presence of bFGF, it is necessary to trypsinize the cells lightly to remove the bFGF (which binds to the extracellular matrix; Bögler et al., 1990).

PURE CULTURES OF TYPE-2 ASTROCYTES

To generate pure cultures of type-2 astrocytes, it is necessary to expose freshly isolated and purified O-2A progenitor cells to 10% FCS (Raff et al., 1983a,b) or other fetal sera (Raff, Abney, et al., 1983). For reasons we do not understand, cultures grown in PDGF + bFGF for extended periods generate many oligodendrocytes when this switch is made, thus precluding the use of cultures expanded in this manner for the generation of large quantities of type-2 astrocytes.

Analysis of Oligodendrocyte Death Induced by Growth Factor Withdrawal or Exposure to Cytotoxic Agents

Cell death in the O-2A lineage has been studied both as a function of withdrawal of survival factors and as a response to cytotoxic agents. In both cases, purified cells are grown at low density (≤ 3000 cells per 13-mm glass coverslip). To study the death of oligodendrocytes, purified progenitor cells are induced first to differentiate by growth in chemically-defined medium in the absence of mitogens for 48 to 72 h. In respect to killing by TNF-α, it is important to note that not all investigators have succeeded in obtaining this killing. For example, we tried for 2 years to get TNF-α to kill oligodendrocytes before we started to see a cytotoxic effect routinely. Once we began conducting experiments on pure cultures, in which O-2A progenitor cells were first immunopurified and then allowed to differentiate, killing was observed routinely. In light of our findings that a variety of agents can protect against this cytotoxicity, we suspect that in mixed cultures contributions from other cells may contribute to protection of oligodendrocytes in a manner that is not reproducible between different laboratories.

MTT STAINING

MTT staining is used to discriminate between live and dead cells. First described 1983 by Mosmann, this is a chemical reaction using MTT [3-(4,5-dimethylthiazol-2yl)-2,5-diphenyltetrazolium bromide, Sigma]. The tetrazolium ring is cleaved by active mitochondria into a dark blue formazan product. The staining can be combined with fluorsecence staining using standard immunofluorescence protocols.

To carry out MTT staining, proceed as follows:

1. Stain living (unfixed) cells only.
2. Add to each coverslip or staining dish one-tenth of volume of MTT solution for 30 to 60 min. (MTT solution: Dissolve 5 mg/ml MTT in PBS. Filter, store in the dark, and use within a week.)
3. Count cells under the microscope using bright-field optics. Live cells will appear dark blue, whereas dead cells will be unstained.

Note: Do not wait too long before analyzing the cells, as the MTT reaction eventually will proceed to crystal formation.

DEATH FROM CYTOTOXIC AGENTS
To study death in response to cytotoxic agents, such as TNF-α, experiments are conducted as follows (Mayer and Noble, 1994):

1. Add TNF-α at the desired concentration to oligodendrocytes growing at low density in chemically defined medium.
2. Leave cultures for 48 h.
3. Label cultures with MTT.
4. To combine MTT labeling with immunofluorescence, cells can be fixed with 4% paraformaldehyde and stained with antigalactocerebroside antibodies, using our standard staining protocols. We have not found this procedure to be entirely satisfactory, as it appears that the MTT reaction product can wash out of cells fixed in this manner. At a minimum, it appears to be necessary to analyze the cultures as rapidly as possible. For experiments in which it is desirable to study direct effects, it is best to use purified cells and simply to label the cultures with MTT and count them without delay.

DEATH FROM WITHDRAWAL OF TROPHIC FACTORS
The study of cell death in response to withdrawal of trophic factors is carried out in a manner similar to the foregoing, except that cells are removed from chemically defined medium and are grown in D-MEM with no additives. If no survival factors are added, essentially all cells die within 48 to 72 h. Cells can be rescued by such proteins as insulin, IGF-1, CNTF, and LIF. In addition, it is possible to rescue cells by addition of cocktails of antioxidants with or without progesterone. Details of these experiments are provided in Mayer and Noble (1994).

Protocol Section V. Preparation of Primary Cultures of Adult Rat Optic Nerve

As described in the text, the properties of O-2A progenitor cells isolated from adult animals are different from those isolated from perinatal animals. The differing biology of the O-2A[adult] progenitor cells makes them intrinsically interesting. It is interesting also to understand how precursor cell properties change in association with aging of an animal. In addition, any attempts to understand damage and repair in the adult animal by using cellular biological analysis require an understanding of those precursor cell populations that are in fact present in adult tissues.

1. Dissect optic nerves from rats that are at least 3 months old. Although 0-2A progenitor cells can be isolated from rats that are 3 to 19 months old, their yield diminishes with age.

2. Remove the chiasm and the meninges and mince the tissue finely, as in instructions for other tissues.

3. Transfer the minced tissue to a vial containing 1 ml collagenase (333 IU/ml; Worthington Biochemical Corporation, Freehold, NJ) in Leibovitz L-15 medium (Gibco) and incubate for 60 to 90 min at 37°C. It is important to note that some batches of collagenase can be toxic to 0-2A lineage cells, an effect that is more readily apparent in adult-derived cultures (perhaps owing to the intrinsically lower cell numbers available).

4. Add 1 ml (30,000 IU/ml) bovine pancreas trypsin type III (Sigma) in CMF D-MEM and incubate the tissue for 20 min at 37°C.

5. Spin for 2 min at $3000 \times g$, remove the supernatant, and incubate the tissue for a further 20 min at 37°C in 1 ml trypsin and 1 ml .05 mM EDTA.

6. To terminate the enzymatic digestion, add 4 ml SBTI-DNase [5200 IU/ml soybean trypsin inhibitor (Sigma), 74 IU/ml bovine pancreas DNase (Sigma), and 3.0 mg/ml BSA fraction V (Sigma) in D-MEM] and triturate the tissue through a 5-ml blowout pipette.

7. Spin the suspension for 2 min at $3000 \times g$ and resuspend the pellet in 1 ml D-MEM + 10% FCS.

8. Dissociate the tissue by gentle trituration through a 1-ml pipette, followed by 23-G, 25-G, and 27-G hypodermic needles attached to a 1-ml syringe.

9. Dilute the suspension further in D-MEM + 10% FCS and plate it in 100-µl drops onto round PLL-coated (20 µg/ml, Sigma) glass coverslips (13-mm diameter) placed on platforms. The presence of 10% FCS in the plating medium prevents most of the debris and myelin

from sticking to the coverslips. Owing to the large amount of debris and myelin in the cell suspension, it is difficult to assess the cell yield accurately. Therefore, plate the cell suspension derived from one pair of adult optic nerves onto 10 to 14 coverslips (50–100 0-2A progenitor cells per coverslip).

10. After 1 to 2 h at 37°C, rinse the coverslips in vials containing Leibovitz L-15 medium (Gibco) and place coverslips in the appropriate culture medium.

11. Change two-thirds of the culture medium twice weekly.

19 Tissue Culture Methods for the Study of Myelination

Naomi Kleitman, Patrick M. Wood, and Richard P. Bunge

Many new insights into the mechanisms of myelination have come from studies of myelinating cells and neuronal populations in tissue culture. This chapter first provides a brief review of the history and the use of myelinating tissue cultures during the last 40 years, then describes methods currently in use in our laboratory to attain myelination reliably in culture. The neuronal preparation we use is derived from the embryonic rat dorsal root ganglion (DRG). As these neurons have both central and peripheral myelinated processes in situ, they have been a uniquely valuable and biologically relevant system for the study of myelination in tissue culture. We describe methods for explant culture of these ganglia and for the isolation of a pure neuronal population attained in vitro by the elimination of dividing nonneuronal cells. Using a variety of techniques, we concurrently develop highly purified populations of Schwann cells and of oligodendrocytes. After reintroduction of these myelinating cell types into the neuronal cultures, specialized media can be used to stimulate myelination. The description of these methods is followed by a review of results of recent experiments using this culture system, results that have provided unexpected new insights into the characteristics of myelinating cells.

At the outset, we point out that, for the purposes of this chapter, we define myelin as the compacted membrane deposited segmentally along an axon capable of inducing myelin formation. A variety of cells form membranous aggregates (either extra- or intracellularly) often called *myelin figures*, which are related to the specific and complex configuration of the myelin sheath only by the fact that the membrane components are compacted. Also, oligodendrocytes without axonal contact often generate membranous sheets or whorls (Podulso and Norton, 1972; Yim et al., 1986), which may be useful in basic studies of membrane assembly. For physiological function in mediating saltatory conduction, however, myelin segments of a characteristic spiraled configuration must be deposited systematically along an axon; it is this configuration that we define here as *myelin*.

A Brief History of Myelin Formation in Culture

The first description of myelin formation in tissue culture appeared in 1955 (Peterson and Murray, 1955). Despite this substantial history, the consistent and predictable attainment of myelination in culture has been achieved in relatively few laboratories. (For an earlier general review see Bunge, 1975.) The culture conditions required are exacting, and generally the cultures must be maintained for extended periods (several weeks) to allow full development of the cellular interactions resulting in myelination. Earlier culture preparations of nondividing cells (such as neurons) often were short-lived (several days), allowing landmark observations on growth cone activity (Harrison, 1907) but only limited observations on mechanisms of development requiring interaction between different cell types. As media definition improved, along with the introduction of more stable substrata, cultures could be maintained for the extended periods required for the neuronal and neuroglial maturation required for myelination. A publication by Peterson and Murray (1955) described the formation of myelin sheaths in long-term explant cultures prepared from embryonic avian spinal ganglia. Two years later, Dr. Walter Hild (1957) described myelinogenesis in central nervous system (CNS) cultures prepared from mammalian embryonic or neonatal tissues. Peterson and Murray (1955) used the then popular Maximow double-coverslip chamber and plasma clots in their first preparations of avian ganglia. Hild's approach was to use a rolling drum into which sealed tubes containing media and coverslips were placed. The tissue was bathed continually with the culture medium as the tube slowly rotated. The introduction of the use of reconstituted rat tail collagen as a substratum for the long-term culture of neural tissue (Bornstein, 1958) represented a considerable improvement on these early techniques. The collagen substrata currently used in our laboratory are discussed in detail later.

A description of the preparations available during the first decade of the study of myelination in culture and the principal uses to which these preparations were put is given in a chapter by Dr. Margaret Murray in Willmer's three-volume treatise (1965) on cells and tissues in culture. These early workers focused on establishing complex preparations in which the cellular interrelationships for which the nervous system is so well-known would be preserved maximally in culture. The neural tissue generally was not

dissociated prior to being placed in culture but was set out as pre-organized explants in which much of the subsequent tissue development occurred within the substance of the explant. Myelination in sensory ganglia was an exception; in these cultures, much of the myelination occurred in outgrowth regions. These early preparations often were referred to as *organotypic*. In ensuing years, these preparations were used only occasionally in the study of the genesis of the myelin sheath (for review, see Bunge et al., 1989). Instead, much of the work using these culture techniques concentrated on the study of agents that might damage neural tissue, particularly those that specifically might damage the myelin sheath. Bornstein (1973) and Seil et al. (1975) (among others) used organotypic myelinated CNS cultures for the study of toxic agents in the serum of animals with experimental allergic encephalomyelitis and also in patients with neurological diseases. At that time, essentially all studies of myelination in neural tissue grown in culture were being undertaken in the Maximow double-coverslip assembly, with modifications of the technique initially used by Peterson and Murray (1955). Although the use of the Maximow system continued until fairly recently in a few laboratories (e.g., see Seil and Agrawal, 1984; Wolff et al., 1986; Balentine et al., 1988), these chambers are expensive and, currently, difficult or impossible to obtain. They are used little in myelination studies at the present time. An extensive review of the physiology of cells and tissues established in tissue culture in Maximow assemblies is provided by Crain (1976).

Some of the contributions of this earlier era include the following. There was a clearer definition of the medium requirements for both peripheral and central myelination in culture, establishing that increased glucose levels (as high as 6 g/L) were beneficial for myelination. In addition to the usual serum requirements, chick embryo extract was found to be required for optimal peripheral myelination in culture (Peterson and Murray, 1960). During this era, it was first demonstrated clearly that interneuronal synaptic contacts and neuromuscular junctions (Fischbach et al., 1974; for review, see Nelson, 1975) could be formed in culture. It was demonstrated also that the serum of patients with a variety of neurological diseases contained elements that were toxic to myelin sheaths in culture and, furthermore, that after damage to myelin sheaths in culture, it was possible to observe the phenomenon of remyelination (Peterson and Murray, 1955; Bornstein, 1973).

A New Culture System

In the period 1975 to 1985, we developed a culture system in which sensory ganglia from rat embryos are used as the source of a stable neuronal population for the study of both central and peripheral myelination in vitro. Because DRG neurons have large axons that course both in the peripheral nervous system (PNS) and the CNS, this single neuronal type has the capability of inducing myelination by either Schwann cells or by oligodendrocytes. As currently employed, the culture system is initiated by plating cell suspensions of dissociated DRGs from 15-day rat embryos onto collagen-coated dishes. These cultures subsequently are treated with antimitotic agents to kill all nonneuronal cells. Purified populations of the desired myelin-forming cells, either Schwann cells or oligodendrocytes, then are added back to the neuronal cultures to obtain either peripheral or central myelination in culture.

This culture system evolved from studies of the use of antimitotic agents to remove the nonneuronal cells from culture dishes containing DRG explants (Wood, 1976). In experimenting with the commonly used antimitotic agent fluorodeoxyuridine (FdU), it was observed that certain treatment regimens effectively suppressed the development of populations of fibroblasts but spared a small number of Schwann cells along with the neuronal population. If the DRGs so treated then were transplanted to a new culture dish to allow a new outgrowth of neurites, the emerging neurites would prompt a renewed period of Schwann cell proliferation. This resulted, in a reasonable percentage of cases, in a DRG culture with an outgrowth populated by Schwann cells and free of fibroblasts. We call this preparation a *Schwann cell progenitor*; it can be used to obtain pure populations of Schwann cells by excising the centrally located aggregate containing the neuronal somata while retaining the Schwann cell-rich outgrowth (see later). Alternatively, if the neuron-Schwann cell cultures are left intact and allowed to mature in appropriate culture media, these cultures provide a richly myelinated outgrowth useful for a number of studies.

This peripheral myelinating system first was established by using whole explants of embryonic ganglia; later, it was modified with the use of dissociation techniques to separate the neuronal somata. Plating the neurons in a dissociated state allowed for the elimination of all nonneuronal cells, resulting in a pure neuronal cell population. If these dissociated neurons were plated out over the entire culture surface, however, the option of later removing them from

the dish by microincision was lost. Therefore, now we routinely use an intermediate approach, dissociating the neuronal somata initially and plating them onto the culture dish such that their attachment is confined to the central one-fourth of the culture vessel (see later). As this neuronal population subsequently undergoes axonal extension, two distinct regions are formed: a central neuronal region and a region of extensive outgrowth wherein axons can interact with added Schwann cells under conditions that allow close observation of the cellular interactions that occur. Substantially more myelin is produced in dissociated preparations than in explant cultures. Once the neuronal population is treated to eliminate nonneuronal cells, one has the option subsequently of adding populations of oligodendrocytes or astrocytes instead of or in addition to Schwann cells. For example, recently we have used this type of preparation to study the influences of astrocytes on oligodendrocyte or Schwann cell myelination (Rosen et al., 1989; Guénard et al., 1994).

This approach, then, uses a single neuronal population to drive the activity of either peripheral or central myelinating cells added to the culture dish. This system has several advantages, including the fact that in neuron-Schwann cell cultures, the absence of fibroblasts eliminates cellular barriers between the myelinating Schwann cell-axon unit and the culture medium. This action allows ready access of antibodies and other probes in the culture medium to the axon-Schwann cell unit and allows studies of the effect of such antibodies on axon-Schwann cell interactions. Surface antigens can be detected immunocytochemically by direct application of antibodies to living cultures without the need for permeabilization. These cultures are suitable also for in situ hybridization techniques to detect messenger RNA synthesis (Fernandez-Valle, et al., 1993). Such experiments are problematical if an ensheathing cellular mantle is allowed to form from fibroblasts in cultures containing neurons and Schwann cells (the in vitro version of the perineurium; Mithen et al., 1982) or from astrocytes in cultures containing neurons and oligodendrocytes (P. Wood, unpublished observations).

In recent studies, we have expanded the culture system and adapted it to the study of adult-derived rat and human Schwann cells (Morrissey et al., 1991, 1995a,b). Prompted by observations that Schwann cells play critical roles in regeneration after injury in the peripheral nervous system and can induce axonal regeneration

in the CNS (for review, see Guénard et al., 1993), our goal was to acquire and test adult Schwann cells that could be used for autotransplantation. Although now we have succeeded in obtaining myelination of DRG axons by human Schwann cells in vitro (described later), human cell population dynamics required some modifications of our Schwann cell acquisition and culture techniques (Morrissey et al., 1995b).

Protocols for Preparing Cultures and Inducing Myelination

Housing the Cultures

The Maximow double coverslip assembly allowed the successful maintenance of small fragments of tissue for several months and permitted ready microscopic visualization of the tissue with excellent optics. However, the maintenance of such cultures required repeated disassembly and reassembly of the chamber, which severely limited the number of cultures available for experimentation. Furthermore, the amount of tissue was limited to that which could be maintained in a single drop of culture medium. To circumvent these problems, we developed a small plastic "minidish" with an area 25 mm in diameter (similar in size to the carrying coverslip of the Maximow double coverslip assembly but with raised edges to better contain the culture medium; Bunge and Wood, 1973). These dishes hold up to 1 ml of medium, but we routinely use 0.25 to 0.5 ml to incubate cultures.

Our initial purpose in modifying the basic Maximow culture approach was to allow for some increase in the amount of medium used and thus allow larger amounts of tissue to be maintained. This purpose had to be balanced against considerations that involved retaining the principle of a limited feed volume: (1) Sometimes, cultures are maintained for extended periods, and medium components may not be available in large quantities; (2) cultured neural tissue may benefit from a degree of self-conditioning of its medium; (3) some cultures appear to develop better with a shallow overlay of medium, presumably because of better gas exchange with the atmosphere; and (4) expensive drugs or scarce antibodies to be supplied in the culture medium are applied most advantageously in a small medium volume. Another practical consideration affect-

ing the size of the culture was that smaller "aliquots" of tissue allow more variables per experiment and more cultures per variable. Finally, we wanted to retain the capability of observing the living explant at the higher magnifications with an inverted compound microscope (which requires a relatively thin supporting plastic or glass culture base).

We have found that an ideal dish size for the study of myelination in culture is approximately 1 inch in diameter. To facilitate ultrastructural analysis, we sought a culture dish that would enable us to fix and process intact cultures for electron microscopy. For this, we required a dish in which cultures could be grown successfully and subsequently could be fixed, dehydrated, and embedded. To attain this kind of culture vessel, we have found it advantageous to make our own small culture dishes from a clear inert plastic film (5 mils thick) made of a fluorocarbon designated Aclar 33C (Allied Fibers and Plastics, Pottsville, PA). The dishes are molded from precut circles of this plastic to provide miniature culture dishes with a 25-mm diameter and walls 4 mm high. Aclar 33C may be molded by pressure-forming with a machined aluminum punch and die. The punch is heated (it is wrapped with heating tape regulated with a rheostat), and the plastic film is molded by pressing the film into the die (which is at room temperature). The temperature of the punch and duration of the pressure application are adjusted to produce symmetrical dishes with flat bottoms. These small Aclar dishes are cleaned by soaking for 3 days either in concentrated (70%) nitric acid or 0.5 M sodium hydroxide in 95% ethanol. They undergo a series of rinses in running tap-distilled water, then are soaked overnight in double-distilled water. The acid-washed dishes should be soaked overnight also in 100% ethanol. All dishes are sterilized in 80% ethanol. Before use, the dishes are dried in a sterile hood and coated with collagen (described later).

Cultures plated in Aclar minidishes are housed in groups of four to six in 100 × 10 mm glass or plastic Petri dishes (figure 19.1) and are monitored at low magnifications with an inverted compound microscope. For high-magnification viewing, long-working-distance objectives may be used, or the minidish can be transferred to sterile plastic Petri dishes fitted on the bottom with No. 1 glass coverslips. Used in this manner, the Aclar dish provides for all the aforementioned advantages and has, in addition, the advantages that (1) its bottom can be cut out after fixation and used as a coverslip to carry the cultures through various staining procedures and (2) the

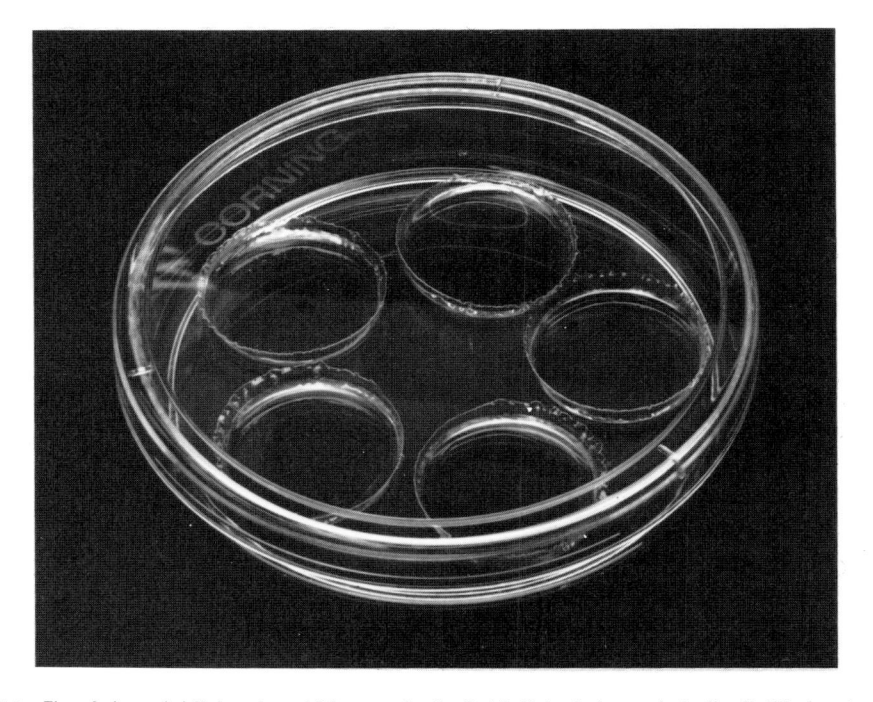

Figure 19.1 Five Aclar minidishes in a 100-mm plastic Petri dish. A drop of sterile distilled water is placed below each Aclar dish to hold it in place.

inert plastic readily peels off the polymerized resins used in electron microscopy. The latter characteristic allows embedment of the tissue for electron microscopy directly in the dish. This type of flat (2- to 3-mm-thick) embedment allows one to review the tissue after it is in plastic and to mark specific regions of the culture (even specific myelin segments) for electron microscopic analysis (Bunge et al., 1989).

Alternatively, we use standard polystyrene plastic culture dishes or multiwell dishes as culture vessels. One should be aware that plastics not specifically designed for tissue-culture use may release a volatile material that can be toxic to neuronal tissue (Mithen et al., 1980), especially when the tissue is incubated in the small desiccators used in our closed culture system (see later). Plastics currently manufactured specifically for tissue-culture use have not been toxic to our cultures, even though one can smell the plastic odor on opening a desiccator. One may also use acid-washed glass or Aclar coverslips inside Aclar minidishes or in multiwell dishes. Coverslips are collagen-coated before being placed into the housing dishes. A serious disadvantage, however, is inherent in using

multiwell dishes for long-term cultures requiring frequent feeding: The frequent handling may lead in time to sporadic infections that, in multiwell dishes, are difficult to contain and eradicate.

Recently, we have modified the disposition of the cultures to allow the efficient application of molecular biological techniques in studies of myelination. Techniques such as those used for in situ hybridization, involving several rinsing steps, frequently led to detachment and loss of the neurons and myelin from collagen-coated dishes or coverslips. For these studies, the dissociated DRG suspensions now are plated onto 12- or 22-mm glass coverslips coated with poly-L-lysine (PLL) and mouse laminin as described later (see the section titled Substratum Preparation). Before use, each coverslip is scrubbed vigorously with Alconox detergent (10% solution), rinsed exhaustively with water, and sterilized in 80% ethanol. The coverslips are placed and maintained in 100 mm Corning tissue-culture dishes lined with 90-mm-diameter circles made of 5-mil-thick Teflon film (Dupont, Wilmington, DE). The use of Teflon promotes retention of the medium on the coverslip and prevents spreading of medium between coverslips. Cultures on 12-mm coverslips can be maintained for several weeks by feeding three times weekly with two drops (100 µl) of medium. Both Schwann cell and oligodendrocyte myelination can be studied by using PLL-laminin-coated coverslips. The small medium volume required makes this system ideal for use in antibody blocking and immunocytochemical studies as well.

For routine maintenance, the culture dishes may be segregated in closed, humidified desiccator jars. A major advantage of this technique is that the evaporation from the culture media which occurs in flow-through carbon dioxide incubators is minimized, permitting long-term maintenance of a low medium-to-tissue ratio. This system also allows for the concurrent use of different culture media with varying serum concentrations that require different gas mixtures. In the event that a mold or fungal infection is introduced, the segregation of cultures helps to minimize the number of cultures affected. The desiccator jars (no. 3118, 160-mm Pyrex, Corning Glass Works, Corning, NY) are cleaned thoroughly with alcohol and then are autoclaved. Sterile water is added to the bottom of the jar to provide a humidified atmosphere. High-vacuum grease (Dow Corning Corp,. Midland, MI) is used to seal ground-glass surfaces. Depending on the type of medium in use (see later), carbon dioxide is added via the glass side arm (normally used for air removal) to

maintain pH 7.2 to 7.4. In this pH range, media containing phenol red will have a salmon color. The amount of carbon dioxide required depends on the concentration of bicarbonate in the particular culture medium. The amount of serum added to a standard medium decreases the amount of carbon dioxide required; therefore, different medium formulations (e.g., Eagle's minimum essential medium versus Dulbecco's modified formulation) differ significantly in their carbon dioxide requirement. After the carbon dioxide is added, the desiccator jars are sealed and placed in a large forced-draft incubator at 37°C.

Cultures used for myelination studies may be housed also in well-humidified, water-jacketed carbon dioxide incubators. For maintenance over several weeks, the cultures should be fed with enough medium and with a frequency (three times weekly) to prevent drying. Conditions of 6% CO_2 atmosphere and 37°C work well for most myelinating cultures.

Substratum Preparation

COLLAGEN SUBSTRATUM

The culture substratum for long-term cultures must be durable, suitable for neuronal outgrowth, and compatible with various types of nonneuronal cell attachment. When used by themselves, substrata such as the popular polyamino acids tend to deteriorate after several weeks in culture, prior to the commencement of the process of myelination. Reconstituted rat tail collagen is, in our experience, the most generally suitable substratum; however, coverslips coated with PLL-laminin can be used as well (see later). We have found no commercial collagen preparation that is satisfactory.

Collagen is prepared by a modification of the method of Bornstein (1958). Because standardization of this procedure has proved to be critical for obtaining consistent culture results, our methods are given here in detail. Tails from 9-month- to 1-year-old male rats are removed, washed, and sterilized carefully with antiseptic soap and 80% alcohol followed by a rinse in sterile distilled water. (Results are more variable if female rats are used.) Then the tails are frozen for 24 h on filter paper in a Petri dish. Thereafter, they are sterilized by immersion in 80% alcohol for 15 min and allowed to dry. Sterility is maintained in all following steps; if the collagen is contaminated, it cannot be sterilized subsequently.

Removing the tendons requires two people. The tail is picked up 1 to 1.5 cm from the small end with a strong hemostat (figure 19.2A). One to two millimeters distal to the point where the hemostat is applied, the skin is abrased crudely with a bone-cutting forceps. The object now is to fracture the vertebrae of the tail without cutting the tendons that run from the pelvic muscle along the entire tail and attach to each vertebra. This process is accomplished by gripping the distal fragment of the tail firmly with the bone forceps, thereby cutting into or through the skin, then rocking the bone forceps to and fro against the hemostat to tear the skin and fracture the vertebrae. As the vertebral fragment is cracked free and pulled away slowly to separate it from the rest of the tail, the attached tendons are pulled out with it and can hang free from the detached fragment (see figure 19.2B). An assistant then cuts the tendons free with fine scissors and places them in a preweighed dish of double-distilled water. Moving 1.5 cm toward the larger end of the tail, the procedure is repeated until the last of the tail is used. The weight of the tendons is determined by reweighing the dish; thus, it is important that no water is lost from the preweighed dish during the addition of tendons. The average yield from one tail is 0.7 to 0.8 g of tendons.

The tendons are extracted by transfer into a sterile aqueous solution of 0.1% acetic acid. The ratio of acetic acid solution to tendon weight is standardized at 150 ml/1 g tendons. The tendons are extracted for 5 days at 4°C with daily agitation to achieve thorough mixing. The tendons swell and release soluble collagen into the extract. The mixture is transferred to sterile 50-ml polycarbonate centrifuge tubes (Nalge no. 3138-0050) and centrifuged at 30,000× g for 30 min, and the supernatant is harvested. Before use, the extract is dialyzed (dialysis tubing no. 8-667D, Fisher Scientific, Pittsburgh, PA) against 50 volumes of sterile double-distilled water for 18 h at 4°C. The collagen is removed from the dialysis bags, aliquoted into sterile containers, and tested for sterility in soy broth. It may be stored for up to several months at 4°C (or indefinitely if frozen at −70°C).

Culture dishes are collagen-coated in a laminar flow hood, and all materials used must be sterile. To collagen-coat, culture dishes are placed in the bottom of a 150-mm Petri dish lined with filter paper. Two drops of dialyzed collagen are applied to each 22-mm dish surface and spread evenly, using a "hockey-stick" type spreader made by flaming a disposable Pasteur pipette. The pipette

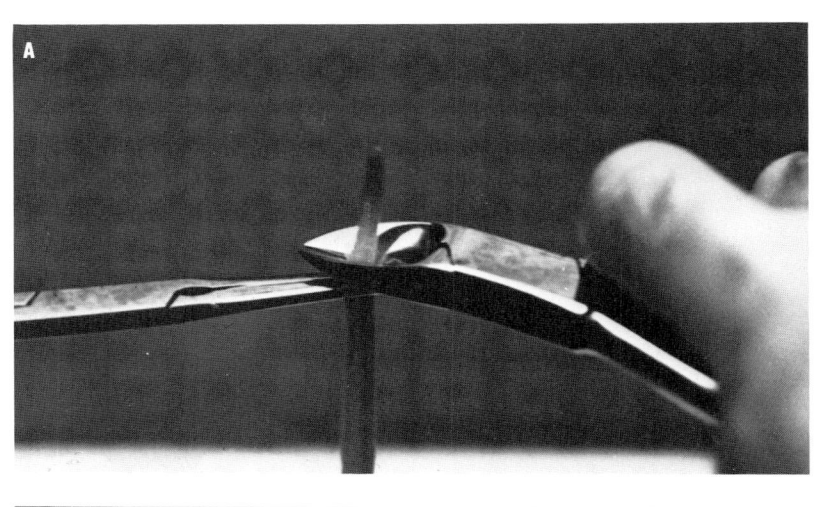

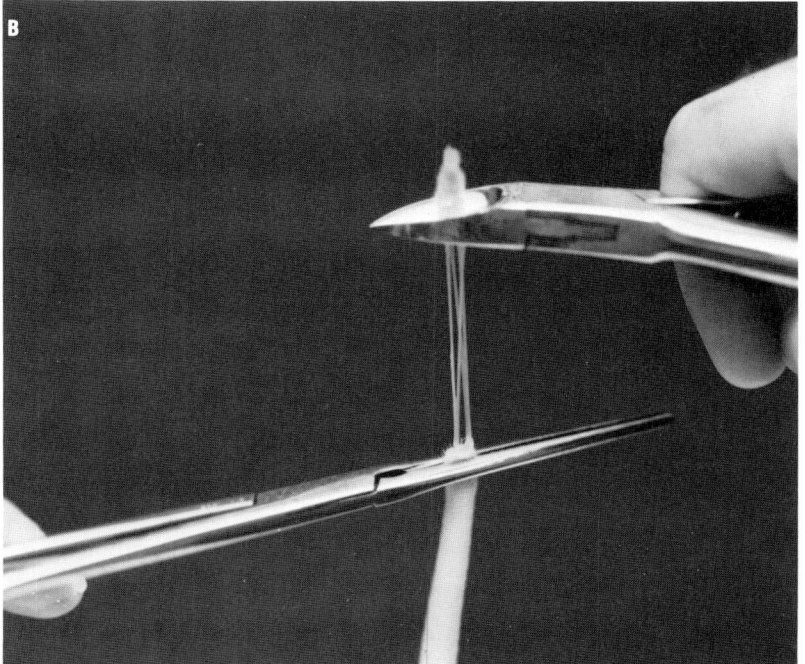

Figure 19.2 Obtaining tendons to prepare collagen. (*A*) A rat tail is grasped with a hemostat 1.5 cm from the tip as bone forceps are applied. The skin is abrased with the forceps, and the tail is fractured by rocking the forceps against the hemostat while cutting superficially into the skin with the forceps. (*B*) After the vertebrae are fractured, the tail fragment is pulled upward, revealing the tendons. Next, the tendons are pulled completely free of the tail, cut, and placed in water as described in the text.

is flamed to close the tip and then, to soften the glass so that it bends at a 45-degree angle, approximately 8 mm from the tip. After spreading the collagen, three drops of concentrated NH_4OH are distributed onto a piece of filter paper lining the bottom of a second 150-mm Petri dish. This dish immediately is inverted over the Petri dish containing the culture dishes, so that the ammonia vapors gel the collagen films below. After the freshly spread collagen has been exposed to ammonia vapor for 2 min, it is allowed to dry completely in the hood. When the collagen film is dried thus, it becomes possible to plate cells in a confined region; because the dried collagen is not easily wettable, a drop of cell suspension placed in the center of the dish remains as placed until the dish is flooded intentionally. Thus, several thousand neurons can be deposited in the disaggregated state but confined to the center of the dish. As will be described in detail later, by the next day the neurons will have attached so that the entire dish surface is flooded with Leibovitz's L-15 medium (see the section titled Other Media), and the culture is refed. The centrally located neurons subsequently develop a neuritic outgrowth that eventually fills the remainder of the dish. (For a discussion of how different collagen surface preparations may vary and the resultant effect on neurite outgrowth, see Roufa et al., 1986.)

POLY-L-LYSINE-LAMININ SUBSTRATUM

Myelinating cultures can also be obtained by using PLL-laminin as a substratum. This substratum is used with glass coverslips only; the coating does not work with Aclar dishes or coverslips. The glass coverslips (12-mm diameter), cleaned and sterilized as described, are placed on the Teflon-lined 100-mm dish. A stock solution containing 20 mg/ml PLL (mol. wt. 30,000–70,000; Sigma, no. P2636) in 0.125 M sodium borate buffer, pH 8.5, is diluted to 0.2 mg/ml PLL with distilled water. The stock PLL solution is filter-sterilized prior to use. Each coverslip is flooded with 150 µl of the diluted PLL solution to cover the glass surface completely. The coverslips are left 45 to 60 min at room temperature in the PLL solution. The coverslips are rinsed three times with 0.05 M sodium carbonate buffer, pH 9.6. The final rinse is replaced with laminin solution. The laminin solution is prepared from frozen (−80°C) mouse laminin aliquots (Collaborative Biomedical Products, Becton Dickinson Labware, Bedford, MA, no. 40232). The frozen aliquot is thawed slowly at 4°C and diluted to 50 µg/ml with ice-cold 0.05 M sodium

carbonate buffer, pH 9.6. All pipettes and pipette tips used for measuring or transferring the laminin solution are prechilled by rinsing with ice-cold water. These precautions are necessary to prevent premature self-assembly or gelation of the concentrated laminin solution. For coating, two drops ($\sim$5 µg of laminin) are placed on each 12-mm coverslip. The coverslips are incubated with the laminin solution for 48 h at 37°C. Before use, the coverslips are rinsed three times with L-15 medium (see the section titled Other Media).

Media Preparation

A variety of media are used in sequence in the purification of neuronal or Schwann cell populations from DRG cultures and to drive Schwann cell function in cultures in which neurons and myelinating cells have been recombined. To avoid repeated freezing and thawing, all these media can be stored in sterile aliquots at -70°C until use, although we routinely refreeze unused portions of the aliquots one time. We do not find it necessary to add antibiotics or antimycotic agents to our culture media if proper sterile technique is observed during medium preparation and handling of cultures.

Standard feed formulations used in the protocols described later are listed in table 19.1. As mentioned, housing isolated culture series in humidified desiccator jars allows for fine control of the carbon dioxide environment, which is critical for the maintenance of a pH of 7.2 to 7.4. Factors affecting the pH of the cultures include the base feed selected, the density of cells per culture, and the concentration of serum in the medium (see earlier section titled Housing the Cultures for more detail). Traditionally, we have used carbon dioxide concentrations ranging from 4% for serum-rich or densely plated cultures to 7% for cultures in defined media. We currently maintain most cultures in water-jacketed carbon dioxide incubators calibrated to 6% CO_2 and 37°C.

MAINTENANCE FEEDS

Our standard maintenance medium is denoted *C feed* and contains either human placental serum (HPS) or fetal bovine serum (FBS). The source species and percentage of serum are denoted in subscripts (H and B, respectively) in table 19.1 and in following descriptions. When purified neuronal preparations are to be carried for some time without added Schwann cells, it is necessary to use a

Table 19.1

	BASE MEDIUM	SERUM	NERVE GROWTH FACTOR	SUPPLEMENTS
Maintenance feeds				
C_{H5}, C_{B5}	E-MEM	5% HPS or FBS	Crude NGF	Glucose (498 mg/dl)
D_{10}	D-MEM	10% FBS	—	—
DM	1:1 D-MEM-Ham's F-12	—	2.5S NGF	Insulin (5 mg/L; Sigma, no. I-5500) Chrompure rat transferrin (10 mg/L; Jackson Immunores, no. 012-000-050) Putrescine (100 µM; Sigma, no. P-7507) Progesterone (20 nM; Sigma, no. P-8783) Sodium selenite (30 nM; Pfaltz & Bauer, no. S-07150)
Fibroblast elimination				
C_F	E-MEM	5% HPS	Crude NGF	Glucose (498 mg/dl) 10 µM uridine (Sigma, no. U-3003) 10 µM FdU (Sigma, no. F-0503)
E_2F	E-MEM	—	2.5S NGF	Glucose (498 mg/dl) DM supplements (see above) 10 µM uridine, 10 µM FdU
Myelinating feeds				
MF (Schwann cells)	E-MEM	15% FBS	Crude NGF	Glucose (498 mg/dl) L-Ascorbic acid (Sigma no. A-4544)
O (oligodendrocytes)	1:1 D-MEM-Ham's F12	2% FBS	Crude NGF	DM supplements (see above)

E-MEM, Eagle's minimum essential medium (Gibco, no. 11095); D-MEM, Dulbecco's minimum essential medium (Gibco, no. 11965); HPS, human placental serum (heat-inactivated; see text for instructions); FBS, fetal bovine serum (heat-inactivated); NGF, nerve growth factor; FDU, fluorodeoxyuridine.

Notes: Crude NGF (used for serum-containing media) is partially purified from mouse salivary glands in our laboratory and used at an empirically determined optimal concentration; purified 2.5S NGF is obtained from Boehringer-Mannheim (no. 100700) and used at 100 ng/ml. NGF, 2.5S, can be substituted for crude NGF in any medium formulation.

Ham's F12, Gibco, no. 11765.

Progesterone is prepared from a stock in ethanol, 0.0012% vol/vol.

serum-containing medium to maintain the health of the neurons. Such cultures often degenerate in C_{B5}; therefore, we use HPS (C_{H5}, see later) for this purpose. Bovine serum also has proved to interfere with the initial purification with antimitotic medium, so traditionally we used HPS (C_{H10}) during this period.

To prepare HPS, we obtain whole placental blood from a local hospital nursery. Individual samples of clotted blood are centrifuged at 1000 rpm for 15 min to compress the clot as much as possible. The supernatants from several tubes then are combined in 10-ml aliquots. A red color indicates severe hemolysis, and such samples are discarded. The aliquots are recentrifuged at 2500 rpm for 15 min, then the clear yellow-orange liquid is transferred to a fresh tube that is frozen at $-70°C$, then heat-inactivated, as described later. After pooling, the sera again are stored at $-70°C$ in 10-ml aliquots. Due to the potential presence of extremely hazardous blood-borne viruses, use of human sera entails an increasing risk to laboratory personnel. To minimize such risks when human sera are used, they are heat-inactivated in a water bath at a temperature sufficient to destroy human immunodeficiency virus and hepatitis viruses (56°C, 30 min) and to inactivate serum complement (desirable in certain antibody experiments).

ANTIMITOTIC FEED

To eliminate fibroblasts or Schwann cells from DRG cultures, C_H is used alternately with C_F (see table 19.1) following the schedule described later. FBS cannot be substituted satisfactorily for HPS in C_F medium. However, we have obtained promising results by alternating C_{B5} medium with a medium containing FdU and no FBS (E_2F; see table 19.1).

DEFINED MEDIUM

Once purified neuronal populations have been established, Schwann cell populations are added back to these cultures, and they are maintained in a serum-free (defined) medium (DM) in which Schwann cell-neuronal interaction is restricted. The composition of DM is listed in table 19.1. In this medium, Schwann cells do not assemble a basal lamina; they incompletely ensheathe neurites, and they do not form myelin. These cultures are "poised" and will begin myelination promptly if the medium is switched to myelinating medium.

MYELINATING FEEDS

The composition of the medium used to obtain myelination varies depending on the cell type being studied. Our standard myelinating feed, suitable for rat Schwann cells, is denoted *MF* (table 19.1). The ascorbic acid is prepared in a 5-mg/ml aqueous stock (filter-sterilized) immediately before medium preparation. Ascorbate is required to permit Schwann cells to produce triple helical collagens and, hence, a basal lamina, which is a necessary prerequisite for Schwann cell myelination (see later).

Ascorbate is not required for obtaining myelination by rat oligo-dendrocytes (Wood and Bunge, 1986b; Eldridge et al., 1989). Instead, DM medium (described earlier), supplemented with 2% heat-inactivated FBS or HPS, is used. This medium is designated *O medium* (see table 19.1). For obtaining myelination by adult-derived human Schwann cells, the medium used is similar to DM, except that Eagle's MEM is substituted for D-MEM in the base medium, human transferrin (Sigma, no. T-2158) is used instead of rat transferrin, and the medium is supplemented with 498 mg/dl glucose, 10 µg/ml ascorbate, 50 nM laminin (Collaborative Biomedical Products, no. 40232), and 0.25% bovine serum albumin (Calbiochem, no. 12660) and antibiotics.

OTHER MEDIA

In the Brockes method for preparing Schwann cells, we use a Dulbecco's medium base with 10% heat-inactivated FBS (D_{10}). Other solutions used in our laboratory as vehicles and rinsing buffers will be referred to as follows: Hank's calcium- and magnesium-free balanced salt solution (Hank's-CMF; Gibco no. 141700), Earle's balanced salt solution (EBSS; Gibco no. 24010), Leibovitz's L-15 medium (L-15; Gibco no. 11415), and L-15 plus 15% to 20% FBS (L-15-FBS; used to stop trypsin action).

Dorsal Root Ganglion Dissection

A 15-day-pregnant rat (the day after insemination is day 0) is anesthetized with ether and tied to a dissection board, and the abdomen is shaved and washed with antiseptic soap and 80% alcohol. The ether exposure is maintained using a nose-cone, taking care to prevent directly contacting the rat's skin with liquid ether. During the dissection, it is convenient to have a second person available to retract the abdominal muscles as the uterus is removed.

To avoid contamination, we use separate sets of sterile forceps and scissors to cut the skin, muscle, and uterus. The skin over the abdomen is incised and retracted laterally; an approximately 3-inch midline incision then is made in the abdominal wall, taking care not to puncture the bowel. The relatively strong muscles near the cervix are grasped with forceps, and the cervix is cut. The uterus is lifted carefully, cutting it free at the ovaries and removing it entirely without contacting the muscles or skin of the mother. The uterus is placed into a sterilized, filter-paper-lined, 150-cm Petri dish and removed to a sterile hood. While still deeply anesthetized, the mother is killed quickly by cutting through the heart.

With sterile scissors, the uterine walls are incised carefully, and the embryos are freed of the disk-shaped placenta and amniotic sac and removed to a 100-mm plastic Petri dish containing several milliliters of L-15 medium. Sterile procedure is observed in this as in all subsequent steps of the procedure. The embryos may be transferred individually to a second plastic Petri dish for dissection.

It is good practice to confirm and note the actual age of the embryos at this point. On day 15 (E15), the crown of the head is characterized by an obvious protrusion over the mesencephalon, whereas the crown is smooth and rounded by day 17. The digits on the forelimbs are defined partly on day 15, whereas the hindlimbs are still paddlelike. Full definition of the digits occurs over the next 48 h, with the forelimbs developing some 12 h ahead of the hindlimbs. The eye is well-developed and fully open at 15 days; the lids do not develop over it until perhaps day 17.5. Long and Burlingame (1938) nicely illustrate these and other developmental markers. Though older embryos may be used, day 15 is preferable for dissociated pure neural cultures because the DRGs usually remain attached to the spinal cord as it is removed from the vertebral column and because the ganglia contain fewer fibroblasts and Schwann cells, thus making purification of neurons a little easier (see later). However, for the preparation of Schwann cell progenitor cultures, day-16 embryos are preferable because they contain more Schwann cells. Older embryos may be used, with a somewhat higher neuronal and Schwann cell yield; however, the dissections are more difficult, fibroblasts are more abundant, and by day 18 the ganglion has a capsule which must be removed painstakingly.

Figure 19.3 illustrates the various stages of the dissection. Under a dissecting microscope, the embryo is laid on its side and decapitated immediately below the skull at the level of the cervical flex-

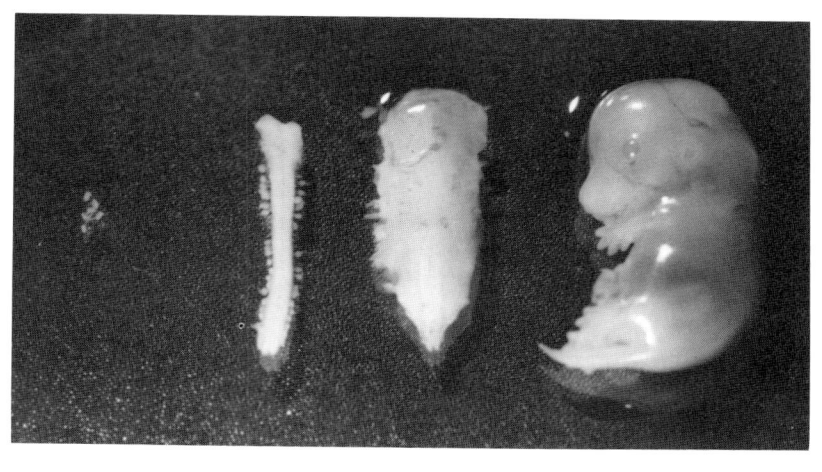

Figure 19.3 Stages of the dorsal root ganglion (DRG) dissection (right to left): day-16 rat embryo; the isolated vertebral column (ventral side is up); the spinal cord and attached DRGs; six isolated DRGs.

ure. The anterior portion of the abdomen and thorax is cut away, along with the limbs. The embryo is then placed on its back, and the ventral side of the spinal column is cleaned carefully of any remaining viscera. One tine of a pair of spring scissors or watch-maker's forceps (Dumont INOX no. 5) is inserted carefully into the rostral end of the spinal column between the vertebral bodies and the spinal meninges. The instrument then is closed to cut through the vertebrae, two or three at a time, proceeding down to the caudal end. The vertebral column is spread gently to loosen the tissue around the spinal cord, but the meninges are left intact. The cord and dura are grasped at the medulla and pulled straight up while the vertebral column is held down with forceps in the other hand. With a little practice and an intact dura mater, it is possible to free the entire spinal cord with its 50 or so attached DRGs from day-15 rats. The cord with attached DRGs is transferred to a 35-mm dish containing L-15. In some cases (especially older embryos), several DRGs will remain within the vertebral column. With proper light-ing, it is possible to retrieve these as well; unless ganglia are scarce, we concentrate mainly on the relatively large cervical and lumbar ganglia.

Once the necessary number of spinal cords and ganglia have been collected in a dish, the large cervical and lumbar ganglia are "plucked" off with no. 5 Biologie forceps. Many ganglia will have substantial lengths of distal roots attached to them; it is advisable to pinch off and discard these roots prior to plucking the ganglia

themselves. The ganglia then are transferred to a new dish of L-15. For embryos older than E18, it is necessary to strip off the capsule to minimize fibroblast contamination. To strip the capsule, very fine undamaged Biologie forceps are an absolute requirement. Once the appropriate number of ganglia are collected, they are ready either to be transferred onto prepared collagen dishes to be used as Schwann cell progenitors (described in the section titled Preparation of Schwann Cells) or to be dissociated (as described in the next section, Preparation of Pure Neuronal Populations) for use in preparing purified neuronal cultures.

Preparation of Pure Neuronal Populations

The sensory ganglia of 15-day rat embryos are plated as mixed populations of dissociated cells. The nonneuronal cells subsequently are eliminated by the use of antimitotic agents. For use in myelination studies, either PNS or CNS glial cells are seeded onto the networks of disaggregated (DRG) neurons approximately 1 week after the final antimitotic treatment (i.e., ~21 days in vitro). Thus, myelinating cells are added back to pure neuronal populations, allowed to expand in number in ascorbate-free medium, and provided with ascorbate to allow myelin sheath formation. Extensive myelination occurs within 7 to 10 days after the addition of ascorbate. The steps involved are described in this and succeeding sections and are summarized in figure 19.4.

DRGs are dissected as described in the preceding section. When enough embryos are available, one may choose to collect only the cervical ganglia to maximize the neuronal yield and minimize the fibroblast number. The ganglia are incubated with 0.25% trypsin (Worthington no. 3707 dissolved in Hank's-CMF) for 45 min at 37°C on a rotary shaker. The trypsin is stopped by the addition of L-15-FBS, the sample is centrifuged at 1000 rpm for 5 min, and the pellet is resuspended in 1 to 2 ml of serum-containing medium and is triturated until the ganglia are dispersed by using a transfer pipette, the tip of which has been reduced by flame polishing to 0.5 to 1.0 mm in bore. The volume is increased to 5 ml, the suspension is mixed and centrifuged as before, and the pellet is resuspended in the desired volume of C_H (1–1.5 ganglia per drop). Approximately 1.5 ganglia in one drop are plated per Aclar minidish. The drop of suspension is placed in the center of a dried ammoniated collagen-coated dish. The drop of cell suspension remains as placed in the

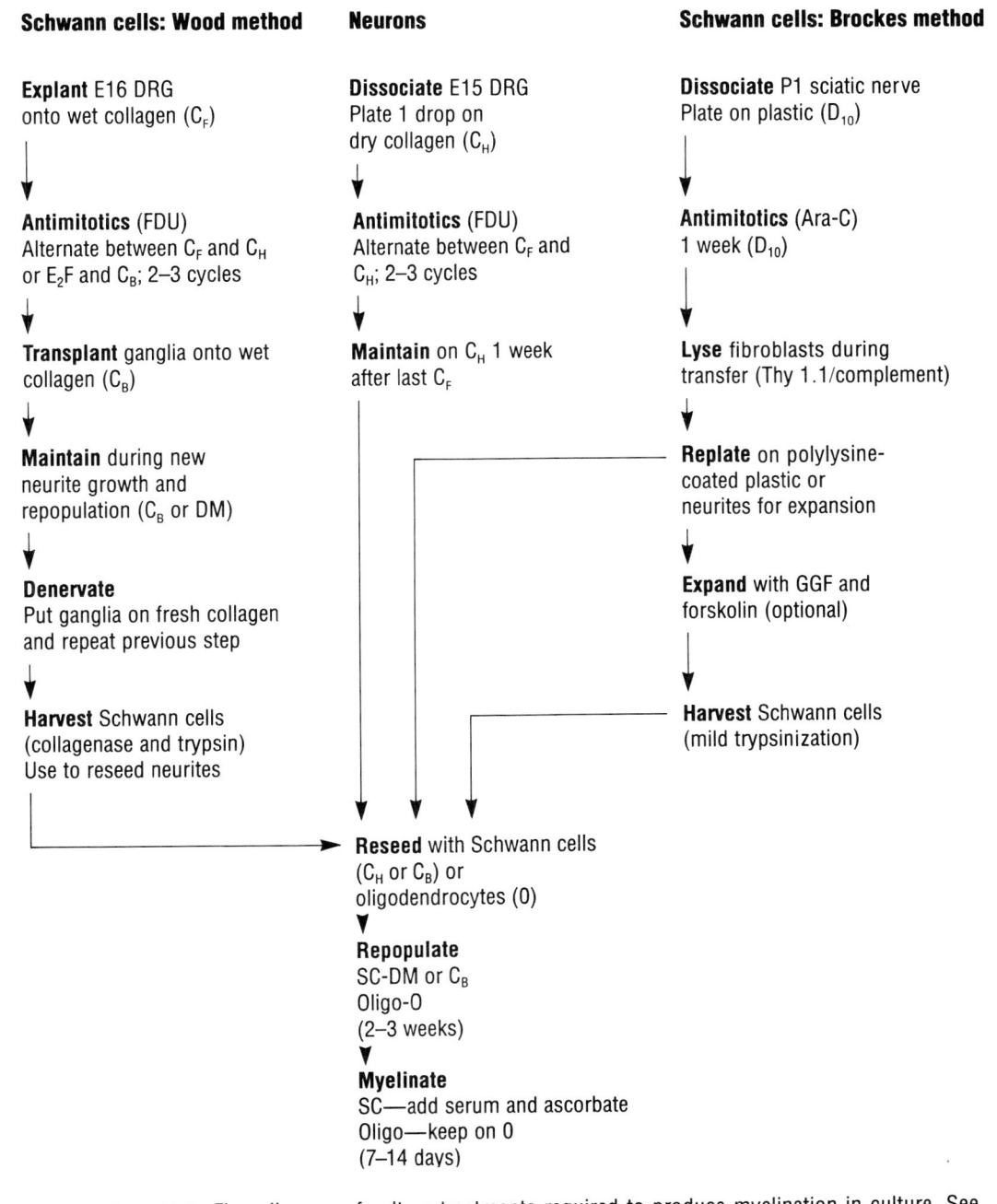

Figure 19.4 Flow diagram of culture treatments required to produce myelination in culture. See the section on Preparation of Pure Neuronal Populations for details.

center of the relatively hydrophobic collagen surface if the cultures are protected carefully from mechanical disturbances. The yield of neurons is 5000 to 7000 per culture.

After the cells have attached to the collagen overnight, the dishes are flooded with 8 to 10 drops of L-15 to wet the rest of the collagen surface. Then the medium is drawn off, and the purification procedure is started by refeeding with C_F. Initially, the cultures contain a mixture of neurons, fibroblasts, Schwann cells, phagocytes, and various other cell types. The cells that are capable of division (essentially all cell types except neurons) are killed by the antimitotic treatment as outlined further. The neurons will survive treatment with antimitotic agents, because almost all of the sensory neuronal population has finished its proliferative phase prior to the time the tissue is taken. The objective of the antimitotic medium is to drive proliferation of the dividing cells in the presence of a drug that is lethal for dividing cells. This action is accomplished by a protocol calling for maintenance medium on days 1, 4 to 6, 8 to 10, and day 12 onward and antimitotic medium on days 2 to 4, 6 to 8, and 10 to 12.

This procedure is more effective when HPS is used than when FBS is used. During this period, considerable cell death is observed as the nonneuronal cells die and much cell debris is evident. After the antimitotic treatment, cultures should be maintained in C feed for at least 1 week to ensure that no residual FdU remains when oligodendrocytes or Schwann cells are added. We refeed cultures every 2 to 3 days. In this and in all our feeding procedures, all the old medium is drained off and replaced quickly with fresh medium. An example of a purified neuronal preparation is shown in figure 19.5A.

The dissociated cultures prepared in this way generally develop in a predictable pattern. After the cultures are flooded with antimitotic medium on the second day in vitro, the nonneuronal cells are killed quickly. By the third to fourth day in vitro, a network of neuritic processes should have formed, and many dying or dead nonneuronal cells may be seen in the central drop area. Thereafter, axons begin to cross the boundary of the central drop and grow toward the edge of the culture. By the third week in vitro, the culture should be mostly free of nonneuronal cells and should consist of a central network of neurons and interconnecting neurites, surrounded by a halo of radially extending bare axons. In a "good" culture, the fascicles of axons will be firmly adherent to the substratum and show few irregularities (i.e., they will appear smooth

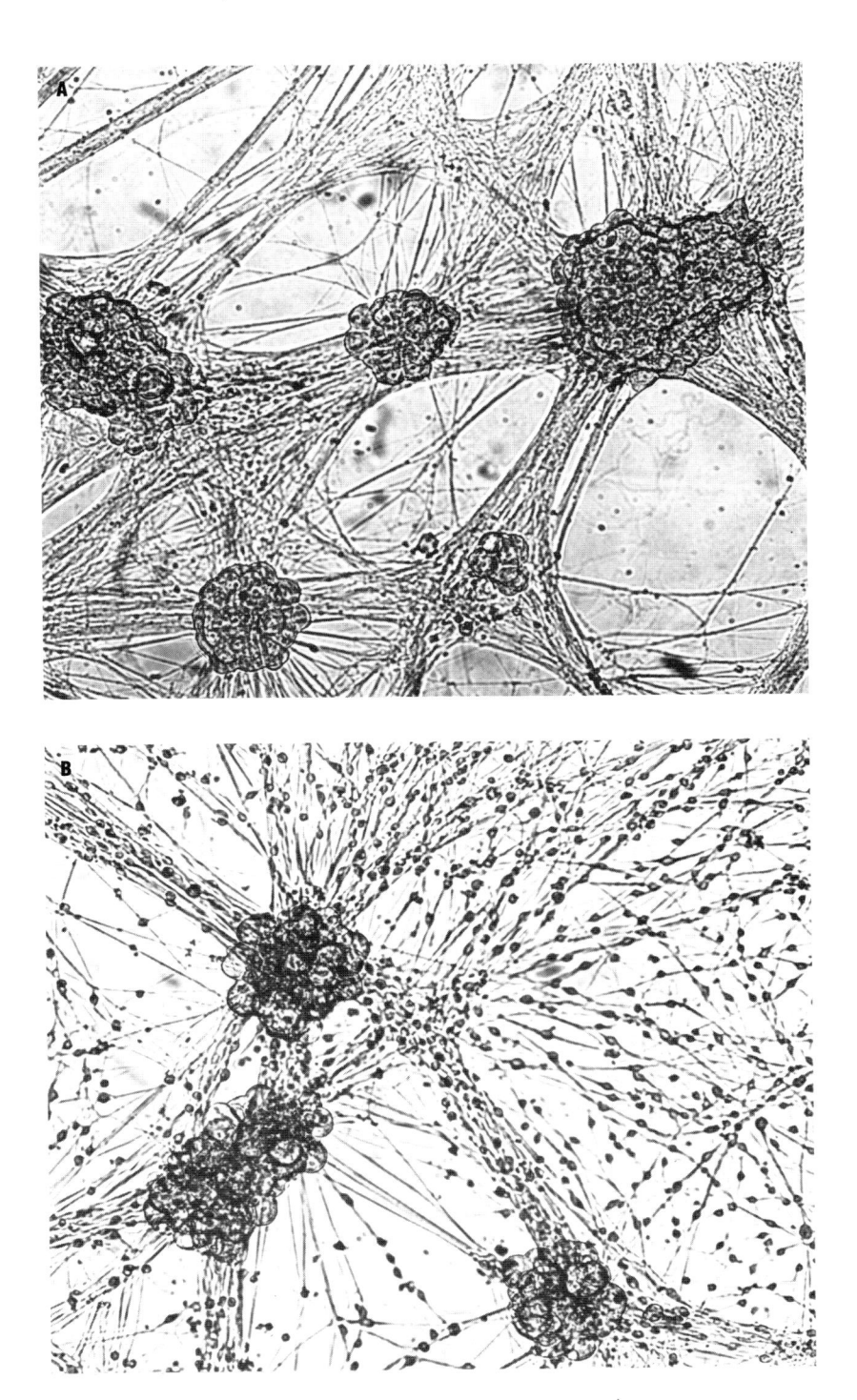

Figure 19.5 (A) Pure dorsal root ganglion neuron culture, 21 days after plating. This photomicrograph of a living culture illustrates the appearance of a central area containing clusters of neuronal somata and developing axonal fascicles. (B) Neuronal culture 10 days after reseeding with purified Schwann cells. This culture was maintained in serum-free defined medium. Note the rounded appearance of the many Schwann cells closely adherent to axons (×112).

and unbroken along their course). The central drop area should have both large- and small-diameter neuronal somata; these somata should exhibit homogeneous cytoplasm containing few or no large granules and should have centrally located nuclei and prominent nucleoli. Some neurons may contain large vacuoles. We have examined such neurons by electron microscopy and found them to exhibit otherwise healthy ultrastructure. They appear to be stable in this condition, and the formation of the vacuoles may be correlated with maintenance in the absence of supporting cells. We consider the occurrence of some vacuolated neurons to be within the norm for this type of preparation.

A problem occasionally seen with dissociated neuronal cultures is that many neurons also die during the course of the antimitotic treatment, for reasons that are not understood clearly at this time. This neuronal die-off typically begins during the second to fourth day of culture and eventually may lead to the loss of the majority of the neurons in some cultures. This pattern can be recognized by the presence of disintegrating axons around the edge of the central drop area and by the presence of atrophic neuronal somata. This phenomenon occurs in approximately 20% of all culture series and is a major cause of variability within those series affected. If this atrophy is severe initially, the amount of myelin formed will vary greatly from one culture to another within the series. We have not been able to correlate this neuronal death with any parameter of the culture conditions, but it may occur less frequently when E_2F medium rather than C_F medium is used as the antimitotic feed.

Preparation of Schwann Cells

Two reliable methods are available for the preparation of pure populations of rodent Schwann cells. The first uses explants of sensory ganglia to provide Schwann cells and stimulate their proliferation; the second uses neonatal sciatic nerve as the source from which Schwann cells are purified.

THE WOOD METHOD

The Wood (1976) approach is to establish embryonic (day-16) rat sensory ganglia as explants and to treat with antimitotic agents. This technique differs from that already described for preparing neuronal cultures in its use of whole ganglion explants (rather than dissociated preparations) from slightly older embryos. The method

presumably depends on the fact that Schwann cells existing as satellite cells within the explants ae less likely to divide than are the fibroblasts that constitute the capsular sheath of the ganglion. Although the initial antimitotic treatment kills many Schwann cells, some do survive and proliferate after transplantation, eventually repopulating the newly forming neuritic outgrowth. The ganglion serves as a source of neuronal outgrowth that drives Schwann cell division, thereby generating large numbers of pure Schwann cells. Yields of up to 250,000 Schwann cells per ganglion have been obtained by this method.

The dissection of the embryos is performed as described. Dried ammoniated collagen-coated dishes are rewetted with L-15, which then is removed and replaced with C_F. A number of ganglia (four to six) are distributed in each dish, and the feed level is lowered so that pressure from the meniscus helps to hold the explants against the collagen surface (but not so low that the dishes dry out). This low medium level is maintained for only the first 18 h to allow firm attachment of the ganglia to the substratum. Subsequently, three 48-h-pulses of antimitotics generally are administered for cultures maintained at 37°C on a schedule calling for antimitotic medium on days 1 to 3, 6 to 8, and 10 to 12 and maintenance medium on days 3 to 6, 8 to 10, and day 12 onward.

Because fibroblasts are never eliminated entirely from the original culture dish and because newly growing neurites are required to stimulate division of the surviving Schwann cells, the neurites are cut at the edge of the explants (containing neurons and surviving Schwann cells) with pieces of broken razor blade (Fine Science Tools, no. 11050-00) held in blade breakers (Fine Science Tools, no. 10052-11). With a No. 5 forceps, the explants are removed from the cultures after careful separation from the underlying collagen substratum (which often harbors residual fibroblasts). The explants are transferred to a new collagen-coated culture dish (three explants per dish) and maintained on C_B. The original culture dishes are discarded. Over the next 2 to 3 weeks, a new outgrowth is established in the new dishes, which spurs the proliferation of the remaining Schwann cell population. The Schwann cells migrate out of the explant along the neurites and divide in response to the axonal mitogen until they fully populate the neurites and cover the surface of the culture dish.

To harvest the surrounding new outgrowth of Schwann cells, the ganglia again are cut out of the cultures, leaving the now pure

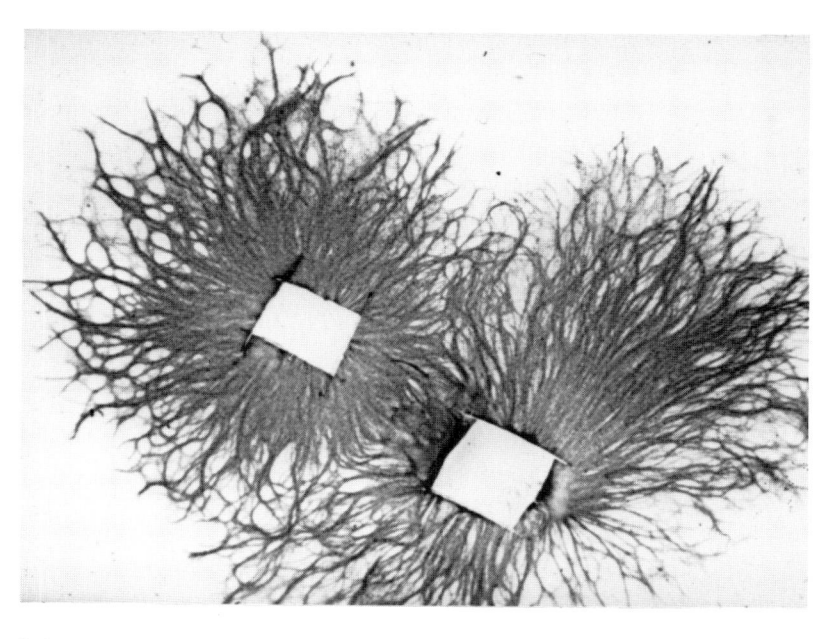

Figure 19.6   Schwann cell beds in a Wood "progenitor culture" after ganglion explants have been removed (toluidine blue stain, ×12).

Schwann cells behind (figure 19.6; for further details, see later). The explants can be transferred again to fresh dishes and allowed to regenerate a new outgrowth of neurites and Schwann cells but, after a number of transplantations, the neurite and Schwann cell yield will decline. The Schwann cells generated in secondary or tertiary transplants are fully functional in that they are capable of going on to myelination.

Two problems that might be encountered using this technique are (1) poor proliferation of Schwann cells following the first transplantation of explants after the antimitotic treatment and (2) fibroblast contamination of the outgrowth zone. To help ensure good Schwann cell growth, only the largest ganglia (i.e., cervical and lumbosacral—not thoracic—ganglia) should be used. Fibroblast contamination can be reduced by careful stripping of roots and connective tissue adhering to the plucked ganglia before they are placed in culture.

THE BROCKES METHOD

The goal of this procedure is to obtain the considerable number of Schwann cells present in the neonatal rat sciatic nerve trunk at a point in development during which the nerve contains relatively

few fibroblasts. This method was published in detail first by Brockes et al. (1979), and we use the procedure essentially as published; however, we review our methods here, as slight modifications have been made. One-day-old rat pups are cold-anesthetized, then killed by decapitation, and their bodies are cleaned thoroughly with 70% alcohol. The hindlimbs are pinned out tautly, the skin over the legs is retracted, and an approximately 1-cm-long segment of sciatic nerve is removed aseptically from each leg by blunt dissection posterior to and parallel to the femur. The nerves are collected in L-15 in a 60-mm Petri dish. When all the nerves have been collected, the L-15 is removed and is replaced with 2 ml of 0.1% collagenase (Worthington CLS, no. 4194) in L-15 for 30 min at 37°C. The medium is removed and is replaced by 2 ml of 0.25% trypsin (Worthington no. 3707) plus 0.1% collagenase and is incubated as before. After the incubation, the nerves are transferred to a centrifuge tube, most of the medium is removed carefully and is replaced by D_{10} to inactivate the trypsin, and the tube is spun at 1500 rpm for 5 min. The pellet is resuspended in 2 ml of D_{10} and is triturated 20 to 40 times, first through a Pasteur pipette, then through a flame-polished pipette to break up the remaining clumps of tissue. One ml of D_{10} is added, the cells are resuspended, and the cell number is estimated with a hemocytometer. Sciatic nerves from 20 pups yield 4 to 5 million cells. We plate the cell suspension onto an uncoated Corning tissue-culture dish (three 60-mm or two 100-mm dishes) prewetted with 1 ml of D_{10}. Prewetting is important to ensure an even distribution of cells.

The next day, the culture medium is replaced with fresh medium containing 10^{-5} M cytosine arabinoside (Sigma, no. C-1768). This treatment kills the fibroblasts, which are driven to divide by the serum in the medium. The cytosine arabinoside–containing medium is changed once after 3 days. The fibroblasts remaining after 5 to 7 days are eliminated mostly by complement mediated lysis during passage using antibodies to Thy-1.1, which is expressed on fibroblasts but not on Schwann cells. For passaging, cells are removed from the culture dish by using 0.05% trypsin–0.02% ethylenediaminetetraacetic acid (EDTA) in Hank's-CMF for up to 5 min at room temperature. L-15-FBS is added to stop the trypsin and rinse the dish as the suspension is transferred to a centrifuge tube. The mixture is spun at 1500 rpm for 5 min, and the pellet is resuspended in a 1-ml solution of anti-Thy 1.1 (hybridoma supernatant; American Type Culture Collection, no. TIB-103), triturated

gently, and incubated in a 7% CO_2 chamber or incubator at 37°C for 30 min. The cells again are spun down and are resuspended in 1 ml rabbit complement (Cappel no. 0012-0602), then are incubated as before. Finally, the solution is diluted with 1 ml of D_{10}, and the cells are plated onto a PLL-coated Petri dish (PLL, mol. wt. 30,000–70,000, Sigma no. P-2636, 0.5 mg/ml, 30 min).

The Schwann cell populations obtained are more than 95% pure and can be used immediately or expanded by using 2 µM forskolin (Sigma, cat. no. F-6886) together with 10 µg/ml glial growth factor (prepared as described in Brockes et al., 1980) or 20 µg/ml pituitary extract (Biomedical Technologies, Inc., no. BT-215). Cells are passaged every 7 to 10 days; Thy 1.1-complement treatment may be repeated during passaging if further purification is needed. Subsequently, these cells can be used for transfer onto DRG neurons, where full functional expression is observed (Porter et al., 1986). Excessive amplification of Schwann cell populations with soluble mitogens is to be avoided because transformation may occur after 11 or 12 passages (4 months; Porter et al., 1986; Langford et al., 1988). In contrast, we have not observed a transformation of Schwann cells that were expanded in contact with living neurites (Wood method).

HARVESTING PERINATAL SCHWANN CELLS
Recovering Schwann cells, prepared using the Brockes method, is relatively straightforward, requiring only a short period (3–5 min) of trypsinization (0.05% trypsin-0.02% EDTA in Hank's-CMF). L-15-FBS is added to stop the trypsin and the cells are centrifuged and resuspended in D_{10} to rinse out remaining trypsin. The centrifugation and resuspension are repeated, and the suspension is plated on PLL-coated plastic or directly onto neurite cultures as described later for the Wood preparation.

Harvesting and replating Schwann cells prepared using the Wood method requires removal of the neuronal cells, digestion of the collagen substratum, and disaggregation of the Schwann cells. Cultures maintained in serum-containing medium should be rinsed once or twice with EBSS. The neurons are cut out of the Schwann cell–neuron cultures as described. (The explants in Schwann cell progenitor cultures may be transplanted to produce new cultures; dissociated neurons usually are discarded.) Six to eight drops of 0.05% collagenase (Worthington CLSPA, no. 5273) in EBSS are added to each culture, and the cultures are incubated in a 6% CO_2

atmosphere for 30 min at 37°C on a rotary shaker. The collagen substratum dissolves, and the Schwann cells aggregate into a mass that is transferred by pipette to a tube containing 10 ml of L-15. The mass of cells is rinsed by gentle trituration with a wide-bore pipette and is harvested by centrifugation (1500 rpm or $200 \times g$ for 5–10 min). The supernatant is discarded, and the pellet is rinsed once in Hank's-CMF and recentrifuged. The pellet then is resuspended in 0.25% trypsin in Hank's-CMF and is incubated at 37°C for 30 min. The trypsin is stopped with L-15-FBS, then is removed after centrifugation. The cells are resuspended in 1 to 2 ml of serum-containing medium and triturated vigorously to break up clumps; some clumps of neurite debris may remain but can be removed subsequently. Because the Schwann cells usually are replated onto other cultures or collagen substrata, it is important to remove all the residual collagenase from the Schwann cell suspension. Therefore, the Schwann cells should be rinsed two more times, and the final Schwann cell pellet should be resuspended in the appropriate level of C_B for reseeding purposes. Drops of this suspension simply are added to neuronal cultures fed with a relatively high volume of C_B.

To determine the approximate number of cells directly, a drop of the final solution can be assessed with a hemocytometer. As a rule of thumb, we use the following estimates. In fully developed progenitor cultures, each ganglion yields 2×10^5 Schwann cells. Repopulated dissociated neuron preparations contain between 1 and 2×10^6 Schwann cells, depending on the length of time since reseeding. A good seeding level for purified neuronal dissociate cultures would be 1.5×10^4 cells. Thus, one good progenitor containing three or four ganglia or one dissociated preparation easily could be used to repopulate 40 new cultures. An example of a repopulated culture is shown in figure 19.5B.

ADULT-DERIVED RAT AND HUMAN SCHWANN CELLS
Looking toward the therapeutic use of Schwann cell populations in nerve repair, a likely application would involve autotransplantation. In such a paradigm, a small biopsy of nerve from a patient could yield a sufficient number of Schwann cells, after purification and proliferation in vitro, to provide sufficient graft material to repair peripheral or central nerve damage not conducive to direct nerve grafting. Such paradigms require the use of adult-derived Schwann cell populations. Until recently, little emphasis had been

placed on the acquisition of Schwann cells from adult animals or from human donors.

Peripheral nerves retrieved from adult rats or human organ donors can be processed to obtain relatively pure populations of Schwann cells, despite the high fibroblast and extracellular matrix content of these nerves. The Schwann cell isolation method was described first by Morrissey et al. (1991), and we are continuing to test modifications of this technique. To dissect sciatic nerves of adult Sprague-Dawley rats, the animals are ether-anesthetized, and their hindlimbs are shaved and cleaned with betadyne and alcohol. In a laminar flow hood, the skin over the legs is incised and retracted. Different sets of sterile scissors are used sequentially (1) to cut the muscles over the femur until the nerve is visible and to expose the nerve from the knee to the spinal column, and (2) to cut the sciatic nerve free, place it in L-15 with 50 units/ml penicillin and 0.05 mg/ml streptomycin, and cut it into pieces some 2 to 3 cm long. We obtain human peripheral nerve with the assistance of the University of Miami Organ Procurement Organization, which retrieves sterile phrenic and intercostal nerves and segments of lumbar plexus and refrigerates them in Belzer's solution until processed.

Both rat and human tissues are processed as follows. Fat and vascular tissue are removed; then with fine forceps grasping the epineurial connective tissue sheath, the perineurium enclosed nerve fascicles are pulled gently from the cut end of the nerves, with fine forceps grasping and pulling the tufted end of the fascicle. This procedure yields a length of clean nerve fascicle that will appear smooth and white, with a circumferential banding pattern. The fascicle is cut into segments (1–4 mm long) with fine scissors. Segments from 10 to 15 cm of nerve are placed into a 100-mm tissue-culture plastic (Corning) dish in 10 ml of D_{10}. A relatively low feed level should be maintained so that the explants will not float off the bottom of the dish and fibroblasts can migrate out of the explants onto the culture surface. The cultures are fed two times per week and are transferred every 10 to 14 days to new dishes by shaking them free and transferring them by pipette to new dishes, leaving behind the adherent fibroblasts. After 4 to 8 weeks of culture (when fibroblast migration has declined), the explants are incubated overnight in a mixture of D-MEM, 1.25 units/ml dispase (Boehringer Mannheim, no. 165-859), 0.05% collagenase (Worthington CLS, no. 4194), and 15% FBS. The following day, the

explants are dissociated by gentle trituration, washed three times, and plated on PLL-coated 100-mm dishes at a density of 1 to 2×10^6 cells per dish in D_{10}.

Purification

We reliably obtain 2×10^4 Schwann cells per milligram (starting wet weight) of rat nerve at a purity of 97% or greater. Most contaminating cells are fibroblasts. Human nerve preparations have yielded on average 3×10^4 cells per milligram, but purity is only 90% to 94%, based on immunostaining for S100 or the low-affinity nerve growth factor receptor (NGFr). Both these antibodies stain Schwann cells but not other cells in these preparations. Human Schwann cell populations can be purified further by fluorescence-activated cell sorting. Following dissociation, cells are allowed to settle overnight on PLL-coated plastic dishes. They are detached from the dish by treatment with 0.05% trypsin–0.02% EDTA in Hank's-CMF for 5 min. The cells are collected, centrifuged, and rinsed three times with D_{10} then they are labeled in suspension (at a concentration of 5×10^6 cells/ml) with a monoclonal antibody that recognizes the human NGFr on the Schwann cells (undiluted culture supernatant from hybridoma cell line HB-8737, American Type Culture Collection) for 30 min on ice. The cell suspension is centrifuged and rinsed two times with D_{10} to remove excess antibody. The pellet is resuspended in a 1:20 dilution of fluorescein-conjugated goat-anti-mouse antibody in L-15 with 0.05% bovine serum albumin at a concentration of 1 to 2×10^6 cells/ml, incubated on ice for 30 min, rinsed, and sorted on a FACSTAR cell sorter with Becton Dickinson software. Following sorting, the cells are centrifuged, resuspended in culture medium, and plated onto neuronal preparations or in plastic dishes for expansion. Small aliquots are taken before and after sorting to assess for purity by immunostaining for NGFr.

Expansion

Adult-derived rat Schwann cells can be expanded by plating the cells on PLL-coated 100-mm dishes at 5×10^5 cells per dish in D_{10} supplemented with 20 µg/ml pituitary extract and 2 µM forskolin (as described for the Brockes method). The division rate and propensity to transform are similar to that seen with Brockes cells (Morrissey et al., 1991). Adult-derived human Schwann cells do not respond to pituitary extract and, for several years, we were unable

to expand these populations. When human fibroblasts contaminating these cultures (even 5% or less) are exposed to serum in the D_{10} medium, they divide rapidly and soon overtake the Schwann cell populations. We have found that a mixture of heregulin (a member of the family of proteins that includes glial growth factor, *neu* differentiation factor, and acetylcholine receptor-inducing activity), cholera toxin, and forskolin will induce human Schwann cells to divide in culture at a level sufficient to maintain the purity of the populations (Levi et al., 1995). The mitogen solution used by Levi and colleagues was 10 nM heregulin $\beta1$ (kindly provided by Genentech), 100 ng/ml cholera toxin (Sigma, no. C3012), and 1 µM forskolin (Sigma, no. F-6886). The triple mitogen method is a modification of one reported by Rutkowski et al. (1992).

Recent experiments show that cholera toxin is not required to stimulate division and to maintain Schwann cell purity when the cells are cultured on ammoniated collagen or on laminin. Therefore, routinely we use heregulin and forskolin alone as mitogens and collagen or laminin as the substratum for growth. A new mitogenic defined medium formulation effective for both rat and human Schwann cells was developed very recently by Li et al. (Li et al., 1996b). This formulation, named *7F*, is composed of a base medium of D-MEM and Ham's F-12 (1:1 vol/vol; see table 19.1 for supplier information), supplemented with seven ingredients: transferrin (10 µg/ml), insulin (5 µg/ml), progesterone (2 nM; Sigma, no. P-7556), α-tocopherol (vitamin E, 5 µg/ml, Gibco, no. 13580), forskolin (2 µM), pituitary extract (20 µg/ml; Biomedical Technologies, Inc., no. BT-215), and heregulin $\beta1$ (2.5 nM; courtesy of Genentech). In a second study, Li et al. (1996b) have identified Gas6, a ligand for the Axl and Rse-Tyro 3 receptor protein tyrosine kinase family, as a mitogen for human Schwann cells, which is synergistic with heregulin and forskolin.

Obtaining Myelination by Schwann Cells

The neuron-Schwann cell coculture is maintained routinely in DM after reseeding for a period of 10 to 14 days (cultures are refed every 2 or 3 days) to allow neurite-driven proliferation to provide enough Schwann cells to populate richly the entire neurite outgrowth. This serum-free medium does not allow the Schwann cells to assemble a basal lamina or adequately to ensheathe the neurites and begin myelination. These Schwann cells, however, are poised

and ready to begin the myelination process on presentation of appropriate medium components. At this point, the culture is transferred to a medium containing both ascorbate and either serum or laminin and BSA (see Other Media) and is refed every 2 or 3 days (Eldridge et al., 1985). Many myelin sheaths are formed beginning by 7 days after the addition of ascorbate, and myelination continues for several weeks (figure 19.7). More recently, we have maintained neuron-Schwann cell cultures in myelinating feed without ascorbate. Such cultures also become poised (i.e., myelination will not occur until ascorbate is added). The first myelin is obtained 5 to 7 days later. Myelinated cultures can be maintained on myelinating feed indefinitely.

Myelin sheathes are visualized easily within living cultures by the use of bright-field illumination. The identification of myelin (especially of the shorter, thinner myelin) is more ambiguous when visualized with phase-contrast optics, particularly in denser areas of the cultures. The accumulation of myelin in the cultures is a gradual process occurring over several weeks. Though older cultures become progressively more uniformly myelinated, variability is seen in the amount of myelin from area to area within a single culture, and variability in the amount of myelin between cultures may be as high as 50%. Variability in the quantity of myelin and its rate of formation can be minimized by careful selection of neuronal cultures with comparable numbers of neurons and with similar distributions of neurons with regard to the degree of clumping and fasciculation.

Initial testing of adult-derived rat Schwann cells showed that myelination could be elicited by the same tissue-culture conditions as those eliciting myelination by perinatally derived Schwann cells. Human Schwann cells, however, failed to myelinate under the same culture conditions, and long-term human cocultures were characterized by an extensive overgrowth of fibroblasts that remained from the initial dissociation procedures (Morrissey et al., 1995a). This overgrowth occurs in part because the human Schwann cells proliferate much more slowly than do rat cells in response to axonal contact. In addition, the DRG neurons in human Schwann cell cocultures were observed to atrophy when exposed to populations of primary human Schwann cells and accompanying fibroblasts, presumably rendering the neurons incapable of supporting myelination. To achieve human adult-derived Schwann cell myelin formation in culture, the human Schwann cell population had to be

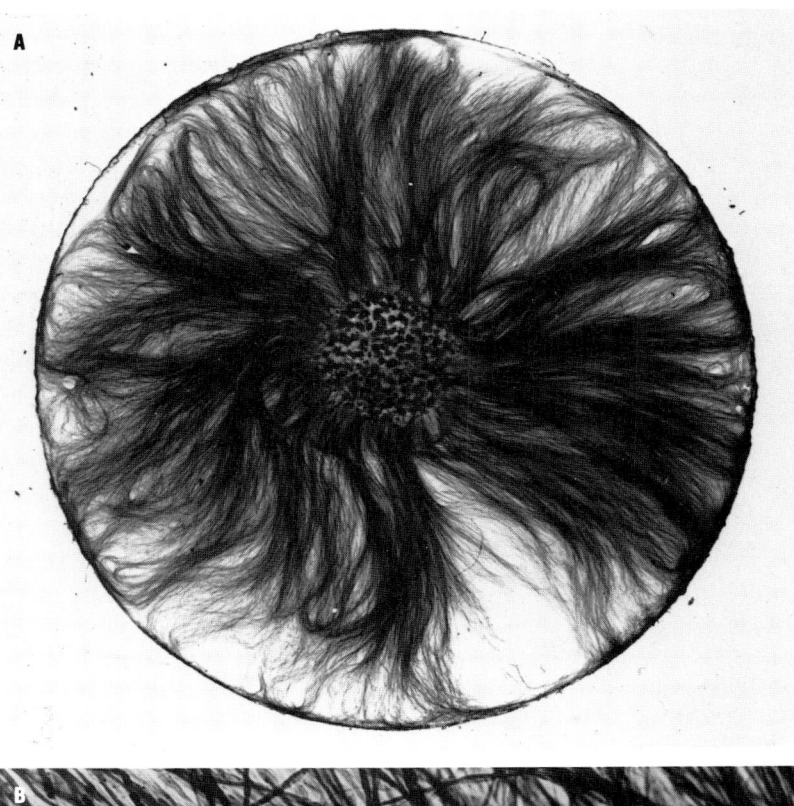

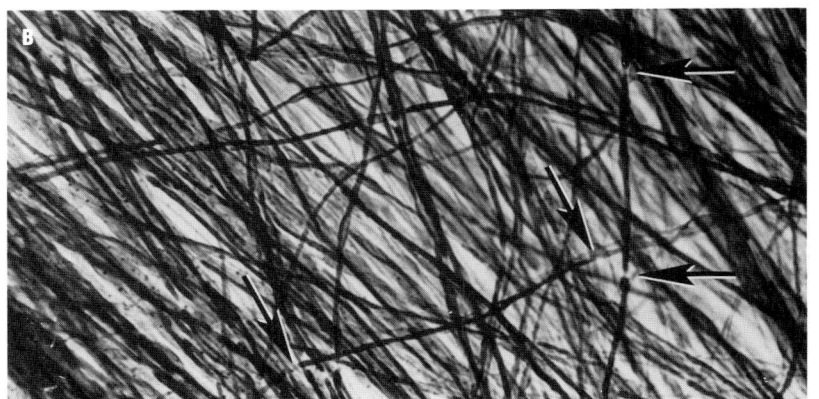

Figure 19.7 (*A*) Heavily myelinated neuron–Schwann cell culture. The dissociated dorsal root ganglion neurons were plated as a drop in the center of the dish. After the antimitotic treatment, Schwann cells were added back, and the culture was maintained in serum and ascorbate until myelin developed (4 weeks after Schwann cell addition). (*B*) Individual sheaths are visible in the area of neurite outgrowth. Two myelin segments are demarcated with small arrows (×320).

maintained with minimal fibroblast contamination. Recently, with the introduction of chemical mitogens that allow us to expand the adult human Schwann cell populations and the use of fluorescence-activated cell sorting to minimize fibroblast contamination, we have demonstrated the development of human peripheral myelin in culture for the first time (Morrissey et al., 1995b). The human Schwann cells could be induced to myelinate by exposure to ascorbate- and serum-containing medium and by exposure to a serum-free medium with added ascorbate and laminin. This serum-free medium also helped to suppress the proliferation of fibroblasts. It should be noted that human myelination occurred more slowly and in much less abundance than that in comparable cultures containing adult rat-derived Schwann cells. We anticipate that refinements of the human Schwann cell coculture system that enhance myelin formation will provide insights into important aspects of human Schwann cell biology.

Obtaining Myelination by Oligodendrocytes

Cultured purified dissociated DRG neurons may be used also to drive the proliferation and differentiation of embryonic CNS glial cells and to support extensive myelination by oligodendrocytes derived from the embryonic glial cells (Wood and Williams, 1984). More recently, we have shown that the same type of neuronal culture supports myelination by oligodendrocytes derived from adult spinal cord tissue (Wood and Bunge, 1986a,b).

The purified dissociated neuronal cultures are prepared essentially as described earlier, except that initially the cells from two DRGs are plated in two drops of C_H medium to cover a larger area of the dish or coverslip. Embryonic CNS glial cells (along with neurons) are obtained as single-cell suspensions after mechanical or enzymatic dissociation of spinal cord fragments dissected from rat embryos on the fourteenth to eighteenth day of gestation. The cord fragments are dissociated by gentle trituration through a pipette with a flame-reduced tip. The resulting suspension is filtered through a 20-μm nylon filter (Small Parts, Inc., Miami Lakes, FL; no. A-CMN-20) and is plated at densities ranging from 30,000 to 100,000 cells per culture onto the dissociated neuronal network. The medium used for dissociation of the cord and maintenance of the cultures throughout is C_{H10} medium (i.e., C medium containing human placental serum at 10%). Extensive myelination is observed

3 to 4 weeks after the glial cells are plated. It should be noted that a vigorous proliferation of glial cells is observed in the first 2 weeks after the plating of the spinal cord cells; a majority of these dividing cells are astrocytes. Increasing numbers of galactocerebroside-positive oligodendrocytes are observed during the second and third weeks, beginning at perhaps 9 days after the plating of the spinal cord glial cells. Galactocerebroside-positive oligodendrocytes themselves do not divide in this type of culture but appear to differentiate from dividing galactocerebroside-negative progenitors. This effect contrasts with the situation that is observed when myelination is obtained with oligodendrocytes from adult animals; adult galactocerebroside-positive oligodendrocytes *do* divide prior to myelination in vitro (see later). Serum is present throughout the periods of proliferation and myelination by embryonic glial cells.

Myelination was observed also when oligodendrocytes prepared from neonatal rat cerebrum by the method of McCarthy and DeVellis (1980) were added to purified dissociated DRG neuronal cultures. Myelination occurred after 3 to 4 weeks. Once again, these cultures become extensively populated with astrocytes, which probably are derived from contaminating cells in the purified oligodendrocyte suspension. Oligodendrocyte percentages were increased in DM (serum-free) medium, but myelination was decreased, possibly as a result of an ongoing attrition of neurons in cultures maintained for long periods in DM medium.

Myelination may be accomplished also by purified oligodendrocytes obtained from adult rats. Spinal cord is dissected from 2- to 3-month-old female Sprague-Dawley rats and is stored in cold (4°C) L-15 medium. The spinal roots and meninges are stripped off, and the entire cord is hemisected, placed in 4 ml of 0.25% trypsin plus 50 µg/ml DNase in EBSS, and sliced into 0.5-mm slices. The tissue then is incubated for 90 min at 37°C on a steadily rotating shaker. At the end of this incubation, 1 ml of ice-cold heat-inactivated serum is added, and the mixture is transferred to a tube and is mixed well. The cord fragments are recovered by centrifugation (300 × g, 5 min). The fragments are triturated through a pipette with a flame-reduced tip (opening 0.5 mm) in 2 ml cold L-15 with 10% heat-inactivated serum. The resulting suspension is diluted to 5 ml and is filtered through a 20-µm pore size nylon filter. This filtered suspension is diluted to 6.5 ml with L-15 + 10% heat-inactivated serum and is mixed thoroughly with 3 ml of 80% Percoll in 0.25 M sucrose buffered with 0.05 M sodium phosphate at pH 7.4. This

mixing and the centrifugation step are carried out in a 10-ml Oak Ridge tube. The final concentration of Percoll in the mixed suspension is 25%. The suspension is centrifuged at $30,000 \times g$ for 45 min. The myelin layer and the upper third of the Percoll gradient beneath the myelin layer contain no cells and are discarded. Oligodendrocytes and other cells are distributed in a 2-cm band that floats just over the red blood cell layer, which is near the bottom of the gradient. This band is harvested, diluted five-fold with L-15-serum, and collected by centrifugation ($500 \times g$, 10 min).

The cell pellet (~ 3 to 4×10^6 cells per spinal cord) thus obtained contains 40% to 50% galactocerebroside-positive oligodendrocytes. This pellet can be resuspended in culture medium and plated directly onto neuronal cultures. However, such cultures become overgrown with nonoligodendroglial cells (including some astrocytes), and the amount of myelin that can be obtained is limited (see Rosen et al., 1989). More extensively myelinated cultures can be obtained if the oligodendrocytes are purified to 90% or greater concentrations. The current method of choice for carrying out this purification involves fluorescence-activated cell sorting.

To this end, the pellet is resuspended in 0.5 ml of hybridoma supernatant containing monoclonal anti-galactocerebroside (GalC) (Ranscht et al., 1982) or anti-O_1 (Sommer and Schachner, 1981). Both antibodies are specific for postmitotic oligodendrocytes. The cells are incubated in this supernatant at 4°C for 30 min and are kept in suspension by gentle trituration every 5 min. Then they are labeled with a fluorochrome-conjugated secondary antibody. If the primary antibody is GalC, labeling with the secondary is accomplished simply by adding a small volume of concentrated antibody to the suspension. The suspension then is incubated at 4°C for an additional 30 min with gentle trituration at 5-min intervals. The labeled cell suspension is diluted to 3 to 4 ml with L-15, filtered through 15 μm Nitex, and sorted by flow cytometry. The cells are sorted in L-15 without other additions. Oligodendrocytes are obtained at a purity of greater than 95% at a yield of 0.5 to 1.0×10^6 cells per cord.

After sorting, the oligodendrocytes can be plated onto the neuronal cultures. Usually, this is done by diluting the sorted cells into the desired volume of a medium we designate as O medium (see table 19.1). Penicillin and streptomycin are added to this medium for the first day after plating. In addition, recombinant basic fibroblast growth factor (R&D Systems, Minneapolis, no. 133-

FB, 5 ng/ml) is added to O medium for the first week after plating. After the first week, the neuron-oligodendrocyte cultures are maintained in O medium without fibroblast growth factor. The addition of 25,000 oligodendrocytes per neuronal culture is sufficient to ensure extensive myelination. A vigorous proliferation of GalC-positive oligodendrocytes can be observed during the second and third weeks after plating. Myelination begins during the third week after the plating of the oligodendrocytes and is heavy by the end of the fourth week (figure 19.8). Living CNS myelin is very difficult to visualize at low magnifications but may be visualized at high power (>500×). Myelin sheaths may be visualized readily and counted after Sudan black staining (see later).

Histological Options

Unstained myelin sheathes are observed best with bright-field optics, taking advantage of the natural birefringence of myelin. When we want to document the appearance of the cultures as they grow by using low-magnification objectives (2.5× and 4×), we use an inverted microscope with a long-working-distance condenser. The unstained living cultures are observed best via nonstandard optics, by closing down the bright-field condenser aperture to increase contrast, or under pseudo-dark-field microscopy (using condenser phase rings with the nonphase low-magnification objectives). The latter is particularly useful for visualizing neuritic outgrowth. At higher magnifications, normal-phase optics also can be used to image other cellular structures.

One major advantage of the culture systems we have described is that at the endpoints of the experiments, the cultures can be fixed easily in the culture dish for a number of different types of analyses. Though we cannot describe protocols for all histological techniques in this chapter, we summarize each and direct the reader to references wherein the detailed protocols are described. In all cases, the cultures may be fixed directly in the Aclar minidishes described earlier. Often, it is convenient to work with a flat preparation, so we cut off the sides of the dishes and treat the bottom of the dish as a coverslip. For the latter type of preparation or for cultures grown on Aclar coverslips, one can cut the culture in half gently and treat each half separately to maximize the number of analyses from a given experiment or to use as control groups for staining procedures.

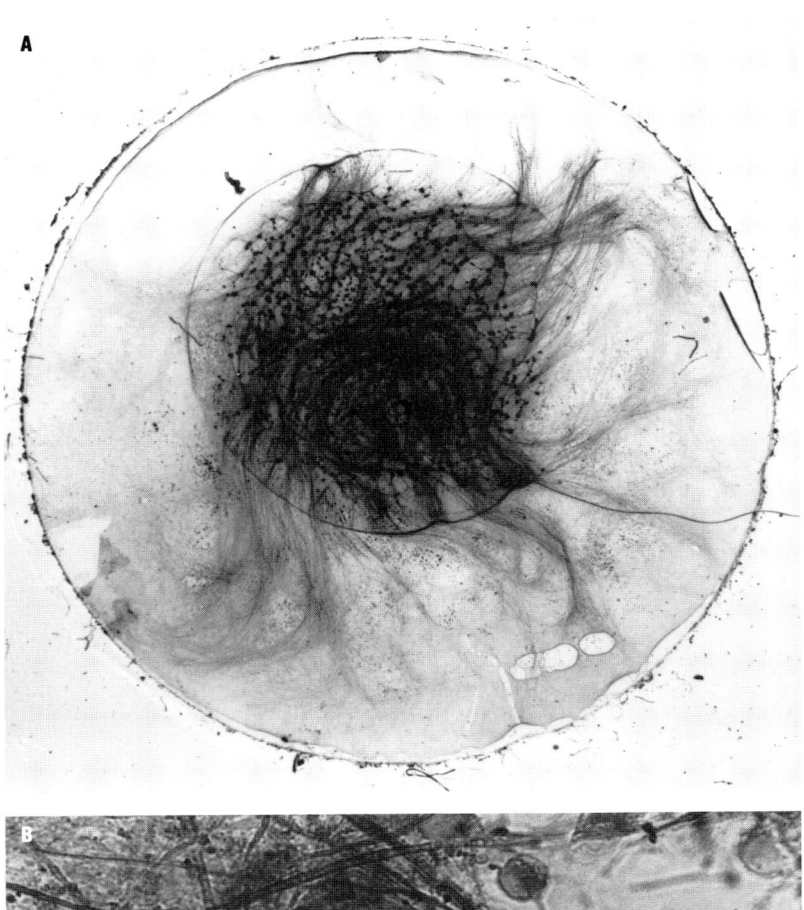

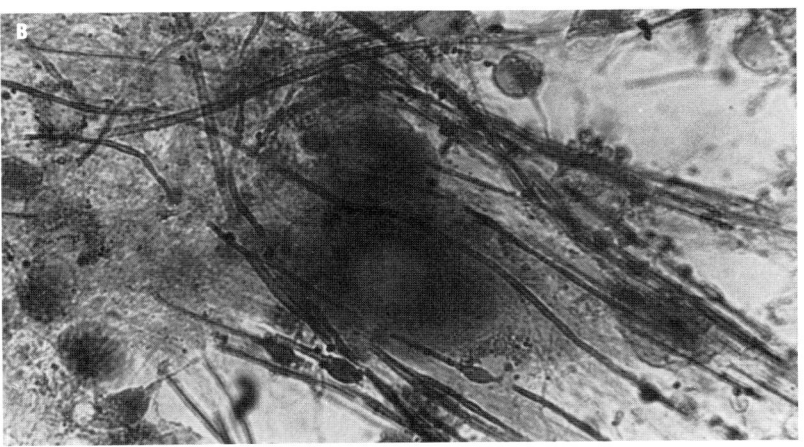

Figure 19.8 Neuron-oligodendrocyte culture. (*A*) Dissociated dorsal root ganglion neurons were plated in two drops in the center of the coverslip and treated with antimitotic agents to remove all Schwann cells and fibroblasts. Oligodendrocytes were purified from suspensions of dissociated adult spinal cord by flow cytometry and were added to the neuronal cultures after the antimitotic treatment. The cultures became extensively myelinated by 4 weeks after the addition of oligodendrocytes ($\times 4$). (*B*) Higher magnification illustrating oligodendrocyte myelin. Though myelination is extensive, the process is not as well-organized as Schwann cell myelination in vitro. Myelin segments are shorter, thinner, and not consecutive ($\times 512$).

ELECTRON MICROSCOPY

When the cultures are grown in the minidishes, the Aclar culture dish becomes the vessel for fixation (2% glutaraldehyde overnight at 4°C), osmification (2% OsO_4, 1 h, room temperature), dehydration, and embedding (Polybed, Polysciences) for electron microscopical preparations. If coverslips were used, they are placed into an Aclar dish for processing. For a detailed protocol and excellent examples of the ultrastructural appearance of myelinating cultures, see M. Bunge et al. (1983) and R. Bunge et al. (1989).

SUDAN BLACK STAINING

Used to visualize lipids, this stain is especially valuable in the study of myelination. The cultures are fixed overnight in 4% paraformaldehyde, osmicated (0.1% OsO_4, 1 h, room temperature), and rinsed. For cultures grown in minidishes, the walls of the dishes are cut off to provide flat coverslips that can be processed further in standard staining racks or Coplin jars. They are dehydrated (25%, 50%, and 70% ethanol), then stained for 1 h in Sudan black (0.5% in 70% ethanol). Subsequently, they are destained for some 30 to 60 s in 70% ethanol, rehydrated, and mounted tissue-side-down onto microscope slides. We use a glycerin jelly mounting medium to preserve the stained sections. Examples of cultures prepared with Sudan black are shown in figures 14.7 and 14.8 and in Wood (1976) and Eldridge et al. (1987).

IMMUNOCYTOCHEMISTRY

The protocols for immunostaining vary, depending on the antibodies used. Coverslips or cut-out minidishes are used to minimize solution volumes. If the coverslip is placed on a hydrophobic surface or on a pedestal so that the fluid is confined by surface tension to the top of the culture, one can use volumes as low as 75 μl. Tissue may be reacted with primary and secondary antibodies before fixation for surface antigens or after fixation (4% paraformaldehyde, 10 min; 4% paraformaldehyde plus 0.1% Triton X-100, 10 min at room temperature) and further permeabilization (2 min each in 50%, 100%, then 50% acetone at 4°C). Generally, antibodies are incubated for 30 to 45 min at room temperature. After rinsing, coverslips are mounted onto slides with mounting solutions, such as Citifluor mountant (Citifluor Limited, London, England). The requirements of different antibody preparations vary so widely that these guidelines are only general; for specific examples of immunostained preparations, see Eldridge et al. (1987).

IN SITU HYBRIDIZATION

The protocol used for in situ hybridization has been described in detail in Fernandez-Valle et al. (1994a). The method presented uses a nonradioactive digoxigenin-linked RNA probe. The reader should consult the reference cited for additional details and for illustrated examples of the labeling obtained.

AUTORADIOGRAPHY

Cultures exposed to radioactive tracers are processed as follows. Cultures are fixed in 4% paraformaldehyde and are dehydrated, and the coverslips (or cut-out minidish bottoms) are mounted tissue-side up on slides with DPX mounting medium. When thoroughly dry (overnight), the slides are dipped in NTB-2 emulsion (2:1 dilution in water, 40°C), dried, and exposed at 4°C (exposure time depending on the tracers used). They are developed for 2.5 min at 15°C in D-19 (Kodak) then rinsed and fixed for 5 min in Kodak fixer. The slides may be counterstained with 0.25% toluidine blue, dehydrated through a series of alcohols and xylene, and coverslipped (in DPX). For an example of tritiated thymidine labeling, see Salzer and Bunge (1980).

Troubleshooting

No matter how closely one follows a given protocol, the culture of mammalian tissues for the lengths of time necessary to observe myelination is a process fraught with pitfalls. The following is a short list of some of the major classes of problems one might encounter and possible remedies for them.

Infection

Three major sources of infection are yeast, bacteria, and mold. Strategies to combat them start with prevention. Cultures should be examined before each feeding, with special attention paid to the color of the culture medium, as yeast and bacterial infections tend to render the cultures more acidic (yellowish).

Yeast looks like small round beads or clumps and generally comes from the person handling the cultures. Though frequent hand washing is sufficient in most cases, some of our workers wear gloves rinsed with alcohol to minimize yeast infections. Keeping one's fingers safely away from the solutions is accomplished best by using a larger dish to hold the one containing the tissue.

Bacteria (which have varied appearances but generally are smaller than yeast) can come also from hands but more likely are spread through contaminated solutions or pipettes. It is essential that laboratory workers know which supplies are sterile and understand that questionable tools and solutions are to be removed from common stocks. We pipette rather than pour from stock bottles, and test medium and collagen solutions by incubating a sample in a sterile soy broth solution prior to use (3 g/dl). Limiting the number of cultures contacted by a single pipette can limit the spread of infection. If caught early, a bacterial infection can be stopped with penicillin-streptomycin (Gibco, no. 15140).

Mold is a problem seen mostly in very-long-term cultures. The spores strike somewhat randomly and, because they are airborne, one infected dish can jeopardize others in the desiccator (or carbon dioxide incubator). The best prevention is being certain that the desiccators are cleaned before an experiment and that no mold begins to grow in the water kept in the bottom of the desiccator to humidify the atmosphere. The outside of the dishes holding the culture dishes should be examined for the branched, linear strands of mold regularly during feeding and should be wiped with 70% alcohol or changed every 2 or 3 weeks. When alcohol is used as disinfectant, surfaces must be allowed to dry completely before they are put back into desiccator, to prevent damage to the cultures from toxic fumes.

Other toxins may enter the system from the use of non-tissue-culture plastics or glassware that retains traces of toxins from previous uses. We keep our tissue-culture supplies and rinsing vessels completely separate from the other laboratory supplies, to protect against contamination.

Stability of Collagen Substrata

The collagen substrata must be stable enough to last through a long experiment. Care and consistency in preparing the collagen is critical, but we have better luck with some batches than with others. Careful record keeping helps us to discover problems early. During feeding of cultures, pipettes should not be allowed to touch the culture surface, as they may gouge the collagen layer.

Collagen may detach from improperly cleaned dishes or coverslips. It is critical that the washing and rinsing procedure previously detailed be followed for Aclar minidishes. The dishes

should not be allowed to sit overly long in wash solutions, as greasy materials may leech out of the rinsing containers and coat the dishes. Aclar and glass coverslips also are acid-cleaned for several days and are rinsed thoroughly in water and soaked in ethanol (100% and 80%) before use. The edges of Aclar dishes and hats may be scored gently with a razor blade before washing to give the collagen anchor points to which to adhere, but care must be taken not to pierce all the way through the plastic film.

Finally, if in the middle of a long experiment the edges of the collagen begin to detach despite all precautions, they can be held in place mechanically with fine insect pins (Fine Science Tools, no. 26 002–15). Successfully securing four to six pins in each dish without ripping up the collagen and while maintaining sterility is a numbingly difficult job and should be attempted only as a last resort.

Fibroblast Contamination

Fibroblast contamination of "pure" Schwann cell cultures can be a big problem in some experimental designs and a minor inconvenience in others. Fibroblasts may remain hidden while cultures are held in serum-free media or antimitotic media, only to burst out into clones that can overtake dishes maintained in richer media. It is best to be certain that Schwann cell populations are as pure as possible before reseeding neuronal populations.

As a rule, Schwann cells prepared by the Brockes method never are rendered 100% fibroblast-free. Some Schwann cell cultures prepared by the Wood method also will contain recalcitrant fibroblasts but, if the cultures are examined carefully during cleanup and maintenance, contamination can be spotted. These flat cells with relatively large nuclei are distinct from Schwann cells in that they do not associate directly with neurites as the Schwann cells invariably do. If the fibroblasts are in a confined area, this area can be microdissected out of the culture.

Tissue Culture Contribution to Our Understanding of Peripheral Myelin

Separation of pure populations of Schwann cells followed by reintroduction of neurons allowed the direct demonstration that axonal contact strongly drives Schwann cell proliferation (Wood and Bunge, 1975). The induced proliferation is dependent on

contact between the axon and Schwann cell and, in rat tissues, is not serum-dependent. (For review, see Ratner et al., 1986, 1987.) An extensive literature reports on a variety of agents that influence Schwann cell proliferation (Porter et al., 1986, 1987; Davis and Stroobant, 1990; see DeVries, 1993, for review). Contact with an axon remains, however, one of the most effective ways to expand Schwann cell populations, as we have discussed earlier.

The ability to establish in tissue culture the components of the peripheral nerve separately and in combination also has allowed extensive documentation of the cellular interactions required for extracellular matrix production and perineurial assembly in the peripheral nerve trunk. Schwann cells in isolation do not deposit basal lamina over their external surfaces, as is characteristic of the fully developed axon–Schwann cell unit. (See M. Bunge et al., 1983, for review.) When axons reestablish contact with these "orphaned" Schwann cells, basal lamina again is assembled over the Schwann cells' abaxonal surface. These in vitro observations mirror those seen in the peripheral nerve trunk in vivo. Recently, researchers have described an exception to the generally accepted rule that neuronal contact is required to stimulate basal lamina assembly; in cultures containing Schwann cells free of axonal contact but with surrounding populations of fibroblasts, a basal lamina is seen deposited over the parts of the Schwann cell surface facing the fibroblasts but not over the surface of the Schwann cells where they are in contact with other Schwann cells (Obremski et al., 1993a).

Perhaps the most remarkable aspect of Schwann cell biology—which in all likelihood would not have been demonstrable except by tissue-culture techniques—is the fact that not only do Schwann cells deposit basal lamina but that an irrevocable linkage is formed between basal lamina production and the ensheathment function of Schwann cells. (For review, see R. Bunge et al., 1985.) A suggestion of this linkage was discussed in one of the earliest papers on myelination in culture (Peterson and Murray, 1965), in which it was observed that when embryo extract was not added to media nourishing sensory ganglion cultures, Schwann cells failed to relate normally to axons; these Schwann cells stained less regularly with a reticular stain that would stain (among other connective tissue components) parts of what we now call *basal lamina*. Moya et al. (1980) noted the linkage between basal lamina deposition over the abaxonal surface of the Schwann cell and the ability of Schwann cells to ensheathe small axons and myelinate larger axons. These

experiments directly demonstrated that the presence of embryo extract in culture medium allowed ensheathment to occur. Several years later, it was demonstrated that if the embryo extract was replaced by vitamin C, Schwann cell myelination was observed (Eldridge et al., 1987) and, furthermore, that this promotion of myelination could be obtained by direct addition of extracellular matrix components (particularly laminin) to the culture medium in the absence of vitamin C (Eldridge et al., 1989). In cocultures with superior cervical ganglion neurons, Schwann cell ensheathment of axons and basal lamina deposition was enhanced by the presence of fibroblasts or fibroblast-conditioned medium (Obremski, et al., 1993a). This finding suggested that the failure of complete ensheathment was secondary to insufficient basal lamina deposition in the absence of the fibroblast factor, a hypothesis supported by the demonstration that exposure of the cocultures to exogenous basal lamina components led to dramatic enhancement of ensheathment and basal lamina deposition (Obremski and M. Bunge, 1995).

These results indicated that basal lamina assembly was required for full expression of Schwann cell function in myelination. Vitamin C is not a requirement for central myelination (Eldridge et al., 1989); the central axon–myelin sheath–oligodendrocyte unit is not surrounded by basal lamina. On the basis of the results with Schwann cells, we now manipulate peripheral myelination in culture by withholding or adding vitamin C (see earlier). This vitamin C requirement also applies to amphibian peripheral nerve culture (Olsen and Bunge, 1986). Interestingly, cultures of amphibian spinal ganglia require vitamin C but not serum; their differentiation actually is inhibited by serum addition to the culture medium.

In light of these findings, the observation that fibroblast presence in populations of human Schwann cells was detrimental to the formation of myelin was unexpected (Morrissey et al., 1995b) and, as yet, unexplained. The fibroblast influence on Schwann cell function may be density-dependent; whereas a limited fibroblast population may stimulate Schwann cell differentiation, a high fibroblast–Schwann cell ratio may hinder Schwann cell function or adversely affect neuronal health.

The ability to poise cultures at the brink of myelination and then to initiate myelination by the addition of ascorbic acid has allowed the demonstration that basal lamina formation is linked to the expression of P0 gene (Fernandez-Valle et al., 1993). These findings strongly suggest that molecular events at the basal

lamina–Schwann cell interface act together with events at the axon–Schwann cell interface to induce or regulate gene expression critical for the progress of myelination. Further work using the neuron–Schwann cell myelinating culture system has suggested that laminin binding to a $\beta 1$ integrin may be an initial event in the regulation of myelination (Fernandez-Valle et al., 1994).

Cultures of neurons plus Schwann cells containing no fibroblasts will differentiate in the appropriate medium to become richly myelinated (as shown), but they do not develop perineurial sheaths. The perineurium is a layer of flattened cells enclosing multiple axon–Schwann cell units and providing a permeability barrier between innermost parts of the nerve (the endoneurium) and the body fluids outside the nerve trunk. It was long debated whether perineurium might be organized from the fibroblasts surrounding nerve trunks or from Schwann cells altered for this particular purpose. The fact that the inner cell layers of the perineurium are covered by basal lamina favored the latter view. The issue was addressed (M. Bunge et al., 1989) by using tissue cultures of neurons plus Schwann cells (of the type we have described) to which fibroblasts were added. Perineurium formed in these cultures only when fibroblasts were added. This experiment could not rule out, however, that the presence of fibroblasts induced the Schwann cells also present to alter their course of differentiation to form perineurium. Most recently, genetic markers were used to infect Schwann cells or fibroblasts prior to addition to the culture system (M. Bunge et al., 1989). This experiment showed that perineurium formed only from fibroblasts; no Schwann cell contributions were seen.

The culture system of purified populations of neurons and Schwann cells also has been used to study the cellular mechanisms of myelin deposition. These studies required direct observations of Schwann cell nuclei during the process of myelin formation; these observations were facilitated by the fact that the culture system has cells in an adequately dissociated state, so that direct observations of single living Schwann cells are possible. The observations were aided also by the ability to synchronize the onset of myelin formation by withholding, then adding, vitamin C (as discussed).

It has been known for several decades that the peripheral myelin sheath is arranged as a spiral of Schwann cell plasma membranes. Just how the spiral deposition of this membrane occurs in the process of myelin formation had, however, not been clarified. It

had been observed by several authors that some movement of the Schwann cell nucleus occurs during myelin formation, which suggested that the Schwann cell may circumnavigate the axon systematically to deposit a trail of plasma membrane that then would be deposited as a spiral. The most likely explanation was that the external lip of the encircling Schwann cell progressed around the axon, carrying the nucleus with it and, thus, accomplishing the remarkable configuration of the mature myelin sheath. A systematic study of Schwann cell nuclear movement during the early stages of myelination in culture, however, clearly implicated the progression of the inner Schwann cell lip over the axon's surface in the deposition of membrane that results in the establishment of myelin segments. The evidence from which this conclusion was derived and other implications for the cellular mechanisms of myelin deposition, are summarized in a recent publication (R. Bunge et al., 1989).

Prior to the time in which the inner Schwann cell lip begins encircling the axon in the process of myelin deposition, the axons large enough to induce myelination are separated from the remaining smaller axons to obtain their own individual Schwann cell ensheathment (Webster et al., 1973; recently reviewed in Kleitman and R. Bunge, 1995). This development of a one-to-one relationship between the larger axons and the Schwann cells gearing up for the process of myelination precedes the spiral deposition of myelin membranes. Observations that one of the distinctive myelin proteins—myelin-associated glycoprotein—already is expressed on Schwann cells at this early stage of development has led Owens and Bunge (1989) to suggest that the Schwann cell surface molecule myelin-associated glycoprotein may be implicated in this early step of axon–Schwann cell relationship that precedes myelinogenesis. Furthermore, the fact that this one-to-one relationship will develop in cultures containing Schwann cells that express very small amounts of the myelin-associated glycolipid GalC suggests that the surface-localized GalC on Schwann cells is not essential for the initial encirclement of an axon by the Schwann cell prior to myelin formation. Earlier experiments had shown that in the presence of antibodies to GalC, the antibody-GalC complex is cycled rapidly from the surface of the cell into internal compartments of the cell, and this activity keeps the GalC concentration on the Schwann cell surface much reduced. Under these conditions, Schwann cells surround the axon but do not proceed with the

spiral deposition of myelin membranes. This suggests that the presence of GalC on the Schwann cell surface is a requirement for the progression of the spiral deposition phase of myelin formation (Ranscht et al., 1987).

These antibody blocking experiments performed during the process of peripheral myelin formation require the presence of substantial levels of antibodies maintained in the culture medium during the several days in which the process of myelination is initiated. Again, the timing is facilitated by the ability to synchronize more or less the beginning of myelin formation in these cultures by the withdrawal and subsequent addition of vitamin C. It is also facilitated (as discussed) by the fact that, in the absence of fibroblasts, no perineurial barriers arise to antibody penetration into the culture system.

This experimental paradigm has been used more recently to elucidate the specific role of L1, the cell adhesion molecule expressed on both Schwann cells and axons, in the process of Schwann cell myelination and in the ensheathment of nonmyelinating axons. Work by Seilheimer et al. (1989) has indicated that antibodies to L1 block the ensheathing activity of nonmyelinating mouse Schwann cells, cocultured in this case with mouse sensory neurons. Using our culture system, Wood et al. (1990) have demonstrated that anti-L1 also blocks the process of myelination. This blockage of Schwann cell function occurs at a very early stage in the interaction between the Schwann cell and axon and occurs in spite of the fact that lamina is deposited in this culture system.

In addition to allowing studies of the role of cell-cell interactions in myelination, the neuron–Schwann cell culture system has been useful in exploring the role of soluble factors. In one such study, it has been demonstrated clearly that the cytokine transforming growth factor–β (TGF-β) acts to suppress myelination strongly and to allow or to promote the differentiation of Schwann cells into a mature nonmyelinating phenotype (Guénard et al., 1995). This study may be more relevant to events occuring in the aftermath of injury or in disease states within the nerve, in which levels of TGF-β are elevated. Studies of the effects of growth factors and cytokines on myelination have been relatively few in number; the dissociated cultures with defined medium composition appear to be a convenient and fruitful way to carry out such studies.

It should be apparent from the foregoing description that dissociated cultures capable of reproducing faithfully the events of

myelination have been and continue to be extremely valuable tools with which to study the cellular and molecular events of myelination. Experiments revealing the mechanisms by which Schwann cells affect neuronal function, such as neurite outgrowth, can be performed by using the same experimental tools. We have shown that the same antibodies to L1 that block myelination also prevent rat retinal ganglion cells from extending neurites onto Schwann cell surfaces (Kleitman et al., 1988). New ways in which the functions of Schwann cells and neurons are interdependent undoubtedly will continue to be revealed. We believe that the use of combined neuron–Schwann cell cultures of the type we have described is an effective experimental approach that will continue to yield new insights into the mechanism of the initiation and completion of the formation of the myelin sheath.

Finally, we mention two ways in which the use of the sensory neuron system has been used to study the interactions and interdependencies of central glial cells, in the process of central myelination. We have developed a technique to prepare oligodendrocytes from mature rat spinal cord (Rosen et al., 1989) and to observe the formation of myelin sheaths by the adult oligodendrocytes. This preparation can be undertaken with the use of either gradient separation of cell types followed by antimitotic treatment or by fluorescence-activated cell sorting (using GalC antibody), as described. When these purified oligodendrocytes are added to pure populations of sensory neurons, some of the oligodendrocytes proliferate in response to a mitogen that depends on axons. The proliferative response is observed in only a portion of the GalC-positive cells added to these cultures and suggests that, among the adult oligodendrocyte population identified by the expression of cell surface GalC, a subset of cells is capable of proliferation and subsequent myelination. This suggests one source of new myelinating cells within the adult CNS.

The availability of this reliably remyelinating CNS experimental paradigm has allowed us to look at the influence of type I astrocytes on oligodendrocyte function in the system (Rosen et al., 1989). Contrary to our expectations, the addition of astrocytes prepared from neonatal rat tissues by the frequently used method of McCarthy and DeVellis (1980) substantially suppressed the expression of oligodendrocyte myelination. Furthermore, it was clear that this suppression of oligodendrocyte function was mediated by substances

released by cocultured astrocytes, inasmuch as it was observed also in cultures that received only conditioned medium from astrocytes.

These experiments demonstrate the advantages of using tissue-culture preparations that allow the exact definition of cell types in the culture dish. In earlier experiments, we had observed that the presence of embryonic astrocytes grown in coculture with first developing oligodendrocytes were not suppressors of oligodendrocyte function and, in fact, seemed to work in harmony with oligodendrocytes in the process of myelination. Yet, when we used more mature astrocytes and tested their ability to influence the remyelinating capacity of adult oligodendrocytes, we found suppression. It is clear from these and other experiments that the complexity of cellular interactions in the CNS is formidable and that understanding how these interactions are regulated will be a challenging task. We are hopeful that the use of culture systems that allow combinations of very precisely defined cell types will be useful in this effort.

Acknowledgments

Work in the authors' laboratories is supported by US Public Health Service–National Institutes of Neurological and Communicative Disorders and Stroke (USPHS-NINCDS) grant NS09923 (RPB), USPHS-NINCDS grant NS28059 (RPB), the National Multiple Sclerosis Society grant RG-2210-B3/1 (PMW), The Miami Project to Cure Paralysis, and the Hollfelder Foundation.

References

Abney, E. R., B. P. Williams, and M. C. Raff (1983) Tracing the development of oligodendrocytes from precursor cells using monoclonal antibodies, fluorescence-activated cell sorting, and cell culture. Dev. Biol. 100: 166–171.

Acheson, A., D. Edgar, R. Timpl, and H. Thoenen (1986) Laminin increases both levels and activity of tyrosine hydroxylase in calf adrenal chromaffin cells. J. Cell Biol. 102: 151–159.

Acheson, A., J. C. Conover, J. P. Fandl, T. M. deChiara, M. Russell, A. Thadani, S. P. Squinto, G. D. Yancopoulos, and R. M. Lindsay (1995) A BDNF autocrine loop in adult sensory neurons prevents cell death. Nature 374: 450–453.

Adams, J. C. (1981) Heavy metal intensification of DAB-based HRP reaction product. J. Histochem. Cytochem. 29: 775.

Adler, R., G. Teitelman, and A. M. Suburo (1976) Cell interactions and the regulation of cholinergic enzymes during neural differentiation in vitro. Dev. Biol. 50: 48–57.

Ahmed, Z., and R. E. Fellows (1987) Determination of the birth date and proliferative state of dissociated cells from fetal rat brain. Brain Res. 465: 77–87.

Akli, S., C. Caillaud, E. Vigne, L. D. Stratford-Perricaudet, L. Poenaru, M. Perricaudet, A. Kahn, and M. Pachanski (1993) Transfer of a foreign gene into the brain using adenovirus vectors. Nature Genet. 3: 224–228.

Alberini, C. M., M. Ghirardi, R. Metz, and E. R. Kandel (1994) C/EBP is an immediate-early gene required for the consolidation of long-term facilitation in *Aplysia*. Cell 76: 1099–1114.

Alder, J., X. P. Xie, F. Valtorta, P. Greengard, and M. Poo (1992) Antibodies to synaptophysin interfere with transmitter secretion at neuromuscular synapses. Neuron 9: 759–768.

Alder, J., H. Kanki, F. Valtorta, P. Greengard, and M. Poo (1995) Overexpression of synaptophysin enhances neurotransmitter secretion at *Xenopus* neuromuscular synapses. J. Neurosci. 15: 511–519.

Alder, J., N. Cho, and M. E. Hatten (1996) Embryonic precursor cells from the rhombic lip are specified to a cerebellar granule neuron identity. Neuron 17: 389–399.

Aletta, J. M., and L. A. Greene (1988) Growth cone configuration and advance: a time-lapse study using video-enhanced differential interference contrast microscopy. J. Neurosci. 8: 1425–1435.

Aletta, J. M., H. Tsao, and L. A Greene (1990) How do neurites grow? Clues from NGF-regulated cytoskeletal phosphoproteins. In: *Trophic Factors and the Nervous System*, L. A. Horrocks, N. A. Neff, and A. J. Yates, eds., pp. 203–218, Raven, New York.

Allen, C. N., R. Brady, J. Swann, N. Hori and D. O. Carpenter (1988) *N*-methyl-D-aspartate (NMDA) receptors are inactivated by trypsin. Brain Res. 458: 147–150.

Aloe, L., and R. Levi-Montalcini (1979) Nerve growth factor–induced transformation of immature chromaffin cells in vivo into sympathetic neurons: effect of antiserum to nerve growth factor. Proc. Natl. Acad. Sci. U.S.A. 76: 1246–1250.

Altman, J. (1972) Postnatal development of the cerebellar cortex in the rat II. Phases in the maturation of Purkinje cells and of the molecular layer. J. Comp. Neurol. 145: 399–464.

Altman, J., and S. A. Bayer (1985a) Embryonic development of the rat cerebellum I. Delineation of the cerebellar primordium and early cell movement. J. Comp. Neurol. 231: 1–26.

Altman, J., and S. A. Bayer (1985b) Embryonic development of the rat cerebellum II. Translocation and regional distribution of the deep neurons. J. Comp. Neurol. 231: 27–41.

Altman, J., and S. A. Bayer (1995) *Atlas of prenatal rat brain development*, pp. 356–357, CRC Press, Boca Raton, FL.

Amaral, D. G. (1987) Memory: anatomical organization of candidate brain regions. In: *Handbook of Physiology*, sec. 1, F. Blum, ed., pp. 211–294, American Physiological Society, Bethesda, MD.

Amaya, E., T. J. Musci, and M. W. Kirschner (1991) Expression of a dominant negative mutant of the FGF receptor disrupts mesoderm formation in *Xenopus* embryos. Cell 66: 257–270.

Amonn, F., U. Baumann, U. N. Wiesmann, K. Hofmann and N. Herschkowitz (1978) Effects of antibiotics on the growth and differentiation in dissociated brain cell cultures. Neuroscience 3: 465–468.

Anderson, D. J. (1993) Molecular control of cell fate in the neural crest: the sympathoadrenal lineage. Annu. Rev. Neurosci. 16: 129–158.

Anderson, D. J., and R. Axel (1986) A bipotential neuroendocrine precursor whose choice of cell fate is determined by NGF and glucocorticoids. Cell 47: 1079–1090.

Anderson, M. J., and M. W. Cohen (1977) Nerve-induced and spontaneous redistribution of ACh receptors on cultured muscle cell groups. J. Physiol. 268: 757–773.

Anderson, M. J., M. W. Cohen, and E. Zorychta (1977) Effects of innervation on the distribution of ACh receptors on cultured cells. J. Physiol. 268: 731–756.

Andreason, G. L, and G. A. Evans (1989) Optimization of electroporation for transfection of mammalian cell lines. Anal. Biochem. 189: 269–275.

Anker, A. L., and Smilkstein, M. J. (1994) Acetaminophen. Concepts and controversies. Emerg. Med. Clin. North Am. 12: 335–349.

Annis, C. M., J. Edmond, and R. T. Robertson (1990) A chemically-defined medium for organotypic slice cultures. J. Neurosci. Methods 32: 63–70.

Annis, C. M., R. T. Robertson, and D. K. O'Dowd (1993) Aspects of early postnatal development of cortical neurons that proceed independently of normally present extrinisc influences. J. Neurobiol. 24: 1460–1480.

Annis, C. M., D. K. O'Dowd, and R. T. Robertson (1994) Activity-dependent regulation of dendritic spine density on cortical pyramidal neurons in organotypic slice cultures. J. Neurobiol. 25: 1483–1493.

Anton, E. S., M. Hadjiargyrou, P. H. Patterson, and W. D. Matthew (1995) CD9 plays a role in Schwann cell migration in vitro. J. Neurosci. 15: 584–595.

Anton, E. S., R. S. Cameron, and P. Rakic (1996) Role of neuron-glial junctional domain proteins in the maintenance and termination of neuronal migration across the embryonic cerebral wall. J. Neurosci. 16: 2283–2293.

Apperson, M. L., I. S. Moon, and M. B. Kennedy (1996) Characterization of densin-180, a new brain-specific synaptic protein of the o-sialoglycoprotein family. J. Neurosci. 16: 6839–6852.

Argiro, V., M. B. Bunge, and M. I. Johnson (1984) Correlation between growth form and movement and their dependence on neuronal age. J. Neurosci. 4: 3051–3062.

Aruoma, O. I., B. Halliwell, B. M. Hoey, and J. Butler (1989) The antioxidant action of *N*-acetylcysteine: its reaction with hydrogen peroxide, hydroxyl radical, superoxide and hypochlorous acid. Free Radic. Biol. Med. 6: 593–597.

Assouline, J. G., E. P. Bosch, and R. Lim (1983) Purification of rat Schwann cells from cultures of peripheral nerve: an immunoselective method using surfaces coated with anti-immunoglobulin antibodies. Brain Res. 277: 389–392.

Audinat, E., T. Knöpfel, and B. H. Gähwiler (1990) Responses to excitatory amino acids of Purkinje cells and neurones of the deep nuclei in cerebellar slice cultures. J. Physiol. (Lond.) 430: 297–313.

Augusti-Tocco, G., and G. Sato (1969) Establishment of functional clonal lines of neurons from mouse neuroblastoma. Proc. Natl. Acad. Sci. U.S.A. 64: 311–315.

Baas, P. W., and M. M. Black (1990) Individual microtubules in the axon consist of domains that differ in both composition and stability. J. Cell Biol. 111: 495–509.

Baas, P. W., M. M. Black, and G. A. Banker (1989) Changes in microtubule polarity orientation during the development of hippocampal neurons in culture. J. Cell. Biol. 109: 3085–3094.

Bading, H., M. M. Segal, N. J. Sucher, H. Dudek, S. A. Lipton, and M. E. Greenberg (1995) N-methyl-D-aspartate receptors are critical for mediating the effects of glutamate on intracellular calcium concentration and immediate early gene expression in cultured hippocampal neurons. Neuroscience 64: 653–664.

Bahr, B. A., R. L. Neve, J. Sharp, A. I. Geller, and G. Lynch (1994) Rapid and stable gene expression in hippocampal slice cultures from a defective HSV-1 vector. Mol. Brain Res. 26: 277–285.

Bailey, C. H., and M. Chen (1988) Long-term memory in *Aplysia* modulates the total number of varicosities of single identified sensory neurons. Proc. Natl. Acad. Sci. U.S.A. 85: 2373–2377.

Bailey, C. H., M. Chen, P. G. Montarolo, E. R. Kandel, and S. Schacher (1992) Inhibitors of protein and RNA synthesis block structural and functional changes accompanying long-term synaptic facilitation and inhibition in *Aplysia* sensory neurons. Neuron 9: 749–758.

Bain, G., T. P. Ramkumar, J. M. Cheng, and D. I. Gottlieb (1993) Expression of the genes coding for glutamic acid decarboxylase in pluripotent cell lines. Brain Res. Mol. Brain Res. 17: 23–30.

Bain, G., W. J. Ray, M. Yao, and D. I. Gottlieb (1994) From embryonal carcinoma cells to neurons: the P19 pathway. Bioessays 16: 343–348.

Bain, G., D. Kitchens, M. Yao, J. E. Huettner, and D. I. Gottlieb (1995) Embryonic stem cells express neuronal properties in vitro. Dev. Biol. 168: 342–357.

Baird, D. H., M. E. Hatten, and C. A. Mason (1992a) Cerebellar target neurons provide a stop signal for afferent neurite extension in vitro. J. Neurosci. 12: 619–634.

Baird, D. H., C. A. Baptista, L. C. Wang, and C. A. Mason (1992b) Specificity of a target cell-derived stop signal for afferent axonal growth. J. Neurobiol. 23: 579–591.

Baird, D. H., E. Trenkner, and C. A. Mason (1996) Functional NMDA receptors are required for the arrest of axon growth by target neurons in vitro. J. Neurosci. 16: 2642–2648.

Balentine, J. D., W. B. Greene, and M. Bornstein (1988) Spinal cord trauma: in search of the meaning of granular axoplasm and vesicular myelin. J. Neuropath. Exp. Neurol. 47: 77–92.

Bamburg, J. R., D. Bray, and K. Chapman (1986) Assembly of microtubules at the tip of growing axons. Nature 321: 788–790.

Bank, M., and S. Schacher (1992) Segregation of presynaptic inputs on an identified target neuron in vitro: structural remodeling visualized over time. J. Neurosci. 12: 2960–2972.

Banker, G. A. (1980) Trophic interactions between astroglial cells and hippocampal neurons in culture. Science 209: 809–810.

Banker, G. A., and W. M. Cowan (1977) Rat hippocampal neurons in dispersed cell culture. Brain Res. 126: 397–342.

Banker, G. A., and W. M. Cowan (1979) Further observations on hippocampal neurons in dispersed cell culture. J. Comp. Neurol. 187: 469–493.

Banker, G. A., and A. B. Waxman (1988) Hippocampal neurons generate natural shapes in cell culture. In: *Intrinsic Determinants of Neuronal Form and Function*, M. M. Black and R. Lasek, eds., pp. 61–82, Alan R. Liss, New York.

Baptista, C. A., M. E. Hatten, R. Blazeski, and C. A. Mason (1994) Cell-cell interactions influence survival and differentiation of purified Purkinje cells in vitro. Neuron 12: 1–20.

Barakat, I., and B. Droz (1988) Inducing effect of skeletal muscle extracts on the appearance of calbindin-immunoreactive dorsal root ganglion cells in culture. Neuroscience 28: 39–47.

Barakat, I., and B. Droz (1989) Calbindin-immunoreactive sensory neurons in dissociated dorsal root ganglion cell cultures of chick embryo: role of culture conditions. Brain Res. 50: 205–216.

Barald, K. F. (1989) Culture conditions affect the cholinergic development of an isolated subpopulation of chick mesencephalic neural crest cells. Dev. Biol. 135: 349–366.

Baratta, J., J. Marienhagen, D. Ha, J. Yu, and R. T. Robertson (1996) Cholinergic innervation of cerebral cortex in organoytpic slice cultures: sustained basal forebrain and transient striatal cholinergic projections. Neuroscience 72: 1117–1132.

Barbin, G., M. Manthorpe, and S. Varon (1984) Purification of the chick eye ciliary neu-ronotrophic factor. J. Neurochem. 42: 1468–1478.

Barde, Y.-A. (1989) Trophic factors and neuronal survival. Neuron 2: 1525–1534.

Barde, Y.-A, D. Edgar, and H. Thoenen (1980) Sensory neurons in culture: changing requirements for survival factors during embryonic development. Proc. Natl. Acad. Sci. U.S.A. 77: 1199–1203.

Barde, Y.-A, D. Edgar, and H. Thoenen (1982) Purification of a new neurotrophic factor from mammalian brain. EMBO J. 1: 549–553.

Barnes, D., and G. Sato (1980) Methods for growth of cultured cells in serum-free medium [review]. Anal. Biochem. 102: 255–270.

Barnett, S. C., A.-M. Hutchins, and M. Noble (1993) Purification of olfactory nerve ensheathing cells from the olfactory bulb. Dev. Biol. 155: 337–350.

Bar-Peled, O., E. Korkotian, M. Segal, and Y. Groner (1996) Constitutive overexpression of Cu/Zn superoxide dismutase exacerbates kainic acid-induced apoptosis of transgenic-Cu/Zn superoxide dismutase neurons. Proc. Natl. Acad. Sci. U.S.A. 93: 8530–8535.

Barres, B. A., L. L. Chun, and D. P. Corey (1988a) Ion channel expression by white matter glia: I. Type 2 astrocytes and oligodendrocytes. Glia 1: 10–30.

Barres, B. A., B. E. Silverstein, D. P. Corey, and L. L. Chun (1988b) Immunological, mor-phological, and electrophysiological variation among retinal ganglion cells purified by panning. Neuron 1: 791–803.

Barres, B. A., W. J. Koroshetz, L. L. Chun, and D. P. Corey (1990) Ion channel expression by white matter glia: the type-1 astrocyte. Neuron 5: 527–544.

Barres, B. A., I. K. Hart, and H. C. Coles (1992) Cell death and the control of survival in the oligodendrocyte lineage. Cell 70: 31–46.

Barres, B. A., R. Schmidt, M. Sendtner, and M. C. Raff (1993) Multiple extracellular sig-nals are required for long-term oligodendrocyte survival. Development 118: 283–295.

Barres, B. A., M. A. Lazar, and M. C. Raff (1994) A novel role for thyroid hormone, gluco-corticoids and retinoic acid in timing oligodendrocyte development. Development 120: 1097–1108.

Barrett, C. P., E. J. Donati, and L. Guth (1984) Differences between adult and neonatal rats in their astroglial response to spinal injury. Exp. Neurol. 84: 374–385.

Bar-Sagi, D., and J. R. Feramisco (1985) Microinjection of the *ras* oncogene protein into PC12 cells induces morphological differentiation. Cell 42: 841–848.

Bartlett, P. F., M. D. Noble, R. M. Pruss, M. C. Raff and S. Rattray (1980) Rat neural anti-gen-2 (Ran-2): a cell surface antigen on astrocytes, ependymal cells, Muller cells and lepto-meninges defined by a monoclonal antibody. Brain Res. 204: 339–351.

Bartlett, P. F., H. H. Reid, K. A. Bailey, and O. Bernard (1989) Immortalization of mouse neural precursor cells by the c-myc oncogene. Proc. Natl. Acad. Sci. U.S.A. 85: 3255–3259.

Bartlett, W. P., and G. A. Banker (1984) An electron microscopic study of the development of axons and dendrites by hippocampal neurons in culture. I. Cells which develop without intercellular contacts. J. Neurosci. 4: 1944–1953.

Batistatou, A., and L. A Greene (1993) Internucleosomal DNA cleavage and neuronal cell survival/death. J. Cell Biol. 122: 523–532.

Battleman, D. S., A. I. Geller, and M. V. Chao (1993) HSV-1 vector-mediated gene transfer of the human nerve growth factor receptor p75hNGFR defines high-affinity NGF binding. J. Neurosci. 13: 941–951.

Bayer, S. (1984) Neurogenesis in the rat neostriatum. Int. J. Dev. Neurosci. 2: 163–175.

Bayer, S. A. (1980) Development of the hippocampal slices maintained in organotypic cultures. J. Comp. Neurol. 190: 87–114.

Beach, R. L., S. L. Bathgate, and C. W. Cotman (1982) Identification of cell types in rat hippocampal slices maintained in organotypic cultures. Dev. Brain Res. 3: 3–20.

Beadle, D., G. Lees, and S. B. Kater (1988) *Cell Culture Approaches to Invertebrate Neu-roscience*, Academic Press, Orlando, FL.

Becker, T. C., R. J. Noel, W. S. Coats, A. M. Gomez-Foix, T. Alam, R. D. Gerard, and C. B. Newgard (1994) Use of recombinant adenovirus for metabolic engineering of mam-malian cells. Methods Cell Biol. 43: 161–189.

Beggs, H. E., P. Soriano, and P. F. Maness (1994) NCAM-dependent neurite outgrowth is inhibited in neurons from Fyn-minus mice. J. Cell Biol. 127: 825–833.

Bekkers, J. M., and C. F. Stevens (1989) NMDA and non-NMDA receptors are co-localized at individual excitatory synapses in cultured rat hippocampus. Nature 341: 230–233.

Bekkers J. M., and C. F. Stevens (1991) Excitatory and inhibitory autaptic currents in isolated hippocampal neurons maintained in cell culture. Proc. Natl. Acad. Sci. U.S.A. 88: 7834–7838.

Belsham, D. D., W. C. Wetsel, and P. L. Mellon (1996) NMDA and nitric oxide act through the cGMP signal transduction pathway to repress hypothalamic gonadotropin-releasing hormone gene expression. EMBO J. 15: 538–547.

Bennett, M. K., and R. H. Scheller (1993) The molecular machinery for secretion is conserved from yeast to neurons. Proc. Natl. Acad. Sci. U.S.A. 90: 2559–2563.

Benson, D. L., and P. A. Cohen (1996) Activity-independent segregation of excitatory and inhibitory synaptic terminals in cultured hippocampal neurons. J. Neurosci. 16: 6424–6432.

Benson, D. L., F. H. Watkins, O. Steward, and G. Banker (1994) Characterization of GABAergic neurons in hippocampal cell cultures. J. Neurocytol. 23: 279–295.

Berg D. W., and G. D. Fischbach (1978). Enrichment of spinal cord cell cultures with motoneurons. J. Cell Biol. 77: 83–98.

Bergold, P. J., P. Casaccia-Bonnefil, Z. Xiu-Liu, and H. J. Federoff (1993) Transsynaptic neuronal loss induced in hippocampal slice cultures by a herpes simplex virus vector expressing the GluR6 subunit of the kainate receptor. Proc. Natl. Acad. Sci. USA 90: 6165–6169.

Bergstrom, T., E. Sjogren-Jansson, S. Jeansson, and E. Lycke (1992) Mapping neuroinvasiveness of the herpes simplex virus type 1 encephalitis-inducing strain 2762 by the use of monoclonal antibodies. Mol. Cell Probes 6: 41–49.

Berthois, Y., J. A. Katzenellenbogen, and B. S. Katzenellenbogen (1986) Phenol red in tissue culture media is a weak estrogen: implications concerning the study of estrogen-responsive cells in culture. Proc. Natl. Acad. Sci. U.S.A. 83: 2496–2500.

Bett, A. J., W. Haddara, L. Prevec, and F. L. Graham (1994) An efficient and flexible system for construction of adenovirus vectors with insertions or deletions in early regions 1 and 3. Proc. Natl. Acad. Sci. USA 91: 8802–8806.

Betz, W. J., and G. S. Bewick (1992) Optical analysis of synaptic vesicle recycling at the frog neuromuscular junction. Science 255: 200–203.

Bignami, A., and D. Dahl (1976) The astroglial response to stabbing. Immunofluorescence studies with antibodies to astrocyte-specific protein (GFA) in mammalian and submammalian vertebrates. Neuropath. Appl. Neurobiol. 2: 99–110.

Bignami, A., L. F. Eng, D. Dahl, and C. T. Uyeda (1972). Localization of the glial fibrillary acidic protein in astrocytes by immunofluorescence. Brain Res. 43: 429–435.

Birgbauer, E., and F. Solomon (1989) A marginal band-associated protein has properties of both microtubule- and microfilament-associated proteins. J. Cell Biol. 109: 1609–1620.

Birren, S. J., and D. J. Anderson (1990) A v-myc- immortalized sympathoadrenal progenitor cell line in which neuronal differentiation is initiated by FGF but not NGF. Neuron 4: 189–201.

Birren, S. J., J. M. Verdi, and D. J. Anderson (1992) Membrane depolarization induces p140trk and NGF responsiveness, but not p75LNGFR, in MAH cells. Science 257: 395–397.

Bixby, J. L., G. B. Grunwald, and R. J. Bookman (1994) Ca^{2+} influx and neurite growth in response to purified N-cadherin and laminin. J. Cell Biol. 127: 1461–1475.

Björklund, A., and U. Stenevi (1984) Intracerebral neural implants: neuronal replacement and reconstruction of damaged circuits. Annu. Rev. Neurosci. 7: 279–308.

Black, M. M., and W. Smith (1988) Regional differentiation of the neuronal cytoskeleton. In: Intrinsic Determinants of Neuronal Form and Function, R. Lasek and M. M. Black, eds., Alan R. Liss, New York.

Blank, N. K., and F. J. Seil (1982) Mature Purkinje cells in cerebellar tissue cultures. An ultra-structural study. J. Comp. Neurol. 208: 169–176.

Blusztajn, J. K., A. Venturini, D. A. Jackson, H. J. Lee, and W. H. Wainer (1992) Acetylcholine synthesis and release is enhanced by dibutyryl cyclic AMP in a neuronal cell line derived from mouse septum. J. Neurosci. 12: 793–799.

Boder, G. B., W. J. Kleinschmidt, R. J. Harley, and D. C. Williams (1983) Visible light inhibits growth of Chinese hamster ovary cells. Eur. J. Cell Biol. 31: 132–136.

Bögler, O., and M. Noble (1991) Studies relating differentiation to a mechanism that measures time in O-2A progenitor cells. Ann. N.Y. Acad. Sci. 633: 505–507.

Bögler, O., and M. Noble (1994) Measurement of time in oligodendrocyte-type-2 astrocyte (O-2A) progenitors is a cellular process distinct from differentiation or division. Dev. Biol. 162: 525–538.

Bögler, O., D. Wren, S. C. Barnett, H. Land, and M. Noble (1990) Cooperation between two growth factors promotes extended self-renewal, and inhibits differentiation, of O-2A progenitor cells. Proc. Natl. Acad. Sci. U.S.A. 87: 6368–6372.

Bonhoeffer, F., and J. Huf (1980) Recognition of cell types by axonal growth cones in vitro. Nature 288: 162–164.

Bonhoeffer, F., and J. Huf (1985) Position-dependent properties of retinal axons and their growth cones. Nature 315: 409–410.

Bornstein, M. B. (1958) Reconstituted-rat tail collagen used as substrate for tissue cultures on coverslips in Maximow slides and roller tubes. Lab. Invest. 7: 134–140.

Bornstein, M. (1973) The immunopathology of demyelinative disorders examined in organotypic cultures of mammalian central nerve tissues. In: *Progress in Neuropathology*, vol. 2, H. Zimmermann, ed., pp. 69–90, Grune & Stratton, New York.

Boss, B. D., I. Gozes, and W. M. Cowan (1987a) The survival of dentate gyrus neurons in dissociated culture. Brain Res. 433: 199–218.

Boss, B. D., K. Turlejski, B. B. Stanfield, and W. M. Cowan (1987b) On the numbers of neurons in fields CA1 and CA3 of the hippocampus of Sprague-Dawley and Wistar rats. Brain Res. 406: 280–287.

Bottenstein, J., I. Hayashi, S. Hutching, H. Masui, J. Mather, D. B. McLure, S. Onasa, A. Rizzino, G. Sato, G. Serraro, R. Wolfe, and R. Wu (1979) Growth of cells in serum-free hormone supplemented media. Methods Enzymol. 58: 94–109.

Bottenstein, J. E. (1985) Growth and differentiation of neural cells in defined media. In: *Cell Culture in the Neurosciences*, J. E. Bottenstein and G. Sato, eds., pp. 3–14, Plenum, New York.

Bottenstein, J. E., and G. H. Sato (1979a) Growth of a rat neuroblastoma cell line in alpha-bungarotoxin save motoneurons from naturally occurring death in the absence of neuromuscular blockade. J. Neurosci. 15: 6453–6460.

Bottenstein, J. E., and G. H. Sato (1979b) Growth of a rat neuroblastoma cell line in serum-free supplemented medium. Proc. Natl. Acad. Sci. U.S.A. 76: 514–517.

Bottenstein, J. E., S. D. Skaper, S. S. Varon, and G. H. Sato (1980) Selective survival of neurons from chick embryo sensory ganglionic dissociates utilizing serum-free supplemented medium. Exp. Cell Res. 125: 183–190.

Bouillet, P., M. Oulad-Abdelghani, S. Vicaire, J. M. Garnier, P. Schuhbaur, P. Dolle, and P. Chambon (1995) Efficient cloning of cDNAs of retinoic acid-responsive genes in P19 embryonal carcinoma cells and characterization of a novel mouse gene, Stra1 (mouse Lerk-2/Eplg2). Dev. Biol. 170: 420–433.

Boulter, J., K. Evans, D. Goldman, G. Martin, P. Mason, S. Stengelin, S. Heinemann, and J. Patrick (1986). Isolation of a cDNA clone coding for a possible neural nicotinic acetylcholine receptor α-subunit. Nature 319: 368–374.

Boulter J., J. Connolly, E. Deneris, D. Goldman, S, Heinemann, and J. Patrick (1987) Functional expression of two neuronal nicotinic acetylcholine receptors identifies a gene family. Proc. Natl. Acad. Sci. U.S.A. 84: 7763–7767.

Boulter, J., A. O'Shea-Greenfield, R. M. Duvoisin, J. G. Connolly, E. Wada, A. Jensen, P. D. Gardner, M. Ballivet, E. S. Deneris and D. McKinnan (1990) α3, α5 and α4: Three members of the rat neuronal nicotinic acetylcholine receptor-related gene family form a gene cluster. J. Biol. Chem. 265: 4472–4482.

Boussif, O., F. Lezoualc'h, M. A. Zanta, M. D. Mergny, D. Scherman, B. Demeneix, and J.-P. Behr (1995) A versatile vector for gene and oligonucleotide transfer into cells in culture and in vivo: polyethyleneimine. Proc. Natl. Acad. Sci. U.S.A. 92: 7297–7301.

Boyne, L. J., K. Martin, S. Hockfield, and I. Fischer (1995) Expression and distribution of phosphorylated MAP1B in growing axons of cultured hippocampal neurons. J. Neurosci. Res. 40: 439–450.

Brandt, B. L. (1974) Clonal cell lines from the rat central nervous system. Nature 249: 224–227.

Braschler, U. F., A. Iannone, C. Spenger, J. Streit, and H.-R. Lüscher (1989) A modified roller tube technique for organotypic cocultures of embryonic rat spinal cord, sensory ganglia and skeletal muscle. J. Neurosci. Methods 29: 121–129.

Bray, D. (1970) Surface movements during the growth of single explanted neurons. Proc. Natl. Acad. Sci. U.S.A. 65: 905–910.

Bray, D. (1973) Branching patterns of individual sympathetic neurons in culture. J. Cell Biol. 56: 702–712.

Bray, D. (1984) Axonal growth in response to experimentally applied tension. Dev. Biol. 102: 379–389.

Bray, D. (1991) Isolated chick neurons for the study of axonal growth. In: *Culturing Nerve Cells*, G. Banker and K. Goslin, eds., The MIT Press, Cambridge, MA.

Bray, D. (1992) Cytoskeletal basis of nerve axon growth. In: *The Nerve Growth Cone*, P. C. Letourneau, S. B. Kater, and E. R. Macagno, eds., Raven, New York.

Bray, D., and K. Chapman (1985) Analysis of microspike movements on the neuronal growth cone. J. Neurosci. 5: 3204–3213.

Brehm, P., Y. Kidokoro, and F. Moody-Corbett (1984) ACh receptor channel properties of *Xenopus* muscle cells in culture. J. Physiol. 357: 203–217.

Brewer, G. J. (1995) Serum-free B27/neurobasal medium supports differentiated growth of neurons from the striatum, substantia nigra, septum, cerebral cortex, cerebellum, and dentate gyrus. J. Neurosci. Res. 42: 674–683.

Brewer, G. J., and C. W. Cotman (1989) Survival and growth of hippocampal neurons in defined medium at low density: advantages of a sandwich culture technique or low oxygen. Brain Res. 494: 65–74.

Brewer G. J., J. R. Torricelli, E. K. Evege, and P. J. Price (1993). Optimized survival of hippocampal neurons in B-27-supplemented Neurobasal, a new serum-free medium combination. J. Neurosci. Res. 35: 567–576.

Bridgman, P. C., and T. S. Reese (1984) The structure of cytoplasm in directly frozen cultured cells. I. Filamentous meshworks and the cytoplasmic ground substance. J. Cell Biol. 99: 1655–1668.

Bridgman, P. C., B. Kachar, and T. S. Reese (1986) The structure of cytoplasm in directly frozen cultured cells. II. Cytoplasmic domains associated with organelle movements. J. Cell Biol. 102: 1510–1521.

Britland, S., E. Perez-Arnaud, P. Clark, B. McGinn, P. Connolly and G. Moores (1992) Micropatterning proteins and synthetic peptides on solid supports: a novel application for microelectronics fabrication technology. Biotechnol. Prog. 8: 155–160.

Brockes, J. P., K. L. Fields, and M. C. Raff (1979) Studies on cultured rat Schwann cells: I. Establishment of purified populations from cultures of peripheral nerve. Brain Res. 165: 105–118.

Brockes, J. P., G. E. Lemke, and D. R. Balzer (1980) Purification and preliminary characterization of glial growth factor from the bovine pituitary. J. Biol. Chem. 255: 8374–8377.

Broughton, S. J., N. S. Kane, B. Arthur, M. Yoder, R. J. Greenspan, and A. Robichon (1996) Endogenously inhibited protein kinase C in transgenic *Drosophila* embryonic neuroblasts down-regulates the outgrowth of type I and II processes of cultured mature neurons. J. Cell. Biochem. 60: 584–599.

Brown, T. H., and A. M. Zador (1990) Hippocampus. In: *The Synaptic Organization of the Brain*, G. M. Shepherd, ed., pp. 346–388, Oxford University, New York.

Bruckenstein, D., M. I. Johnson, and D. Higgins (1989) Age-dependent changes in the capacity of rat sympathetic neurons to form dendrites in tissue culture. Brain Res. Dev. Brain Res. 46: 21–32.

Bruckner, P., I. Horler, M. Mendler, Y. Houze, K. H. Winterhalter, S. G. Eich-Bender, and M. A. Spycher (1989) Induction and prevention of chondrocyte hypertrophy in culture. J. Cell Biol. 109: 2537–2545.

Brummendorf, T., and F. G. Rathjen (1995) *Cell Adhesion Molecules 1: Immunoglobulin Superfamily*, Academic Press, London.

Bruns, D., and R. Jahn (1995) Real-time measurement of transmitter release from single synaptic vesicles. Nature 377: 62–65.

Buchanan, J., Y. A. Sun, and M-m. Poo (1989) Studies of nerve-muscle interactions in *Xenopus* cell culture: fine structure of early functional contacts. J. Neurosci. 9: 1540–1554.

Buckmaster, E. A., and A. M. Tolkovsky (1994) Expression of the cyclic AMP-dependent protein kinase (PKA) catalytic subunit from a herpes simplex virus vector extends the survival of rat sympathetic neurons in the absence of NGF. Eur. J. Neurosci. 6: 1316–1327.

Bulloch, A. G., and N. I. Syed (1992) Reconstruction of neural networks in culture. Trends Neurosci. 15: 422–427.

Bunge, R. P. (1975) Changing uses of nerve tissue culture 1950–1975. In: *The Nervous System: I. The Basic Neurosciences*, D. B. Tower, ed., pp. 31–42, Raven, New York.

Bunge, R. P., and P. Wood (1973) Studies on the transplantation of spinal cord tissue in the rat: II. Development of a culture system for hemisections of embryonic spinal cord. Brain Res. 57: 261–276.

Bunge, R. P., M. B. Bunge, and E. R. Peterson (1965) An electron microscopic study of cultured rat spinal cord. J. Cell Biol. 24: 163–191.

Bunge, R. P., M. B. Bunge, and C. F. Eldridge (1985) Linkage between axonal ensheathment and basal lamina production by Schwann cells. Annu. Rev. Neurosci. 9: 305–328.

Bunge, R. P., M. B. Bunge, and M. Bates (1989) Movements of the Schwann cell nucleus implicate progression of the inner (axon-related) Schwann cell process during myelination. J. Cell Biol. 109: 273–284.

Bunge, M. B., A. K. Williams, P. M. Wood, et al. (1980) Comparison of nerve cell and nerve cell plus Schwann cell cultures, with particular emphasis on basal lamina and collagen formation. J. Cell Biol. 84: 184–202.

Bunge, M. B., R. P. Bunge, D. J. Carey, C. J. Cornbrooks, C. F. Eldridge, A. K. Williams and P. M. Woods (1983) Axonal and nonaxonal influences on Schwann cell development. In: *Developing and Regenerating Vertebrate Nervous Systems*, P. W. Coates, R. R. Markwald, and A. D. Kenny, eds., pp. 71–105, Alan R. Liss, New York.

Bunge, M. B., P. M. Wood, L. B. Tynan, M. L. Bates and J. R. Sanes (1989) Perineurium originates from fibroblasts: demonstration in vitro with a retroviral marker. Science 243: 229–231.

Burden-Gulley, S. M., H. R. Payne, and V. Lemmon (1995) Growth cones are actively influenced by substrate-bound adhesion molecules. J. Neurosci. 15: 4370–4381.

Burgeson, R. E., M. Chiquet, R. Deutzmann, P. Ekblom, J. Engel, H. Kleinman, G. R. Martin, G. Maneguzzi, M. Paulsson, S. Sarkar and N. J. Cowan (1994) A new nomenclature for the laminins. Matrix Biol. 14: 209–211.

Burgoyne, R. D., M. A. Cambray-Deakin, S. A. Lewis, S. Sarkar, and N. J. Cowan (1988) Differential distribution of beta-tubulin isotypes in cerebellum. EMBO J. 7: 2311–2319.

Burgunder, J. M., A. Varriale, and B. H. Lauterburg (1989) Effect of *N*-acetylcysteine on plasma cysteine and glutathione following paracetamol administration. Eur. J. Clin. Pharmacol. 361: 27–131.

Burmeister, D. W., and D. J. Goldberg (1988) Micropruning: the mechanism of turning of *Aplysia* growth cones at substrate borders in vitro. J. Neurosci. 8: 3151–3159.

Burmeister, D. W., R. J. Rivas, and D. J. Goldberg (1991) Substrate-bound factors stimulate engorgement of lamellipodia during neurite elongation. Cell Motil. Cytoskel. 19: 255–268.

Burstein, D. E., and L. A. Greene (1982) Nerve growth factor has both mitogenic and non-mitogenic actions. Dev. Biol. 94: 477–482.

Buzsaki, G., and J. J. Chrobak (1995) Temporal structure in spatially organized neuronal ensembles: a role for interneuronal networks [review]. Curr. Opin. Neurobiol. 5: 504–510.

Caceres, A., G. Banker, O. Steward, L. Binder and M. Payne (1984) MAP2 is localized to the dendrites of hippocampal neurons which develop in culture. Brain Res. 315: 314–318.

Caceres, A., G. A. Banker, and L. Binder (1986) Immunocytochemical localization of tubulin and microtubule-associated protein 2 during the development of hippocampal neurons in culture. J. Neurosci. 6: 714–722.

Caeser, M., T. Bonhoeffer, and J. Bolz (1989) Cellular organization and development of slice cultures from rat visual cortex. Exp. Brain Res. 77: 234–244.

Caillaud, C., S. Akli, E. Vigne, A. Koulakoff, M. Perricaudet, L. Poenaru, A. Kahn, and Y. Berwald-Netter (1993) Adenoviral vector as a gene delivery system into cultured rat neuronal and glial cells. Eur. J. Neurosci. 5: 1287–1291.

Calof, A. L., and L. F. Reichardt (1984) Motoneurons purified by cell sorting respond to two distinct activities in myotube-conditioned medium. Dev. Biol. 106: 194–210.

Calvet, M. C., J. Calvet, R. Camacho, and D. Eude (1983) The dendritic trees of Purkinje cells: a computer assisted analysis of HRP labeled neurons in organotypic cultures of kitten cerebellum. Brain Res. 280: 199–215.

Camardo, J., E. Proshansky, and S. Schacher (1983) Identified *Aplysia* neurons form specific chemical synapses in culture. J. Neurosci. 3: 2614–2620.

Campenot, R. B. (1977) Local control of neurite development by nerve growth factor. Proc. Natl. Acad. Sci. U.S.A. 74: 4516–4519.

Campenot, R. B. (1982a) Development of sympathetic neurons in compartmentalized cultures: II. Local control of neurite survival by nerve growth factor. Dev. Biol. 93: 13–21.

Campenot, R. B. (1982b) Development of sympathetic neurons in compartmentalized cultures: I. Local control of neurite growth by nerve growth factor. Dev. Biol 93: 1–12.

Campenot, R. B. (1992) Compartmented culture analysis of nerve growth. In: *Cell-Cell Interactions: A Practical Approach*, B. R. Stevenson, W. J. Gallin, and D. L. Paul, eds., pp. 275–298, IRL Press, Oxford.

Campenot, R. B. (1994) NGF and the local control of nerve terminal growth [review]. J. Neurobiol. 25: 599–611.

Camu W., and C. E. Henderson (1992) Purification of embryonic rat motoneurons by panning on a monoclonal antibody to the low-affinity NGF receptor. J. Neurosci. Methods 44: 59–70.

Carbonetto, S., D. Evans, and P. Cochard (1987) Nerve fiber growth in culture on tissue substrata from central and peripheral nervous systems. J. Neurosci. 7: 610–620.

Carlstedt, T., C.-J. Dalsgaard, and C. Molander (1987) Regrowth of lesioned dorsal root nerve fibres into the spinal cord of neonatal rats. Neurosci. Lett. 74: 14–18.

Carnahan, J. F., and P. H. Patterson (1991) Isolation of the progenitor cells of the sympathoadrenal lineage from embryonic sympathetic ganglia with the SA monoclonal antibodies. J. Neurosci. 11: 3520–3530.

Carnahan, J. F., D. R. Patel, and J. A. Miller (1994) Stem cell factor is a neurotrophic factor for neural crest-derived chick sensory neurons. J. Neurosci. 14: 1433–1440.

Carr, V. M., and S. B. Simpson, Jr. (1978) Proliferative and degenerative events in the early development of chick dorsal root ganglia: I. Normal development. J. Comp. Neurol. 182: 727–740.

Carraway, K. L., and S. J. Burden (1995) Neuregulins and their receptors. Curr. Opin. Neurobiol. 5: 606–612.

Carrell, A., and M. T. Burroughs (1910) Cultivation of adult tissues and organs outside of the body. J.A.M.A. 55: 1379–1381.

Carroll, S. L., I. Silos-Santiago, S. E. Frese, K. G. Ruit, J. Milbrandt, and W. D. Snider (1992) Dorsal root ganglion neurons expressing trk are selective to NGF deprivation in utero. Neuron 9: 779–788.

Carter, S. B. (1965) Principles of cell motility: the direction of cell movement and cancer invasion. Nature 208: 1183–1187.

Carter, S. B. (1967) Haptotactic islands. A method for confining single cells to study individual cell reactions and clone formation. Exp. Cell Res. 48: 189–193.

Casaccia-Bonnefil, P., E. Benedikz, H. Shen, A. Stelzer, D. Edelstein, M. Geschwind, M. Brownlee, H. J. Federoff, and P. J. Bergold (1993) Localized gene transfer into organotypic hippocampal slice cultures and acute hippocampal slices. J. Neurosci. Meth. 5: 341–351.

Cashman, N. R., H. D. Durham, J. K. Blusztajn, K. Oda, T. Tabira, I. T. Shaw, S. Dahrouge, and J. P. Antel (1992) Neuroblastoma x spinal cord (NSC) hybrid cell lines resemble developing motor neurons. Dev. Dyn. 194: 209–221.

Castellucci, V. F., H. Blumenfeld, P. Goelet, and E. R. Kandel (1989) Inhibitor of protein synthesis blocks long-term behavioral sensitization in the isolated gill-withdrawal reflex in *Aplysia*. J. Neurobiol. 20: 1–9.

Catarsi, S., and P. Drapeau (1993) Tyrosine-kinase dependent selection of transmitter response is induced by neuronal contact. Nature 363: 353–355.

Catterall, WA (1981) Studies of voltage-sensitive sodium channels in cultured cells using ion-flux and ligand-binding methods. In: *Excitable Cells in Tissue Culture*, P. G. Nelson and M. Lieberman, eds., pp. 279–317, Plenum, New York.

Cepko, C. L. (1989) Immortalization of neural cells via retrovirus-mediated oncogene transduction. Annu. Rev. Neurosci. 12: 47–65.

Cepko, C. (1992) In: *Current Protocols in Molecular Biology*. Volume I. Supplement 17. 9.11.9–9.11.10. Current Protocols.

Chalazonitis, A., and G. D. Fischbach (1980) Elevated potassium induces morphological differentiation of dorsal root ganglionic neurons in dissociated cell culture. Dev. Biol. 78: 173–183.

Chalmers, G. R., L. J. Fisher, K. Niijima, P. H. Patterson, and F. H. Gage (1995) Adrenal chromaffin cells transdifferentiate in response to basic fibroblast growth factor and show directed outgrowth to a nerve growth factor source in vivo. Exp. Neurol. 133 (1): 32–42.

Chao, C. C., S. Hu, and P. K. Peterson (1995) Glia, cytokines, and neurotoxicity [review]. Crit. Rev. Neurobiol. 9: 189–205.

Chard, P. S., J. Jordan, C. J. Marcuccilli, R. J. Miller, J. M. Leiden, R. P. Roos, and G. D. Ghadge (1995) Regulation of excitatory transmission at hippocampal synapses by calbindin D28k. Proc. Natl. Acad. Sci. U.S.A. 92: 5144–5148.

Charlton, H. M., A. N. Barclay, and A. F. Williams (1983) Detection of neuronal tissue from brain grafts with anti-Thy-1.1 antibody. Nature 305: 825–828.

Chedotal, A., and C. Sotelo (1992) Early development of olivocerebellar projections in the fetal rat using CGRP immunocytochemistry. Eur. J. Neurosci. 4: 1159–1179.

Chen, C., and H. Okayama (1987) High-efficiency transformation of mammalian cells by plasmid DNA. Mol. Cell. Biol. 7: 2745–2752.

Cheng, B., and M. P. Mattson (1995) PDGFs protect hippocampal neurons against energy deprivation and oxidative injury: evidence for induction of antioxidant pathways. J. Neurosci. 15: 7095–7104.

Chiocca, E. A., B. B. Choi, W. Cai, N. A. DeLuca, P. A. Schaffer, M. DiFiglia, X. O. Breakefield, and R. L. Martuza (1990) Transfer and expression of the lacZ gene in rat brain neurons mediated by herpes simplex virus mutants. The New Biologist 2: 739–746.

Chiquet, M., and J. G. Nicholls (1987) Neurite outgrowth and synapse formation by identified leech neurons in culture. J. Exp. Biol. 132: 191–206.

Choi, D. W., and S. M. Rothman (1990) The role of glutamate neurotoxicity in hypoxic-ischemic neuronal death. Annu. Rev. Neurosci. 12: 171–182.

Choi, H. K., L. A. Won, P. J. Kontur, D. N. Hammond, A. P. Fox, B. H. Wainer, P. C. Hoffman, and A. Heller (1991) Immortalization of embryonic mesencephalic dopaminergic neurons by somatic cell fusion. Brain Res. 552: 67–76.

Choi, H. K., L. Won, J. D. Roback, B. H. Wainer, and H. Heller (1992) Specific modulation of dopamine expression in neuronal hybrid cells by primary cells from different brain regions. Proc. Natl. Acad. Sci. U.S.A. 89: 8943–8947.

Choi, H. K., L. Won, and A. Heller (1993) Dopaminergic neurons grown in three-dimensional reaggregate culture for periods of up to one year. J. Neurosci. Methods 46: 233–244.

Chomczynski P., and N. Sacchi (1987). Single-step method of RNA isolation by acid guanidinium thiocyanate-phenol-chloroform extraction. Anal. Biochem. 162: 156–159.

Chow, I., and M-m. Poo (1984) Formation of electrical coupling between embryonic *Xenopus* muscle cells in culture. J. Physiol. 346: 181–194.

Chow, I., and M-m Poo (1985) Release of acetylcholine from embryonic neurons upon contact with muscle cell. J. Neurosci. 5: 1076–1082.

Christakos, S., W. B. Rhoten, and S. C. Feldman (1987) Rat CaBP-D28K: purification, quantitation, immunocytochemical localization, and comparative aspects. In *Methods in Enzymology*, Vol. 139, A. R. Means and P. M. Conn, eds., pp. 534–551, Academic Press, New York.

Chuang, W., and C. F. Lagenaur (1990) Central nervous system antigen P84 can serve as a substrate for neurite outgrowth. Dev. Biol 137: 219–232.

Cid-Arregui, A., H. M. De, and C. G. Dotti (1995) Mechanisms of neuronal polarity. Neurobiol. Aging 16: 239–243.

Clark, P., S. Britland, and P. Connolly (1993) Growth cone guidance and neuron morphology on micropatterned laminin surfaces. J. Cell. Sci. 105: 203–212.

Claude, P., I. M. Parada, K. A. Gordon, et al. (1988) Acidic fibroblast growth factor stimulates adrenal chromaffin cells to proliferate and to extend neurites, but is not a long-term survival factor. Neuron 1: 783–790.

Clendening, B., and R. I. Hume (1990) Cell interactions regulate dendritic morphology and responses to neurotransmitters in embryonic chick sympathetic preganglionic neurons in vitro. J. Neurosci. 10: 3992–4005.

Cohan, C. S., P. G. Haydon, and S. B. Kater (1985) Single channel activity differs in growing and non-growing growth cones of isolated identified neurons of *Helisoma*. J. Neurosci. Res. 13: 285–300.

Cohan, C. S., J. A. Connor, and S. B. Kater (1987) Electrically and chemically mediated increases in intracellular calcium in neuronal growth cones. J. Neurosci. 7: 3588–3599.

Cohen, M. W., E. Rodriguez-Marin, and E. M. Wilson (1987) Distribution of synaptic specializations along isolated motor units formed in *Xenopus* nerve-muscle cultures. J. Neurosci. 7: 2849–2861.

Cohen, R. I., R. Marmur, W. T. Norton, M. F. Mehler, and J. A. Kessler. (1996) Nerve growth factor and neurotrophin-3 differentially regulate the proliferation and survival of developing rat brain oligodendrocytes. J. Neurosci. 16: 6433–6442.

Cohen-Cory, S., C. F. Dreyfus, and I. B. Black (1991) NGF and excitatory neurotransmitters regulate survival and morphogenesis of cultured cerebellar Purkinje cells. J. Neurosci. 11: 462–471.

Coles, H. S. R., J. F. Burne, and M. C. Raff (1993) Large-scale normal death in the developing rat kidney and its reduction by epidermal growth factor. Development 118: 777–784.

Collier, T. J., M. J. Gallagher, and C. D. Sladek (1993) Cryopreservation and storage of embryonic rat mesencephalic dopamine neurons for one year: comparison to fresh tissue in culture and neural grafts. Brain Res. 623: 249–256.

Collins, F. (1978) Axon inititation by ciliary neruons in culture. Dev. Biol. 65: 50–57.

Contestabile, A., and F. Fonnum (1983) Cholinergic and GABAergic forebrain projections to the habenula and nucleus interpeduncularis: surgical and kainic acid lesions. Brain Res. 275: 287–297.

Contestabile, A. L., A. Villani Fasolo, M. F. Franzoni, et al. (1987). Topography of cholinergic and substance P pathways in the habenulo-interpeduncular system of the rat. An immunocytochemical and microchemical approach. Neuroscience 21: 253–270.

Costero, I., and C. M. Pomerat (1951) Cultivation of neurons from the adult human cerebral and cerebellar cortex. Am. J. Anat. 89: 405–467.

Costâchel, O., L. Fadei, and E. Badea (1969) Tumor cell suspension culture on non adhesive substratum. Zeit. Krebsforsch. 72: 24–31.

Cotten, M., E. Wagner, K. Zatloukal, S. Phillips, D. T. Curiel, and M. L. Birnstiel (1992) High-efficiency receptor-mediated delivery of small and large (48 kilobase) gene constructs using the endosome-disrupting activity of defective or chemically inactivated adenovirus particles. Proc. Natl. Acad. Sci. USA 89: 6094–6098.

Couturier, S., D. Bertrand, J. M. Matter, M. C. Hernandez, S. Bertrand, N. Millar, S. Vallera, T. Barkas, and M. Ballivet (1990a) A neuronal nicotinic acetylcholine receptor subunit (α7) is developmentally regulated and forms a homo-oligomeric channel blocked by a-BTX. Neuron 5: 847–856.

Couturier, S., L. Erkman, S. Valera, D. Rungger, S. Bertrand, J. Boulter, M. Ballivet, and D. Bertrand (1990b) α5, α3, non- α3. Three clustered avian genes encoding neuronal nicotinic receptor-related subunits. J. Biol. Chem. 265: 17560–17567.

Covault, J., J. M. Cunningham, and J. R. Sanes (1987) Neurite outgrowth on cryostat sections of innervated and denervated skeletal muscle. J. Cell Biol. 105: 2479–2488.

Craig, A. M., and G. Banker (1994) Neuronal polarity. Annu. Rev. Neurosci. 17: 267–310.

Craig, A. M., C. D. Blackstone, R. L. Huganir, and G. Banker (1993) The distribution of glutamate receptors in cultured rat hippocampal neurons: postsynaptic clustering of AMPA-selective subunits. Neuron 10: 1055–1068.

Craig, A. M., C. D. Blackstone, R. L. Huganir, and G. Banker (1994a) Selective clustering of glutamate and gamma-aminobutyric acid receptors opposite terminals releasing the corresponding neurotransmitters. Proc. Natl. Acad. Sci. U.S.A. 91: 12373–12377.

Craig, A. M., O. Steward, and G. Banker (1994b) Use of HSV-1 amplicon vectors to study RNA and protein targeting in cultured hippocampal neurons. Gene Ther. 1(suppl. 1): S72.

Craig, A. M., R. J. Wyborski, and G. Banker (1995) Preferential addition of newly synthesized membrane protein at axonal growth cones. Nature 375: 592–594.

Craig, A. M., G. Banker, W. Chang, M. E. McGrath, and S. E. Serpinskaya (1996) Clustering of gephyrin at GABAergic but not glutamatergic synapses in cultured rat hippocampal neurons. J. Neurosci. 16: 3166–3177.

Crain, S. M. (1976) *Neurophysiologic Studies in Tissue Culture*, Raven Press, New York.

Crawford, G. D. F., W. D. Le, R. G. Smith, W. J. Xie, E. Stefani, and S. H. Appel (1992) A novel N18TG2 x mesencephalon cell hybrid expresses properties that suggest a dopaminergic cell line of substantia nigra origin. J. Neurosci. 12: 3392–3398.

Crino, P. B., and J. Eberwine (1996) Molecular characterization of the dendritic growth cone regulated MRNA transport and local protein synthesis. Neuron 17: 1173–1187.

Crossin, K. L., S. Hoffman, S.-S. Tan, and G. M. Edelman (1989) Cytotactin and its proteoglycan ligand mark structural and functional boundaries in somatosensory cortex of the early postnatal mouse. Dev. Biol. 136: 381–392.

Cuello, A. C. (1983) *Immunohistochemistry*, Wiley, New York.

Cunningham, M. E., R. M. Stephens, D. R. Kaplan, and L. A. Green (1997) Autophosphorylation of activation loop tyrosines regulates signaling by the Trk NGF receptor. J. Biol. Chem. 272: 10957–10967.

Cunningham, M. E., J. Kitajewski, and L. A. Green (in press) Efficient generation of stable recombinant pheochromocytoma (PCIZ) cell lines using a recombinant retrovirus (LNC). In: *Neurotrophin Receptor Methods and Protocols*, R. A. Rush, ed., Humana Press, Clifton, NJ.

Dagle, J. M., J. A. Walder, and D. L. Weeks (1990) Targeted degredation of mRNA in *Xenopus* oocytes and embryos directed by modified oligonucleotides: studies of An2 and cyclin in embryogenesis. Nucleic Acids Res. 18: 4751–4757.

Dai, J., and M. P. Sheetz (1995) Axon membrane flows from the growth cone to the cell body. Cell 83: 693–701.

Dai, Z., and H. B. Peng (1995) Presynaptic differentiation induced in cultured neurons by local application of basic fibroblast growth factor. J. Neurosci. 15: 5466–5475.

Dambska, M., M. Laure-Kamionowska, and B. Schmidt-Sidor (1989) Early and late neuropathological changes in perinatal white matter damage. J. Child Neurol. 4: 291–2948.

Dan, Y., Y. Lo, and M-m. Poo (1995) Plasticity of developing neuromuscular synapses [review]. Prog. Brain Res. 105: 211–215.

Dash, P. K., B. Hochner, and E. R. Kandel (1990) Injection of the cAMP-responsive element into the nucleus of *Aplysia* sensory neurons blocks long-term facilitation. Nature 345: 718–721.

Davenport, R. W., P. Dou, V. Rehder, and S. B. Kater (1993) A sensory role for neuronal growth cone filopodia. Nature 361: 721–724.

Davenport, R. W., E. Thies, and P. G. Nelson (1996) Cellular localization of guidance cues in the establishment of retinotectal topography. J. Neurosci. 16: 2074–2085.

Davidson, B. L., E. D. Allen, K. F. Kozarsky, J. M. Wilson, and B. J. Roessler (1993) A model system for in vivo gene transfer into the central nervous system using an adenoviral vector. Nature Genet. 3: 219–223.

Davies, A. L. (1989) Neurotrophic factor bioassay using dissociated neurons. In: *Nerve Growth Factors*, R. A. Rush, ed., Wiley, Chichester, UK.

Davies, A. M. (1987) Molecular and cellular aspects of patterning sensory neurone connections in the vertebrate nervous system. Development 101: 185–208.

Davis, J. B., and P. Stroobant (1990) Platelet-derived growth factors and fibroblast growth factors are mitogens for rat Schwann cells. J. Cell Biol. 110: 1353–1360.

Davis, L., G. A. Banker, and O. Steward (1987) Selective dendritic transport of RNA in hippocampal neurons in culture. Nature 330: 477–479.

Davis, L., B. Burger, G. A. Banker, and O. Steward (1990) Dendritic transport: quantitative analysis of the time course of somatodendritic transport of recently synthesized RNA. J. Neurosci. 10: 3056–3068.

Dawson, V. L., V. M. Kizushi, P. L. Huang, S. H. Snyder, and T. M. Dawson (1996) Resistance to neurotoxicity in cortical cultures from neuronal nitric oxide synthase-deficient mice. J. Neurosci. 16: 2479–2487.

Debanne, D., B. H. Gähwiler, and S. M. Thompson (1994) Asynchronous pre- and post-synaptic activity induces associative long-term depression in area CA1 of the rat hippocampus in vitro. Proc. Natl. Acad. Sci. USA 91: 1148–1152.

Debanne, D., N. C. Guérineau, B. H. Gähwiler, and S. M. Thompson (1995) Physiology and pharmacology of unitary synaptic connections between pairs of cells in areas CA3 and CA1 of rat hippocampal slice cultures. J. Neurophysiol. 73: 1282–1294.

DeHoop, M. J., L. A. Huber, H. Stenmark, E. Williamson, M. Zerial, R. G. Parton, and C. G. Dotti (1994) The involvement of the small GTP-binding protein rab5a in neuronal endocytosis. Neuron 13: 11–22.

Deitch, J. S., and G. A. Banker (1993) An electron microscopic analysis of hippocampal neurons developing in culture: early stages in the emergence of polarity. J. Neurosci. 13: 4301–4315.

Delfs, J., J. Friend, and S. Ishimoto (1989) Ventral and dorsal horn acetylcholinesterase neurons are maintained in organotypic cultures of postnatal rat spinal cord explants. Brain Res. 488: 31–42.

Delree, P., P. Leprince, J. Schoenen, and G. Moonen (1989) Purification and culture of adult rat dorsal root ganglia neurons. J. Neurosci. Res. 23: 198–206.

DeLuca, N. A., A. M. McCarthy, and P. A. Schaffer (1985) Isolation and characterization of deletion mutants of herpes simplex virus type 1 in the gene encoding immediate-early regulatory protein ICP4. J. Virol. 56: 558–570.

Deneris, E. S., J. Boulter, L. W. Swanson, J. Patrick, and S. Heinemann (1989) β3: A new member of nicotinic acetylcholine receptor gene family is expressed in brain. J. Biol. Chem. 264: 6268–6272.

Denis-Donini, S., J. Glowinski, and A. Prochiantz (1984) Glial heterogeneity may define the three-dimensional shape of mouse mesencephalic dopaminergic neurones. Nature 307: 641–643.

Dessi, F., H. Pollard, J. Moreau, Y. Ben-Ari, and C. Charriaut-Marlangue (1995) Cytosine arabinoside induces apoptosis in cerebellar neurons in culture. J. Neurochem. 64: 1980–1987.

Detrick, R. J., D. Dickey, and C. R. Kitner (1990) The effects of N-cadherin misexpression on morphogenesis in *Xenopus* embryos. Neuron 4: 493–506.

DeVries, G. H. (1993) Schwann cell proliferation. In: *Peripheral Neuropathy, 3rd ed.*, P. J. Dyck, P. K. Thomas, J. W. Griffin, et al., eds., pp. 290–298, Saunders, Philadelphia.

Di, P. U., G. Rougon, E. A. Novotny, and J. L. Barker (1987) Dopaminergic neurons from embryonic mouse mesencephalon are enriched in culture through immunoreaction

with monoclonal antibody to neural specific protein 4 and flow cytometry. Proc. Natl. Acad. Sci. U.S.A. 84: 7334–7338.

Dichter, M. A. (1978) Rat cortical neurons in cell culture: culture methods, cell morphology, electrophysiology, and synapse formation. Brain Res. 149: 279–293.

Dimpfel, W., R. T. Huang, and E. Habermann (1977) Gangliosides in nervous tissue cultures and binding of 125I-labeled tetanus toxin, a neuronal marker. J. Neurochem. 29: 329–334.

diPorzio U., G. Rougon, E. A. Novotny, and J. L. Barker (1987) Dopaminergic neurons from embryonic mouse mesencephalon are enriched in culture through immunoreaction with monoclonal antibody to neural specific protein 4 and flow cytometry. Proc. Natl. Acad. Sci. U.S.A. 84: 7334–7338.

Dirks, W., M. Wirth, and H. Hauser (1993) Dicistronic transcription units for gene expression in mammalian cells. Gene 128: 247–249.

Distler, P. G., and R. T. Robertson (1992) Development of AChE-positive neuronal projections from basal forebrain to cerebral cortex in organotypic slice cultures. Dev. Brain Res. 67: 181–196.

Distler, P. G., and R. T. Robertson (1993) Formation of synapses between basal forebrain afferents and cerebral cortex neurons: an electron microscopic study in organotypic slice cultures. J. Neurocytol. 22: 627–643.

Dobson, A. T., T. P. Margulis, E. Sedarati, J. G. Stevens, and L. T. Feldman (1990) A latent, nonpathogenic HSV1-derived vector stably expresses β-galactosidase in mouse neurons. Neuron. 5: 353–360.

Doherty, P., L. H. Rowett, S. E. Moore, D. A. Mann and F. S. Walsh (1991) Neurite outgrowth in response to transfected N-CAM and N-cadherin reveals fundamental differences in neuronal responsiveness to CAMs. Neuron. 6: 247–258.

Dong, J. F., A. Detta, M. H. Bakker, and E. R. Hitchcock (1993) Direct interaction with target-derived glia enhances survival but not differentiation of human fetal mesencephalic dopaminergic neurons. Neuroscience 56: 53–60.

Dotti, C. G., and K. Simons (1990) Polarized sorting of viral glycoproteins to the axon and dendrites of hippocampal neurons in culture. Cell 62: 63–72.

Dotti, C. G., C. A. Sullivan, and G. A. Banker (1988) The establishment of polarity by hippocampal neurons in culture. J. Neurosci. 8: 1454–1468.

Doupe, A. J., S. C. Landis, and P. H. Patterson (1985a) Environmental influences in the development of neural crest derivatives: glucocorticoids, growth factors, and chromaffin cell plasticity. J. Neurosci. 5: 2119–2142.

Doupe, A. J., S. C. Landis, and P. H. Patterson (1985b) Small intensely fluorescent (SIF) cells in culture: role of glucocorticoidsand growth factors in their development and phenotypic interconversions with other neural crest derivatives. J. Neursoci. 5: 2143–2160.

Doyle, A., and J. B. Griffiths (1993) *Cell and Tissue Culture: Laboratory Procedures*, Wiley, New York.

Drapeau, P. (1990) Loss of channel modulation by transmitter and protein kinase C during innervation of an identified leech neuron. Neuron 4: 875–882.

Drescher, U., C. Kremoser, C. Handwerker, J. Loschinger, M. Noda, and F. Bonhoeffer (1995) In vitro guidance of retinal ganglion cell axons by RAGS, a 25 kDa tectal protein related to ligands for Eph receptor tyrosine kinases. Cell 82: 359–370.

Dröge, W., D. Mannel, W. Falk, H. Schmidt, S. Panknin, and W. Dotterer (1983) The optimal activation of cytotoxic t lymphocytes requires metabolically intact stimulator cells not only for the activation of the interleukin 2-producing helper cells. J. Immunol. 131: 520–528.

Dröge, W., C. Pottmeyer-Gerber, H. Schmidt, and S. Nick (1986) Glutathione augments the activation of cytotoxic T lymphocytes in vivo. Immunobiology 172: 151–156.

Dugerian, S., F. Bahls, J. Richmond, et al. (1993) Roles for arachidonic acid and GTP-binding proteins in synaptic transmission. J. Physiol. Paris 87: 123–137.

During, M. J., J. R. Naegele, K. L. O'Malley, and A. I. Geller (1994) Long-term behavioral recovery in Parkinsonian rats by an HSV vector expressing tyrosine hydroxylase. Science 266: 1399–1403.

Duvoisin R. M., E. S. Deneris, J. Patrick, and S. Heinemann (1989) The functional diversity of the neuronal nicotinic receptors is increased by a novel subunit: $\beta 4$. Neuron. 3: 487–496.

Dyatlov, V. A., A. V. Platoshin, D. A. Lawrence, and D. O. Carpenter (1996) Mercury (Hg^{2+}) enhances the depressant effect of kainate on Ca-inactivated potassium current in telencephalic cells derived from chick embryos. Toxicol. Appl. Pharmacol. 138: 285–297.

Ebendal, T. (1989) Use of collagen gels to bioassay nerve growth factor activity. In: *Nerve Growth Factors*, R. A. Rush, ed., Wiley, Chichester, UK.

Ebendal, T., and C. O. Jacobson (1977) Tissue explants affecting extension and orientation of axons in cultured chick embryo ganglia. Exp. Cell Res. 105: 379–387.

Eccleston, A., and D. R. Silberberg (1985) Fibroblast growth factor is a mitogen for oligo-dendrocytes in vitro. Dev. Brain Res. 21: 315–318.

Eckenstein, F. P., F. Esch, T. Holbert, R. W. Blacher, and R. Nishi (1990) Purification and characterization of a trophic factor for embryonic peripheral neurons: comparison with fibroblast growth factors. Neuron 4: 623–631.

Eckenstein, F. P., K. Kuzis, R. Nishi, W. R. Woodward, C. Meshul, L. Sherman, and G. Ciment (1994) Cellular distribution, subcellular localization and possible functions of basic and acidic fibroblast growth factors. Biochem. Pharmacol. 47: 103–110.

Edgar, D., R. Timpl, and H. Thoenen (1984) The heparin-binding domain of laminin is responsible for its effects on neurite outgrowth and neuronal survival. EMBO J. 3: 1463–1468.

Edmondson, J. C., and M. E. Hatten (1987) Glial-guided granule neuron migration in vitro: A high-resolution time-lapse video microscopic study. J. Neurosci. 7: 1928–1934.

Edstrom, A., P. A. Ekstrom, and D. Tonge (1996) Axonal outgrowth and neuronal apopto-sis in cultured adult mouse dorsal root ganglion preparations: effects of neuro-trophins, of inhibition of neurotrophin actions and of prior axotomy. Neuroscience 75: 1164–1175.

Eide, F. F., D. H. Lowenstein, and L. F. Reichardt (1993) Neurotrophins and their receptors —current concepts and implications for neurologic disease. Exp. Neurol. 121: 200–214.

Eisenbarth, G. S., F. S. Walsh, and M. Nirenberg (1979) Monoclonal antibody to a plasma membrane antigen of neurons. Proc. Natl. Acad. Sci. U.S.A. 76: 4913–4917.

Eldridge, C. F., M. B. Bunge, and R. P. Bunge (1985) Serum ascorbic acid regulates myelin formation and basal lamina assembly by Schwann cells in vitro. Soc. Neurosci. Abstr. 11: 986.

Eldridge, C. F., M. B. Bunge, R. P. Bunge, and P. M. Wood (1987) Differentiation of axon-related Schwann cells in vitro: I. Ascorbic acid regulates basal lamina assembly and myelin formation. J. Cell Biol. 105: 1023–1034.

Eldridge, C. F., M. B. Bunge, and R. P. Bunge (1989) Differentiation of axon-related Schwann cells in vitro: II. Control of myelin formation by basal lamina. J. Neurosci. 9: 625–638.

Eliot, L. S., E. R. Kandel, and R. D. Hawkins (1994) Modulation of spontaneous transmitter release during depression and posttetanic potentiation of *Aplysia* sensory-motor neuron synapses isolated in culture. J. Neurosci. 14: 3280–3292.

Engel, U., and G. Wolswijk (1996) Oligodendrocyte-type-2 astrocyte (o-2a) progenitor cells derived from adult rat spinal cord: in vitro characteristics and response to pdgf, bfgf and nt-3. GLIA 16: 16–26.

Enokido, Y., T. Araki, S. Aizawa, and H. Hatanaka (1996) p53 involves cytosine arabinoside-induced apoptosis in cultured cerebellar granule neurons. Neurosci. Lett. 203: 1–4.

Erickson, G. F., and W. B. Watkins (1981) Long term primary monolayer culture of adult murine magnocellular neurons. Endocrinology 108: 1810–1814.

Ernsberger, U., D. Edgar, and H. Rohrer (1989a) The survival of early chick sympathetic neurons in vitro is dependent on a suitable substrate but independent of NGF. Dev. Biol 135: 250–262.

Ernsberger, U., M. Sendtner, and H. Rohrer (1989b) Proliferation and differentiation of embryonic chick sympathetic neurons: effects of ciliary neurotrophic factor. Neuron 2: 1275–1284.

Esch, T. (1995) The effect of adhesion molecules on the development of polarity in cultured rat hippocampal neurons. Soc. Neurosci. Abstr. 21.

Eshhar, N., R. S. Petralia, C. A. Winters, A. S. Niedzielski, and R. J. Wenthold (1993) The segregation and expression of glutamate receptor subunits in cultured hippocampal neurons. Neuroscience 57: 943–964.

Evans, M. J., and M. H. Kaufman (1981) Establishment in culture of pluripotential cells from mouse embryos. Nature 292: 154–156.

Evers, J., M. Laser, and Y. A. Sun (1989) Studies of nerve-muscle interactions in *Xenopus* cell culture: analysis of early synaptic events. J. Neurosci. 9: 1523–1539.

Eves, E. M., M. S. Tucker, J. D. Roback, M. Downen, M. R. Rosner, and B. H. Wainer (1992) Immortal rat hippocampal cell lines exhibit neuronal and glial lineages and neurotrophin gene expression. Proc. Natl. Acad. Sci. U.S.A. 89: 4373–4377.

Eylar, E., C. Rivera-Quinones, C. Molina, I. Baez, F. Molina, C. M. Mercado (1993) *N*-acetylcysteine enhances T cell functions and T cell growth in culture. Int. Immunol. 5: 97–101.

Fallon, J. R. (1985) Preferential outgrowth of central nervous system neurites on astrocytes and Schwann cells as compared with nonglial cells in vitro. J. Cell Biol. 100: 198–207.

Falls, D. L., K. M. Rosen, G. Corfas, W. S. Lane and G. D. Fischbach (1993) ARIA, a protein that stimulates acetylcholine receptor synthesis, is a member of the neu ligand family. Cell 72: 801–815.

Fann, M.-J., and P. H. Patterson (1993) A novel approach to screen for cytokine effects on neuronal gene expression. J. Neurochem. 61: 1349–1355.

Farlie, P. G., R. Dringen, S. M. Rees, G. Kannourakis, and O. Bernard (1995) bcl-2 Transgene expression can protect neurons against developmental and induced cell death. Proc. Natl. Acad. Sci. U.S.A. 92: 4397–4401.

Fawcett, J. W. (1992) Intrinsic neuronal determinants of regeneration. Trends Neurosci. 15: 5–8.

Fawcett, J. W., E. Housden, L. Smith-Thomas, and R. L. Meyer (1989) The growth of axons in three-dimensional astrocyte cultures. Dev. Biol. 135: 449–458.

Federoff, S., and A. Vernadakis (1986) *Astrocytes*, Academic Press, Orlando, FL.

Felgner, P. L., T. R. Gadek, M. Holm, R. Roman, H. W. Chan, M. Wenz, J. P. Northrop, G. M. Ringold, and M. Danielsen (1987) Lipofection: a highly efficient, lipid-mediated DNA-transfection procedure. Proc. Natl. Acad. Sci. USA 84: 7413–7417.

Fernandez-de-Miguel, F., and P. Drapeau (1995) Synapse formation and function: insights from identified leech neurons in culture [review]. J. Neurobiol. 27: 367–379.

Fernandez-Valle, C., N. Fregien, P. M. Wood, and M. B. Bunge (1993a) Expression of the protein zero myelin gene in axon-related Schwann cells is linked to basal lamina formation. Development 119: 867–880.

Fernandez-Valle, C., L. A. Gwynn, P. M. Wood (1994) Anti β-1 integrin antibody inhibits Schwann cell myelination. J. Neurobiol. 25: 1207–1226.

Ferrari G., and L. A. Greene (1994) Proliferative inhibition by dominant-negative *ras* rescues naive and neuronally-differentiated PC12 cells from apoptotic death. EMBO J. 13: 5922–5928.

Fidelus, R. K. (1988) The generation of oxygen radicals: a positive signal for lymphocyte activation. Cell Immunol. 113: 175–182.

Fidelus, R. K., and M. F. Tsan (1986) Enhancement of intracellular glutathione promotes lymphocyte activation by mitogen. Cell. Immunol. 97: 155–163.

Fidelus, R. K., P. Ginouves, D. Lawrence, and M. F. Tsan (1987) Modulation of intracellular glutathione concentrations alters lymphocyte activation and proliferation. Exp. Cell Res. 170: 269–275.

Field, S. J., R. S. Johnson, R. M. Mortensen, et al. (1992) Growth and differentiation of embryonic stem cells that lack an intact c-*fos* gene. Proc. Natl. Acad. Sci. U.S.A. 89: 9306–9310.

Fields, K. L. (1979) Cell type-specific antigens of cells of the central and peripheral nervous system. Curr. Top. Dev. Biol. 13(1): 237–257.

Fields, K. L. (1985) Neuronal and glial surface antigens on cells in culture. In: *Cell Culture in the Neurosciences*, J. E. Bottenstein and G. Sato, eds., pp. 45–93, Plenum, New York.

Fields, R. D., C. Yu, and P. G. Nelson (1991) Calcium, network activity, and the role of NMDA channels in synaptic plasticity in vitro. J. Neurosci. 11: 134–146.

Fink, D. J., L. R. Sternberg, P. C. Weber, M. Mata, W. F. Goins, and J. C. Glorioso (1992) In vivo expression of β-galactosidase in hippocampal neurons by HSV-mediated gene transfer. Human Gene Therapy 3: 11–19.

Fink, D. J., N. A. DeLuca, W. F. Goins, and J. C. Glorioso (1996) Gene transfer to neurons using herpes simplex virus-based vectors. Annu. Rev. Neurosci. 19: 265–287.

Finley, M. F., N. Kulkarni, and J. E. Huettner (1995) Synapse formation and establishment of polarity by neurons derived from P19 embryonic carcinoma cells. Soc. Neurosci. Abstr. 21: 1287.

Finley, M. F., N. Kulkarni, and J. E. Huettner (1996) Synapse formation and establishment of neuronal polarity by P19 embryonic carcinoma cells and embryonic stem cells. J. Neurosci. 16: 1056–1065.

Fischbach, G. D. (1972) Synapse formation between dissociated nerve and muscle cells in low-density cell cultures. Dev. Biol. 28: 407–429.

Fischbach, G. D., and P. G. Nelson (1977) Cell culture in neurobiology. In: *Handbook of Physiology*, J. M. Brookhart and V. B. Mountcastle, eds., pp. 719–774, American Physiology Society, Bethesda, MD.

Fischbach, G., M. Henkart, S. Cohen, A. Breuer, J. Whysner and F. Neal (1974) Studies on the development of neuromuscular junctions in cell culture. In: *Synaptic Transmission and Neuronal Interaction*, M. V. Bennett, ed., pp. 259–283, Raven, New York.

Fischman, C. M., M. C. Udey, M. Kurtz, and J. J. Wedner (1981) Inhibition of lectin-induced lymphocyte activation by 2-cyclohexene-1-one: decreased intracellular glutathione inhibits and early event in the activation sequence. J. Immunol. 127: 2257.

Fishell, G., and M. E. Hatten (1991) Astrotactin provides a receptor system for CNS neuronal migration. Development 113: 755–765.

Fishell, G., C. A. Mason, and M. E. Hatten (1993) Dispersion of neural progenitors within the germinal zones of the forebrain. Nature 362: 636–638.

Fisher, K. J., H. Choi, J. Burda, S.-J. Chen, and J. M. Wilson (1996) Recombinant adenovirus deleted of all viral genes for gene therapy of cystic fibrosis. Virology 217: 11–22.

Fisher, T. E., S. Levy, and L. K. Kaczmarek (1994) Transient changes in intracellular calcium associated with a prolonged increase in excitability in neurons of *Aplysia californica*. J. Neurophysiol. 71: 1254–1257.

Fishman, R., and M. E. Hatten (1993) Multiple receptor systems promote CNS neuronal migration. J. Neurosci. 13: 3485–3495.

Fleischer, S., and B. Fleischer (1989) Biomembranes. Methods Enzymol. 171: 397–604.

Fletcher, T. L., and G. A. Banker (1989) The establishment of polarity by hippocampal neurons: the relationship between the stage of a cell's development in situ and its subsequent development in culture. Dev. Biol. 136: 446–454.

Fletcher, T. L., P. Cameron, P. DeCamilli, and G. Banker (1991) The distribution of synapsin I and synaptophysin in hippocampal neurons developing in culture. J. Neurosci. 11: 1617–1626.

Fletcher, T. L., P. DeCamilli, and G. Banker (1994) Synaptogenesis in hippocampal cultures: evidence indicating that axons and dendrites become competent to form synapses at different stages of neuronal development. J. Neurosci. 14: 6695–6706.

Folkman, J., and A. Moscona (1978) Role of cell shape in growth control. Nature 273: 345–349.

Fonnum F., and A. Contestabile (1984) Colchicine neurotoxicity demonstrates the cholinergic projection from the supracomissural septum to the habenula and the nucleus interpeduncularis in the rat. J. Neurochem. 43: 881–884.

Forscher, P., and S. J. Smith (1988) Actions of cytochalasins on the organization of actin filaments and microtubules in a neuronal growth cone. J. Cell Biol. 107: 1505–1516.

Forscher, P., L. K. Kaczmarek, J. A. Buchanan, and S. J. Smith (1987) Cyclic AMP induces changes in distribution and transport of organelles within growth cones of *Aplysia* bag cell neurons. J. Neurosci. 7: 3600–3611.

Forsythe, I. D., and G. L. Westbrook (1988) Slow excitatory postsynaptic currents mediated by *N*-methyl-D-aspartate receptors on cultured mouse central neurones. J. Physiol. (Lond.) 396: 515–533.

Fraefel, C., S. Song, F. Lim, P. Lang, L. Yu, Y. Wang, P. Wild, and A. I. Geller (1996) Helper virus-free transfer of herpes simplex virus type 1 plasmid vectors into neural cells. J. Virol. 70: 7190–7197.

Fraichard, A., O. Chassande, G. Bilbaut, C. Dehay, P. Savatier, and J. Samarut (1995) In vitro differentiation of embryonic stem cells into glial cells and functional neurons. J. Cell Sci. 108: 3181–3188.

Franklin, J. L., and E. M. J. Johnson (1994) Elevated intracellular calcium blocks programmed neuronal death. Ann. N.Y. Acad. Sci. 747: 195–204.

Franklin, R. J., and W. F. Blakemore (1995) Glial-cell transplantation and plasticity in the O-2A lineage—implications for CNS repair. Trends Neurosci. 18: 151–156.

French-Constant, C., R. H. Miller, J. F. Burne, and M. C. Raff (1988) Evidence that migratory oligodendrocyte-type-2 astrocyte (O-2A) progenitor cells are kept out of the rat retina by a barrier at the eye-end of the optic nerve. J. Neurocytol. 17: 13–25.

Freshney, R. I. (1987) *Culture of Animal Cells: A Manual of Basic Technique.* 2nd ed., Liss, New York.

Freshney, R. I. (1994) *Culture of Animal Cells: A Manual of Basic Technique.* 3rd ed., Wiley-Liss, New York.

Friedrich, G., and P. Soriano (1991) Promoter traps in embryonic stem cells: a genetic screen to identify and mutate developmental genes in mice. Genes Dev. 5: 1513–1523.

Frodl, E. M., W. M. Duan, H. Sauer, A. Kupsch, and P. Brundin (1994) Human embryonic dopamine neurons xenografted to the rat: effects of cryopreservation and varying regional source of donor cells on transplant survival, morphology and function. Brain Res. 647: 286–298.

Frotscher, M., and B. H. Gähwiler (1988) Synaptic organization of intracellularly stained CA3 pyramidal neurons in slice cultures of rat hippocampus. Neurosci. 24: 541–551.

Fu, W. M., J. C. Liou, Y. H. Lee, and H. C. Liou (1995) Potentiation of neurotransmitter release by activation of presynaptic glutamate receptors at developing neuromuscular synapses of *Xenopus*. J. Physiol. (Lond.) 489: 813–823.

Fujimori, T., S. Miyatani, and M. Takeichi (1990) Ectopic expression of *N*-cadherin perturbs histogenesis in *Xenopus* embryos. Development 110: 97–104.

Fulton, B. P., J. F. Burne, and M. C. Raff (1991) Glial cells in the rat optic nerve: the search for the type-2 astrocytes. Ann. N.Y. Acad. Sci. 633: 27–34.

Funte, L. R., and P. G. Haydon (1993) Synaptic target contact enhances presynaptic calcium influx by activating cAMP-dependent protein kinase during synaptogenesis. Neuron 10: 1069–1078.

Furshpan E. J., and D. D. Potter (1989) Seizure-like activity and cellular damage in rat hippocampal neurons in cell culture. Neuron. 3: 199–207.

Furshpan, E. J., P. R. MacLeish, P. H. O'Lague, and D. D. Potter (1976) Chemical transmission between rat sympathetic neurons and cardiac myocytes developing in microcultures: evidence for cholinergic, adrenergic, and dual-function neurons. Proc. Natl. Acad. Sci. U.S.A. 73: 4225–4229.

Furshpan, E. J., S. C. Landis, S. G. Matsumoto, and D. D. Potter (1986a) Synaptic functions in rat sympathetic neurons in microcultures: I. Secretion of norepinephrine and acetylcholine. J. Neurosci. 6: 1061–1079.

Furshpan, E. J., D. D. Potter, and S. G. Matsumoto (1986b) Synaptic functions in rat sympathetic neurons in microcultures: III. A Purinergic effect on cardiac myocytes. J. Neurosci. 6: 1099–1107.

Futerman, A. H., and G. A. Banker (1996) The economics of neurite outgrowth—the addition of new membrane to growing axons. Trends Neurosci. 19: 144–149.

Gabellini, N., M.-C. Minozzi, A. Leon, and R. Dal Toso (1992) Nerve growth factor transcriptional control of c-fos promoter transfected in cultured spinal sensory neurons. J. Cell Biol. 118: 131–138.

Gage, F. H., P. W. Coates, T. D. Palmer, H. G. Kuhn, L. J. Fisher, J. O. Suhonen, D. A. Peterson, S. T. Suhr, and J. Ray (1995a) Survival and differentiation of adult neuronal progenitor cells transplanted to the adult brain. Proc. Natl. Acad. Sci. U.S.A. 92: 11879–11883.

Gage, F. H., J. Ray, and L. J. Fisher (1995b) Isolation, characterization, and use of stem cells from the CNS. Annu. Rev. Neurosci. 18: 159–192.

Gage, P. J., B. Sauer, M. Levine, and J. C. Glorioso (1992) A cell-free recombination system for site-specific integration of multigenic shuttle plasmids into the herpes simplex virus type 1 genome. J. Virol. 66: 5509–5515.

Gähwiler, B. H. (1978) Mixed cultures of cerebellum and inferior olive: generation of complex spikes in Purkinje cells. Brain Res. 145: 168–172.

Gähwiler, B. H. (1981a) Morphological differentiation of nerve cells in thin organotypic cultures derived from rat hippocampus and cerebellum. Proc. R. Soc. Lond. B. Biol. Sci. 211: 287–290.

Gähwiler, B. H. (1981b) Organotypic monolayer cultures of nervous tissue. J. Neurosci. Methods 4: 329–342.

Gähwiler, B. H. (1984a) Development of the hippocampus in vitro: cell types, synapses, and receptors. Neuroscience 11: 751–760.

Gähwiler, B. H. (1984b) The hypothalamo-hypophyseal system in culture. In: *Neuronal Communications*, B. J. Meyer and S. Kramer, eds., pp. 145–154, A. A. Balkema, Cape Town, Rotterdam.

Gähwiler, B. H. (1984c) Slice cultures of cerebellar, hippocampal and hypothalamic tissue. Experientia 40: 235–243.

Gähwiler, B. H. (1988) Organotypic cultures of neural tissue. TINS 11: 484–489.

Gähwiler, B. H., and D. A. Brown (1985a) Functional innervation of cultured hippocampal neurones by cholinergic afferents from cocultured septal explants. Nature 313: 577–579.

Gähwiler, B. H., and D. A. Brown (1985b) $GABA_B$-receptor-activated K^+ current in voltage-clamped CA3 pyramidal cells in hippocampal cultures. Proc. Natl. Acad. Sci. U.S.A. 82(5): 155–162.

Gähwiler, B. H., and F. Hefti (1984) Guidance of acetylcholinesterase containing fibres by target tissue in cocultured brain slices. Neuroscience 13: 681–689.

Gähwiler, B. H., and T. Knöpfel (1990) Cultures of brain slices. In: *Preparations of Vertebrate Central Nervous System in Vitro*, H. Jahnsen, ed., chapt. 4, pp. 77–100. John Wiley & Sons Ltd., Chichester.

Gähwiler, B. H., and I. Llano (1989) Sodium and potassium conductances in somatic membranes of rat Purkinje cells from organotypic cerebellar cultures. J. Physiol. (Lond.) 417: 105–122.

Gähwiler, B. H., A. Enz, and F. Hefti (1987) Nerve growth factor promotes development of the rat septo-hippocampal cholinergic projection in vitro. Neurosci. Lett. 75: 6–10.

Gähwiler, B. H., D. A. Brown, A. Enz, and T. Knöpfel (1989) Development of the septo-hippocampal projection in vitro. In: *Central Cholinergic Synaptic Transmission*, M. Frotscher and U. Misgeld, eds., pp. 236–250, Birkhäuser Verlag, Basel.

Gähwiler, B. H., L. Rietschin, T. Knöpfel, and A. Enz (1990) Continuous presence of nerve growth factor is required for maintenance of cholinergic septal neurons in organotypic slice cultures. Neuroscience 36: 27–31.

Galiana, E., I. Borde, P. Marin, M. Rassoulzadegan, F. Cuzin, F. Gros, P. Rouget, and C. Evrard (1990) Establishment of permanent astroglial cell lines, able to differentiate in vitro, from transgenic mice carrying the polyoma virus large T gene: an alternative approach to brain cell immortalization. J. Neurosci. Res. 26: 269–277.

Gao, W. Q., and M. E. Hatten (1993) Neuronal differentiation rescued by implantation of weaver granule cell precursors into wild-type cerebellar cortex. Science 260: 367–369.

Gao, W. Q., and M. E. Hatten (1994) Immortalizing oncogenes subvert the control of granule cell lineage in developing cerebellum. Development 120: 1059–1070.

Gao, W. Q., N. Heintz, and M. E. Hatten (1991) Cerebellar granule cell neurogenesis is regulated by cell-cell interactions in vitro. Neuron 6: 705–715.

Gao, W. Q., X. L. Liu, and M. E. Hatten (1992) The weaver gene encodes a nonautonomous signal for CNS neuronal differentiation. Cell 68: 841–854.

Gao, W. Q., J. L. Zheng, and M. Karihaloo (1995) Neurotrophin-4/5 (NT-4/5) and brain-derived neurotrophic factor (BDNF) act at later stages of cerebellar granule cell differentiation. J. Neurosci. 15(4): 2656–2667.

Garber, B. B. (1977) Cell aggregation and recognition in the self-assembly of brain tissues. In: *Cell, Tissue and Organ Cultures in Neurobiology*, S. Federoff, ed., pp. 515–537, Academic Press, New York.

Garber, B. B., and A. A. Moscona (1972) Reconstruction of brain tissue from cell suspensions: II. Specific enhancement of aggregation of embryonic cerebral cells by supernatant from homologous cell cultures. Dev. Biol. 27: 235–243.

Garcia, I., I. Martinou, Y. Tsujimoto, and J.-C. Martinou (1992) Prevention of programmed cell death of sympathetic neurons by the bcl-2 proto-oncogene. Science 258: 302–304.

Gard, A. L., and S. E. Pfeiffer (1989) Oligodendrocyte progenitors isolated directly from developing telencephalon at a specific phenotypic stage: myelinogenic potential in a defined environment. Development 106: 119–132.

Gard, A. L., and S. E. Pfeiffer (1990) Two proliferative stages of the oligodendrocyte lineage (A2B5 + O4- and O4 + GalC-) under different mitogenic control. Neuron. 5: 615–625.

Gasser, U. E., and M. E. Hatten (1990a) Neuron-glia interactions of rat hippocampal cells in vitro: glial-guided neuronal migration and neuronal regulation of glial differentiation. J. Neurosci. 10: 1276–1285.

Gasser, U. E., and M. E. Hatten (1990b) Central nervous system neurons migrate on astroglial fibres from heterotypic brain regions in vitro. Proc. Natl. Acad. Sci. U.S.A. 87: 4543–4547.

Gebicke-Haerter, P. J., J. Bauer, A. Schobert, and H. Northoff (1989) Lipopolysaccharide-free conditions in primary astrocyte cultures allow growth and isolation of microglial cells. J. Neurosci. 9: 183–194.

Gehrmann, J., Y. Matsumoto, and G. W. Kreutzberg (1995) Microglia: intrinsic immun-effector cell of the brain. Brain Res. Rev. 20: 269–287.

Geisert, E. E., and A. M. Stewart (1991) Changing interactions between astrocytes and neurons during CNS maturation. Dev. Biol. 143: 335–345.

Geller, A. I., and X. O. Breakefield (1988) A defective HSV1 vector expresses Escherichia coli beta-galactosidase in cultured neurons. Science 241: 1667–1669.

Geller, A. I., M. J. During, J. W. Haycock, A. Freese, and R. Neve (1993) Long-term increases in neurotransmitter release from neuronal cells expressing a constitutively active adenylate cyclase from a herpes simplex virus type 1 vector. Proc. Natl. Acad. Sci. USA 90: 7603–7607.

Geller, H. M., and M. Dubois-Dalcq (1988) Antigenic and functional characterization of a rat central nervous system–derived cell line immortalized by a retrovinal vector. J. Cell Biol. 107: 1977–1986.

Geppert M., Y. Goda, R. E. Hammer, C. Li, T. W. Rosahl, C. F. Stevens, and T. C. Sudhof (1994) Synaptotagmin I: a major Ca^{2+} sensor for transmitter release at a central synapse. Cell 79: 717–727.

Gerdes, H. H., and C. Kaether (1996) Green fluorescent protein: applications in cell biology. FEBS Lett. 389: 44–47.

Gerfen, C. H. (1992) The neostriatal mosaic: multiple levels of compartmental organization in the basal ganglia. Annu. Rev. Neurosci. 15: 285–320.

Gerfin-Moser, A., and H. Monyer (1994) In situ hybridization on organotypic slice cultures. In: *In Situ Hybridization Protocols for the Brain: Biological Technique Series*, W. Wisden and B. J. Morris, eds., pp. 50–54, Academic Press, London.

Geschwind, M. D., J. A. Kessler, A. I. Geller, and H. J. Federoff (1994) Transfer of nerve growth factor gene into cell lines and cultured neurons using a defective herpes sim-

plex virus vector. Transfer of the NGF gene into cells by a HSV-1 vector. Mol. Brain Res. 24: 327–335.

Ghosh, A. (1996) Cortical development: with an eye on neurotrophins. Curr. Biol. 6: 130–133.

Ghosh, A., J. Carnahan, and M. E. Greenberg (1994) Requirement for BDNF in activity-dependent survival of cortical neurons. Science 263: 1618–1623.

Gimlich, R. (1991) Fluorescent dextran clonal markers. In: *Methods in Cell Biology*, vol. 36, B. K. Kay and H. B. Peng, eds., p. 285, Academic Press, New York.

Giulian, D., and T. J. Baker (1986) Characterization of ameboid microglia isolated from developing mammalian brain. J. Neurosci. 6: 2163–2178.

Giulian, D., M. Corpuz, S. Chapman, M. Mansouri, and C. Robertson (1993) Reactive mononuclear phagocytes release neurotoxins after ischemic and traumatic injury to the central nervous system. J. Neurosci. Res. 36: 681–693.

Giulian, D., J. Li, S. Bartel, J. Broker, X. Li, and J. B. Kirkpatrick (1995) Cell surface morphology identifies microglia as a distinct class of mononuclear phagocyte. J. Neurosci. 15: 7712–7726.

Glanzman, D. L., E. R. Kandel, and S. Schacher (1989) Identified target motor neuron regulates neurite outgrowth and synapse formation of *Aplysia* sensory neurons in vitro. Neuron 3: 441–450.

Glanzman, D. L., E. R. Kandel, and S. Schacher (1990) Target-dependent structural changes accompanying long-term synaptic facilitation in *Aplysia* neurons. Science 249: 799–802.

Glanzman, D. L., E. R. Kandel, and S. Schacher (1991) Target-dependent morphological segregation of *Aplysia* sensory outgrowth in vitro. Neuron 7: 703–713.

Goldberg, D. J. (1988) Local role of Ca^{2+} in formation of veils in growth cones. J. Neurosci. 8: 2596–2605.

Goldberg, D. J., and D. W. Burmeister (1986) Stages in axon formation: observations of growth of *Aplysia* axons in culture using video-enhanced contrast-differential interference contrast microscopy. J. Cell Biol. 103: 1921–1931.

Goldberg, D. J., and D. W. Burmeister (1992) Microtubule-based filopodium-like protrusions form after axotomy. J. Neurosci. 12: 4800–4807.

Goldberg, D. J., and S. Schacher (1987) Differential growth of the branches of a regenerating bifurcate axon is associated with differential transport of organelles. Dev. Biol. 124: 35–40.

Goldman, D., E. Deneris, W. Luyten, A. Kochnar, J. Patrick, and S. Heinemann (1987) Members of a nicotinic acetylcholine receptor gene family are expressed in different regions of the mammalian central nervous system. Cell 48: 965–973.

Goldman-Wohl, D. S., E. Chan, D. Baird, and N. Heintz (1994) Kv3.3b: A novel shaw type potassium channel expressed in terminally differentiated cerebellar Purkinje cells and deep cerebellar nuclei. J. Neurosci. 14: 511–522.

Goldstein, M. N., and D. Pinkel (1957) Long-term tissue culture of neuroblastoma. J. Natl. Cancer Inst. 20: 467–477.

Gomperts, S. N. (1996) Clustering membrane proteins: it's all coming together with the PSD-95/SAP90 protein family. Cell 84: 659–662.

Good, N. E., G. D. Winget, W. Winter, T. N. Connolly, S. Izawa and R. M. M. Singh (1966) Hydrogen ion buffers for biological research. Biochemistry 5: 467–477.

Gordon-Weeks, P. R., S. G. Mansfield, C. Alberto, M. Johnstone, and F. Moya (1993) A phosphorylation epitope on MAP 1B that is transiently expressed in growing axons in the developing rat nervous system. Eur. J. Neurosci. 5: 1302–1311.

Gorin, P. D., and E. M. Johnson (1979) Experimental autoimmune model of nerve growth factor deprivation: effects on developing peripheral sympathetic and sensory neurons. Proc. Natl. Acad. Sci. U.S.A. 76: 5382–5386.

Gorman, C. M, and B. H. Howard (1983) Expression of recombinant plasmids in mammalian cells is enhanced by sodium butyrate. Nucl. Acids Res. 11: 7631–7648.

Goslin, K., and G. Banker (1989) Experimental observations on the development of polarity by hippocampal neurons in culture. J. Cell Biol. 108: 1507–1516.

Goslin, K., and G. Banker (1990) Rapid changes in the distribution of GAP-43 correlate with the expression of neuronal polarity during normal development and under experimental conditions. J. Cell Biol. 110: 1319–1331.

Goslin, K., D. J. Schreyer, J. H. P. Skene, and G. Banker (1988) Development of neuronal polarity: GAP43 distinguishes axonal from dendritic growth cones. Nature 336: 672–680.

Goslin, K., E. Birgbauer, G. Banker, and F. Solomon (1989) The role of cytoskeleton in organizing growth cones: a microfilament-associated growth cone component depends upon microtubules for its localization. J. Cell Biol. 109: 1621–1631.

Goslin, K., D. J. Schreyer, J. H. P. Skene, and G. Banker (1990) Changes in the distribution of GAP-43 during the development of neuronal polarity. J. Neurosci. 10: 588–602.

Gossen, M. and H. Bujord (1992) Tight control of gene expression in mammalian cells by tetracycline responsive promoters. Proc. Natl. Acad. Sci. USA 89: 5547–5551.

Gottesfeld Z., and D. M. Jakobowitz (1979) Cholinergic projection from the septal-diagonal band area to the habenular nuclei. Brain Res. 176: 391–394.

Gotz, B., A. Scholze, A. Clement, A. Joester, K. Schutte, F. Wigger, R. Frank, E. Spiess, P. Ekblom, and A. Faissner (1996) Tenascin-C contains distinct adhesive, anti-adhesive, and neurite outgrowth promoting sites for neurons. J. Cell Biol. 132: 681–699.

Graham, F. L., and A. J. Van der Eb (1973) A new technique for the assay of infectivity of human adenovirus 5 DNA. Virology 52: 456–467.

Gratzner, H. G. (1982) Monoclonal antibody to 5-bromo and 5-qiododeoxyuridine: a new reagent for detection of DNA replication. Science, 318: 474–475.

Greenberg, S. S., A. Johns, J. Kleha, J. Xie, Y. Wang, J. Bianchi, and K. Conley (1994) Phenol red is a thromboxane A2/prostaglandin H2 receptor antagonist in canine lingual arteries and human platelets. J. Pharmacol. Exp. Ther. 268: 1352–1361.

Greene, L. A. (1978) Nerve growth factor prevents the death and stimulates neuronal differentiation of clonal PC12 pheochromocytoma cells in serum-free medium. J. Cell Biol. 78: 747–755.

Greene, L. A. (1984) The importance of both early and delayed responses in the mechanism of action of nerve growth factor. Trends Neurosci. 7: 91–94.

Greene, L. A., and D. R. Kaplan (1995) Early events in neurotrophin signalling via trk and p75 receptors. Curr. Opin. Neurobiol. 5: 579–587.

Greene, L. A., and G. Rein (1977) Release storage and uptake of catecholamines by a clonal cell line of nerve growth factor (NGF) responsive pheocytoma cells. Brain Res. 129: 247–263.

Greene, L. A., and A. Rukenstein (1989) The quantitative assay of nerve growth factor with PC12 cells. In: Nerve Growth Factors (IBRO Handbook Series Methods in the Neurosciences, Vol. 12, R. A. Rush, ed., pp. 139–147, Wiley, New York.

Greene, L. A., and A. S. Tischler (1976) Establishment of a noradrenergic clonal line of rat adrenal pheochromocytoma cells which respond to nerve growth factor. Proc. Natl. Acad. Sci. U.S.A. 73: 2424–2428.

Greene, L. A., and A. S. Tischler (1982) PC12 pheochromocytoma cells in neurobiological research. Adv. Cell. Neurobiol. 3: 373–414.

Greene, L. A., W. Shain, A. Chalazonitis, X. Breakfield, J. Minna, H. G. Coon and M. Nirenberg (1975) Neuronal properties of hybrid neuroblastoma X sympathetic ganglion cells. Proc. Natl. Acad. Sci. U.S.A. 72: 4923–4927.

Greene, L. A., D. E. Burstein, and M. M. Black (1982) The role of transcription-dependent priming in nerve growth factor promoted neurite outgrowth. Dev. Biol. 91: 305–316.

Greene, L. A., J. M. Aletta, A. Rukenstein, and S. H. Green (1987) PC12 pheochromocytoma cells: culture, NGF treatment and experimental exploitation. In: Methods in Enzymology: 147. Peptide Growth Factors (part B), D. Barnes and D. A. Sirbasku, eds., pp. 207–216, Academic Press, New York.

Green, S., R. E. Rydel, J. L. Connolly, and L. A. Greene (1986) PC12 mutants possessing low- but not high-affinity NGF receptors neither respond to, nor internalize NGF. J. Cell. Biol. 102: 830–843.

Gregory, W. A., J. C. Edmondson, M. E. Hatten, and C. A. Mason (1988) Cytology and neuron-glial apposition of migrating cerebellar granule cells in vitro. J. Neurosci. 8: 1728–1738.

Grinnell, F., M. Milam, and P. A. Srere (1972) Studies on cell adhesion: II. Adhesion of cells to surfaces of diverse chemical composition and inhibition of adhesion by sulfhydryl binding reagents. Arch. Biochem. Biophys. 153: 193–198.

Groves, A. K., S. C. Barnett, R. J. M. Franklin, A. J. Crang, M. Mayer, W. F. Blakemore, and M. Noble (1993) Repair of demyelinated lesions by transplantation of purified O-2A progenitor cells. Nature 362: 453–455.

Gu, X., and N. C. Spitzer (1995) Distinct aspects of neuronal differentiation encoded by frequency of spontaneous Ca^{2+} transients. Nature 375: 784–787.

Guénard, V., L. A. Gwynn, and P. M. Wood (1994) Astrocytes inhibit Schwann cell proliferation and myelination of dorsal root ganglion neurons in vitro. J. Neurosci. 14: 2980–2992.

Guénard, V., L. A. Gwynn, and P. M. Wood (1995) Transforming growth factor-beta blocks myelination but not ensheathment axons by Schwann cells in vitro. J. Neurosci. 15: 419–428.

Guerrero, I., A. Pellicer, and D. Burstein (1986) Activated N-ras gene induces neuronal differentiation of PC12 rat pheochromocytoma cells. J. Cell Physiol. 129: 71–76.

Gundersen, R. W. (1987) Response of sensory neurites and growth cones to patterned substrata of laminin and fibronectin in vitro. Dev. Biol. 121: 423–431.

Gundersen, R. W. (1988) Interference reflection microscopic study of dorsal root growth cones on different substrates: assessment of growth cone-substrate contacts. J. Neurosci. Res. 21: 298–306.

Gundersen, R. W., and J. N. Barrett (1980) Characterization of the turning response of dorsal root neurites toward nerve growth factor. J. Cell Biol. 87: 546–554.

Guroff, G. (1985) PC12 cells as a model of neuronal differentiation. In: *Cell Culture in the Neurosciences*, J. E. Bottenstein and G. Sato, eds., pp. 245–272, Plenum, New York.

Guthrie, P. B., R. E. Lee, V. Rehder, et al. (1994) Self-recognition: a constraint on the formation of electrical coupling in neurons. J. Neurosci. 14: 1477–1485.

Haga, T., E. M. Ross, H. J. Anderson, and A. G. Gilman (1977) Adenylate cyclase permanently uncoupled from hormone receptors in a novel variant of S49 mouse lymphoma cells. Proc. Natl. Acad. Sci. U.S.A. 74: 2016–2020.

Halegoua S., R. C. Armstrong, and N. E. Kremer (1991) Dissecting the mode of action of nerve growth factor. Curr. Top. Microbiol. Immunol. 165: 119–170.

Halfter, W., D. F. Newgreen, J. Sauter, and U. Schwarz (1983) Oriented axon outgrowth from avian embryonic retinae in culture. Dev. Biol. 95: 56–64.

Halliwell, B. (1988) Albumin an important extracellular antioxidant? Biochem. Pharmacol. 37: 569–571.

Halpain, S., and G. S. Withers (1995) A phosphorylation state-dependent antibody defines isoforms of MAP2 with distinctive subcellular localization and developmental expression. Soc. Neurosci. Abstr. 21: 81.

Ham, J., C. Babij, J. Whitfield, C. M. Pfarr, D. Lallemand, M. Yaniv, and L. L. Rubin (1995) A c-Jun dominant negative mutant protects sympathetic neurons against programmed cell death. Neuron 14: 927–939.

Hamburger V. (1948) Mitotic patterns in the spinal cord of the chick embryo. J. Comp. Neurol. 88: 221–283.

Hamilos, D. L., and J. J. Wedner (1985) The role of glutathione in lymphocyte activation: I. Comparison of inhibitory effects of buthionine sulfoximine and 2-cyclohexene-1-one by nuclear size transformation. J. Immunol. 135: 2740.

Hamilos, D. L., P. Zelarney, and J. J. Mascali (1989) Lymphocyte proliferation in glutathione-depleted lymphocytes: direct relationship between glutathione availability and the proliferative response. Immunopharmacology 18: 223.

Hammang, J. P., E. E. Baetge, R. R. Behringer, R. L. Brinster, R. D. Palmiter, and A. Messing (1990) Immortalized retinal neurons derived from SV40 T-antigen-induced tumors in transgenic mice. Neuron 4: 775–782.

Hammond, D. N., G. W. Moll, G. L. Robertson, and E. Chelmicka-Schorr (1986) Hypo-dipsic hypernatremia with normal osmoregulation of vasopressin. N. Engl. J. Med. 315: 433–436.

Hamprecht, B. (1977) Structural, electrophysiological, biochemical, and pharmacological properties of neuroblastoma-glioma cell hybrids in cell culture [review]. Int. Rev. Cytol. 49: 99–170.

Hamprecht, B., T. Glaser, G. Reiser, E. Bayer and F. Propst (1985) Culture and characteristics of hormone-responsive neuroblastoma X glioma hybrid cells. Methods Enzymol. 109: 316–341.

Hankin, M. H., and C. F. Lagenaur (1994) Cell adhesion molecules in the early developing mouse retina: retinal neurons show preferential outgrowth in vitro on L1 but not N-CAM. J. Neurobiol. 25: 472–487.

Hanks, J. H. (1955) Balanced salt solutions, inorganic requirements and pH control. In: *An Introduction to Cell and Tissue Culture*, W. F. Scherer, ed., p. 5, Burgess Publishing Co., Minneapolis, MN.

Harada, A., K. Oguchi, S. Okabe, J. Kuno, S. Terada, T. Oshima, R. Sato-Yoshitake, Y. Takei, T. Noda, and N. Hirokawa (1994) Altered microtubule organization in small-calibre axons of mice lacking tau protein. Nature 369: 488–491.

Hardy, M., D. Younkin, C. M. Tang, J. Pleasure, Q. Y. Shi, M. Williams, and D. Pleasure (1994) Expression of non-NMDA glutamate receptor channel genes by clonal human neurons. J. Neurochem. 63: 482–489.

Harlow, E., and D. Lane (1988) *Antibodies: a laboratory manual*, Cold Spring Harbor, NY: Cold Spring Harbor Laboratory.

Harris, G. L., L. P. Henderson, and N. Spitzer (1988) Changes in densities and kinetics of delayed rectifier potassium channels during neuronal differentiation. Neuron 1: 739–750.

Harris, K. M., and P. A. Rosenberg (1993) Localization of synapses in rat cortical cultures. Neuroscience 53: 495–508.

Harris, P. J. (1986) Cytology and immunocytochemistry. Methods Cell Biol. 27: 243–262.

Harrison, R. G. (1907) Observations on the living developing nerve fiber. Anat. Rec. 1: 116–118.

Harrison, R. G. (1910) The outgrowth of the nerve fiber as a mode of protoplasmic movement. J. Exp. Zool. 9: 787–846.

Harrison, R. G. (1912) The cultivation of tissues in extraneous media as a method of morphogenetic study. Anat. Rec. 6: 181–193.

Harrison, R. G. (1914) The reaction of embryonic cells to solid structures. J. Exp. Zool. 17: 521–544.

Hasty, D. L., and E. D. Hay (1978) Freeze-fracture studies of the developing cell surface: II. Particle-free membrane blisters on glutaraldehyde-fixed corneal fibroblasts are arte-facts. J. Cell Biol. 78: 756–768.

Hatten, M. E. (1985) Neuronal regulation of astroglial morphology and proliferation in vitro. J. Cell Biol. 100: 384–396.

Hatten, M. E., and N. Heintz (1995) Mechanisms of neural patterning and specification in the developing cerebellum. Annu. Rev. Neurosci. 18: 385–408.

Hatten, M. E., and R. L. Sidman (1978) Plant lectins detect age and region-specific differences in cell surface carbohydrates and cell reassociation behavior of embryonic mouse cerebellar cells. J. Supramol. Struct. 7: 267–278.

Hatten, M. E., R. K. H. Liem, and C. A. Mason (1986) Weaver mouse cerebellar granule neurons fail to migrate on wild type astroglial processes in vitro. J. Neurosci. 6: 2676–2683.

Hatten, M. E., R. K. H. Liem, M. L. Shelanski, and C. A. Mason (1991) Astroglia in CNS injury. Glia 4: 233–243.

Hawkins, R. D., E. R. Kandel, and S. A. Siegelbaum (1993) Learning to modulate transmitter release: themes and variations in synaptic plasticity [review]. Annu. Rev. Neurosci. 16: 625–665.

Hawrot, E., and P. H. Patterson (1979) Long-term culture of dissociated sympathetic neurons. Methods Enzymol. 58: 574–583.

Hawver, D., and S. Schacher (1993) Selective fasciculation as a mechanism for the formation of specific chemical connections between *Aplysia* neurons in vitro. J. Neurobiol. 24: 368–383.

Haydon, P. G., D. P. McCobb, and S. B. Kater (1984) Serotonin selectively inhibits growth cone motility and synaptogenesis of specific identified neurons. Science 226: 561–564.

Heffner, C. D., A. G. Lumsden, and D. D. O'Leary (1990) Target control of collateral extension and directional axon growth in the mammalian brain. Science 247: 217–220.

Heidemann, S. R. (1996) Cytoplasmic mechanisms of axonal and dendritic growth in neurons. Int. Rev. Cytol. 165: 235–296.

Hendelman, W. J., and K. C. Marshall (1980) Axonal projection patterns visualized with horseradish peroxidase in organized cultures of cerebellum. Neuroscience 5: 1833–1846.

Hendelman, W. J., K. C. Marshall, A. S. Aggerwal, and J. M. Wojtowicz (1977) Organization of pathways in cultures of mouse cerebellum. In: *Cell, Tissue and Organ Cultures in Neurobiology*, S. Fedoroff and L. Hertz, eds., pp. 539–554, Academic Press, New York.

Herkenham M, and W. J. H. Nauta (1979) Efferent connections of the habenular nuclei in the rat. J. Comp. Neurol. 187: 19–48.

Herman, B., and J. J. Lamasters (1993) *Optical Microscopy Emerging Methods and Applications*, Academic Press, San Diego.

Heuser, J. E., T. S. Reese, M. J. Dennis, Y. Jan, L. Jan, and L. Evans (1979) Synaptic vesicle exocytosis captured by quick freezing and correlated with quantal transmitter release. J. Cell Biol. 81: 275–300.

Higgins, D., A. Waxman, and G. Banker (1988) The distribution of microtubule-associated protein 2 changes when dendritic growth is induced in rat sympathetic neurons in vitro. Neuroscience 24: 583–592.

Higgins, D., P. J. Lein, D. J. Osterhout, and M. I. Johnson (1991) Tissue culture of mammalian autonomic neurons. In: *Culturing Nerve Cells*, G. Banker and K. Goslin, eds., The MIT Press, Cambridge, MA.

Hild, W. (1957) Myelinogenesis in cultures of mammalian central nervous tissue. Z. Zellforsch. 46: 71.

Hild, W. (1977) Characteristic of neurons in tissue culture. In: *Cell, Tissue, and Organ Cultures in Neurobiology*, S. Fedoroff and L. Hertz, eds., pp. 99–118, Academic Press, New York.

Hild, W., and I. Tasaki (1962) Morphological and physiological properties of neurons and glial cells in tissue culture. J. Neurosci. 277–304.

Hille, B. (1994) Modulation of ion-channel function by G-protein-coupled receptors. Trends Neurosci. 17: 531–536.

Hirano, Y., and Y. Kidokoro (1989) Heparin and heparan sulfate partially inhibit induction of acetylcholine receptor accumulation by nerve in *Xenopus* culture. J. Neurosci. 9: 1555–1561.

Hitt, M., A. J. Bett, L. Prevec, and F. L. Graham (1994) Construction and propagation of human adenovirus vectors. In: *Cell Biology. A Laboratory Handbook*, Vol. 1. J. E. Celis, ed., Academic Press, New York.

Ho, D. Y. (1994) Amplicon-based herpes simplex virus vectors. Methods Cell Biol. 43: 191–210.

Ho, D. Y., and E. S. Mocarski (1988) Beta-galactosidase as a marker in the peripheral and nervous tissues of the herpes simplex virus infected mouse. Virology 174: 279–283.

Ho, D. Y., E. S. Mocarski, and R. M. Sapolsky (1993) Altering central nervous system physiology with a defective herpes simplex virus vector expressing the glucose transporter gene. Proc. Natl. Acad. Sci. U.S.A. 90: 3655–3659.

Ho, D. Y., S. L. Fink, M. S. Lawrence, T. J. Meier, T. C. Saydam, R. Dash, and R. M. Sapolsky (1995) Herpes simplex virus vector system: analysis of its in vivo and in vitro cytopathic effects. J. Neurosci. Methods 57: 205–215.

Ho, D. Y., J. R. McLaughlin, and R. M. Sapolsky (1996) Inducible gene expression from defective herpes simplex virus vectors using the tetracycline-responsive promoter system. Mol. Brain Res. 41: 200–209.

Hoch, D. B., and R. Dingledine (1986) GABAergic neurons in rat hippocampal culture. Brain Res. 390: 53–64.

Hockberger, P. E., H.-Y. Tseng, and J. A. Connor (1989) Development of rat cerebellar Purkinje cells: electrophysiological properties following acute isolation and in long-term culture. J. Neurosci. 9: 2258–2271.

Hofman, F. M., R. I. von Hanwehr, C. A. Dinarello, S. B. Mizel, D. Hinton, and J. E. Merrill (1986) Immunoregulatory molecules and IL2 receptors identified in multiple sclerosis brain. J. Immunol. 136: 3239–3245.

Hogan, B., F. Costantini, and E. Lacy (1986) *Manipulating the Mouse Embryo*, pp. 48–61, Cold Spring Harbor Laboratory, Cold Spring Harbor, NY.

Hogue, M. J. (1947) Human fetal brain cells in tissue culture: their identification and motility. J. Exp. Zool. 106: 85–107.

Holtzman, D., H. Nguyen, S. Zamvil, and J. Olson (1982) In vitro cellular respiration at elevated temperatures in developing rat cerebral cortex. Brain Res. 256: 401–405.

Holz, G. G., K. Dunlap, and R. M. Kream (1988) Characterization of the electrically evoked release of substance P from dorsal root ganglion neurons: methods and dihydropyridine sensitivity. J. Neurosci. 8: 463–471.

Honegger, P. (1985) Biochemical differentiation in serum-free aggregating brain cell cultures. In: *Cell Culture in the Neurosciences*, J. E. Bottenstein and G. Sato, eds., pp. 223–243, Plenum, New York.

Honegger, P., D. Lenoir, and P. Favrod (1979) Growth and differentiation of aggregating fetal brain cells in a serum-free defined medium. Nature 282: 305–308.

Honig, M. G., and R. I. Hume (1986) Fluorescent carbocyanine dyes allow living neurons of identified origin to be studied in long-term cultures. J. Cell Biol. 103: 171–187.

Honig, M. G, and J. Kueter (1995) The expression of cell adhesion molecules on the growth cones of chick cutaneous and muscle sensory neurons. Dev. Biol. 167: 563–583.

Honig, M. G., and J. Y. Zou (1995) The effects of target tissues on the outgrowth of chick cutaneous and muscle sensory neurons. Dev. Biol. 167: 549–562.

Hopp, L., and C. H. Bunker (1993) Lipophilic impurity of phenol red is a potent cation transport modulator. J. Cell. Physiol. 157: 594–602.

Horikawa, H., and W. Armstrong (1988) A versatile means of intracellular labelling: injection of biocytin and its detection with avidin conjugates. J. Neurosci. Methods 25: 1–11.

Hory-Lee, F., and E. Frank (1995) The nicotinic blocking agents d-tubocurare and alpha-bungarotoxin save motoneurons from naturally occurring death in the absence of neuromuscular blockade. J. Neurosci. 15: 6453–6460.

Hotary, K. B., and K. W. Tosney (1996) Cellular interactions that guide sensory and motor neurites identified in an embryo slice preparation. Dev. Biol. 176: 22–35.

Houser C. R., G. D. Crawford, R. P. Barber, P. M. Salvaterra, and J. E. Vaughn (1983) Organizational and morphological characteristics of cholinergic neurons: an immunocytochemical study with a monoclonal antibody to choline acetyltransferase. Brain Res. 266: 97–119.

Hsiang, J., B. H. Wainer, I. A. Shalaby, P. C. Huffman, A. Heller and B. R. Heller (1987) Neurotrophic effects of hippocampal target cells on developing septal cholinergic neurons in culture. Neuroscience 21: 333–343.

Hsiang, J., S. D. Price, A. Heller, P. C. Hoffman, and B. H. Wainer (1988) Ultrastructural evidence for hippocampal target cell-mediated trophic effects on septal cholinergic neurons in reaggregating cell cultures. Neuroscience 26: 417–431.

Hubert, J. F., A. Vincent, and F. Labrie (1986) Estrogenic activity of phenol red in rat anterior pituitary cells in culture. Biochem. Biophys. Res. Commun. 141: 885–891.

Huck, S. (1983) Serum-free medium for cultures of the postnatal mouse cerebellum: only insulin is essential. Brain Res. Bull. 10: 667–674.

Huettner, J. E., and R. W. Baughman (1986) Primary culture of identified neurons from the visual cortex of postnatal rats. J. Neurosci. 6: 3044–3060.

Huettner, J. E., and R. W. Baughman (1988) The pharmacology of synapses formed by identified corticocollicular neurons in primary cultures of rat visual cortex. J. Neurosci. 8: 160–175.

Hughes, A. (1953) The growth of embryonic neurites. A study on cultures of chick neural tissue. J. Anat. (Lond.) 87: 150–162.

Hunter, K. E., and M. E. Hatten (1995) Radial glial cell transformation to astrocytes is bidirectional: Regulation by a diffusible factor in embryonic forebrain. Proc. Natl. Acad. Sci. 92: 2061–2065.

Huntington's Disease Collaborative Research Group (1993) A novel gene containing a trinucleotide repeat that is expanded and unstable on Huntington's disease chromosomes. Cell 72: 971–983.

Hyman, C., M. Junasz, C. Jackson, P. Write, N. Y. Ip, and R. M. Lindsay (1994) Overlapping and distinct actions of the neurotrophins BDNF, NT-3 and NT-4/5 on cultured dopaminergic and GABAergic neurons of the ventral mesencephalon. J. Neurosci. 14: 335–347.

Iacopino, A. M., and S. Christakos (1990) Specific reduction of calcium-binding protein (28 kilodalton calbindin-D) gene expression in aging and neurodegenerative diseases. Proc. Natl. Acad. Sci. U.S.A. 87: 4078–4082.

Iacovitti, L., M. I. Johnson, T. H. Joh, and R. P. Bunge (1982) Biochemical and morphological characterization of sympathetic neurons grown in a chemically-defined medium. Neuroscience 7: 2225–2239.

Ibarolla, N., M. Mayer, A. Rodriguez-Pena, and M. Noble (1996) Evidence for the existence of two timing mechanisms in oligodendrocyte development. Dev. Biol. 180: 1–21.

Ignelzi, M. A. J., D. R. Miller, P. Soriano, and P. F. Maness (1994) Impaired neurite outgrowth of src-minus cerebellar neurons on the cell adhesion molecule L1. Neuron 12: 873–884.

Ikeda, S. R., D. M. Lovinger, B. A. McCool, and D. L. Lewis (1995) Heterologous expression of metabotropic glutamate receptors in adult rat sympathetic neurons: subtype-specific coupling to ion channels. Neuron 14: 1029–1038.

Ikonen, E., R. G. Parton, W. Hunziker, K. Simons, and C. G. Dotti (1993) Transcytosis of the polymeric immunoglobulin receptor in cultured hippocampal neurons. Curr. Biol. 3: 635–644.

Inouye, S. (1986) *Video Microscopy*, Plenum, New York.

Ip, N. Y., and G. D. Yancopoulos (1996) The neurotrophins and CNTF two families of collaborative neurotrophic factors. Annu. Rev. Neurosci. 19: 491–515.

Ip, N. Y., Y. Li, G. D. Yancopoulos, and R. M. Lindsay (1993) Cultured hippocampal neurons show responses to BDNF, NT-3, and NT-4, but not NGF. J. Neurosci. 13: 3394–3405.

Ishitani, R., and D. M. Chuang (1996) Glyceraldehyde-3-phosphate dehydrogenase antisense oligodeoxynucleotides protect against cytosine arabinonucleoside-induced apoptosis in cultured cerebellar neurons. Proc. Natl. Acad. Sci. U.S.A. 93: 9937–9941.

Ishizaki, Y., J. F. Burne, and M. C. Raff (1994) Autocrine signals enable chondrocytes to survive in culture. J. Cell Biol., 126: 1069–1077.

Jacobson, M. (1982) Origin of the nervous system in amphibians. In: *Neuronal Development*, N. C. Spitzer, ed., p. 424, Plenum, New York.

Jaeger, C. B., R. Kapoor, and R. Llinás (1988) Cytology and organization of rat cerebellar organ cultures. Neuroscience 26: 509–538.

Jahr, C. E., and C. F. Stevens (1987) Glutamate activates multiple single-channel conductances in hippocampal neurons. Nature 325: 522–525.

James, I. F., and J. N. Wood (1992) A catalogue of neuronal properties expressed by cell lines. In: *Neuronal Cell Lines: A Practical Approach*, J. N. Wood, ed., pp. 249–254, Oxford University, New York.

Jareb, M., and G. Banker (1995) The polarized sorting of membrane proteins expressed in cultured hippocampal neurons using viral vectors. Mol. Biol. Cell 6: 2339.

Jessell, T. M., R. E. Siegel, and G. D. Fischbach (1979) Induction of acetylcholine receptors on cultured skeletal muscle by a factor extracted from brain and spinal cord. Proc. Natl. Acad. Sci. U.S.A. 76: 5397–5401.

Jiao, S., L. Cheng, J. A. Wolff, and N.-S. Yang (1993) Particle bombardment-mediated gene transfer and expression in rat brain tissues. Bio/Technology 11: 497–502.

Johnson, E. M., Jr., P. D. Gorin, L. D. Brandeis, and J. Pearson (1980) Dorsal root ganglion neurons are destroyed by exposure in utero to maternal antibodies to nerve growth factor. Science 219: 916–918.

Johnson, E. M., Jr., K. M. Rich, and H. K. Yip (1986) The role of NGF in sensory neurons in vivo. Trends Neurosci. 9: 33–37.

Johnson, J. E., Y. A. Barde, M. Schwab, and H. Thoenen (1986) Brain-derived neurotrophic factor supports the survival of cultured rat retinal ganglion cells. J. Neurosci. 6: 3031–3038.

Johnson, M. D. (1994) Electrophysiological and histochemical properties of postnatal rat serotonergic neurons in dissociated cell culture. Neuroscience 63: 775–787.

Johnson, M. I., and V. Argiro (1983) Techniques in the tissue culture of rat sympathetic neurons. Methods Enzymol. 103: 334–347.

Johnson, P. A., and T. Friedmann (1994) Replication-defective recombinant herpes simplex virus vectors. Methods Cell Biol. 43: 211–230.

Johnson, P. A., A. Miyanohara, F. Levine, T. Cahill, and T. Friedmann (1992a) Cytotoxicity of a replication-defective mutant of herpes simplex virus type 1. J. Virol. 66: 2952–2965.

Johnson, P. A., K. Yoshida, F. H. Gage, and T. Friedmann (1992b) Effects of gene transfer into cultured CNS neurons with a replication-defective herpes simplex virus type 1 vector. Mol. Brain Res. 12: 95–102.

Johnson, P. A., M. J. Wang, and T. Friedmann (1994) Improved cell survival by the reduction of immediate-early gene expression in replication-defective mutants of herpes simplex virus type 1 but not by mutation of the virion host shutoff function. J. Virol. 68: 6347–6362.

Jomary, C., T. A. Piper, G. Dickson, L. A. Couture, A. E. Smith, M. J. Neal, and S. E. Jones (1994) Adenovirus-mediated gene transfer to murine retianl cells in vitro and in vivo. FEBS Lett. 347: 117–122.

Jones, K. A., and R. W. Baughman (1988) Both NMDA and non-NMDA subtypes of glutamate receptors are concentrated at synapses on cerebral cortical neurons in culture. Neuron 7: 593–603.

Jones-Villeneuve, E. M. V., M. W. McBurney, K. A. Rogers, and V. I. Kalnins (1982) Retinoic acid induces embryonal carcinoma cells to differentiate into neurons and glial cells. J. Cell Biol. 94: 253–262.

Kaang, B.-K., E. R. Kandel, and S. G. N. Grant (1993) Activation of cAMP-responsive genes by stimuli that produce long-term facilitation in *Aplysia* sensory neurons. Neuron 10: 427–435.

Kaczmarek, L. K., M. Finbow, J. P. Revel, and F. Strumwasser (1979) The morphology and coupling of *Aplysia* bag cells within the abdominal ganglion and in cell culture. J. Neurobiol. 10: 535–550.

Kaech, S., J. B. Kim, M. Cariola, and E. Ralston (1996) Improved lipid-mediated gene transfer into primary cultures of hippocampal neurons. Mol. Brain Res. 35: 344–348.

Kain, S. R., M. Adams, A. Kondepudi, T. T. Yang, W. W. Ward, and P. Kitts (1995) Green fluorescent protein as a reporter of gene expression and protein localization. Biotechniques 19: 650–655.

Kanai, Y., and N. Hirokawa (1995) Sorting mechanisms of tau and MAP2 in neurons: suppressed axonal transit of MAP2 and locally regulated microtubule binding. Neuron 14: 421–432.

Kandel, E. R. (1976) *Cellular Basis of Behavior*, W. H. Freeman, San Francisco.

Kandel, E. R., T. Abrams, L. Bernier, et al. (1983) Classical conditioning and sensitization share aspects of the same molecular cascade in *Aplysia*. Cold Spring Harb. Symp. Quant. Biol. 48: 821–830.

Kandel, E. R., J. Schwartz, and T. M. Jessell. (1991) *Principles of Neural Science*. 3rd ed., Applteon and Lange, Norwalk, CT.

Kapfhammer, J. P., and J. A. Raper (1987) Collapse of growth cone structure on contact with specific neurites in culture. J. Neurosci. 7: 201–212.

Kaplan, D. R., and R. M. Stephens (1994) Neurotrophin signal transduction by the Trk receptor. J. Neurobiol. 25: 1404–1417.

Kaplan, F. S., C. T. Brighton, M. J. Boytim, M. E. Selzer, V. Lee, K. Spindler, D. Silberberg and J. Black (1986) Enhanced survival of rat neonatal cerebral cortical neurons at subatmospheric oxygen tensions in vitro. Brain Res. 384: 199–203.

Kaplitt, M. G., A. D. Kwong, S. P. Kleopoulos, C. V. Mobbs, S. D. Rabkin, and D. W. Pfaff (1994a) Preproenkephalin promoter yields region-specific and long-term expression in adult brain after direct in vivo gene transfer via a defective herpes simplex viral vector. Proc. Natl. Acad. Sci. U.S.A. 91: 8979–8983.

Kaplitt, M. G., J. G. Pfaus, S. P. Kleopoulos, B. A. Hanlon, S. D. Rabkin, and D. W. Pfaff (1991) Expression of a functional foreign gene in adult mammalian brain following in vivo transfer via a herpes simplex virus type 1 defective viral vector. Mol. Cell. Neurosci. 2: 320–330.

Kaplitt, M. G., P. Leone, R. J. Samulski, X. Xiao, D. W. Pfaff, K. L. O'Malley, and M. J. During (1994b) Long-term gene expression and phenotypic correction using adeno-associated virus vectors in the mammalian brain. Nature Genet. 8: 148–153.

Kapoor, R., C. B. Jaeger, and R. Llinás (1988) Electrophysiology of the mammalian cerebellar cortex in organ culture. Neuroscience 26: 493–507.

Kater, S. B., and M. P. Mattson (1988) Extrinsic and intrinsic regulators of neurite outgrowth and synaptogenesis in isolated, identified *Helisoma* neurons in culture. In: *Cell Culture Approaches to Invertebrate Neuroscience*, D. Beadle, G. Lees, and S. B. Kater, eds., Academic Press, Orlando, FL.

Kato, A. C., G. Touzeau, D. Bertrand, and C. R. Bader (1985) Human spinal cord neurons in dissociated monolayer cultures: morphological, biochemical, and electrophysiological properties. J. Neurosci. 5: 2750–2761.

Katz, L. C., A. Burkhalter, and W. J. Dreyer (1984) Fluorescent latex microspheres as a retrograde neuronal marker for in vivo and in vitro studies of visual cortex. Nature 310: 498–500.

Katz, P. S., and I. B. Levitan (1993) Quisqualate and ACPD are agonists for a glutamate-activated current in identified *Aplysia* neurons. J. Neurophysiol. 69: 143–150.

Kawamoto, J. C., and J. N. Barrett (1986) Cryopreservation of primary neurons for tissue culture. Brain Res. 384: 84–93.

Kay, A. R., and R. K. S. Wong (1986) Isolation of neurons suitable for patch clamping from different brain regions. J. Neurosci. Methods 16: 227–238.

Kay, B. K., L. M. Schwartz, U. Rutishauser, T. H. Qiu, and H. B. Peng (1988) Patterns of N-CAM expression during myogenesis in *Xenopus* laevis. Development 103: 463–471.

Keller, F., and S. Schacher (1990) Neuron-specific membrane glycoproteins promoting neurite fasciculation in *Aplysia californica*. J. Cell Biol. 111: 2637–2650.

Kelly, R. B. (1993) Storage and release of neurotransmitters. Cell Neuron Suppl. 72(10): 43–53.

Kennedy, T. E., and M. Tessier-Lavigne (1995) Guidance and induction of branch formation in developing axons by target-derived diffusible factors [review]. Curr. Opin. Neurobiol. 5: 83–90.

Kerr, C. W., L. J. Lee, A. A. Romero, N. D. Stull, and L. Iacovitti (1994) Purification of dopamine neurons by flow cytometry. Brain Res. 665: 300–306.

Kessler, M., M. Baudry, and G. Lynch (1987) Use of cystine to distinguish glutamate binding from glutamate sequestration. Neurosci. Lett. 81: 221–226

Kidokoro, Y., and M. Saito (1988) Early cross-striation formation in twitching *Xenopus* myocytes in cultures. Proc. Natl. Acad. Sci. U.S.A. 85: 1978–1982.

Kidokoro, Y., and E. Yeh (1982) Initial synaptic transmission at the growth cone in *Xenopus* nerve-muscle cultures. Proc. Natl. Acad. Sci. U.S.A. 79: 6727–6731.

Kilpatrick, T. J., L. J. Richards, and P. F. Bartlett (1995) The regulation of neural precursor cells within the mammalian brain. Mol. Cell Neurosci. 6: 2–15.

Kim, J. H., S. U. Kim, and S. Kito (1984) Immunocytochemical demonstration of beta-endorphin and beta-lipotropin in cultured human spinal ganglion neurons. Brain Res. 304: 192–196.

Kim, Y. T., and C. F. Wu (1987) Reversible blockage of neurite development and growth cone formation in neuronal cultures of a temperature-sensitive mutant of *Drosophila*. J. Neurosci. 7: 3245–3255.

Kimelberg, H. K. (1988) *Glial Cell Receptors*, Raven, New York.

Kimelman, D., and A. Maas (1992) Induction of dorsal and ventral mesoderm by ectopically expressed *Xenopus* basic fibroblast growth factor. Development 114: 261–269.

Kimhi, Y. (1981) Nerve cells in clonal systems. In: *Excitable Cells in Tissue Culture*, M. Lieberman, ed., pp. 173–245, Plenum, New York.

Kirschenbaum, B., M. Nedergaard, A. Preuss, K. Barami, R. A. Fraser, and S. A. Goldman (1994) In vitro neuronal production and differentiation by precursor cells derived from the adult human forebrain. Cerebral Cortex 4: 576–589.

Kita, H., and W. Armstrong (1991) A biotin-containing N-(2 aminoethyl)biotinamide for intracellular labelling and neuronal tracing studies: comparison with biocytin. J. Neurosci. Methods 37: 141–146.

Kleiman, R., G. Banker, and O. Steward (1993a) Inhibition of protein synthesis alters the subcellular distribution of mRNA in neurons but does not prevent dendritic transport of RNA. Proc. Natl. Acad. Sci. U.S.A. 90: 11192–11196.

Kleiman, R., G. Banker, and O. Steward (1993b) Subcellular distribution of rRNA and poly(A) RNA in hippocampal neurons in culture. Brain Res. Mol. Brain Res. 20: 305–312.

Kleinfeld, D., K. H. Kahler, and P. E. Hockberger (1988) Controlled outgrowth of dissociated neurons on patterned substrates. J. Neurosci. 8: 4098–4120.

Kleitman, N., and R. P. Bunge (1995) The Schwann cell: morphology and development. In: *The Axon*, S. G. Waxman, J. D. Kocsis, and P. K. Stys, eds., pp. 97–115, Oxford University, New York.

Kleitman, N., D. K. Simon, M. Schachner, and R. P. Bunge (1988) Growth of embryonic retinal neurites elicited by contact with Schwann cell surfaces is blocked by antibodies to L1. Exp. Neurol. 102: 298–306.

Knöpfel, T., H. J. Kasper, B. Köhler, Z. Zglinski, L. Zeller, and B. H. Gähwiler (1988) Optical recording of neuronal activity in organotypic slice cultures. Soc. Neurosci. Abstr. 14: 247.

Knöpfel, T., L. Rietschin, and B. H. Gähwiler (1989) Organotypic cocultures of rat locus coeruleus and hippocampus. Eur. J. Neurosci. 1: 678–689.

Knöpfel, T., E. Audinat, and B. H. Gähwiler (1990a) Climbing fiber responses in olivo-cerebellar slice cultures. I. Microelectrode recordings from Purkinje cells. Eur. J. Neurosci. 2: 726–732.

Knöpfel, T., S. Charpak, D. A. Brown, and B. H. Gähwiler (1990b) Cytosolic free calcium in hippocampal CA3 pyramidal cells. In: *Understanding the Brain Through the Hippocampus. The Hippocampal Region as a Model for Studying Brain Structure and Function*, J. Storm-Mathisen, J. Zimmer, and O. P. Ottersen, eds., Progr. Brain Res., vol. 83, pp. 189–195, Elsevier Science Publishers B.V., Amsterdam, New York, Oxford.

Knöpfel, T., I. Vranesic, B. H. Gähwiler, and D. A. Brown (1990c) Muscarinic and a-adrenergic depression of the slow Ca^{2+} activated potassium conductance in hippocampal CA3 pyramidal cells is not mediated by a reduction of depolarization-induced cytosolic Ca^{2+} transients. Proc. Natl. Acad. Sci. U.S.A. 87: 4083–4087.

Knowles, R. B., J. H. Sabry, M. E. Martone, J. J. Deernick, M. H. Ellisman, G. J. Bassell, and K. S. Kosik (1996) Translocation of RNA granules in living neurons. J. Neurosci. 16: 7812–7820.

Kofuji, P., M. Hofer, K. J. Millen, et al. (1996) Functional analysis of the weaver mutant GIRK2 K^+ channel and rescue of weaver granule cells. Neuron 16: 941–952.

Komuro, H., and P. Rakic (1996) Intracellular Ca^{2+} fluctuations modulate the rate of neuronal migration. Neuron 17: 275–285.

Kornau, H. C., L. T. Schenker, M. B. Kennedy, and P. H. Seeburg (1995) Domain interaction between NMDA receptor subunits and the postsynaptic density protein PSD-95. Science 269: 1737–1740.

Korsching, S. (1993) The neurotrophic factor concept: a reexamination. J. Neurosci. 133: 2739–2748.

Korte, M., O. Griesbeck, C. Gravel, P. Carroll, V. Staiger, H. Theonen, and T. Bonhoeffer (1996) Virus-mediated gene transfer into hippocampal CA1 region restores long-term potentiation in brain-derived neurotrophic factor mutant mice. Proc. Natl. Acad. Sci. USA 93: 12547–12552.

Koseki, C., D. Herzlinger, and Q. Al-Awqati (1992) Apoptosis in metanephric development. J. Cell Biol. 119: 1327–1333.

Kosik, K. S., A. Ferreira, and N. LeClerc (1993) Manipulating neuronal genes in cell culture: antisense suppression and baculoviral expression. Ins and outs of genes: knockouts and transfers. Soc. Neurosci. short course, pp. 41–48.

Kraszewski, K., O. Mundigl, L. Daniell, C. Verderio, M. Matteoli, and P. Decamilli (1995) Synaptic vesicle dynamics in living cultured hippocampal neurons visualized with CY3-conjugated antibodies directed against the lumenal domain of synaptotagmin. J. Neurosci. 15: 4328–4342.

Kreis, T., and R. Vale (1994) *Guidebook to the Extracellular Matrix and Adhesion Proteins*, Oxford University, New York.

Krieglstein, K., M. Rufer, C. Suter-Crazzolara, and K. Unsicker (1995) Neural functions of the transforming growth factors beta. Int. J. Dev. Neurosci. 13: 301–315.

Kriegstein, A. R., and M. A. Dichter (1983) Morphological classification of rat cortical neurons in cell culture. J. Neurosci. 3: 1634–1647.

Krushel, L. A., J. A. Connolly, and D. vonder Kooy (1989) Pattern formation in the mammalian forebrain: patch neurons from the rat striatum selectively reassociate in vitro. Brain Res. Dev. Brain Res. 47: 137–142.

Kuhar, S., L. Feng, S. Vidan, E. R. Ross, M. E. Hatten, and N. Heintz (1993) Developmentally regulated cDNAs define four stages of cerebellar granule neuron differentiation. Development 112: 97–104.

Kuhn, T. B., E. T. Stoeckli, M. A. Condrau, et al. (1991) Neurite outgrowth on immobilized axonin-1 is mediated by a heterophilic interaction with L1(G4). J. Cell Biol. 115: 1113–1126.

Kullberg, R. W., T. L. Lentz, and M. W. Cohen (1977) Development of the myotomal neuromuscular junction in *Xenopus laevis*: an electrophysiological and fine-structural study. Dev. Biol. 60: 101–129.

Kupfermann, I., and T. J. Carew (1974) Behavior patterns of *Aplysia californica* in its natural environment. Behav. Biol. 12: 317–337.

Kuromi, H., B. Brass, and Y. Kidokoro (1985) Formation of acetylcholine receptor clusters at neuromuscular junction in *Xenopus* cultures. Dev. Biol. 109: 165–176.

Lagenaur, C., and V. Lemmon (1987) An L1-like molecule, the 8D9 antigen, is a potent substrate for neurite extension. Proc. Natl. Acad. Sci. U.S.A. 84: 7753–7757.

Lamoureux, P., R. E. Buxbaum, and S. R. Heidemann (1989) Direct evidence that growth cones pull. Nature 340: 159–162.

Landis, D. M., and T. S. Reese (1981) Membrane structure in mammalian astrocytes: a review of freeze-fracture studies on adult, developing, reactive and cultured astrocytes. J. Exp. Biol. 95: 35–48.

Landis, D. M., L. A. Weinstein, and T. S. Reese (1987) Substructure in the postsynaptic density of Purkinje cell dendritic spines revealed by rapid freezing and etching. Synapse 1: 552–558.

Landis, S. C. (1994) Development of sympathetic neurons: neurotransmitter plasticity and differentiation factors. Prog. Brain Res. 100: 19–23.

Langanger, G., J. De May, and H. Adam (1983) 1,4-Diazobicyclo-(2,2,2)-octane (DABCO) retards the fading of immunofluorescence preparations. [German]. Mikroskopie 40: 237–241.

Langford, L. A., S. Porter, and R. P. Bunge (1988) Immortalized rat Schwann cells produce tumors in vivo. J. Neurocytol. 17: 521–529.

Largent, B. L., R. G. Sosnowski, and R. R. Reed (1993) Directed expression of an oncogene to the olfactory neuronal lineage in transgenic mice. J. Neurosci. 13: 300–312.

LaSalle, G. L. G., J. J. Robert, S. Berrard, V. Ridoux, L. D. Stratford-Perricaudet, M. Perricaudet, and J. Mallet (1993) An adenovirus vector for gene transfer into neurons and glia in the brain. Science 259: 988–990.

Lasher, R. S., and I. S. Zagon (1972) The effect of potassium on neuronal differentiation in cultures of dissociated newborn rat cerebellum. Brain Res. 41: 482–488.

Latov, N., G. Nilaver, E. A. Zimmerman, W. G. Johnson, A. J. Silverman, R. Defendini, and L. Cote (1979) Fibrillary astrocytes proliferate in response to brain injury. Dev. Biol. 72: 381–384.

Lawrence, J. B., and R. H. Singer (1985) Quantitative analysis of in situ hybridization methods for the detection of actin gene expression. Nucleic Acids Res. 13: 1777–1799.

Lawrence, M. S., D. Y. Ho, G. H. Sun, G. K. Steinberg, and R. M. Sapolsky (1996a) Overexpression of Bcl-2 with herpes simplex virus vectors protects CNS neurons against neurological insults in vitro and in vivo. J. Neurosci. 16: 486–496.

Lawrence, M. S., G. H. Sun, D. M. Kunis, et al. (1996b) Overexpression of the glucose transporter gene with a herpes simplex viral vector protects striatal neurons against stroke. J. Cereb. Blood Flow Metab. 16: 181–185.

Lawson, S. (1992) Morphological and biochemical cell types of sensory neurons. In: *Sensory Neurons: Diversity, Development, and Plasticity*, S. A. Scott, ed., pp. 27–59, Oxford University, New York.

LeDouarin, N. (1982) *The Neural Crest*, Cambridge University, New York.

Lee, M. K., J. B. Tuttle, L. I. Rebhun, D. W. Cleveland, and A. Frankfurter (1990) The expression and post translational modification of a neuron-specific beta-tubulin isotype during chick embryogenesis. Cell Motil. Cytoskeleton 17: 118–132.

Leifer, D., S. A. Lipton, C. J. Barnstable, and R. H. Masland (1984) Monoclonal antibody to Thy-1 enhances regeneration of processes by rat retinal ganglion cells in culture. Science 224: 303–306.

Lein P., M. Johnson, X. Guo, D. Rueger, and D. Higgins (1995) Osteogenic protein-1 induces dendritic growth in rat sympathetic neurons. Neuron 15: 597–605.

Lein, P., X. Guo, A. M. Hedges, D. Rueger, M. Johnson, and D. Higgins (1996) The effects of extracellular matrix and osteogenic protein-1 on the morphological differentiation of rat sympathetic neurons. Int. J. Dev. Neurosci. 14: 203–215.

Lein, P. J., and D. Higgins (1989) Laminin and a basement membrane extract have different effects on axonal and dendritic outgrowth from embryonic rat sympathetic neurons in vitro. Dev. Biol. 136: 330–345.

Lein, P. J., D. Higgins, D. C. Turner, L. A. Flier, and V. P. Terranova (1991) The NC1 domain of type IV collagen promotes axonal growth in sympathetic neurons through interaction with the alpha 1 beta 1 integrin. J. Cell Biol. 113: 417–428.

Lein, P. J., G. A. Banker, and D. Higgins (1992) Laminin selectively enhances axonal growth and accelerates the development of polarity by hippocampal neurons in culture. Brain Res. Dev. Brain Res. 69: 191–197.

Leivo, I., and E. Engvall (1988) Merosin, a protein specific for basement membranes of Schwann cells, striated muscle, and trophoblast, is expressed late in nerve and muscle development. Proc. Natl. Acad. Sci. U.S.A. 85: 1544–1548.

Lemmon, V., S. M. Burden, H. R. Payne, G. J. Elmslie, and M. L. Hlavin (1992) Neurite growth on different substrates: permissive versus instructive influences and the role of adhesive strength. J. Neurosci. 12: 818–826.

Lenn, N. J., and S. A. Bayer (1986) Neurogenesis in subnuclei of the rat interpeduncular nucleus and medial habenula. Brain Res. Bull. 16: 219–224.

Leonard, D. G. B., E. B. Ziff, and L. A. Greene (1987) Identification and characterization of mRNAs regulated by nerve growth factor in PC12 cells. Mol. Cell. Biol. 7: 3156–3167.

Lester R. A. J., and J. A. Dani (1995) Acetylcholine receptor desensitization induced by nicotine in rat medial habenula neurons. J. Neurophysiol. 74: 195–206.

Letourneau, P. C. (1975a) Possible roles for cell-to-substratum adhesion in neuronal morphogenesis. Dev. Biol. 44: 77–91.

Letourneau, P. C. (1975b) Cell-to-substratum adhesion and guidance of axonal elongation. Dev. Biol. 44: 92–101.

Letourneau, P. C. (1979) Cell-substratum adhesion of neurite growth cones, and its role in neurite elongation. Exp. Cell Res. 124: 127–138.

Letourneau, P. C. (1992) Integrins and *N*-cadherin are adhesive molecules involved in growth cone migration. In: *The Nerve Growth Cone*, P. C. Letourneau, S. B. Kater, and E. R. Macagno, eds., Raven, New York.

Letourneau, P. C., M. L. Condic, and D. M. Snow (1994) Interactions of developing neurons with the extracellular matrix. J. Neurosci. 14: 915–928.

Levallois, C., M. C. Calvet, J. M. Kamenka, D. Petite, and A. Privat (1995) Primary dissociated cultures of human brainstem cells: a useful tool for their characterization and neuroprotection study. Cell Biology and Toxicology 11: 155–160.

Levi, A., and S. Alemá (1991) The mechanism of action of nerve growth factor. Annu. Rev. Pharmacol. Toxicol. 31: 205–228.

Levi, A. D., R. P. Bunge, J. A. Lofgren, L. Meima, F. Hefti, K. Nikolics, and M. X. Sliwkowski (1995) The influence of heregulins on human Schwann cell proliferation. J. Neurosci. 15: 1329–1340.

Levi-Montalcini, R. (1950). The origin and development of the visceral system in the spinal cord of the chick embryo. J. Morphol. 86: 253–283.

Levi-Montalcini, R. (1982) Developmental neurobiology and the natural history of nerve growth factor. Annu. Rev. Neurosci. 5: 341–362.

Levi-Montalcini, R. (1987) The nerve growth factor 35 years later. Science 237: 1154–1162.

Levi-Montalcini, R., and P. U. Angeletti (1963) Essential role of the nerve growth factor in the survival and maintenance of dissociated sensory and sympathetic nerve cells in vitro. Dev. Biol. 7: 653–659.

Levi-Montalcini, R., and P. U. Angeletti (1968) Nerve growth factor. Physiol. Rev. 48: 534–569.

Levine, J. M., and P. Flynn (1986) Cell surface changes accompanying the neural differentiation of an embryonal carcinoma cell line. J. Neurosci 6: 3374–3384.

Levine, R. B., and J. C. Weeks (1996) Cell culture approaches to understanding the actions of steroid hormones on the insect nervous system. Dev. Neurosci. 18: 73–86.

Levison, S. W., and K. D. McCarthy (1991) Astroglia in culture. In: *Culturing Nerve Cells* (1st ed.), G. Banker and K. Goslin, eds., pp. 309–336, The MIT Press, Cambridge, MA.

Leviton, A., and Paneth, N. (1990) White-matter damage in preterm newborns—an epidemiologic perspective. Early Hum. Dev. 24: 1–22.

Lewis, W. H., and M. R. Lewis (1912) The cultivation of sympathetic nerves from the intestine of chick embryos in saline solutions. Anat. Rec. 6: 7–31.

Li, R.-H., J. Chen, G. Hammonds, H. Phillips, M. Armanini, P. Wood, R. Burge, P. J. Godowski, M. X. Sliwkowski and J. P. Mather (1996a) Identification of Gas6 as a growth factor for human Schwann cells. J. Neurosci. 16: 2012–2019.

Li, R.-H., M. X. Sliwkowski, J. Lo, and J. P. Mather (1996b) Establishment of Schwann cell lines from normal adult and embryonic rat dorsal root ganglia. J. Neurosci. Methods 67: 57–69.

Liesi, P., and J. M. Wright (1996) Weaver granule neurons are rescued by calcium channel antagonists and antibodies against a neurite outgrowth domain of the B2 chain of laminin. J. Cell Biol. 134: 477–486.

Liljeström, P., and H. Garoff (1991) A new generation of animal cell expression vectors based on the semliki forest virus replicon. BioTechnology 9: 1356–1361.

Lillien, L., and P. Claude (1985) Nerve growth factor is a mitogen for cultured chromaffin cells. Nature 317: 632–634.

Lin., C. H., and P. Forscher (1993) Cytoskeletal remodeling during growth cone-target interactions. J. Cell. Biol. 121: 1369–1383.

Lin, C. H., and P. Forscher (1995) Growth cone advance is inversely proportional to retrograde F-actin flow. Neuron 14: 763–771.

Lin, C. H., E. M. Espreafico, M. S. Mooseker, and P. Forscher (1996) Myosin drives retrograde F-actin flow in neuronal growth cones. Neuron 16: 769–782.

Lin, W., and B. G. Szaro (1995) Neurofilaments help maintain normal morphologies and support elongation of neurites in *Xenopus laevis* cultured embryonic spinal cord neurons. J. Neurosci. 15: 8331–8344.

Lin, X. Y., and D. L. Glanzman (1994a) Long-term potentiation of *Aplysia* sensorimotor synapses in cell culture: regulation by postsynaptic voltage. Proc. R. Soc. Lond. B. Biol. Sci. 255: 113–118.

Lin, X. Y., and D. L. Glanzman (1994b) Hebbian induction of long-term potentiation of *Aplysia* sensorimotor synapses: partial requirement for activation of an NMDA-related receptor. Proc. R. Soc. Lond. B. Biol. Sci. 255: 215–221.

Lindsay R. M., S. J. Wiegand, C. A. Altar, and P. S. DiStefano (1994) Neurotrophic factors: from molecule to man. Trends Neurosci. 17: 182–190.

Lindvall, O., H. Widner, S. Rehncrona, P. Brundin, P. Odin, B. Gustavi, R. Frackowiak, K. L. Leenders, G. Sawle and J. C. Rothwell (1992) Transplantation of fetal dopamine neurons in Parkinson's disease: one year clinical and neurophysiological observations in two patients with putaminal implants. Ann. Neurol. 31: 155–165.

Lioy, J., W. Z. Ho, J. R. Cutilli, R. A. Polin, and S. D. Douglas (1993) Thiol suppression of human immunodeficiency virus type 1 replicaton in primary cord blood monocyte-derived macrophages in vitro. J. Clin. Invest. 91: 495–498.

Listerud, M., A. B. Brussard, P. Devay, D. R. Colman, and L. W. Role (1991) Functional contribution of neuronal AChR subunits revealed by antisense oligonucleotides. Science 254: 1518–1521.

Liu, G., and R. W. Tsien (1995) Properties of synaptic transmission at single hippocampal synaptic boutons. Nature 375: 404–408.

Liu, Y., E. R. Chapman, and D. R. Storm (1991) Targeting of neuromodulin (GAP-43) fusion proteins to growth cones in cultured rat embryonic neurons. Neuron 6: 411–420.

Liuzzi, F. J., and R. J. Lasek (1987) Astrocytes block axonal regeneration in mammals by activating the physiological stop pathway. Science 237: 642–645.

Llano, I., A. Marty, J. W. Johnson, P. Ascher, and B. H. Gähwiler (1988) Patch-clamp recording of amino acid-activated responses in "organotypic" slice cultures. Proc. Natl. Acad. Sci. U.S.A. 85: 3221–3225.

Llano, I., B. H. Gähwiler, and A. Marty (1992) Voltage and transmitter gated channels in Purkinje cells from organotypic cerebellar cultures. In: *The Cerebellum Revisited*, R. Llinás and C. Sotelo, eds., pp. 182–200, Springer Verlag, New York.

Lo, D. C., A. K. McAllister, and L. C. Katz (1994) Neuronal transfection in brain slices using particle-mediated gene transfer. Neuron 13: 1263–1268.

Lo, M. M., M. K. Conrad, C. Mamalak, and M. J. Kadan (1988) Retroviral-mediated gene transfer Applications in neurobiology. Mol. Neurobiol. 2: 155–182.

Loeb, D. H., and L. A. Greene (1993) Transfection with trk restores "slow" NGF binding, efficient NGF uptake, and multiple NGF responses to NGF-nonresponsive PC12 cell mutants. J. Neurosci. 13: 2929–2929.

Loeb, D. M., J. Maragos, D. Martin-Zanca, M. V. Chao, L. F. Parada, and L. A. Green (1991) The trk proto-oncogene rescues NGF responsiveness in mutant NGF-responsive PC12 cell lines. Cell 66: 961–966.

Loeb, D. M., R. M. Stephens, T. Copeland, D. R. Kaplan, and L. A. Green (1994) A Trk NGF receptor point mutation affecting interaction with PLCg1 abolishes NGF-promoted peripherin induction, but not neurite outgrowth. J. Biol. Chem. 269: 8901–8910.

Loffner, F., S. M. Lohmann, B. Walckhoff, U. Walter, and B. Hamprecht (1986) Immuno-cytochemical characterization of neuron-rich primary cultures of embryonic rat brain cells by established neuronal and glial markers and by monospecific antisera against cyclic nucleotide-dependent protein kinases and the synaptic vesicle protein synapsin I. Brain Res. 363: 205–221.

Lohof, A. M. (1994) Regulation of Neurite Growth and Synaptic Activity by Neurotrophins. Doctoral dissertation, Columbia University, New York.

Lohof, A. M., M. Quillan, Y. Dan, and M-m. Poo (1992) Asymmetric modulation of cytosolic cAMP activity induces growth cone turning. J. Neurosci. 12: 1253–1261.

Lom, B., K. E. Healy, and P. E. Hockberger (1993) A versatile technique for patterning biomolecules onto glass coverslips. J. Neurosci. Methods 50: 385–397.

Long, J. A., and P. L. Burlingame (1938) The development of the external form of the rat with observations on the origin of the extraembryonic coelom and fetal membranes. Univ. Calif. Publ. Zool. 43: 143–184.

Lopez-Garcia, J. C., O. Arancio, E. R. Kandel, and D. Baranes (1996) A presynaptic locus for long-term potentiation of elementary synaptic transmission at mossy fiber synapses in culture. Proc. Natl. Acad. Sci. U.S.A. 93: 4712–4717.

Lopez-Lozano, J. J., M. F. Notter, D. M. Gash, and J. F. Leary (1989) Selective flow cytometric sorting of viable dopamine neurons. Brain Res. 486: 351–356.

Louis, J. C., E. Magal, S. Takayama, and S. Varon (1993) CNTF protection of oligodendrocytes against natural and tumor necrosis factor-induced death. Science 259: 689–692.

Louis, J. C., K. Langley, P. Anglard, M. Wolf, and G. Vincendon (1983) Long-term culture of neurones from human cerebral cortex in serum-free medium. Neurosci. Lett. 41: 313–319.

Lowenstein, P. R., S. Fournel, D. Bain, P. Tomasec, P. M. Clissold, M. G. Castro, and A. L. Epstein (1994a) Simultaneous detection of amplicon and HSV-1 helper encoded proteins reveals that neurons and astrocytoma cells do express amplicon-borne transgenes in the absence of synthesis of virus immediate early proteins. Mol. Brain Res. 30: 169–175.

Lowenstein, P. R., E. E. Morrison, D. Bain, P. Hodge, C. M. Preston, P. Clissold, N. D. Stow, T. A. McKee, and M. G. Castro (1994b) Use of recombinant vectors derived from herpes simplex virus 1 mutant tsK for short-term expression of transgenes encoding cytoplasmic and membrane anchored proteins in postmitotic polarized cortical neurons and glial cells in vitro. Neuroscience 60: 1059–1077.

Lu, B., and H. J. Federoff (1995) Herpes simplex virus type 1 amplicon vectors with glucocorticoid-inducible gene expression. Human Gene Therapy 6: 419–428.

Lu, B., M. Yokoyama, C. F. Dreyfus, and I. B. Black (1991) Depolarizing stimuli regulate nerve growth factor gene expression in cultured hippocampal neurons. Proc. Natl. Acad. Sci. U.S.A. 88: 6289–6292.

Lu, B., P. Greengard, and M-m. Poo (1992) Exogenous synapsin I promotes functional maturation of developing neuromuscular synapses. Neuron 8: 521–529.

Lucas, J. H., L. E. Czisny, and G. W. Gross (1986) Adhesion of cultured mammalian central nervous system neurons to flame-modified hydrophobic surfaces. In Vitro Cell. Dev. Biol. 22: 37–43.

Luduena, M. A. (1973) The growth of spinal ganglion neurons in serum-free medium. Dev. Biol. 33: 470–476.

Lukas, W., and K. A. Jones (1994) Cortical neurons containing calretinin are selectively resistant to calcium overload and excitotoxicity in vitro. Neuroscience 61: 307–316.

Lumsden, A. G., and A. M. Davies (1983) Earliest sensory nerve fibres are guided to peripheral targets by attractants other than nerve growth factor. Nature 306: 786–788.

Lumsden, A. G., and A. M. Davies (1986) Chemotropic effect of specific target epithelium in the developing mammalian nervous system. Nature 323: 538–539.

Lumsden, C. E. (1968) Nervous Tissue in Culture. In: *The Structure and Function of Nervous Tissue*, G. H. Bourne ed., pp 67–140, Academic Press, New York.

Luo Y., D. Raible, and J. A. Raper (1993) Collapsin: a protein in the brain that induces the collapse and paralysis of neuronal growth cones. Cell 75: 217–227.

MacLeish, P. R., C. J. Barnstable, and E. Townes-Anderson (1983) Use of a monoclonal antibody as a substrate for mature neurons in vitro. Proc. Natl. Acad. Sci. U.S.A. 80: 7014–7018.

MacPherson, P. A., and M. W. McBurney (1995) P19 embryonal carcinoma cells: a source of cultured neurons amenable to genetic manipulation. Methods Enzymol. 7: 222–237.

Maggi, R., F. Pimpinelli, L. Martini, and F. Piva (1995) Inhibition of luteinizing hormone-releasing hormone secretion by delta-opioid agonists in GT1-1 neuronal cells. Endocrinology 136: 5177–5181.

Magistretti, J., M. Decurtis, A. Vescovi, R. Galli, and A. Gritti (1996) Long-term survival of cortical neurones from adult guinea-pig maintained in low-density cultures. Neuroreport 7: 1559–1564.

Mahanthappa, N. K., and P. H. Patterson (1992a) Thy-1 involvement in neurite outgrowth: perturbation by antibodies, phospholipase C, and mutation. Dev. Biol. 150: 47–59.

Mahanthappa, N. K., and P. H. Patterson (1992b) Thy-1 multimerization is correlated with neurite outgrowth. Dev. Biol. 150: 60–71.

Mahanthappa, N. K., F. H. Gage, and P. H. Patterson (1990) Adrenal chromaffin cells as multipotential neurons for autografts. Prog. Brain Res. 82: 33–39.

Maiese, K., I. Boniece, D. DeMeo, and J. A. Wagner (1993) Peptide growth factors protect against ischemia in culture by preventing nitric oxide toxicity. J. Neurosci. 13: 3034–3040.

Mains, R. E., and P. H. Patterson (1973) Primary cultures of dissociated sympathetic neurons: I. Establishment of long-term growth in culture and studies of differentiated properties. J. Cell Biol. 59: 329–345.

Maisonpierre P. C., L. Belluscio, S. Squinto, N. Ip, M. Furth, R. Lindsay, and G. Yanco-poulos (1990) Neurotrophin-3: a neurotrophic factor related to NGF and BDNF. Science 247: 1446–1451.

Malenka, R. C. (1994) Synaptic plasticity in the hippocampus: LTP and LTD. Cell 78: 535–538.

Malenka, R. C., and R. A. Nicoll (1993) NMDA-receptor-dependent synaptic plasticity: multiple forms and mechanisms. Trends Neurosci. 16: 521–527.

Malgaroli, A., A. E. Ting, B. Wendland, A. Bergamaschi, A. Villa, R. W. Tsien, and R. H. Scheller (1995) Presynaptic component of long-term potentiation visualized at individual hippocampal synapses. Science 268: 1624–1628.

Mandell, J. W., and G. A. Banker (1996) A spatial gradient of tau protein phosphorylation in nascent axons. J. Neurosci. 16: 5727–5740.

Maniatis, T., E. F. Fritsch, and J. Sambrook (1982) *Molecular Cloning: A Laboratory Manual*, Cold Spring Harbor Laboratory, Cold Spring Harbor, NY.

Mann, R., R. C. Mulligan, and D. Baltimore (1983) Construction of a retrovirus packaging mutant and its use to produce helper-free defective retrovirus. Cell 33: 153–159.

Mansour, S. L., K. R. Thomas, C. Deng, and M. R. Capecchi (1990) Introduction of a lacz reporter gene into the mouse int-2 locus by homologous recombination. Proc. Natl. Acad. Sci. U.S.A. 87: 7688–7692.

Manthorpe, M., E. Engvall, E. Ruoslahti, F. M. Longo, G. E. Davis, and S. Varon (1983) Laminin promotes neuritic regeneration from cultured peripheral and central neurons. J. Cell Biol. 97: 1882–1890.

Manthorpe, M., R. Fagnani, S. D. Skaper, and S. Varon (1986a) An automated colorimetric microassay for neuronotrophic factors. Brain Res. 390: 191–198.

Manthorpe, M., S. D. Skaper, L. R. Williams, and S. Varon (1986b) Purification of adult rat sciatic nerve ciliary neuronotrophic factor. Brain Res. 367: 282–286.

Marangos, P. J., and D. E. Schmechel (1987) Neuron specific enolase, a clinically useful marker for neurons and neuroendocrine cells. Annu. Rev. Neurosci. 10: 269–295.

Marchand, R., and L. Lajoie (1986) Histogenesis of the striopallidal system in the rat. Neurogenesis of its neurons. Neuroscience 17: 573–590.

Marconi, P., D. Krisky, T. Oligino, P. L. Poliani, R. Ramakrishnan, W. F. Goins, D. J. Fink, and J. C. Glorioso (1996) Replication-defective herpes simplex virus vectors for gene transfer in vivo. Proc. Natl. Acad. Sci. U.S.A. 93: 11319–11320.

Marshall, C. J. (1995) Specificity of tyrosine receptor signaling: transient versus sustained extracellular signal-regulated kinase activation. Cell 80: 179–186.

Marshall, J., R. Molloy, G. W. Moss, J. R. Howe, and T. E. Hughes (1995) The jellyfish green fluorescent protein: a new tool for studying ion channel expression and function. Neuron 14: 211–215.

Martin, D. L., V. Madelian, and W. Shain (1989) Spontaneous and beta-adrenergic receptor-mediated taurine release from astroglial cells do not require extracellular calcium. J. Neurosci. Res. 23: 191–197.

Martin, D. P., R. E. Schmidt, P. S. DiStefano, O. H. Lowry, J. G. Carter and E. M. Johnson, Jr. (1988) Inhibitors of protein synthesis and RNA synthesis prevent neuronal death caused by nerve growth factor deprivation. J. Cell Biol. 106: 829–844.

Martin, F. C., and C. A. Wiley (1995) A serum-free, pyruvate-free medium that supports neonatal neural/glial cultures. J. Neurosci. Res. 41: 246–258.

Martin, G. R. (1981) Isolation of a pluripotent cell line from early mouse embryos cultured in medium conditioned by teratocarcinoma stem cells. Proc. Natl. Acad. Sci. U.S.A. 78: 7634–7638.

Martinou, I., P. A. Fernandez, M. Missotten, E. White, B. Allet, R. Sadoul, and J. C. Martinou (1995) Viral proteins E1B19K and p35 protect sympathetic neurons from cell death induced by NGF deprivation. J. Cell Biol. 128: 201–208.

Martinou, J. C., A. Le Van Thai, G. Cassar, F. Roubinet and M. J. Weber (1989). Characterization of two factors enhancing choline acetyltransferase activity in cultures of purified rat motoneurons. J. Neurosci. 9: 3645–3656.

Martinou, J. C., I. Martinou and A. C. Kato (1992) Cholinergic differentiation factor (CDF/LIF) promotes survival of isolated rat embryonic motoneurons in vitro. Neuron 8: 737–744.

Marusich, M. F., K. Pourmehr, and J. S. Weston (1986) The development of an identified subpopulation of avian sensory neurons is regulated by interaction with the periphery. Dev. Biol. 118: 505–510.

Mason, C. A. (1986) Afferent axon development in mouse cerebellum: embryonic axon forms and onset of expression of synapsin I. Neuroscience 19: 1319–1333.

Mason, C. A., and E. Gregory (1984) Postnatal maturation of cerebellar mossy and climbing fibers: transient expression of dual features on single axons. J. Neurosci. 4: 1715–1735.

Mason, C. A., J. C. Edmondson, and M. E. Hatten (1988) The extending astroglial process: development of glial cell shape, the growing tip, and interactions with neurons. J. Neurosci. 8: 3124–3134.

Mason, C. A., S. Christakos, and S. M. Catalano (1990) Early climbing fibers interactions with Purkinje cells in postnatal mouse cerebellum. J. Comp. Neurol. 297: 77–90.

Mathewson, A. J., and M. Berry (1985) Observations on the astrocyte response to a cerebral stab wound in adult rats. Brain Res. 327: 61–69.

Matsuzawa, M., R. S. Potember, D. A. Stenger, and V. Krauthamer (1993) Containment and growth of neuroblastoma cells on chemically patterned substrates. J. Neurosci. Methods 50: 253–260.

Matsuzawa, M., F. F. Weight, R. S. Potember, and P. Liesi (1996) Directional neurite outgrowth and axonal differentiation of embryonic hippocampal neurons are promoted by a neurite outgrowth domain of the B2-chain of laminin. Int. J. Dev. Neurosci. 14: 283–295.

Matthews, W. B., ed. (1991) *McAlpine's Multiple Sclerosis* (2nd ed.), Churchill Livingstone, London.

Mattson, M. P., and S. B. Kater (1989) Development and selective neurodegeneration in cell cultures from different hippocampal regions. Brain Res. 19(490): 110–125.

Mattson, M. P., and B. Rychlik (1990) Cell culture of cryopreserved human fetal cerebral cortical and hippocampal neurons: neuronal development and responses to trophic factors. Brain Res. 522: 204–214.

Mattson, M. P., R. E. Lee, M. E. Adams, P. B. Guthrie, and S. B. Kater (1988) Interactions between entorhinal axons and target hippocampal neurons: a role for glutamate in the development of hippocampal circuitry. Neuron 1: 865–876.

Mattson, M. P., B. Rychlik, and B. Cheng (1992) Degenerative and axon outgrowth—altering effects of phencyclidine in human fetal cerebral cortical cells. Neuropharmacology 31: 279–291.

Mattson, M. P., M. A. Lovell, K. Furukawa, and W. R. Markesbery (1995) Neurotrophic factors attenuate glutamate-induced accumulation of peroxides, elevation of intracellular Ca^{2+} concentration, and neurotoxicity and increase antioxidant enzyme activities in hippocampal neurons. J. Neurochem. 65: 1740–1751.

Matus, A., R. Bernhardt, R. Bodmer, and D. Alaimo (1986) Microtubule-associated protein 2 and tubulin are differently distributed in the dendrites of developing neurons. Neuroscience 17: 371–389.

Maue, R. A., R. Ventimiglia, P. E. Mather, R. M. Lindsay, and G. R. Franger (1995) Selective induction of Na channel gene expression in embryonic striatal neurons in vitro in response to BDNF, NT-3 and NT-4/5. Soc. Neurosci. Abstr. 21: 1051.

Maximow, A. (1925) Tissue cultures of young mammalian embryos. Contr. Embryol. Carnegie Inst. 16: 47–114.

Maxwell, G. D., M. E. Forbes, and D. S. Christie (1988) Analysis of the development of cellular subsets present in the neural crest using cell sorting and cell culture. Neuron 1: 557–568.

Mayer, M., and M. Noble (1992) The inhibition of oligodendrocytic differentiation of O-2A progenitors caused by basic fibroblast growth factor is overridden by astrocytes. Glia 8: 12–19.

Mayer, M., and M. Noble (1994) N-acetyl-L-cysteine is a pluripotent protector against cell death and enhancer of trophic-factor mediated cell survival in vitro. Proc. Natl. Acad. Sci. U.S.A. 91: 7496–7500.

Mayer, M., K. Bhakoo, and M. Noble (1994) Ciliary neurotrophic factor and leukemia inhibitory factor promote the generation, survival and maturation of oligodendrocytes in vitro. Development 120: 143–153.

Mayford, M., A. Barzilai, F. Keller, S. Schacher, and E. R. Kandel (1992) Modulation of an NCAM-related adhesion molecule with long-term synaptic plasticity in *Aplysia*. Science 256: 638–644.

McAllister, A. K., D. C. Lo, and L. C. Katz (1995) Neurotrophins regulate dendritic growth in developing visual cortex. Neuron 15: 791–803.

McBurney, M. W., and B. J. Rogers (1982) Isolation of male embryonal carcinoma cells and their chromosome replication patterns. Dev. Biol. 89: 503–508.

McBurney, M. W., E. M. Jones-Villeneuve, M. K. Edwards, and P. J. Anderson (1982) Control of muscle and neuronal differentiation in a cultured embryonal carcinoma cell line. Nature 299: 165–167.

McBurney, M. W., K. R. Reuhl, A. I. Ally, S. Nasipuri, J. C. Bell, and J. Craig (1988) Differentiation and maturation of embryonal carcinoma-derived neurons in culture. J. Neurosci. 8: 1063–1073.

McCaffery, C. A., T. R. Raju, and M. R. Bennett (1984) Effects of cultured astroglia on the survival of neonatal rat retinal ganglion cells in vitro. Dev. Biol. 104: 441–448.

McCarthy, K., and J. deVellis (1980) Preparation of separate astroglial and oligodendroglial cell cultures from rat cerebral tissue. J. Cell. Biol. 85: 890–902.

McCarthy, K. D., and L. M. Partlow (1976) Neuronal stimulation of (^{3}H)thymidine incorporation by primary cultures of highly purified non-neuronal cells. Brain Res. 114: 415–426.

McCormick, D. A., and D. A. Prince (1987) Acetylcholine causes a rapid nicotinic exitation in the medial habenula nucleus of guinea-pig, in vitro. J. Neurosci. 7: 742–752.

McCormick, D. A., B. W. Connors, J. W. Lighthall, and D. A. Prince (1985) Comparative electrophysiology of pyramidal and sparsely spiny neurons of the neocortex. J. Neurophysiol. 54: 782–806.

McGrory, W. J., D. S. Bautista, and F. L. Graham (1988) A simple technique for the rescue of early region 1 mutations into infectious human adenovirus type 5. Virology 163: 614–617.

McKeehan, W. L., W. G. Hamilton, and R. G. Ham (1976) Selenium is an essential trace nutrient for growth of WI-38 diploid human fibroblasts. Proc. Natl. Acad. Sci. U.S.A. 73: 2023–2027.

McKenna, N. M., and Y. L. Wang (1989) Culturing cells on the microscope stage. Methods Cell Biol. 29: 195–205.

McKiernan, C. J., P. F. Stabila, and I. G. Macara (1996) Role of the Rab3A-binding domain in targeting of rabphilin-3A to vesicle membranes of PC12 cells. Mol. Cell. Biol. 16: 4985–4995.

McKinnon, R. D., T. Matsui, M. Dubois-Dalcq, and S. A. Aaronson (1990) FGF modulates the PDGF-driven pathway of oligodendrocyte development. Neuron 5: 603–614.

McNaughton, B. L. (1993) The mechanism of expression of long-term enhancement of hippocampal synapses: current issues and theoretical implications. Annu. Rev. Physiol. 55: 375–396.

Mehler, M. F., R. Marmur, R. Gross, P. C. Mabie, Z. Zhang, A. Papavasiliou, J. E. Kessler (1995) Cytokines regulate the cellular phenotype of developing neural lineage species. Int. J. Dev. Neurosci. 13: 213–240.

Meister, A., and M. E. Anderson (1983) Glutathione. Annu Rev. Biochem. 52: 711–760.

Meister, A., M. E. Anderson, and O. Hwang (1986) Intracellular cysteine and glutathione delivery systems. J. Am. Coll. Nutr. 5: 137–151.

Meldrum, B., and J. Garthwaite (1990) Excitatory amino acid toxicity and neuro-degenerative disease. Trends Pharmacol. Sci. 11: 179–387.

Mellon, P. L., J. J. Windle, P. C. Goldsmith, C. A. Padula, J. L. Roberts and R. I. Weiner (1990) Immortalization of hypothalamic GnRH neurons by genetically targeted tu-morigenesis. Neuron 5: 1–10.

Mennerick, S., J. Que, A. Benz, and C. F. Zorumski (1995) Passive and synaptic properties of hippocampal neurons grown in microcultures and in mass cultures. J. Neuro-physiol. 73: 320–332.

Merrill, J. E. (1991) Effects of interleukin-1 and tumor necrosis factor-a on astrocytes, microglia, oligodendrocytes and glial precursors in vitro. Dev. Neurosci. 13: 130–137.

Merrill, J. E., and G. M. Jonakait (1995) Interactions of the nervous and immune systems in development, normal brain homeostasis, and disease. FASEB J. 9: 611–618.

Merz, D. C., and P. Drapeau (1994) Segmental specificity of neuronal recognition during synapse formation between identified leech neurons. J. Neurosci. 14: 4125–4129.

Messer, A. (1981) Primary monolayer cultures of the rat corpus striatum: morphology and properties related to acetylcholine and gamma-aminobutyrate. Neuroscience 6: 2677–2687.

Messer, A., and D. M. Smith (1977) In vitro behavior of granule cells from Staggerer and Weaver mutants of mice. Brain Res. 130: 13–23.

Messer, A., G. L. Snodgrass, and P. Maskin (1984) Enhanced survival of cultured cerebellar Purkinje cells by plating on antibody to Thy-1. Cell. Mol. Neurobiol. 4: 285–290.

Mettling, C., A. Gouin, M. Robinson, et al. (1995) Survival of newly postmitotic moto-neurons is transiently independent of exogenous trophic support. J. Neurosci. 15: 3128–3137.

Meyer-Franke, A., M. R. Kaplan, F. W. Pfrieger, and B. A. Barres (1995) Characterization of the signaling interactions that promote the survival and growth of developing retinal ganglion cells in culture. Neuron 15: 805–819.

Miale, I., and R. L. Sidman (1961) An autoradiographic analysis of histogenesis in the mouse cerebellum. Expl. Neurol. 4: 277–296.

Mihm, S., J. Ennen, U. Pessara, R. Kurth, and W. Droge (1991) Inhibition of HIV-1 repli-cation and NF-kappaB activity by cysteine and cysteine derivatives. AIDS 5: 497–503.

Milbrandt, J. (1987) A nerve growth factor-induced gene encodes a possible transcrip-tional regulatory factor. Science 238: 797–799.

Miller, A. D., and C. Buttimore (1986) Redesign of retrovirus packaging cell lines to avoid recombination leading to helper virus production. Mol. Cell. Biol. 6: 2895–2902.

Miller, A. D., and G. J. Rosman (1989) Improved retroviral vectors for gene transfer and expression. Biotechniques 7: 980–990.

Miller, R. H., S. David, E. R. Patel, and M. C. Raff (1985) A quantitative immunohisto-chemical study of macroglial cell development in the rat optic nerve: in vivo evidence for two distinct astrocyte lineages. Dev. Biol. 111: 35–43.

Miller, R. H., E. R. Abney, S. David, C. Ffrench-Constant, R. Lindsay, R. Patel, J. Stone, and M. C. Raff (1986) Is reactive gliosis a property of a distinct subpopulation of astro-cytes? J. Neurosci. 6: 22–29.

Mirsky, R., L. M. Wendon, P. Black, C. Stolkin, and D. Bray (1978) Tetanus toxin: a cell surface marker for neurons in culture. Brain Res. 148: 251–259.

Mithen, F. A., M. Cochran, M. I. Johnson, and R. P. Bunge (1980) Neurotoxicity of poly-styrene containers detected in a closed tissue culture system. Neurosci. Lett. 17: 107–111.

Mithen, F. A., H. C. Agrawal, E. H. Eylar, M. A. Fishman, W. Blank, and R. P. Bunge (1982) Studies with antisera against peripheral nervous system myelin and myelin basic proteins: I. Effects of antiserum upon living cultures of nervous tissue. Brain Res. 250: 321–331.

Miyashiro, K., M. Dichter, and J. Eberwine (1994) On the nature and differential distribution of mRNAs in hippocampal neurites: implications for neuronal functioning. Proc. Natl. Acad. Sci. U.S.A. 91: 10800–10804.

Montarolo, P. G., P. Goelet, V. F. Castellucci, J. Morgan, E. R. Kandel, and S. Schacher (1986) A critical period of macromolecular synthesis in long-term heterosynaptic facilitation in *Aplysia*. Science 234: 1249–1254.

Montarolo, P. G., E. R. Kandel, S. Schacher (1988) Long-term heterosynaptic inhibition in *Aplysia*. Nature 333: 171–174.

Moore, M. W., R. D. Klein, I. Farinas, et al. (1996) Renal and neuronal abnormalities in mice lacking GDNF. Nature 382: 76–79.

Moreira, J. E., T. S. Reese, and B. Kachar (1996) Freeze-substitution as a preparative technique for immunoelectronmicroscopy: evaluation by atomic force microscopy. Microsc. Res. Tech. 33: 251–261.

Morimoto, T., X. Wang, and M-m. Poo (1998) Overexpression of synaptotagmin modulate short-term synaptic plasticity at developing neuromuscular synapses. Neuroscience 82: 969–978.

Moriyoshi, K., L. J. Richards, C. Akazawa, D. D. O'Leary, and S. Nakanishi (1996) Labeling neural cells using adenoviral gene transfer of membrane-targeted GFP. Neuron 16: 255–260.

Morrison, M. E., and C. A. Mason (1998) Granule neuron regulation of Purkinje cell development: striking a balance between neurotrophin and glutamate signalling. under revision

Morrissey, T. K., N. Kleitman, and R. P. Bunge (1991) Isolation and functional characterization of Schwann cells derived from adult peripheral nerves. J. Neurosci. 11: 2433–2442.

Morrissey, T. K., R. P. Bunge, and N. Kleitman (1995a) Human Schwann cells in vitro: I. Failure to differentiate and support neuronal health under coculture conditions that promote full function of rodent cells. J. Neurobiol. 28: 171–189.

Morrissey, T. K., N. Kleitman, and R. P. Bunge (1995b) Human Schwann cells in vitro: II. Myelination of sensory axons following extensive purification and heregulin-induced expansion. J. Neurobiol. 28: 190–201.

Mortensen, R. M., M. Zubiaur, E. J. Neer, and J. G. Seidman (1991) Embryonic stem cells lacking a functional inhibitory G-protein subunit (alpha i2) produced by gene targeting of both alleles. Proc. Natl. Acad. Sci. U.S.A. 88: 7036–7040.

Moscona, A. A. (1965) Recombination of dissociated cells and the development of cell aggregates. In: *The Biology of Cells and Tissues in Culture*, vol. 1, E. N. Willmer, ed., pp. 489–529, Academic Press, New York.

Mosmann, T. (1983) Rapid colorimetric assay for cellular growth and survival: application to proliferation and cytotoxicity assays. J. Immunol. Methods 65: 55–63.

Mouginot, D., and B. H. Gähwiler (1994) Characterization of synaptic connections between cortex and deep nuclei of the rat cerebellum in vitro. Neuroscience 64: 699–712.

Moya, F., M. B. Bunge, and R. P. Bunge (1980) Schwann cells proliferate but fail to differentiate in defined medium. Proc. Natl. Acad. Sci. U.S.A. 77: 6902–6906.

Mulle C., and J. P. Changeux (1990) A novel type of nicotinic receptor in the rat central nervous system characterized by patch clamp techniques. J. Neurosci. 10: 169–175.

Mulle C., D. Choquet, H. Korn, and J. P. Changeux (1992) Calcium influx through nicotinic receptor in rat neurons: its relevance to cellular regulation. Neuron 8: 135–143.

Muller S. R., P. D. Sullivan, D. O. Clegg, and S. C. Feinstein (1990) Efficient transfection and expression of heterologous genes in PC12 cells. DNA Cell Biol. 9: 221–229.

Munir, M., L. Lu, Y. H. Wang, et al. (1996) Pharmacological and immunological characterization of N-methyl-D-aspartate receptors in human NT2-N neurons. J. Pharmaol. Exp. Ther. 276: 819–828.

Muñoz-Blay, T., C. V. Benedict, P. T. Picciano, and S. Cohen (1987) Substrate requirements for the isolation and purification of thymic epithelial cells. J. Exp. Pathol. 3: 251–258.

Murphy, G. G., and D. L. Glanzman (1996) Enhancement of sensorimotor connections by conditioning-related stimulation in Aplysia depends upon postsynaptic Ca^{2+}. Proceedings of the National Academy of Sciences of the United States of America 93: 9931–9936.

Murray, M. R. (1965) Nervous tissues in vitro. In: *Cells and Tissues in Culture: Methods, Biology and Physiology*, vol. 2, E. N. Willmer, ed., pp. 373–455. Academic, New York.

Muzyczka, N. (1992) Use of adeno-associated virus as a general transduction vector for mammalian cells. Curr. Topics Microbiol. Immunol. 158: 97–129.

Nakai, J. (1956) Dissociated dorsal root ganglia in tissue culture. Am. J. Anat. 99: 81–130.

Nakai, J. (1960) Studies on the mechanism determining the course of nerve fibers in tissue culture. II. The mechanism of fasciculation. Z. Zellforsch. Mikrosk. Anat. 52: 427–449.

Nakai. J., and Y. Kawasaki (1959) Studies on the mechanism determining the course of nerve fibers in tissue culture: 1. The reaction of the growth cone to various obstructions. Zeit. Zellforsch. 51: 108–122.

Naldini, L., U. Blömer, P. Gallay, D. Ory, R. Mulligan, F. H. Gage, I. M. Verma, and D. Trono (1996) In vivo gene delivery and stable transduction of nondividing cells by a lentiviral vector. Science 272: 263–267.

Neale, E. A., R. L. MacDonald, and P. G. Nelson (1978) Intracelluar horseradish peroxidase injection for correlation of light and electron microscopic anatomy and synaptic physiology of cultured mouse spinal cord neurons. Brain Res. 152: 265–282.

Neale, E. A., W. H. Oertel, L. M. Bowers, and V. K. Weise (1983) Glutamate decarboxylase immunoreactivity and gamma-[^{3}H] aminobutyric acid accumulation within the same neurons in dissociated cell cultures of cerebral cortex. J. Neurosci. 3: 376–382.

Neely, M. D., and M. Gesemann (1994) Disruption of microfilaments in growth cones following depolarization and calcium influx. J. Neurosci. 14: 7511–7520.

Nef, P., C. Oneyser, C. Alliod, S. Couturier, and M. Balliuet (1988) Genes expressed in the brain define three distinct neuronal nicotinic acetylcholine receptors. EMBO J. 7: 595–601.

Nelson, P. G. (1975) Nerve and muscle cells in culture. Physiol. Rev. 55: 1–11.

Nelson, P. G., R. D. Fields, C. Yu, and Y. Liu (1993) Synapse elimination from the mouse neuromuscular junction in vitro: a non-Hebbian activity-dependent process. J. Neurobiol. 24: 1517–1530.

Niehrs, C., R. Keller, K. W. Y. Cho, and E. M. De Robertis (1993) The homeobox gene goosecoid controls cell migration in *Xenopus* embryos. Cell 72: 491–503.

Nieminen, K., B. A. Suarez-Isla, and S. I. Rapoport (1988) Electrical properties of cultured dorsal root ganglion neurons from normal and trisomy 21 human fetal tissue. Brain Res. 474: 246–254.

Nieuwkoop, P. D., and J. Faber (1967) *Normal Table of Xenopus laevis* (Daudin), North Holland, Amsterdam.

Niijima, K., G. R. Chalmers, D. A. Peterson, L. J. Fisher, P. H. Patterson, and F. H. Gage (1995) Enhanced survival and neuronal differentiation of adrenal chromaffin cells co-grafted into the striatum with NGF-producing fibroblasts. J. Neurosci. 15: 1180–1194.

Nikolic, M., H. Dudek, Y. T. Kwon, Y. F. M. Ramos, and L. T. Tsai (1996) The cdk5/p35 kinase is essential for neurite outgrowth during neuronal differentiation. Genes Dev. 10: 816–825.

Nishi, R. (1994a) Neurotrophic factors: two are better than one. Science 19 (265): 1052–1053.

Nishi, R. (1994b) Target-derived molecules that influence the development of neurons in the avian ciliary ganglion. J. Neurobiol. 25: 612–619.

Nishi, R., and D. K. Berg (1981) Two components from eye tissue that differentially stimulate the growth and development of ciliary ganglion neurons in cell cultures. J. Neurosci. 1: 505–513.

Noakes, P. G., M. Gautam, J. Mudd, J. R. Sanes, and J. P. Merlie (1995) Aberrant differentiation of neuromuscular junctions in mice lacking s-laminin/laminin beta 2. Nature 374: 258–262.

Noble, M., and K. Murray (1984) Purified astrocytes promote the division of a bipotential glial progenitor cell. EMBO J. 3: 2243–2247.

Noble, M., J. Fok-Seang, and J. Cohen (1984) Glia are a unique substrate for the in vitro growth of central nervous system neurons. J. Neurosci. 4: 1892–1903.

Noble, M., K. Murray, P. Stroobant, M. D. Waterfield, and P. Riddle (1988) Platelet-derived growth factor promotes division and motility, and inhibits premature differentiation, of the oligodendrocyte- type-2 astrocyte progenitor cell. Nature 333: 560–562.

Noda M., K. Minoru, A. Ogura, D. Liu, T. Amano, T. Takano and Y. Ikawa (1985) Sarcoma viruses carrying *ras* oncogenes induce differentiation-associated properties in a neuronal cell line. Nature 318: 73–75.

Northrup, J. K., P. C. Sternweiss, M. D. Smigel, et al. (1980) Purification of the regulatory component of adenylate cyclase. Proc. Natl. Acad. Sci. U.S.A. 77: 6516–6520.

Novelli, A., J. A. Reilly, P. G. Lysko, and R. C. Henneberry (1988) Glutamate becomes neurotoxic via the *N*-methyl-D-aspartate receptor when intracellular energy levels are reduced. Brain Res. 451: 205–212.

Nowakowski, R., and P. Rakic (1979) The mode of migration of neurons to the hippocampus. A Golgi and electron microscope analysis in foetal rhesus monkey. J. Neurocytol. 8: 697–718.

Nowycky, M. (1992) Voltage-gated ion channels in dorsal root ganglion neurons. In: *Sensory Neurons: Diversity, Development, and Plasticity*, S. A. Scott, ed., pp. 97–115, Oxford University, New York.

Nye, J. E., R. Kopan, and R. Axel (1994) An activated notch suppresses neurogenesis and myogenesis but not gliogenesis in mammalian cells. Development 120: 2421–2430.

O'Brien R. J., and G. D. Fischbach (1986a). Excitatory synaptic transmission between interneurons and motoneurons in chick spinal cord cell cultures. J. Neurosci. 6: 3284–3289.

O'Brien, R. J., and G. D. Fischbach (1986b) Isolation of embryonic chick motoneurons and their survival in vitro. J. Neurosci. 6: 3265–3274.

O'Brien, R. J., and G. D. Fischbach (1986c) Modulation of embryonic chick motoneuron glutamate sensitivity by interneurons and agonists. J. Neurosci. 6: 3290–3296.

Obremski, V. J., and M. B. Bunge (1995) Addition of purified basal lamina molecules enables Schwann cell ensheathment of sympathetic neurites in culture. Dev. Biol. 168: 124–137.

Obremski, V. J., M. I. Johnson, and M. B. Bunge (1993a) Fibroblasts are required for Schwann cell basal lamina deposition and ensheathment of unmyelinated sympathetic neurites in culture. J. Neurocytol. 22: 102–117.

Obremski, V. J., P. M. Wood, and M. B. Bunge (1993b) Fibroblasts promote Schwann cell basal lamina deposition and elongation in the absence of neurons in culture. Dev. Biol. 160: 119–134.

O'Connor, T., J. Duerr, and E. Bentley (1990) Pioneer growth cone steering decisions mediated by single filopodial contacts in situ. J. Neurosci. 10: 3935–3946.

O'Donnell-Tormey, J., C. F. Nathan, K. Lanks, C. J. DeBoer and J. De La Harpe (1987) Secretion of pyruvate. An antioxidant defense of mammalian cells. J. Exp. Med. 165: 500–514.

O'Dowd, D. K. (1995) Voltage-gated currents and firing properties of embryonic *Drosophila* neurons grown in a chemically defined medium. J. Neurobiol. 7: 113–126.

O'Dowd, D. K., and R. W. Aldrich (1988) Voltage-clamp analysis of sodium channels in wild-type and mutant *Drosophila* neurons. J. Neurosci. 8: 3633–3643.

O'Dowd, D. K., J. R. Gee, and M. A. Smith (1995) Sodium current density correlates with expression of specific alternatively spliced sodium channel mRNAs in single neurons. J. Neurosci. 15: 4005–4012.

Oh, T. H., and G. J. Markelonis (1982) Chicken serum transferrin duplicates the myotrophic effects of sciatin on cultured muscle cells. J. Neurosci. Res. 8: 535–545.

Oka, A., M. J. Belliveau, P. A. Rosenberg, and J. J. Volpe (1993) Vulnerability of oligodendroglia to glutamate: pharmacology, mechanism and prevention. J. Neurosci. 13: 1441–1453.

Okabe, S., K. Forsberg-Nilsson, C. A. Spiro, M. Segal, and R. D. G. McKay (1996) Development of neuronal precursor cells and functional postmitotic neurons from embryonic stem cells in vitro. Mech. Dev. 59: 89–102.

Okun, L. M. (1981) Identification and isolation in vitro of neurons marked in situ by retrograde transport. In: *New Approaches in Developmental Neurobiology*, pp. 109–121, Society for Neuroscience, Bethesda, MD.

Olkkonen, V. M., P. Liljeström, P. Dupree, H. Garoff, and K. Simons (1994) Expression of exogenous proteins in mammalian cells with the semliki forest virus vector. Methods Cell Biol. 43: 43–53.

Olsen, C., and R. P. Bunge (1986) Requisites for growth and myelination of urodele sensory neurons in tissue culture. J. Exp. Zool. 238: 373–384.

O'Malley, M. B., and P. R. MacLeish (1993) Monoclonal antibody substrates facilitate long-term regenerative growth of adult primate retinal neurons. J. Neurosci. Methods 47: 61–71.

Oppenheim, R. W. (1996) Neurotrophic survival molecules for motorneurons: an embarrassment of riches. Neuron 17: 195–197.

Orgel, L. E. (1973) Aging of clones of mammalian cells [review]. Nature 243: 441–445.

Orr, D. J., and R. A. Smith (1988) Neuronal maintenance and neurite extension of adult mouse neurones in non-neuronal cell-reduced cultures is dependent on substratum coating. J. Cell Sci. 91: 555–561.

Osborn, M., and K. Weber (1982) Immunofluorescence and immunocytochemical procedures with affinity purified antibodies: tubulin-containing structures. Methods Cell Biol. 24: 97–132.

Osborne, N. N., and D. W. Beaton (1985) Occurrence of serotonin-accumulating neurones in cultures of retina from the human foetus. Neurosci. Lett. 55: 229–232.

Østergaard, K. (1993) Organotypic slice cultures of rat striatum-I. A histochemical and immunocytochemical study of acetylcholinesterase, choline acetyltransferase, glutamate decarboxylase and GABA. Neuroscience 53: 679–693.

Othberg, A., P. Odin, A. Ballagi, A. Ahgren, K. Funa, and O. Lindvall (1995) Specific effects of platelet derived growth factor (PDGF) on fetal rat and human dopaminergic neurons in vitro. Exp. Brain Res. 105: 111–122.

Otte, A. P., P. L. McGrew, J. Olate, N. M. Nathanson, and R. T. Moon (1992) Expression and potential functions of G-protein subunits in embryos of *Xenopus laevis*. Development 116: 141–146.

Owens, G. C., and R. P. Bunge (1989) Evidence for an early role for myelin-associated glycoprotein in the process of myelination. Glia 2: 119–128.

Ozaki, M., K. Matsumura, S. Kaneko, M. Satoh, Y. Watanabe, and T. Aoyama (1993) A vaccinia virus vector for efficiently introducing into hippocampal slices. Biochem. Biophys. Res. Commun. 193: 653–660.

Pagano, R. E. (1989) A fluorescent derivative of ceramide: physical properties and use in studying the Golgi apparatus of animal cells. Methods Cell Biol. 29: 75–85.

Palay, S. F., and V. Chan-Palay (1974) *Cerebellar Cortex, Cytology and Organization*, Springer-Verlag, Berlin.

Papa, M., and M. Segal (1996) Morphological plasticity in dendritic spines of cultured hippocampal neurons. Neuroscience 71: 1005–1011.

Paquet, L., B. Massie, and R. E. Mains (1996) Proneuropeptide Y processing in large dense core vesicles: manipulation of prohormone convertase expression in sympathetic neurons using adenoviruses. J. Neurosci. 16: 964–973.

Paramore, C. G., D. A. Turner, and R. D. Madison (1992) Fluorescent labeling of dissociated fetal cells for tissue culture. J. Neurosci. Methods 44: 7–17.

Patel, A. J., P. Seaton, and A. Hunt (1988) A novel way of removing quiescent astrocytes in a culture of subcortical neurons grown in a chemically defined medium. Brain Res. 470: 283–288.

Patel, M. N., and J. O. McNamara (1995) Selective enhancement of axonal branching of cultured dentate gyrus neurons by neurotrophic factors. Neuroscience 69: 763–770.

Paterson, T., and R. D. Everett (1990) A prominent serine-rich region in Vmw175, the major regulatory protein of herpes simplex virus type 1 is not essential for virus growth in tissue culture. J. Gen. Virol. 71: 1775–1783.

Patterson, M. K., Jr. (1979) Measurement of growth and viability of cells in culture. Methods Enzymol. 58: 141–152.

Patterson, P. H. (1978) Environmental determination of autonomic neurotransmitter functions. Annu. Rev. Neurosci. 1: 1–17.

Patterson, P. H. (1990) Control of cell fate in a vertebrate neurogenic lineage. Cell 62: 1035–1038.

Patterson, P. H., and H. Nawa (1993) Neuronal differentiation factors/cytokines and synaptic plasticity. Cell 72 (suppl.): 123–137.

Patterson, P. H., L. F. Reichardt, and L. L. Y. Chun (1975) Biochemical studies on the development of primary sympathetic neurons in cell culture. Cold Spring Harb. Symp. Quant. Biol. 40: 389–397.

Patterson, S. L., L. M. Grover, P. A. Schwartzkroin, and M. Bothwell (1992) Neurotrophin expression in rat hippocampal slices: a stimulus paradigm inducing LTP in CA1 evokes increases in BDNF and NT-3 mRNAs. Neuron 9: 1081–1088.

Paul, J. (1965) *Cell and Tissue Culture*, Williams and Wilkins, Baltimore.

Payne, H. R., S. M. Burden, and V. Lemmon (1992) Modulation of growth cone morphology by substrate-bound adhesion molecules. Cell Motil. Cytoskeleton 21: 65–73.

Peacock, J. H., D. F. Rush, and L. H. Mathers (1979) Morphology of dissociated hippocampal cultures from fetal mice. Brain Res. 169: 231–246.

Pear, W. S., M. L. Scott, and G. P. Nolan (1996) Generations of High titer, helper-free retroviruses by transient transfection. In: *Methods in Molecular Medicine: Gene Therapy Protocols*, P. Robbins, ed.

Pear, W. S., G. P. Nolan, M. L. Scott, and D. Baltimore (1993) Production of high-titer helper-free retroviruses by transient transfection. Proc. Natl. Acad. Sci. U.S.A. 90: 8392–8396.

Penfold, M. E., P. Armati, and A. L. Cunningham (1994) Axonal transport of herpes simplex virions to epidermal cells: evidence for a specialized mode of virus transport and assembly. Proc. Natl. Acad. Sci. U.S.A. 91: 6529–6533.

Peng, H. B., L. P. Baker, and Q. Chen (1991) Tissue culture of *Xenopus* neurons and muscle cells as a model for studying synaptic induction. In: *Methods in Cell Biology*, vol. 36, B. K. Kay and H. B. Peng, eds., p. 511, Academic Press, New York.

Peng, H. B., P. C. Bridgman, S. Nakajiima, A. Greenberg, and Y. Nakajima (1979) A fast development of presynaptic function and structure of the neuromuscular junction in *Xenopus* tissue culture. Brain Res. 361: 200–211.

Peter, N., B. Aronoff, F. Wu, and S. Schacher (1994) Decrease in growth cone–neurite fasciculation by sensory or motor cells in vitro accompanies downregulation of *Aplysia* cell adhesion molecules by neurotransmitters. J. Neurosci. 14: 1413–1421.

Peterson, E. R., and M. R. Murray (1955) Myelin sheath formation of avian spinal ganglia. Am. J. Anat. 96: 319.

Peterson, E. R., and M. R. Murray (1960) Modification of development in isolated dorsal root ganglia by nutritional and physical factors. Dev. Biol. 21: 461–476.

Peterson, E. R., and M. R. Murray (1965) Patterns of peripheral demyelination in culture. Ann. N. Y. Acad. Sci. 122: 39–50.

Petite, D., and M. C. Calvet (1995) Cryopreserved neuronal cells in long-term cultures of dissociated rat cerebral cortex: survival and morphometric characteristics as revealed by immunocytochemistry. Brain Research 669: 263–274.

Petroski, R. E., and H. M. Geller (1994) Selective labeling of embryonic neurons cultured on astrocyte monolayers with 5(6)-carboxyfluorescein diacetate (CFDA). J. Neurosci. Methods 52: 23–32.

Pettit, D. L., S. Perlman, and R. Malinow (1994) Potentiated transmission and prevention of further LTP by increased CaMKII activity in postsynaptic hippocampal slice neurons. Science 266: 1881–1885.

Pettit, D. L., T. Koothan, D. Liao, and R. Malinow (1995) Vaccinia virus transfection of hippocampal slice neurons. Neuron 14: 685–688.

Pfeiffer, S. W., B. Betschart, J. Cook, P. Mancini, and R. Morris (1977) Glial cell lines. In: *Cell, Tissue, and Organ Cultures in Neurobiology*, S. Federoff and L. Hertz, eds., pp. 287–346, Academic Press, New York.

Phillips, H. J. (1973) Dye exclusion tests for cell viability. In: *Tissue Culture: Methods and Applications*, P. F. Kruse and M. K. Patterson, eds., pp. 406–408, Academic Press, New York.

Pincus, D. W., E. M. DiCicco-Bloom, and I. B. Black (1990) Vasoactive intestinal peptide regulates mitosis, differentiation and survival of cultured sympathetic neuroblasts. Nature 343: 564–567.

Pittman, R. N. (1985) Release of plasminogen activator and a calcium-dependent metalloprotease from cultured sympathetic and sensory neurons. Dev. Biol. 110: 91–101.

Pittman, R. N., and H. M. Buettner (1989) Degradation of extracellular matrix by neuronal proteases. Dev. Neurosci. 11: 361–375.

Pittman R. N., S. Wang, A. J. DiBenedetto, and J. Mills (1993) A system for characterizing cellular and molecular events in programmed neuronal cell death. J. Neurosci. 13: 3669–3680.

Platika, D., M. H. Boulos, L. Baizer, and M. C. Fishman (1985) Neuronal traits of clonal cell lines derived by fusion of dorsal root ganglia neurons with neuroblastoma cells. Proc. Natl. Acad. Sci. U.S.A. 82: 3499–3503.

Pleasure, S. J., C. Page, and V. M. Lee (1992) Pure, postmitotic, polarized human neurons derived from NTera 2 cells provide a system for expressing exogenous proteins in terminally differentiated neurons. J. Neurosci. 12: 1802–1815.

Podulso, S., and W. Norton (1972) Isolation and some chemical properties of oligodendroglia from calf brain. J. Neurochem. 19: 727–736.

Poltorak, M., M. Isono, W. J. Freed, G. V. Ronnett, and S. H. Snyder (1992) Human cortical neuronal cell line (HCN-1): further in vitro characterization and suitability for brain transplantation. Cell Transplantation 1: 3–15.

Pomerat, C. M., and I. Costero (1956) Tissue culture of cat cerebellum. Am. J. Anat. 99: 211–248.

Pomerat, C. M., W. J. Hendelman, and C. W. Raiborn (1967) Dynamic activities of nervous tissue in vitro. In: *The Neuron*, H. Hyden, ed., pp. 119–173, Elsevier, New York.

Pontén, J., and L. Stolt (1980) Proliferation control in cloned normal and malignant human cells. Exp. Cell Res. 129: 367–375.

Porter, S., L. Glaser, and R. P. Bunge (1987) Release of autocrine growth factor by primary and immortalized Schwann cells. Proc. Natl. Acad. Sci. U.S.A. 83: 7768–7771.

Porter, S., M. B. Clark, L. Glaser, and R. P. Bunge (1986) Schwann cells stimulated to proliferate in the absence of neurons retain full functional capability. J. Neurosci. 6: 3070–3078.

Posse, D. C., D. E. Vance, R. B. Campenot, and J. E. Vance (1995) Axonal synthesis of phosphaticylcholine is required for axonal growth in rat sympathetic neurons. J. Cell. Biol. 128: 913–918.

Powell, S. K., R. J. Rivas, E. Rodriguez-Boulan, and M. E. Hatten (1997) Development of polarity in cerebellar granule neurons. J. Neurobiol. 32: 223–236.

Price, J., and R. O. Hynes (1985) Astrocytes in culture synthesize and secrete a variant form of fibronectin. J. Neurosci. 5: 2205–2211.

Pringle, N., E. J. Collarini, M. J. Mosley, et al. (1989) DGF A chain homodimers drive proliferation of bipotential (O-2A) glial progenitor cells in the developing rat optic nerve. EMBO J. 8: 1049–1056.

Privat, A., and M. J. Drian (1976) Postnatal maturation of rat Purkinje cells cultivated in the absence of two afferent systems: an ultrastructural study. J. Comp. Neurol. 166: 201–244.

Raff, M. C. (1989) Glial cell diversification in the rat optic nerve. Science 243: 1450–1455.

Raff, M. C. (1992) Social controls on cell survival and cell death. Nature 356: 397–400.

Raff, M. C., K. L. Fields, S. I. Hakomori, R. Mirsky, R. M. Pruss and J. Winter (1979) Cell-type-specific markers for distinguishing and studying neurons and the major classes of glial cells in culture. Brain Res. 174: 283–308.

Raff, M. C., E. R. Abney, J. Cohen, C. Lindsay and M. Noble (1983a) Two types of astrocytes in cultures of developing rat white matter: differences in morphology, surface properties and growth characteristics. J. Neurosci. 3: 1289–1300.

Raff, M. C., R. H. Miller, and M. Noble (1983b) A glial progenitor cell that develops in vitro into an astrocyte or an oligodendrocyte depending on the culture medium. Nature 303: 390–396.

Raff, M. C., R. H. Miller, and M. Noble (1983c) Glial cell lineages in the rat optic nerve. Cold Spring Harb. Symp. Quant. Biol. 48: 569–572.

Raff, M. C., E. R. Abney, and J. Fok-Seang (1985) Reconstitution of a developmental clock in vitro: a critical role for astrocytes in the timing of oligodendrocyte differentiation. Cell 42: 61–69.

Raff, M. C., L. E. Lillien, W. D. Richardson, J. F. Burne, and M. D. Noble (1988) Platelet-derived growth factor from astrocytes drives the clock that times oligodendrocyte development in culture. Nature 333: 562–565.

Raff, M. C., B. A. Barres, J. F. Burne, H. S. Coles, Y. Ishizaki, and M. D. Jacoloson (1993) Programmed cell death and the control of cell survival: lessons from the nervous system. Science 262: 695–700.

Rakic, P. (1975) Role of cell interaction in development of dendritic patterns. Adv. Neurol. 12: 117–134.

Rakic, P. (1988) Specification of cerebral cortical areas. Science 241: 170–176.

Ramón y Cajal, S. (1889) Sobre las fibras nerviosas de la capa granulosa del cerebelo. Rev. Trim. de Histol. Norm. y Pathol. 3 & 4.

Ramón y Cajal, S. (1890) A quelle epoque apparaissent les expansions des celles nerveuses de la moelle epineiere de polet?. Anat. Anz. 5: 609–613.

Ranscht, B., P. A. Clapshaw, J. Price, et al. (1982) Development of oligodendrocytes and Schwann cells studied with a monoclonal antibody against galactocerebroside. Proc. Natl. Acad. Sci. U.S.A. 79: 2709–2713.

Ranscht, B., P. M. Wood, and R. P. Bunge (1987) Inhibition of in vitro peripheral myelin formation by monoclonal anti-galactocerebroside. J. Neurosci. 7: 2936–2947.

Rao, A., and A. M. Craig (1997) Activity regulates the synatic localization of the NMDA receptor in hippocampal neurons. Neuron 19: 801–812.

Rao, A., E. Kim, M. Sheng, and A. M. Craig (1997) Heterogeneity in the molecular composition of excitatory postsynaptic sites during development of hippocampal neurons in culture. J. Neurosci. 18: 1217–1229.

Rao, M. S., P. H. Patterson, and S. C. Landis (1992) Multiple cholinergic differentiation factors are present in footpad extracts: comparison with known cholinergic factors. Development 116: 731–744.

Raper, J. A., and J. P. Kapfhammer (1990) The enrichment of a neuronal growth cone collapsing activity from embryonic chick brain. Neuron 4: 21–29.

Rashbass, J., M. V. Taylor, and J. B. Gurdon (1992) The DNA-binding protein E12 cooperates with XMyoD in the activation of muscle-specific gene expression in *Xenopus* embryos. EMBO J. 11: 2981–2990.

Ratner, N., R. P. Bunge, and L. Glaser (1986) Schwann cell proliferation in vitro. An overview. Ann. N.Y. Acad. Sci. 486: 170–181.

Ratner, N., P. Wood, L. Glaser, and R. P. Bunge (1987) Further characterization of the neuronal cell surface protein mitogenic for Schwann cells. In: *Glial-Neuronal Communication in Development and Regeneration*, H. H. Althaus and W. Seifert, eds., pp. 685–698, Springer-Verlag, Heidelberg.

Rauvala, H., A. Vanhala, E. Castren, R. Nolo, E. Raulo, J. Merenmies, and P. Panula (1994) Expression of HB-GAM (heparin-binding growth-associated molecules) in the pathways of developing axonal processes in vivo and neurite outgrowth in vitro induced by HB-GAM. Brain Res. Dev. Brain Res. 79: 157–176.

Ray, J., D. Peterson, M. Schinstine, and F. H. Gage (1993) Proliferation, differentiation, and long-term culture of primary hippocampal neurons Proc. Natl. Acad. Sci. U.S.A. 90: 3602–3606.

Rayport, S. G., and S. Schacher (1986) Synaptic plasticity in vitro: cell culture of identified *Aplysia* neurons mediating short-term habituation and sensitization. J. Neurosci. 6: 759–763.

Ready, D. F., and J. G. Nicholls (1979) Identified neurons isolated from the leech CNS make selective connections in culture. Nature 281: 67–69.

Rees, R. P., and T. S. Reese (1981) New structural features of freeze-substituted neuritic growth cones. Neuroscience 6: 247–254.

Rehder, V., and S. B. Kater (1992) Regulation of growth cone filopodia by intracellular calcium. J. Neurosci. 12: 3175–3186.

Reichardt, L. F., and P. H. Patterson (1977) Neurotransmitter synthesis and uptake by isolated rat sympathetic neurons developing in microcultures. Nature 270: 147–151.

Reichardt, L. F., and K. J. Tomaselli (1991) Extracellular matrix molecules and their receptors: functions in neural development. Annu. Rev. Neurosci. 14: 531–570.

Reier, P. J., L. J. Stensaas, and L. Guth (1983) The astrocytic scar as an impediment to regeneration in the central nervous system. In: *Spinal Cord Reconstruction*, C. C. Kao, R. P. Bunge, and P. J. Reier, eds., pp. 163–195, Raven, New York.

Reitzer, L. J., B. M. Wice, and D. Kennell (1979) Evidence that glutamine, not sugar, is the major energy source for cultured HeLa cells. J. Biol. Chem. 254: 2669–2676.

Renfranz, P. J., M. G. Cunningham, and R. D. McKay (1991) Region-specific differentiation of the hippocampal stem cell line HiB5 upon implantation into the developing mammalian brain. Cell 66: 713–729.

Reynolds, B. A., and S. Weiss (1992) Generation of neurons and astrocytes from isolated cells of the adult mammalian central nervous system. Science 255: 1707–1710.

Reynolds, J. N., P. J., Ryan, A. Prasad, and G. D. Paterno (1994) Neurons derived from embryonal carcinoma (P19) cells express multiple GABA-A receptor subunits and fully functional GABA-A receptors. Neurosci. Lett. 165: 129–132.

Ribera, A. B., and N. C. Spitzer (1989) A critical period of transcription required for differentiation of the action potential of spinal neurons. Neuron 2: 1055–1062.

Ribera, A. B., and N. C. Spitzer (1992) Developmental regulation of potassium channels and the impact on neuronal differentiation. In: *Ion Channels*, vol. 3, T. Narahashi, ed., p. 1, Plenum, New York.

Richardson, W. D., N. Pringle, M. Mosley, B. Westermark, and M. Dubois Dalcq (1988) A role for platelet-derived growth factor in normal gliogenesis in the central nervous system. Cell 53: 309–319.

Rivas, R. J., and M. E. Hatten (1995) Motility and cytoskeletal organization of migrating cerebellar granule neurons. J. Neurosci. 15: 981–989.

Rivas, R. J., D. W. Burmeister, and D. J. Goldberg (1992) Rapid effects of laminin on the growth cone. Neuron 8: 107–115.

Robards, A. W., and U. B. Sleytr (1985) *Low Temperature Methods in Biological Electron Microscopy*, Elsevier, New York.

Roberts, J. L. (1988) In situ hybridization and related techniques to study cell-specific gene expression in the nervous system. Soc. Neurosci.

Robertson, E. J. (1987) Embryo-derived stem cell lines. In: *Teratocarcinoma and Embryonic Stem Cells: A Practical Approach*, IRL Press, Washington, DC.

Robertson, R. T., J. Zimmer, and B. H. Gähwiler (1989) Dissection procedures for preparation of slice cultures. In: *A Dissection and Tissue Culture. Manual of the Nervous System*, A. Shahar, J. de Vellis, A. Vernadakis, and B. Haber, eds., pp. 1–15, Alan R. Liss, Inc., New York.

Robertson, R. T., C. M. Annis, and B. H. Gähwiler (1991) Production of organotypic slice cultures of neural tissue using the roller tube technique. In: *Cellular and Molecular Neurobiology: A Practical Approach*, H. Wheal and J. Chad, eds., pp. 39–56, IRL Press, Oxford.

Roederer, M., F. J. Staal, P. A. Raju, L. Swelsa, L. A. Herzenberg, and L. A. Herzenberg (1990) Cytokine-stimulated human immunodeficiency virus replication is inhibited by *N*-acetyl-L-cysteine. Proc. Natl. Acad. Sci. U.S.A. 87: 4884–4888.

Roederer, M., P. A. Raju, F. J. Staal, L. A. Herzenberg, and L. A. Herzenberg (1991a) *N*-acetylcysteine inhibits latent HIV expression in chronically-infected cells. AIDS Res. Hum. Retroviruses 7: 491–496.

Roederer, M., F. J. Stall, H. Osada, L. A. Herzenberg, and L. A. Herzenberg (1991b) CD4 and CD8 T cells with high intracellular glutathione levels are selectively lost as the HIV infection progresses. Int. Immunol. 3: 933–937.

Roederer, M., S. W. Ela, F. J. Staal, L. A. Herzenberg, and L. A. Herzenberg. (1992) N-acetylcysteine: a new approach to anti-HIV therapy. AIDS Res. Hum. Retroviruses 8: 209–217.

Rogers, A. W. (1979) *Techniques of Autoradiography*, Elsevier, New York.

Rogers, S. L., P. C. Letourneau, and I. V. Pech (1989) The role of fibronectin in neural development. Dev. Neurosci. 11: 248–265.

Rohrer, H., and H. Thoenen (1987) Relationship between differentiation and terminal mitosis: chick sensory and ciliary neurons differentiate after terminal mitosis of precursor cells, whereas sympathetic neurons continue to divide after differentiation. J. Neurosci. 7: 3739–3748.

Role L. W., R. J. Matossian, R. J. O'Brien, and G. D. Fischbach (1985) On the mechanism of Ach receptor accumulation at newly formed synapses on chick myotubes. J. Neurosci. 5: 2197–2204.

Role, L. W., D. G. Roufa, and G. D. Fischbach (1987) The distribution of ACh receptor clusters and sites of transmitter release along chick ciliary ganglion neurite-myotube contacts in culture. J. Cell Biol. 104: 371–379.

Romijn, H. J. (1988) Development and advantages of serum-free, chemically defined nutrient media for culturing of nerve tissue. Biol Cell 63: 263–268.

Romijn, H. J., H. von Huizon, and P. S. Wolters (1984) Towards an improved serum-free, chemically defined medium for long-term culturing of cerebral cortex tissue. Neurosci. Biobehav. Rev. 8: 301–334.

Romijn, H. J., B. M. de Jong, and J. M. Ruijter (1988) A procedure for culturing rat neo-cortex explants in a serum-free nutrient medium. J. Neurosci. Methods 23: 75–83.

Ronnett, G. V., L. D. Hester, J. S. Nye, K. Connors, and S. H. Snyder (1990) Human cortical neuronal cell line: establishment from a patient with unilateral megalencephaly. Science 248: 603–605.

Ronnett, G. V., L. D. Hester, J. S. Nye, and S. H. Snyder (1994) Human cerebral cortical cell lines from patients with unilateral megalencephaly and Rasmussen's encephalitis. Neuroscience 63: 1081–1099.

Rose, G. (1954) A separable and multipurpose tissue culture chamber. Texas Rep. Biol. Med. 12: 1074–1083.

Rosen, C. L., R. P. Bunge, M. D. Ard, and P. M. Wood (1989) Type 1 astrocytes inhibit adult rat oligodendrocyte function in vitro. J. Neurosci. 9: 3371–3379.

Rosen, K. M., E. D. Lamperti, and L. Villa-Komaroff (1990) Optimizing the Northern blot procedure. Bio. Techniques 8: 398–403.

Rosenberg, P. A., and M. A. Dichter (1989) Extracellular cAMP accumulation and degradation in rat cerebral cortex in dissociated cell culture. J. Neurosci. 9: 2654–2663.

Rosenberg P. A., S. Amin, and M. Leitner (1992) Glutamate uptake disguises neurotoxic potency of glutamate agonists in cerebral cortex in dissociated cell culture. J. Neurosci. 12: 56–61.

Ross, E. M., A. C. Howlett, K. M. Ferguson, and A. G. Gilman (1978) Reconstitution of hormone-sensitive adenylate cyclase activity with resolved components of the enzyme. J. Biol. Chem. 253: 6401–6412.

Rossant, J., and M. McBurney (1982) The developmental potential of a euploid male teratocarcinoma cell line after blastocyst injection. J. Embryol. Exp. Morphol. 67: 167.

Roth, M. G. (1994) SV40 virus expression vectors. In: *Methods in Cell Biology*, Vol 43: *Protein Expression Animal Cells*, M. G. Roth ed. pp. 113–136, Academic Press, New York.

Roth, M. G. ed. (1994) *Methods in Cell Biology*, vol, 43: *Protein Expression in Animal Cells*, Academic Press, New York.

Rothman, S. (1984) Synaptic release of excitatory amino acid neurotransmitter mediates anoxic neuronal death. J. Neurosci. 4: 1884–1891.

Rothman, S., and W. M. Cowan (1979) A scanning electron microscopic study of the in vitro development of dissociated hipocampal cells. J. Comp. Neurol. 195: 141–155.

Rothman, S. M., and J. W. Olney (1987) Excitotoxicity and the NMDA receptor. Trends Neurosci. 10: 299–302.

Rothman, T. P., M. D. Gershon, and H. Holtzer (1978) The relationship of cell division to the acquisition of adrenergic characteristics by developing sympathetic ganglion cell precursors. Dev. Biol. 65: 322–341.

Rotman, B., and B. W. Papermaster (1966) Membrane properties of living mammalian cells as studied by enzymatic hydrolysis of fluorogenic esters. Proc. Natl. Acad. Sci. U.S.A. 55: 134–141.

Roufa, D., M. B. Bunge, M. I. Johnson, and C. J. Cornbrooks (1986) Variation in content and function of non-neuronal cells in the outgrowth of sympathetic ganglia from embryos of differing age. J. Neurosci. 6: 790–802.

Rousselet, A., L. Fetler, B. Chamak, and A. Prochiantz (1988) Rat mesencephalic neurons in culture exhibit different morphological traits in the presence of media conditioned on mesencephalic or striatal astroglia. Dev. Biol. 129: 495–504.

Rubin, L. L., et al. (1991) A cell culture model of the blood-brain barrier. J. Cell Biol. 115: 1725–1735.

Rudnicki, M. A., and M. W. McBurney (1987) Cell culture methods and induction of differentiation of embryonal carcinoma cell lines. In: *Teratocarcinoma and Embryonic Stem Cells. A Practical Approach*, E. J. Robertson, ed., pp. 19–50, IRL Press, Washington, DC.

Ruit, K. G., J. L. Elliott, P. A. Osborne, Q. Yan, and W. D. Snider (1992) Selective dependence of mammalian dorsal root ganglion neurons on nerve growth factor during embryonic development. Neuron 8: 573–587.

Ruiz i Altaba, A., and D. Melton (1989) Involvement of the *Xenopus* homeobox gene Xhox3 in pattern formation along the anterior-posterior axis. Cell 57: 317–326.

Rukenstein, A., and L. A. Greene (1983) The quantitative bioassay of nerve growth factor: use of frozen "primed" PC12 pheochromocytoma cells. Brain Res. 263: 177–180.

Rukenstein, A., R. Rydel, and L. A. Greene (1991) Multiple agents rescue PC12 cells from serum-free cell death by translation- and transcription-independent mechanisms. J. Neurosci. 11: 2552–2563.

Ruthel, G., and G. Banker (1998) Actin-dependent anterograde movement of growth cone-like structures along growing hippocampal axons: A novel form of actin transport? Cell Motil. Cytoskel.: in press.

Rutkowski, J. L., G. I. Tennekoon, and J. E. McGillicuddy (1992) Selective culture of mitotically active human Schwann cells from adult sural nerve. Ann. Neurol. 6: 580–586.

Rutkowski, J. L., C. J. Kirk, M. A. Lerner, and G. I. Tennekoon (1995) Purification and expansion of human Schwann cells in vitro. Nature Med. 1: 80–83.

Ryan, T. A., and S. J. Smith (1995) Vesicle pool mobilization during action potential firing at hippocampal synapses. Neuron 14: 983–989.

Ryan, T. A., H. Reuter, B. Wendland, F. E. Schweizer, R. W. Tsien, and S. J. Smith (1993) The kinetics of synaptic vesicle recycling measured at single presynaptic boutons. Neuron 11: 713–724.

Ryan, T. A., S. J. Smith, and H. Reuter (1996) The timing of synaptic vesicle endocytosis. Proc. Natl. Acad. Sci. U.S.A. 93: 5567–5571.

Ryder, E. F., E. Y. Snyder, and C. L. Cepko (1990) Establishment and characterization of multipotent neural cell lines using retrovirus vector–mediated oncogene transfer. J. Neurobiol. 21: 356–375.

Saez, J. C., J. A. Kessler, M. V. Bennett, and D. C. Spray (1987) Superoxide dismutase protects cultured neurons against death by starvation. Proc. Natl. Acad. Sci. U.S.A. 84: 3056–3059.

Salvaterra, P. M., N. Bournias-Vardiabasis, T. Nair, G. Hou, and C. Lieu (1987) In vitro neuronal differentiation of *Drosophila* embryo cells. J. Neurosci. 7: 10–22.

Salzer, J. L., and R. P. Bunge (1980) Studies of Schwann cell proliferation: I. An analysis in tissue culture of proliferation during development, Wallerian degeneration, and direct injury. J. Cell Biol. 84: 739–752.

Sambrook, J., E. F. Fritsch, and T. Maniatis (1989) *Molecular Cloning: A Laboratory Manual*, Cold Spring Harbor Laboratory, Cold Spring Harbor, NY.

Sanes, D. H., and M-m. Poo (1989) In vitro analysis position and lineage dependent selectivity in the formation of neuromuscular synapses. Neuron 2: 1237–1244.

Sanes, J. R. (1989) Analyzing cell lineage with a recombinant retrovirus. Trends Neurosci. 12: 21–28.

Saneto, R. P., and J. DeVellis (1985) Characterization of cultured rat oligodendrocytes proliferating in a serum-free chemically defined medium. Proc. Natl. Acad. Sci. U.S.A. 82: 3509–3513.

Sato, M., L. Lopez-Mascaraque, C. D. Heffner, and D. D. O'Leary (1994) Action of a diffusible target-derived chemoattractant on cortical axon branch induction and directed growth. Neuron 13: 791–803.

Savoca, R., U. Ziegler, and P. Sonderegger (1995) Effects of L-serine on neurons in vitro. J. Neurosci. Methods 61: 159–167.

Sawai, S., A. Shimono, K. Hanaoka, and H. Kondoh (1991) Embryonic lethality resulting from disruption of both *N-myc* alleles in mouse zygotes. New Biologist 3: 861–869.

Sayer, R. J., M. J. Friedlander, and S. J. Redman (1990) The time course and amplitude of EPSPs evoked at synapses between pairs of CA3/CA1 neurons in the hippocampal slice. J. Neurosci. 10: 826–836.

Scanziani, M., D. Debanne, M. Mller, B. H. Gähwiler, and S. M. Thompson (1994) Role of excitatory amino acid and GABA$_B$ receptors in the generation of epileptiform activity in disinhibited hippocampal slice cultures. Neuroscience 61: 823–832.

Schacher, S. (1985) Differential synapse formation and neurite outgrowth at two branches of the metacerebral cell of *Aplysia* in dissociated cell culture. J. Neurosci. 5: 2028–2034.

Schacher, S., and P. G. Montarolo (1991) Target-dependent structural changes in sensory neurons of *Aplysia* accompany long-term heterosynaptic inhibition. Neuron 6: 679–690.

Schacher, S., and E. Proshansky (1983) Neurite regeneration by *Aplysia* neurons in dissociated cell culture: modulation by *Aplysia* hemolymph and the presence of the initial axonal segment. J. Neurosci. 3: 2403–2413.

Schacher, S., P. G. Montarolo, and E. R. Kandel (1990) Selective short- and long-term effects of serotonin, small cardioactive peptide, and tetanic stimulation on sensorimotor synapses of *Aplysia* in culture. J. Neurosci. 10: 3286–3294.

Schacher, S., E. R. Kandel, and P. G. Montarolo (1993) cAMP and arachidonic acid simulate long-term structural and functional changes produced by neurotransmitters in *Aplysia* sensory neurons. Neuron 10: 1079–1088.

Schachner, M. (1990) Boundaries during normal and abnormal brain development: in vivo and in vitro studies of glia and glycoconjugates. Exp. Neurol. 109: 35–56.

Schaeffer, E., J. Alder, P. Greengard, and M-m. Poo (1994) Synapsin IIa accelerates functional development of neuromuscular synapses. Proc. Natl. Acad. Sci. U.S.A. 91: 3882–3886.

Schaffner, A. E., P. A. St. John, and J. L. Barker (1987) Fluorescence-activated cell sorting of embryonic mouse and rat motoneurons and their long-term survival in vitro. J. Neurosci. 7: 3088–3104.

Schaffner, A. E., J. L. Barker, D. A. Stenger, and J. J. Hickman (1995) Investigation of the factors necessary for growth of hippocampal neurons in a defined system. J. Neurosci. Methods 62: 111–119.

Schilling, K., M. H. Dickinson, J. A. Connor and J. I. Morgan (1991) Electrical activity in cerebellar cultures determines Purkinje cell dendritic growth patterns. Neuron 7: 891–902.

Schindler, M., M. L. Allen, M. R. Olinger, and J. F. Holland (1985) Automated analysis and survival selection of anchorage-dependent cells under normal growth conditions. Cytometry 6: 368–374.

Schlessinger, A. R., W. M. Cowan, and L. W. Swanson (1978) The time of origin of neurons in Ammon's horn and the associated retrohippocampal fields. Anat. Embryol. (Berl.) 154: 153–173.

Schmidt, M. F., and S. B. Kater (1993) Fibroblast growth factors, depolarization, and sub-stratum interact in a combinatorial way to promote neuronal survival. Dev. Biol. 158: 228–237.

Schubert, D. (1984) *Developmental Biology of Cultured Nerve, Muscle, and Glia*. Wiley, New York.

Schubert, D., S. Humphreys, C. Baroni, and M. Cohn (1969) In vitro differentiation of a mouse neuroblastoma. Proc. Natl. Acad. Sci. U.S.A. 64: 316–323.

Schubert, D., S. Humphreys, F. Jacob, and F. Vitry (1971) Induced differentiation of a neuroblastoma. Dev. Biol. 25: 514–546.

Schubert, D., S. Heinemann, W. Carlisle, H. Tarikas, B. Kimes, J. Patrick, J. H. Steinbach, W. Culp, and B. L. Brandt (1974) Clonal cell lines from the rat central nervous system. Nature 249: 224–227.

Schubert, D., H. Kimura, and P. Maher (1992) Growth factors and vitamin E modify neu-ronal glutamate toxicity. Proc. Natl. Acad. Sci. U.S.A. 89: 8264–8267.

Schuch, U., M. J. Lohse, and M. Schachner (1989) Neural cell adhesion molecules influ-ence second messenger systems. Neuron 3: 13–20.

Schulze-Osthoff, K., A. C. Bakker, B. Vanhaesebroeck, R. Beyaert, W. A. Jacob, and W. Fiers (1992) Cytotoxic activity of tumor necrosis factor is mediated by early damage of mitochondrial functions. J. Biol. Chem. 2647: 5317–5323.

Schulze-Osthoff, K., R. Beyaert, V. Vandevoorde, G. Haegeman, and W. Fiers (1993) Depletion of the mitochondrial electron transport abrogates the cytotoxic and gene inductive effects of TNF. EMBO J. 12: 3095–3104.

Schwab, M. E., and P. Caroni (1988) Oligodendrocytes and CNS myelin are nonpermissive substrates for neurite growth and fibroblast spreading in vitro. J. Neurosci. 8: 2381–2393.

Schweitzer, E. S., and R. B. Kelly (1985) Selective packaging of human growth hormone into synaptic vesicles in a rat neuronal PC12 cell line J. Cell Biol. 101: 667–676.

Scolding, N. J., J. P. Zajicek, N. Wood, and D. A. Compston (1994) The pathogenesis of demyelinating disease. Prog Neurobiol 43: 143–173.

Scott, B., and J. Lew (1986) Neurons in cell culture survive freezing. Effect on electric membrane properties. Exp. Cell Res. 162: 566–573.

Scott, B. S. (1982) Adult neurons in cell culture: electrophysiological characterization and use in neurobiological research. Prog. Neurobiol. 19: 187–211.

Scott, B. S., and K. C. Fisher (1970) Potassium concentration and number of neurons in cultures of dissociated ganglia. Exp. Neurol. 27: 16–22.

Scott, B. S., T. L. Petit, L. E. Becker, and B. A. Edwards (1979) Electric membrane prop-erties of human DRG neurons in cell culture and the effect of high K medium. Brain Res. 178: 529–544.

Scott, S. A. (1992) *Sensory Neurons: Diversity, Development, and Plasticity*. Oxford University, New York.

Seecof, R. L., N. Alleaume, R. L. Teplitz, and I. Gerson (1971) Differentiation of neurons and myocytes in cell cultures made from *Drosophila* gastrulae. Exp. Cell Res. 69: 161–173.

Seeds, N. W. (1983) Neuronal differentiation in reaggregate cell cultures. In: *Advances in Cellular Neurobiology*, S. Federoff and L. Hertz, eds., pp. 57–80, Academic Press, New York.

Seeley, P. J., and L. A. Greene (1983) Short latency, local actions of nerve growth factor on growth cones. Proc. Nat. Acad. Sci. U.S.A. 80: 2789–2793.

Segal, M. (1983) Rat hippocampal neurons in culture: responses to electrical and chemical stimuli. J. Neurophysiol. 50: 1249–1264.

Segal, M. M. (1991) Epileptiform activity in microcultures containing one excitatory hippocampal neuron. J. Neurophysiol. 65: 761–770.

Segal, M. M. (1994) Endogenous bursts underlie seizure-like activity in solitary excitatory hippocampal neurons in microcultures. J. Neurophysiol. 72: 1874–1884.

Segal, M. M., and E. J. Furshpan (1990) Epileptiform activity in microcultures containing small numbers of hippocampal neurons. J. Neurophysiol. 64: 1390–1399.

Seiger, A., and L. Olson (1977) Quantitation of fibre growth in transplanted central monoamine neurons. Cell Tissue Res. 179: 285–316.

Seil, F., M. Smith, and A. Leiman (1975) Myelination inhibiting and neuroelectric blocking factors in experimental allergic encephalomyelitis (EAE). Science 187: 951–953.

Seil, F. J., and H. C. Agrawal (1984) Serum antimyelin factors in experimental allergic encephalomyelitis and multiple sclerosis. Prog. Clin. Biol. Res. 146: 199–206.

Seiler, N. (1981) Polyamine metabolism and function in brain. Neurochem. Res. 3: 95–110.

Seiler, N., S. Sarhan, and B. F. Roth-Schechter (1984) Polyamines and the development of isolated neurons in cell culture. Neurochem. Res. 9: 871–886.

Seilheimer, B., E. Persohn, and M. Schachner (1989) Antibodies to the L1 adhesion molecule inhibit Schwann cell ensheathment of neurons in vitro. J. Cell Biol. 109: 3095–3103.

Selak, I , J. M. Foidart, and G. Moonen (1985a) Laminin promotes cerebellar granule cells migration in vitro and is synthesized by cultured astrocytes. Dev. Neurosci. 7: 278–285.

Selak, I., S. D. Skaper, and S. Varon (1985b) Pyruvate participation in the low molecular weight trophic activity for central nervous system neurons in glia-conditioned media. J. Neurosci. 5: 23–28.

Selmaj, K., C. S. Raine, B. Canella, and C. F. Brosnan (1991) Identification of lymphotoxin and tumor necrosis factor in multiple sclerosis lesions. J. Clin. Invest. 87: 949–954.

Selmaj, K. W., and C. S. Raine (1988) Tumour necrosis factor mediates myelin and oligodendrocyte damage in vitro. Ann. Neur. 23: 339–346.

Sensenbrenner, M., and P. Mandel (1974) Behavior of neuroblasts in the presence of glial cells, fibroblasts and meningeal cells in culture. Exp. Cell Res. 87: 159–167.

Sensenbrenner, M., K. Maderspach, L. Latzkovits, and G. G. Jaros (1978) Neuronal cells from chick embryo cerebral hemispheres cultivated on polylysine-coated surfaces. Dev. Neurosci. 1: 90–101.

Sensenbrenner, M., J. C. Deloulme, and C. Gensburger (1994) Proliferation of neuronal precursor cells from the central nervous system in culture. Rev. Neurosci. 5: 43–53.

Serafini, T., T. E. Kennedy, M. J. Galko, et al. (1994) The netrins define a family of axon outgrowth-promoting proteins homologous to C. elegans UNC-6. Cell 78: 409–424.

Seress, L., and C. E. Ribak (1988) The development of GABAergic neurons in the rat hippocampal formation. An immunocytochemical study. Dev. Brain Res. 44: 197–209.

Shafer, T. J. (1991) Transmitter, ion channel and receptor properties of pheochromocytoma (PC12) cells: a model for neurotoxicological studies. Neurotoxicology 12: 473–492.

Shafit-Zagardo, B., C. Peterson, and J. E. Goldman (1988) Rapid increases in glial fibrillary acidic protein mRNA and protein levels in the copper-deficient, brindled mouse. J. Neurochem. 51: 1258–1266.

Shain, W., J. A. Connor, V. Madelian, and D. L. Martin (1989) Spontaneous and beta-adrenergic receptor-mediated taurine release from astroglial cells are independent of manipulations of intracellular calcium. J. Neurosci. 9: 2306–2312.

Sharp, D. J., W. Yu, and P. W. Baas (1995) Transport of dendritic microtubules establishes their nonuniform polarity orientation. J. Cell Biol. 130: 93–103.

Sharpe, P. T. (1988) Methods of Cell Separation, Elsevier, New York.

Shaw, G., and D. Bray (1977) Movement and extension of isolated growth cones. Exp. Cell Res. 104: 55–62.

Shen, M., and P. Leder (1992) Leukemia inhibitory factor is expressed by the pre-implantation uterus and selectively blocks primitive ectoderm formation in vitro. Proc. Natl. Acad. Sci. U.S.A. 89: 8240–8244.

Shen, X. Y., S. Billings-Gagliardi, R. L. Sidman, and M. K. Wolf (1986) Myelin deficient (schimld) mutant allele: morphological comparison with shiverer (shi) allele in a B6C3 mouse stock. Brain Res. 360: 235–247.

Sheng, M. (1996) PDZs and receptor/channel clustering—rounding up the latest suspects. Neuron 17: 575–578.

Shepherd, G. M. (1991) Sensory transduction: entering the mainstream of membrane signaling. Cell 67: 845–851.

Shihabuddin, L. S., J. P. Brunschwig, V. R. Holets, M. B. Bunge, and S. R. Whittemore (1996) Induction of mature neuronal properties in immortalized neuronal precursor cells following grafting into the neonatal CNS. J. Neurocytol. 25: 101–111.

Shotten, D. (1993) *Electronic Light Microscopy: Techniques in Modern Biomedical Microscopy*, Wiley-Liss, New York.

Shoukimas, G., and J. Hinds (1978) The development of the cerebral cortex in the embryonic mouse: an electron microscopic serial section analysis. J. Comp. Neurol. 179: 795–830.

Sidman, R. L., and P. Rakic (1973) Neuronal migration with special reference to developing human brain: a review. Brain Res. 62: 1–35.

Silver, J., S. E. Lorenz, D. Washten, and J. Coughin (1982) Axonal guidance during development of the great cerebral commissures: descriptive and experimental studies, in vivo, on the role of preformed glial pathways. J. Comp. Neurol. 210: 10–29.

Simons, M., E. Ikonen, P. J. Tienari, A. Cidarregui, U. Monning, K. Beyreuther and C. G. Dotti (1995) Intracellular routing of human amyloid protein precursor—axonal delivery followed by transport to the dendrites. J. Neurosci. Res. 41: 121–128.

Singer, R. H., J. B. Lawrence, and C. Villnave (1986) Optimization of in situ hybridization using isotopic and non-isotopic detection methods. Biotechniques 4: 230–250.

Skene, J. H. P. (1989) Axonal growth-associated proteins. Annu. Rev. Neurosci. 12: 127–156.

Skoff, R. P., and P. E. Knapp (1991) Division of astroblasts and oligodendroblasts in postnatal rodent brain: evidence for separate astrocyte and oligodendrocyte lineages. Glia 4: 165–174.

Skoff, R. P., D. L. Price, and A. Stocks (1976a) Electron microscopic autoradiographic studies of gliogenesis in rat optic nerve: I. Cell proliferation. J. Comp. Anat. 169: 291–311.

Skoff, R. P., D. L. Price, and A. Stocks (1976b) Electron microscopic autoradiographic studies of gliogenesis in rat optic nerve: II. Time of origin. J. Comp. Anat. 169: 313–323.

Slack, R. S., and F. D. Miller (1996) Viral vectors for modulating gene expression in neurons. Curr. Opin. Neurobiol. 6: 576–583.

Slack, R. S., I. S. Skerjanc, B. Lach, J. Craig, K. Jardine, and M. W. McBurney (1995) Cells differentiating into neuroectoderm undergo apoptosis in the absence of functional retinoblastoma family proteins. J. Cell Biol. 129: 779–788.

Slack, R. S., D. J. Belliveau, M. Rosenberg, J. Atwal, H. Lochmuller, R. Aloyz, A. Haghighi, B. Lach, P. Seth, E. Cooper, and F. D. Miller (1996) Adenovirus-mediated gene transfer of the tumor suppressor, p53, induces apoptosis in postmitotic neurons. J. Cell Biol. 135: 1085–1096.

Small, R., P. Riddle, and M. Noble (1987) Evidence for migration of oligodendrocyte-type-2 astrocyte progenitor cells into the developing rat optic nerve. Nature 328: 155–157.

Smilkstein, M. J., G. L. Knapp, K. W. Kulig, and B. H. Rumack (1988) Efficacy of oral N-acetylcysteine in the treatment of acetaminophen overdose. N. Engl. J. Med. 319: 1557–1562.

Smith, C. L. (1994a) Cytoskeletal movements and substrate interactions during the initiation of neurite outgrowth by sympathetic neurons in vitro. J. Neurosci. 14: 384–398.

Smith, C. L. (1994b) The initiation of neurite outgrowth by sympathetic neurons grown in vitro does not depend on assembly of microtubules. J. Cell Biol. 127: 384–398.

Smith, G. M., R. H. Miller, and J. Silver (1986) Changing role of forebrain astrocytes during development, regenerative failure and induced regeneration upon transplantation. J. Comp. Neurol. 251: 23–43.

Smith, G. M., U. Rutishauser, J. Silver, and R. H. Miller (1990) Maturation of astrocytes in vitro alters the extent and molecular basis of neurite outgrowth. Dev. Biol. 138: 377–390.

Smith, J. E., and T. S. Reese (1980) Use of aldehyde fixatives to determine the rate of synaptic transmitter release. J. Exp. Biol. 89: 19–29.

Smith, R. G., K. Vaca, J. McManaman, S. H. Appel (1986) Selective effects of skeletal muscle extract fractions on motoneuron development in vitro. J. Neurosci. 6: 439–447.

Smolich, B. D., and J. Papkoff (1994) Regulated expression of Wnt family members during neuroectodermal differentiation of P19 embryonal carcinoma cells: overexpression of Wnt-1 perturbs normal differentiation-specific properties. Dev. Biol. 166: 300–310.

Snider, W. D. (1994) Functions of the neurotrophins during nervous system development: what the knockouts are teaching us. Cell 77: 627–638.

Snow, D. M., D. A. Steindler, and J. Silver (1990) Molecular and cellular characterization of the glial roof plate of the spinal cord and optic tectum: a possible role for the proteoglycan in the development of an axon barrier. Dev. Biol. 138: 359–376.

Snyder, E. Y., and S. U. Kim (1979) Hormonal requirements for neuronal survival in culture. Neurosci. Lett. 13: 225–230.

Snyder, E. Y., D. L. Deitcher, C. Walsh, S. Arnold-Aldea, E. A. Hartwieg, and C. L. Cepko (1992) Multipotent neural cell lines can engraft and participate in development of mouse cerebellum. Cell 68: 33–51.

Sommer, I., and M. Schachner (1981) Monoclonal antibodies (O_1 to O_4) to oligodendrocyte cell surfaces. An immunocytological study in the central nervous system. Dev. Biol. 83: 311–327.

Sommer, L., N. Shah, M. Rao, and D. J. Anderson (1995) The cellular function of MASH1 in autonomic neurogenesis. Neuron 15: 1245–1258.

Sotelo, C. (1975) Anatomic, physiological and biochemical studies of the cerebellum from mutant mice. II Morphological study of the cerebellar cortical neurons and circuits in the weaver mouse. Brain Res. 94: 19–44.

Soto, A. M., and C. Sonnenschein (1985) The role of estrogen on the proliferation of human breast tumor cells (MCF-7). J. Steroid Biochem. 23: 87–94.

Spaete, R. R., and N. Frenkel (1982) The herpes simplex virus amplicon: a new eukaryotic defective-virus cloning-amplifying vector. Cell 30: 285–304.

Spenger, C., C. Hyman, L. Studer, M. Egli, L. Evtouchenko, C. Jackson, A. Dahl-Jorgensen, R. M. Lindsay, and R. W. Seiler (1995) Effects of BDNF on dopaminergic, serotonergic, and GABAergic neurons in cultures of human fetal ventral mesencephalon. Exp. Neurol. 133: 50–63.

Spira, M. E., D. Benbassat, and A. Dormann (1993) Resealing of the proximal and distal cut ends of transected axons: electrophysiological and ultrastructural analysis. J. Neurobiol. 24: 300–316.

Spitzer, N. C. (1991) A developmental handshake: neuronal control of ionic currents and their control of neuronal differentiation. J. Neurobiol. 22: 659–673.

Spitzer, N. C. (1994) Spontaneous Ca^{2+} spikes and waves in embryonic neurons: signaling systems for differentiation. Trends Neurosci. 17: 115–118.

Spitzer, N. C., and J. E. Lamborghini (1976) The development of the action potential mechanism of amphibian neurons isolated in cell culture. Proc. Natl. Acad. Sci. U.S.A. 73: 1641–1645.

Spitzer, N. C., E. Olson, and X. Gu (1995) Spontaneous calcium transients regulate neuronal plasticity in developing neurons. J. Neurobiol. 26: 316–324.

St. John, P. A. (1990) Cell culture of identified mammalian motoneurons by fluorescence-activated cell sorting. Unpublished manuscript.

St. John, P. A. (1991) Toxicity of "DiI" for embryonic rat motoneurons and sensory neurons in vitro. Life Sci. 49: 2013–2021.

St. John, P. A., L. Kam, S. W. Turner, H. G. Craighead, Milsaacson, J. N. Turner, and W. Shain (1997) Preferential glial cell attachment to microcontact printed surfaces. J. Neurosci. Methods 75: 171–177.

Staal, F. J. T., M. Roederer, L. A. Herzenberg, and L. A. Herzenberg (1990) Intracellular thiols regulate NF-kB activation and HIV transcription. Proc. Natl. Acad. Sci. U.S.A. 87: 9943–9947.

Stahl, B., B. Muller, Y. von Boxberg, E. C. Cox, and F. Bonhoeffer (1990) Biochemical characterization of a putative axonal guidance molecule of the chick visual system. Neuron 5: 735–743.

Stahl, N., and G. D. Yancopoulos (1993) The alphas, betas and kinases of cytokine receptor complexes. Cell 74: 587–590.

Staines, W. A., D. J. Morassutti, K. R. Reuhl, A. I. Ally, and M. W. McBurney (1994) Neurons derived from P19 embryonal carcinoma cells have varied morphologies and neurotransmitters. Neuroscience 58: 735–751.

Steindler, D. A., N. G. F. Cooper, A. Faissner, and M. Schachner (1989) Boundaries defined by adhesion molecules during development of the cerebral cortex: the J1/ tenascin glycoprotein in the mouse somatosensory cortical barrel field. Dev. Biol. 131: 243–260.

Steindler, D. A., T. F. O'Brien, E., Laywell, K. Harrington, A. Faissner, and M. Schachner (1990) Boundaries during normal and abnormal brain development. In vivo and in vitro studies of glia and glycoconjugates. Exp. Neurol. 109: 35–36.

Stemple, D. L., and D. J. Anderson (1992) Isolation of a stem cell for neurons and glia from the mammalian neural crest. Cell 71: 973–985.

Stemple, D. L., N. K. Mahanthappa, and D. J. Anderson (1988) Basic FGF induces neuronal differentiation, cell division, and NGF dependence in chromaffin cells: a sequence of events in sympathetic development. Neuron 1: 517–525.

Stephens, R. M., D. M. Loeb, T. D. Copeland, T. Pawson, L. A. Greene, and D. R. Kaplan (1994) Trk receptors use redundant signal transduction pathways involving SHC and PLC-g1 to mediate NGF responses. Neuron 12: 691–705.

Stergaard, K. (1993) Organotypic slice cultures of the rat striatum: I. A histochemical and immunocytochemical study of acetylcholinesterase, choline acetyltransferase, glutamate decarboxylase and GABA. Neuroscience 53: 679–693.

Sternberger, L. A. (1986) *Immunocytochemistry*, Wiley, New York.

Stewart, W. W. (1978) Functional connections between cells as revealed by dye-coupling with a highly fluorescent naphthalamide tracer. Cell 14: 741–759.

Stoop, R., and M-m. Poo (1995) Potentiation of transmitter release by ciliary neurotrophic factor requires somatic signaling. Science 267: 695–699.

Stoppini, L., P. A. Buchs, D. Muller (1991) A simple method for organotypic cultures of nervous tissue. J. Neurosci. Methods 37: 173–182.

Stow, N. D. (1981) Cloning of a DNA fragment from the left-hand terminus of the adenovirus type 2 genome and its use in site-directed mutagenesis. J. Virol. 37: 171–180.

Straus, W. (1982) Imidazole increases the sensitivity of the cytochemical reaction for peroxidase with diaminobenzidine at a neutral pH. J. Histochem. Cytochem. 30: 491–493.

Streit, P., S. M. Thompson, and B. H. Gähwiler (1989) Anatomical and physiological properties of GABAergic neurotransmission in organotypic slice cultures of rat hippocampus. Eur. J. Neurosci. 1: 603–615.

Strubing, C., G. Ahnert-Hilger, J. Shan, B. Wiedenmann, J. Hescheler, and A. M. Wolous (1995) Differentiation of pluripotent embryonic stem cells into the neuronal lineage in vitro gives rise to mature inhibitory and excitatory neurons. Mech. Dev. 53: 275–287.

Suda, Y., M. Suzuki, Y. Ikawa, and S. Aizawa (1987) Mouse embryonic stem cells exhibit indefinite proliferative potential. J. Cell. Physiol. 133: 197–201.

Sugiyama, K., A. Brunori, and M. L. Mayer (1989) Glial uptake of excitatory amino acids influences neuronal survival in cultures of mouse hippocampus. Neuroscience 32: 779–791.

Sullivan, K. F., J. C. Havercroft, P. S. Machlin, and D. W. Cleveland (1986) Sequence and expression of the chicken beta 5- and beta 4-tubulin genes define a pair of divergent beta-tubulins with complementary patterns of expression. Mol. Cell. Biol. 6: 4409–4418.

Sun, Y.-a., and M-m. Poo (1987) Evoked release of acetylcholine from the growing, embryonic neuron. Proc. Natl. Acad. Sci. U.S.A. 84: 2540–2544.

Suri, C., B. P. Fung, A. S. Tischler, and D. M. Chikaraishi (1993) Catecholaminergic cell lines from the brain and adrenal glands of tyrosine hydroxylase-SV40 T antigen transgenic mice. J. Neurosci. 13: 1280–1291.

Suthanthiran, M., M. E. Anderson, V. K. Sharma, and A. Meister (1990) Glutathione regulates activation-dependent DNA synthesis in highly purified normal human T

lymphocytes stimulated via the CD2 and CD3 antigens. Proc. Natl. Acad. Sci. U.S.A. 87: 3343–3347.

Swanson, L. W., C. Kohler, and A. Bjorkland (1987) In: *The Limbic Region: I. The Septo-hippocampal System*, pp. 125–277, Elsevier, New York.

Syed, N. I., A. G. M. Bulloch, and K. Lukowiak (1990) In vitro reconstruction of the respiratory central pattern generator of the mollusk *Lymnaea*. Science 250: 282–285.

Szczupak, L., S. Jordan, and W. B. J. Kristan, Jr. (1993) Segment-specific modulation of the electrophysiological activity of leech *Retzius* neurons by acetylcholine. J. Exp. Biol. 183: 115–135.

Takahashi, T., Y. Nakajima, K. Hirosawa, S. Nakajma, and K. Onodera (1987) Structure and physiology of developing neuromuscular synapses in culture. J. Neurosci. 7: 473–481.

Takamiya, Y., S. Kohsaka, S. Toya, M. Otani, and Y. Tsukada (1988) Immunohisto-chemical studies on the proliferation of reactive astrocytes and the expression of cytoskeletal proteins following brain injury in rats. Dev. Brain Res. 38: 201–210.

Takei, K., O. Mundigl, L. Daniell, and P. DeCamilli (1996) The synaptic vesicle cycle: a single vesicle budding step involving clathrin and dynamin. J. Cell Biol. 133: 1237–1250.

Takeichi, M. (1988) The cadherins: cell-cell adhesion molecules controlling animal morphogenesis. Development 102: 639–655.

Tamayose, K., T. Hirai, and T. Shimada (1996) A new strategy for large-scale preparation of high-titer recombinant adeno-associated virus vectors by using packaging cell lines and sulfonated cellulose column chromatography. Human Gene Therapy 7: 507–513.

Tanaka, E. M., and M. W. Kirschner (1991) Microtubule behavior in the growth cones of living neurons during axon elongation. J. Cell Biol. 115: 345–363.

Tanaka, J., H. Sadanari, H. Sato, and S. Fukuda (1991) Sodium butyrate-inducible replication of human cytomegalovirus in a human epithelial cell line. Virology 185: 271–280.

Taniguchi, N., T. Higashi, Y. Sakamoto, and A. Meister (1989) *Glutathione Centennial: Molecular Properties and Clinical Implications*, Academic Press, New York.

Taschenberger, H., and R. Grantyn (1995) Several types of Ca^{2+} channels mediate glutamatergic synaptic responses to activation of single Thy-1-immunolabeled rat retinal ganglion neurons. J. Neurosci. 15: 2240–2254.

Tatsuoka, H., and T. S. Reese (1989) New structural features of synapses in the anteroventral cochlear nucleus prepared by direct freezing and freeze-substitution. J. Comp. Neurol. 290: 343–357.

Taylor, D. L., and E. D. Salmon (1989) Basic fluorescence microscopy. Methods Cell Biol. 29: 207–237.

Temple, S., and M. C. Raff (1985) Differentiation of of a bipotential glial progenitor cell in single cell microculture. Nature 313: 223–225.

Temple, S., and M. C. Raff (1986) Clonal analysis of oligodendrocyte development in culture: evidence for a developmental clock that counts cell divisions. Cell 44: 773–779.

Temple, S., and X. Qian (1995) bFGF, neurotrophins, and the control or cortical neurogenesis. Neuron 15: 249–252.

Teng, K. K., and L. A. Greene (1993) Depolarization maintains neurites and priming of PC12 cells after nerve growth factor withdrawal. J. Neurosci. 13: 3124–3135.

Teng, K. K., and L. A. Greene (1994) Cultured PC12 cells: a model for neuronal function and differentiation. In: *Cell Biology: A Laboratory Handbook*, vol. 1, J. E. Celis, ed., pp. 218–224, Academic Press, San Diego.

Terasaki, M., J. Song, J. R. Wong, M. J. Weiss, and L. B. Chen (1984) Localization of endoplasmic reticulum in living and glutaraldehyde-fixed cells with fluorescent dyes. Cell 38: 101–108.

Tessier-Lavigne, M., M. Placzek, A. G. Lumsden, et al. (1988) Chemotropic guidance of developing axons in the mammalian central nervous system. Nature 336: 775–778.

Thomas, W. E., F. L. Jordan, and J. G. Townsel (1987) The status of the study of invertebrate neurons in tissue culture phylum Arthropoda. Comp. Biochem. Physiol. Physiol. 87: 215–222.

Thompson, D. E., and R. L. Franks (1978) Xenopus *Care and Culture*, Carolina Biological Supply Company, Burlington, NC.

Tiedge, H., and J. Brosius (1996) Translational machinery in dendrites of hippocampal neurons in culture. J. Neurosci. 16: 7171–7181.

Timpl, R., H. Rohde, P. G. Robey, S. I. Rennard, J. M. Foidart, and G. R. Martin (1979) Laminin a glycoprotein from basement membranes. J. Biol. Chem. 254: 9933–9937.

Tokunaga A., and K. Otani (1978) Fine structure of the medial habenular nucleus in the rat. Brain Res. 150: 600–606.

Tomozawa, Y., and S. H. Appel (1986) Soluble extracts enhance development of mesencephalic dopaminergic neurons in vitro. Brain Res. 399: 111–124.

Tong, G., R. C. Malenka, and R. A. Nicoll (1996) Long-term potentiation in cultures of single hippocampal granule cells: a presynaptic form of plasticity. Neuron 16: 1147–1157.

Toran-Allerand, D. (1976) Gogi-Cox modifications for the impregnation of whole mount preparations of organotypic cultures of the CNS. Brain Res. 118: 293–298.

Toran-Allerand, D. (1990) Long-term organotypic culture of central nervous system in Maximow assemblies. In: *Methods in Neuroscience.* Vol. 2: *Cell Culture*, P. M. Conn, ed., pp. 257–296, Academic Press, New York.

Townsel, J. G., and W. E. Thomas (1987) On the status of the study of invertebrate neurons in tissue culture—phyla Mollusca and Annelida. Comp. Biochem. Physiol. Physiol. 86: 199–207.

Traub, R. D., and R. K. S. Wong (1982) Cellular mechanism of neuronal synchronization in epilepsy. Science 216: 745–747.

Trenkner, E., and R. Sidman (1977) Histogenesis of mouse cerebellum in microwell cultures: cell reaggregation and migration, fiber and synapse formation. J. Cell Biol. 75: 915–940.

Trojanowski, J. Q., M. A. Obrocka, and V. M. Lee (1983) A comparison of eight different chromogen protocols for the demonstration of immunoreactive neurofilaments or glial filaments in rat cerebellum using the peroxidase-antiperoxidase method and monoclonal antibodies. J. Histochem. Cytochem. 31: 1217–1223.

Troy, C. M., L. A. Greene, and M. L. Shelanski (1992) Neurite outgrowth in peripherin-depleted cells. J. Cell Biol. 117: 1085–1092.

Tschan, T., I. Hoerler, Y. Houze, K. H. Winterhalter, C. Richter, and P. Bruckner (1990) Resting chondrocytes in culture survive without growth factors, but are sensitive to toxic oxygen metabolites. J. Cell Biol. 111: 257–260.

Turetsky, D. M., J. E. Huettner, D. I. Gottlieb, M. P. Goldberg, and D. W. Choi (1993) Glutamate receptor-mediated currents and toxicity in embryonal carcinoma cells. J. Neurobiol. 24: 1157–1169.

Turner, R. W., L. L. Borg, and N. I. Syed (1995) A technique for the primary dissociation of neurons from restricted regions of the vertebrate CNS. J. Neurosci. Methods 56: 57–70.

Tuttle, J. B., and W. D. Steers (1992) Nerve growth factor responsiveness of cultured major pelvic ganglion neurons from the adult rat. Brain Res. 588: 29–40.

Ulloa, L., F. J. Diez-Guerra, J. Avila, and J. Diaz-Nido (1994) Localization of differentially phosphorylated isoforms of microtubule-associated protein 1B in cultured rat hippocampal neurons. Neuroscience 61: 211–223.

Unsicker, K., B. Krisch, U. Otten, and H. Thoenen (1978) Nerve growth factor induced fiber outgrowth from isolated rat adrenal chromaffin cells: impairment by glucocorticoids. Proc. Natl. Acad. Sci. U.S.A. 75: 3498–3502.

Ure, D. R., and R. B. Campenot (1994) Leukemia inhibitor factor and nerve growth factor are retrogradely transported and processed by cultured rat sympathetic neurons. Dev. Biol. 162: 339–347.

Ure, D. R., R. B. Campenot, and A. Acheson (1992) Cholinergic differentiation of rat sympathetic neurons in culture: effects of factors applied to distal neurites. Dev. Biol. 154: 388–395.

Usdin, T. B., and G. D. Fischbach (1986) Purification and characterization of a polypeptide from chick brain that promotes the accumulation of acetylcholine receptors in chick myotubes. J. Cell Biol. 103: 493–507.

Utzschneider, D. A., D. R. Archer, and J. D. Kocsis (1994) Transplantation of glial cells enhances action potential conduction of amyelinated spinal cord axons in the myelin-deficient rat. Proc. Natl. Acad. Sci. U.S.A. 91: 53–57.

Valentino, K. L., J. H. Eberwine, and J. D. Barchas (1987) *In Situ Hybridization: Applications to Neurobiology*, Oxford University, New York.

Vallorta, F., N. Iezzi, F. Benfenati, B. Lu, M. M. Poo, and P. Greengard (1995) Accelerated structural maturation induced by synapsin I at developing neuromuscular synapses of *Xenopus* laevis. Eur. J. Neurosci. 7: 261–270.

VanBuskirk, R., T. Corcoran, and J. A. Wagner (1985) Clonal variants of PC12 pheochromocytoma cells with defects in cAMP-dependent protein kinases induce ornithine decarboxylase in response to nerve growth factors but not to adenosine agonists. Mol. Cell. Biol. 5: 1984–1992.

van de Boor, M., G. L. Guit, and A. M. Schreuder (1989) Early detection of delayed myelination in preterm infants. Pediatrics 84: 407–411.

Veis, D. J., C. M. Sorenson, J. R. Shutter, and S. J. Korsmeyer (1993) Bcl-2-deficient mice demonstrate fulminant lymphoid apoptosis, polycystic kidneys and hypopigmented hair. Cell 75: 229–240.

Venstrom, K. A., and L. F. Reichardt (1993) Extracellular matrix: 2. Role of extracellular matrix molecules and their receptors in the nervous system. FASEB J. 7: 996–1003.

Ventimiglia, R., B. E. Jones, and A. Möller (1995a) A quantitative method for morphometric analysis in neuronal cell culture: unbiased estimation of neuron area and number of branch points. J. Neurosci. Methods 57: 63–66.

Ventimiglia, R., P. E. Mather, B. E. Jones, and R. M. Lindsay (1995b) The neurotrophins BDNF, NT-3 and NT-4/5 promote survival and morphological and biochemical differentiation of striatal neurons in vitro. Eur. J. Neurosci. 7: 213–222.

Verdi, J. M., and D. J. Anderson (1994) Neurotrophins regulate sequential changes in neurotrophin receptor expression by sympathetic neuroblasts. Neuron 13: 1359–1372.

Verna, J. M. (1985) In vitro analysis of interactions between sensory neurons and skin: evidence for selective innervation of dermis and epidermis. J. Embryol. Exp. Morphol. 86: 53–70.

Vicario-Abejon, C., M. G. Cunningham, and R. D. McKay (1995a) Cerebellar precursors transplanted to the neonatal dentate gyrus express features characteristic of hippocampal neurons. J. Neurosci. 15: 6351–6363.

Vicario-Abejon, C., K. K. Johe, T. G. Hazel, D. Collazo, and R. D. McKay (1995b) Functions of basic fibroblast growth factor and neurotrophins in the differentiation of hippocampal neurons. Neuron 15: 105–114.

Vidal, L., B. Heller, L. Won, and A. Heller (1995) Quantitation of dopaminergic neurons in 3-dimensional reaggregate tissue culture by computer-assisted image analysis. J. Neurosci. Methods 56: 89–98.

Vielmetter, J., B. Stolze, F. Bonhoeffer, and C. A. Stuermer (1990) In vitro assay to test differential substrate affinities of growing axons and migratory cells. Exp. Brain Res. 81: 283–287.

Vitkovic, L. (1992) GAP-43 expression in macroglial cells: potential functional significance. Perspect. Dev. Neurobiol. 1: 39–43.

Vize, P. D., A. Hemmati-Brivanlou, R. M. Harland, and D. A. Melton (1991) Assays for gene function in developing *Xenopus* embryos. Methods Cell Biol. 36: 368.

Vogel, K. S., and J. A. Weston (1988) A subpopulation of cultured avian neural crest cells has transient neurogenic potential. Neuron 1: 569–577.

Vogel, Z., A. J. Sytkowski, and M. W. Nirenberg (1972) Acetylcholine receptors of muscle grown in vitro. Proc. Natl. Acad. Sci. U.S.A. 69: 3180–3184.

Vogt, L., R. J. Giger, U. Ziegler, B. Kunz, A. Buchstaller, W. T. J. M. C. Hermens, M. G. Kaplitt, M. R. Rosenfeld, D. W. Pfaff, J. Verhaagen, and P. Sonderegger (1996) Continuous renewal of the axonal pathway sensor apparatus by insertion of new sensor molecules into the growth cone membrane. Curr. Biol. 6: 1153–1158.

Voigt, P., Y. J. Ma, D. Gonzalez, W. H. Fahrenbach, W. C. Westel, K. Berg-Vonder Emde, K. G. Taylor, M. E. Costa and N. G. Seidah (1996) Neural and glial-mediated effects of

growth factors acting via tyrosine kinase receptors on luteinizing hormone-releasing hormone neurons. Endocrinology 137: 2593–2605.

Wada, K., M. Ballivet, J. Boulter, J. Connolly, E. Wada, E. S. Deneris, L. W. Swanson, S. Heinemann, and J. Patrick (1988) Functional expression of a new pharmacological subtype of brain nicotinic acetylcholine receptor. Science 240: 330–334.

Wada, E., K. Wada, J. Boulter, E. Deneris, S. Heinemann, J. Patrick, and S. W. Swanson (1989) Distribution of $alpha_2$, $alpha_3$, $alpha_4$, and $beta_2$, neuronal nicotinic acetylcholine receptor subunit mRNAs in the central nervous system: a hybridization histochemical study in the rat. J. Comp. Neurol. 284: 314–335.

Waggoner, A., R. DeBiasio, P. Conrad, et al. (1989) Multiple spectral parameter imaging. Methods Cell Biol. 30: 449–478.

Wagner, E., K. Zatloukal, M Cotten, H. Kirlappos, K. Mechtler, D. T. Curiel, and M. L. Birnstiel (1992) Coupling of adenovirus to transferrin-polylysine/DNA complexes greatly enhances receptor-mediated gene delivery and expression of transfected genes. Proc. Natl. Acad. Sci. U.S.A. 89: 6099–6103.

Wakade, A. R. (1982) Proliferation of cultured glial cells from embryonic chick sympathetic ganglia: inhibition by horse serum. Exp. Cell Res. 140: 779–784.

Wakade, A. R., and H. Thoenen (1984) Interchangeability of nerve growth factor and high potassium in the long-term survival of chick sympathetic neurons in serum-free culture medium. Neurosci. Lett. 45: 71–74.

Wakade, A. R., D. Edgar, and H. Thoenen (1982) Substrate requirement and media supplements necessary for the long-term survival of chick sympathetic and sensory neurons cultured without serum. Exp. Cell Res. 140: 71–78.

Walch-Soliman, C., R. Jahn, and T. C. Sudhof (1993) Neurotransmitter release. Curr. Opin. Neurobiol. 3: 329–336.

Walicke, P., W. M. Cowan, N. Ueno, A. Baird and R. Guillemin (1986a) Fibroblast growth factor promotes survival of dissociated hippocampal neurons and enhances neurite extension. Proc. Natl. Acad. Sci. U.S.A. 83: 3012–3016.

Walicke, P., S. Varon, and M. Manthrope (1986b) Purification of a human red blood cell protein supporting the survival of cultured CNS neurons, and its identification as catalase. J. Neurosci. 6: 1114–1121.

Wallace, T. L., and E. M. Johnson (1989) Cytosine arabinoside kills postmitotic neurons: evidence that deoxycytidine may have a role in neuronal survival that is independent of DNA synthesis. J. Neurosci. 9: 115–124.

Walsh, C., C. L. Cepko (1990) Cell lineage and cell migration in the developing cortex. Experientia 46: 940–947.

Walter, J., B. Kern-Veits, J. Huf, et al. (1987) Recognition of position-specific properties of tectal cell membranes by retinal axons in vitro. Development 101: 685–696.

Wang, L. C., D. H. Baird, M. E. Hatten, and C. A. Mason (1994) Astroglial differentiation is required for support of neurite outgrowth. J. Neurosci. 14: 3195–3207.

Wang, S., and T. Hazelrigg (1994) Implications for bcd mRNA localization from spatial distribution of exu protein in *Drosophila* oogenesis. Nature 369: 400–403.

Wang, Y. L., and D. L. Taylor (1989) *Fluorescence Microscopy of Living Cells in Culture Part A. Fluorescent Analogs, Labeling Cells, and Basic Microscopy*, Academic Press, San Diego.

Warren, S., and R. Chute (1972) Pheochromocytoma. Cancer 29: 327–331.

Watson, A., E. Ensor, A. Symes, J. Winter, G. Kendall, and D. Latchman (1995) A minimal CGRP gene promoter is inducible by nerve growth factor in adult rat dorsal root ganglion neurons but not in PC12 phaeochromocytoma cells. Eur. J. Neurosci. 7: 394–400.

Webb, B., M. B. Heaton, M. A. King, and D. W. Walker (1995) A method for labeling embryonic rat medial septal region projection neurons, in vitro, using fluorescent tracers. Brain Res. Bull. 37: 317–323.

Webster, H. D., J. R. Martin, and M. F. O'Connell (1973) The relationships between interphase Schwann cells and axons before myelination: a quantitative electron microscopic study. Dev. Biol. 32: 401–416.

Weintraub, H., R. Davis, S. Tapscott, M. Thayer, M. Krause, R. Benezia, T. K. Blackwell, D. Turner, R. Rupp and S. Hollenberg (1991) The myoD gene family: nodal point during specification of the muscle cell lineage. Science 251: 761–766.

Weiss, M. L., and P. Cobbett (1992) Intravenous injection of Evans Blue labels magnocellular neuroendocrine cells of the rat supraoptic nucleus in situ and after dissociation. Neuroscience 48: 383–395.

Weisz, O. A., and C. E. Machamer (1994) Use of recombinant vaccinia virus vectors for cell biology. Meth. Cell Biol. 43: 137–159.

Weldon, P. R., and M. W. Cohen (1979) Development of synaptic ultrastructure at neuromuscular contacts in an amphibian cell culture system. J. Neurocytol. 8: 239–259.

Werner, M., S. Madreperla, P. Lieberman, and R. Adler (1990) Expression of transfected genes by differentiated, postmitotic neurons and photoreceptors in primary cell cultures. J. Neurosci. Res. 25: 50–57.

Westbrook, G. L. (1993) Glutamate receptors and excitotoxicity. Res. Publ. Assoc. Res. Nerv. Ment. Dis. 71: 35–50.

Westermark, B. (1978) Growth control in miniclones of human glial cells. Exp. Cell Res. 111: 295–299.

Wetts, R., and S. E. Fraser (1991) Microinjection of fluorescent tracers to study neural cell lineages. Development 2 (suppl): 1–8.

Whetsell, W. O., and R. Schwarcz (1989) Prolonged exposure to submicromolar concentrations of quinolinic acid causes excitotoxic damage in organotypic cultures of rat corticostriatal system. Neurosci. Lett. 97: 271–275.

White, W. F., S. R. Snodgrass, and M. Dichter (1980) Identification of GABA neurons in rat cortical cultures by GABA uptake autoradiography. Brain Res. 190(1): 139–152.

Whittemore, S. R., and E. Y. Snyder (1996) Physiological relevance and functional potential of central nervous system–derived cell lines. Mol. Neurobiol. 12: 13–38.

Whittemore, S. R., and L. A. White (1993) Target regulation of neuronal differentiation in a temperature-sensitive cell line derived from medullary raphe. Brain Res. 615: 27–40.

Wijnholds, J., K. Chowdhury, R. Wehr, and P. Gruss (1995) Segment-specific expression of the neuronatin gene during early hindbrain development. Dev. Biol. 171: 73–84.

Wilkemeyer, M. F., K. L. Smith, M. M. Zarei, T. A. Benke, J. W. Swann, K. J. Angelides, and R. C. Eisensmith (1996) Adenovirus-mediated gene transfer into dissociated and explant cultures of rat hippocampal neurons. J. Neurosci. Res. 43: 161–174.

Williams, D. K., and C. S. Cohan (1995) Calcium transients in growth cones and axons of cultured Helisoma neurons in response to conditioning factors. J. Neurobiol. 27: 60–75.

Williams, E. J., P. Doherty, G. Turner, R. A. Reid, J. J. Hemperly, and F. S. Walsh (1992) Calcium influx into neurons can solely account for cell contact-dependent neurite outgrowth stimulated by transfected L1. J. Cell Biol. 119: 883–892.

Williams, E. J., F. S. Walsh, and P. Doherty (1994a) Tyrosine kinase inhibitors can differentially inhibit integrin-dependent and CAM-stimulated neurite outgrowth. J. Cell Biol. 124: 1029–1037.

Williams, E. J., J. Furness, F. S. Walsh, and P. Doherty (1994b) Activation of the FGF receptor underlies neurite outgrowth stimulated by L1, N-CAM, and N-cadherin. Neuron 13: 583–594.

Williams, E. J., B. Mittal, F. S. Walsh, and P. Doherty (1995a) FGF inhibits neurite outgrowth over monolayers of astrocytes and fibroblasts expressing transfected cell adhesion molecules. J. Cell. Sci. 108: 3523–3530.

Williams, E. J., B. Mittal, F. S. Walsh, and P. Doherty (1995b) A Ca^{2+}/calmodulin kinase inhibitor, KN-62, inhibits neurite outgrowth stimulated by CAMs and FGF. Mol. Cell. Neurosci. 6: 69–79.

Withers, G. S., J. M. George, G. A. Banker, and D. F. Clayton (1994) Delayed localization of synelfin (synuclein, nacp) to presynaptic terminals in cultured rat hippocampal neurons. Brain Research 87–94.

Withers, G. S., S. E. Fahrbach, and G. E. Robinson (1995) Effects of experience and juvenile hormone on the organization of the mushroom bodies of honey bees. J. Neurobiol. 26: 130–144.

Withers, G. S., D. Higgins, D. Rueger, and G. Banker (1996) Receptivity of osteogenic protein-1 (OP-1) induced dendrites to axonal innervation. Soc. Neurosci. Abstracts: 22: 768.8.

Wolburg, H., J. Neuhaus, U. Kniesel, B. Krauss, E. M. Schmid, M. Ocalan, C. Farrell, and W. Risau (1994) Modulation of tight junction structure in blood-brain barrier endothelial cells. Effects of tissue culture, second messengers and cocultured astrocytes. J. Cell Sci. 107: 1347–1357.

Wolf, M. K., and M. Dubois-Dalcq (1970) Anatomy of cultured mouse cerebellum: I. Golgi and electron microscopic demonstrations of granule cells, their afferent and efferent synapses. J. Comp. Neurol. 140: 261–280.

Wolinsky, E. J., S. C. Landis, and P. H. Patterson (1985) Expression of noradrenergic and cholinergic traits by sympathetic neurons cultured without serum. J. Neurosci. 5: 1497–1508.

Wolswijk, G. (in press) Perinatal to adult transitions in precursor populations of the oligodendrocyte-type-2 astrocyte (O-2A) lineage. Handbook Exp. Immunol.

Wolswijk, G., and M. Noble (1989) Identification of an adult-specific glial progenitor cell. Development 105: 387–400.

Wolswijk, G., and M. Noble (1992) Cooperation between PDGF and FGF converts slowly dividing O-2A adult progenitor cells to rapidly dividing cells with characteristics of their perinatal counterparts. J. Cell Biol. 118: 889–900.

Wolswijk, G., P. Riddle, and M. Noble (1990) Co-existence of perinatal and adult forms of a glial progenitor cell during development of the rat optic nerve. Development 109: 691–698.

Wolswijk, G., P. N. Riddle, and M. Noble (1991) Platelet-derived growth factor is mitogenic for O-2A adult progenitor cells. Glia 4: 495–503.

Won, L., S. Price, B. H. Wainer, P. C. Hoffmann, J. P. Bolam, P. Greengaard, and A. Heller (1989) Correlated light and electron microscopic study of dopaminergic neurons and their synaptic junctions with DARPP-32-containing cells in three-dimensional reaggregate tissue culture. J. Comp. Neurol. 289: 165–177.

Wong, G. H. W., J. H. Elwell, L. W. Oberley, and D. V. Goeddel (1989) Manganous superoxide dismutase is essential for cellular resistance to cytotoxicity of tumor necrosis factor. Cell 58: 923–931.

Wood, P. M. (1976) Separation of functional Schwann cells and neurons from normal peripheral nerve tissue. Brain Res. 115: 361–375.

Wood, P. M., and R. P. Bunge (1975) Evidence that sensory axons are mitogenic for Schwann cells. Nature 256: 662–664.

Wood, P. M., and R. P. Bunge (1984) Biology of the oligodendrocyte. In: *Oligodendroglia*, W. Norton, ed., pp. 1–46, Plenum, New York.

Wood, P. M., and R. P. Bunge (1986a) Evidence that axons are mitogenic for oligodendrocytes isolated from adult animals. Nature 320: 756–758.

Wood, P. M., and R. P. Bunge (1986b) Myelination of cultured dorsal root ganglion neurons by oligodendrocytes obtained from adult rats. J. Neurol. Sci. 74: 153–169.

Wood, P. M., and A. K. Williams (1984) Oligodendrocyte proliferation and CNS myelination in cultures containing dissociated embryonic neuroglia and dorsal root ganglion neurons. Dev. Brain Res. 12: 225–241.

Wood, P. M., E. Okada, and R. P. Bunge (1980) The use of networks of dissociate rat dorsal root ganglion neurons to induce myelination by oligodendrocytes in culture. Brain Res. 196: 247–252.

Wood, P. M., M. Schachner, and R. P. Bunge (1990) Inhibition of Schwann cell myelination in vitro by antibody to the L1 adhesion molecule. J. Neurosci. 10: 3635–3645.

Woolf, N. J., and L. L. Butcher (1985) Cholinergic systems in the rat brain: II. Projections to the interpeduncular nucleus. Brain Res. Bull. 14: 63–83.

Wray, S., B. H. Gähwiler, and H. Gainer (1988) Slice cultures of LHRH neurons in the presence and absence of brainstem and pituitary. Peptides 9: 1151–1175.

Wray, S., K. Kusano, and H. Gainer (1991) Maintenance of LHRH and oxytocin neurons in slice explants cultured in serum-free media: effects of tetrodotoxin on gene expression. Neuroendocrinology 54: 327–339.

Wren, D., G. Wolswijk, and M. Noble (1992) In vitro analysis of origin and maintenance of O-2A adult progenitor cells. J. Cell Biol. 116: 167–176.

Wright, E. M., K. S. Vogel, and A. M. Davies (1992) Neurotrophic factors promote the maturation of developing sensory neurons before they become dependent on these factors for survival. Neuron 9: 139–150.

Wright, N. J., and Y. Zhong (1995) Characterization of K$^+$ currents and the cAMP-dependent modulation in cultured *Drosophila* mushroom body neurons identified by lacZ expression. J. Neurosci. 15: 1025–1034.

Wu, C. F., N. Suzuki, and M-m. Poo (1983) Dissociated neurons from normal and mutant *Drosophila* larval central nervous system in cell culture. J. Neurosci. 3: 1888–1899.

Wu, D.-Y., and D. J. Goldberg (1993) Regulated tyrosine phosphorylation at the tips of growth cone filopodia. J. Cell Biol. 123: 653–664.

Wu, F., and S. Schacher (1994) Pre- and postsynaptic changes mediated by two second messengers contribute to the expression of long-term heterosynaptic inhibition in *Aplysia*. Neuron 12: 407–421.

Wu, G. Y., D. J. Zou, T. Koothan, and H. T. Cline (1995) Infection of frog neurons with vaccinia virus permits in vivo expression of foreign proteins. Neuron 14: 681–684.

Wu, X., Y. Leduc, M. Cynader, and F. Tufaro (1995) Examination of conditions affecting the efficiency of HSV-1 amplicon packaging. J. Virol. Meth. 52: 219–229.

Wysocki, L. J., and V. L. Sato (1978) Panning for lymphocytes: a method for cell selection. Proc. Natl. Acad. Sci. U.S.A. 75: 2844–2848.

Wyszynski, M., J. Lin, A. Rao, E. Nigh, A. H. Beggs, A. M. Craig, and M. Sheng (1997) Competitive binding of alpha-actinin and calmodulin to the NMDA receptor. Nature 385: 439–442.

Xia, Z., M. Dickens, J. Raingeaud, R. J. Davis, and M. E. Greenberg (1995) Opposing effects of ERIC and JNK-p 38 MAP kinases on apoptosis. Science 270: 1326–1331.

Xia, Z., H. Dudek, C. K. Miranti, and M. E. Greenberg (1996) Calcium influx via the NMDA receptor induces immediate early gene transcription by a MAP kinase/ERK-dependent mechanism. J. Neurosci. 16: 5425–5436.

Xiang, H., D. W. Hochman, H. Saya, T. Fujiwara, P. A. Schwartzkroin, and R. S. Morrison (1996) Evidence for P53-mediated modulation of neuronal viability. J. Neurosci. 16: 6753–6765.

Xie, Z. P., and M-m. Poo (1983) Initial events in the formation of neuromuscular synapse: rapid induction of acetylcholine release from embryonic neuron. Proc. Natl. Acad. Sci. U.S.A. 83: 7069–7073.

Xu, H., H. Federoff, J. Maragos, L. F. Parada, and J. A. Kessler (1994) Viral transduction of trkA into cultured nodose and spinal motor neurons conveys NGF responsiveness. Dev. Biol. 163: 152–161.

Yamada, K., B. S. Spooner, and N. K. Wessells (1970) Axon growth: roles of microfilaments and microtubules. Proc. Natl. Acad. Sci. U.S.A. 66: 1206–1212.

Yamada, K. A., J. M. Dubinsky, and S. M. Rothman (1989) Quantitative physiological characterization of a quinoxalinedione non-NMDA receptor antagonist. J. Neurosci. 9: 3230–3236.

Yamamori, T., K. Fukada, R. Aebersold, K. Korsching, M.-J., Farnand, and P. H. Patterson (1989) The cholinergic neuronal differentiation factor from heart cells is identical to leukemia inhibitory factor. Science 246: 1412–1416.

Yang, J., L. L. Thio, D. B. Clifford, and C. F. Zorumski (1993) Electrophysiological properties of identified postnatal rat hippocampal pyramidal neurons in primary culture. Brain Res. Dev. Brain Res. 71: 19–26.

Yao, M., G. Bain, and D. I. Gottlieb (1995) Neuronal differentiation of P19 embryonal carcinoma cells in defined media J. Neurosci. Res. 41: 792–804.

Yavin, E., and Z. Yavin (1974) Attachment and culture of dissociated cells from rat embryo cerebral hemispheres on polylysine-coated surface. J. Cell Biol. 62: 540–546.

Yavin, Z., and E. Yavin (1980) Survival and maturation of cerebral neurons on poly(L-lysine) surfaces in the absence of serum. Dev. Biol. 75: 454–459.

Yeh, H. J., I. Silos-Santiago, Y. X. Wang, R. J. George, W. D. Snider, and T. F. Deuel (1993) Developmental expression of the platelet-derived growth factor alpha-receptor gene in mammalian central nervous system. Proc. Natl. Acad. Sci. U.S.A. 90: 1952–1956.

Yeh, P., J. F. Dedieu, C. Orsini, E. Vigne, P. Denefle, and M. Perricaudet (1996) Efficient dual transcomplementation of adenovirus E1 and E4 regions from a 293-derived cell line expressing a minimal E4 functional unit. J. Virol. 70: 559–565.

Yim, S. H., S. Szuchet, and P. E. Polak (1986) Cultured oligodendrocytes. A role for cell-substratum interaction in phenotypic expression. J. Biol. Chem. 261: 11808–11815.

Yong, V. W., H. Horie, and S. U. Kim (1988) Comparison of six different substrata on the plating efficiency, differentiation, and survival of human dorsal root ganglion neurons in culture. Dev. Neurosci. 10: 222–230.

Zackenfels, K., R. W. Oppenheim, and H. Rohrer (1995) Evidence for an important role of IGF-I and IGF-II for the early development of chick sympathetic neurons. Neuron 14: 731–741.

Zaczek, R., M. Balm, S. Arlis, H. Drucker and J. T. Coyle (1987) Quisqualate-sensitive, chloride-dependent transport of glutamate into rat brain synaptosomes. J. Neurosci. Res. 18: 425–431.

Zafirov, S., B. Heimrich, and M. Frotscher (1994) Dendritic development of dentate granule cells in the absence of their specific extrinsic afferents. J. Comp. Neurol. 345: 472–480.

Zeevalk, G. D., L. L. Cederqvist, and K. M. Lyser (1982) The ultrastructure of human fetal sympathetic ganglion cells in serum-free medium. Brain Res. 256: 248–252.

Zhang, H., and R. H. Miller (1996) Density-dependent feedback inhibition of oligodendrocyte precursor expansion. J. Neurosci. 16: 6886–6895.

Zhang, H. G., R. H. French-Constant, and M. B. Jackson (1994a) A unique amino acid of the *Drosophila* GABA receptor with influence on drug sensitivity by two mechanisms. J. Physiol. 479: 65–75.

Zhang, Q., and C. A. Mason (1998) Developmental regulation of mossy fiber afferent interactions with target granule cells Dev. Biol. (in press)

Zhang, Z. W., S. Vijayaraghavan, and D. K. Berg (1994) Neuronal acetylcholine receptors that bind alpha-bungarotoxin with high affinity function as ligand-gated ion channels. Neuron 12: 167–177.

Zheng, C., N. Heintz, and M.E. Hatten (1996) CNS gene encoding Astrotactin, which supports neuronal migration along glial fiber. Science 272: 417–419.

Zheng, J., R. E. Buxbaum, and S. R. Heidemann (1994) Measurements of growth cone adhesion to culture surfaces by micromanipulation. J. Cell Biol. 127: 2049–2060.

Zheng, J. Q., M. Felder, J. Connor, and M-m. Poo (1994) Turning of nerve growth cones induced by neurotransmitters. Nature 368: 140–144.

Zheng, J. Q., J. Wan, and M-m. Poo (1996) Essential role of filopodia in chemotropic turning of nerve growth cone induced by a glutamate gradient. J. Neurosci. 16: 1140–1149.

Zhou, X. F., and R. Rush (1995) Sympathetic neurons in neonatal rats require endogenous neurotrophin-3 for survival. J. Neurosci. 15: 6521–6530.

Zhu, H., F. Wu, and S. Schacher (1994) *Aplysia* cell adhesion molecules and serotonin regulate sensory cell–motor cell interactions during early stages of synapse formation in vitro. J. Neurosci. 14: 6886–6900.

Zhuang, Y., C. G. Kim, S. Bartelmez, P. Cheng, M. Groudine, and H. Weintrauls (1992) Helix-loop-helix transcription factors E12 and E47 are not essential for skeletal or neurogenesis. Proc. Natl. Acad. Sci. U.S.A. 89: 12132–12136.

Zimmer, J., and B. H. Gähwiler (1984) Cellular and connective organization of slice cultures of the rat hippocampus and fascia dentata. J. Comp. Neurol. 228: 432–446.

Zimmer, J., and B. H. Gähwiler (1987) Growth of hippocampal mossy fibers: A lesion and coculture study of organotypic slice cultures. J. Comp. Neurol. 264: 1–13.

Ziv, N. E., and M. E. Spira (1993) Spatiotemporal distribution of Ca^{2+} following axotomy and throughout the recovery process of cultured *Aplysia* neurons. Eur. J. Neurosci. 5: 657–668.

Ziv, N. E., and S. J. Smith (1996) Evidence for a role of dendritic filopodia in synaptogenesis and spine formation. Neuron 17: 91–102.

Zolotukhin, S., M. Potter, W. W. Hauswirth, J. Guy, and N. Muzyczka (1996) A "humanized" green flurescent protein cDNA adapted for high-level expression in mammalian cells. J. Virol. 70: 4646–4654.

Zoran, M. J., R. T. Doyle, and P. G. Haydon (1990) Target-dependent induction of secretory capabilities in an identified motoneuron during synaptogenesis. Dev. Biol. 138: 202–213.

Zoran, M. J., R. T. Doyle, and P. G. Haydon (1991) Target contact regulates the calcium responsiveness of the secretory machinery during synaptogenesis. Neuron 6: 145–151.

Index